Computational Vision and Medical Image Processing

VipIMAGE 2011

Editors

João Manuel R.S. Tavares & R.M. Natal Jorge
Faculdade de Engenharia da Universidade do Porto
Porto, Portugal

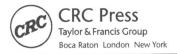

CRC Press
Taylor & Francis Group
Boca Raton London New York

CRC Press is an imprint of the
Taylor & Francis Group, an **informa** business

A BALKEMA BOOK

CRC Press
Taylor & Francis Group
6000 Broken Sound Parkway NW, Suite 300
Boca Raton, FL 33487-2742

First issued in paperback 2018

CRC Press/Balkema is an imprint of the Taylor & Francis Group, an informa business

© 2012 by Sarah Redshaw

Typeset by Vikatan Publishing Solutions (P) Ltd., Chennai, India

No claim to original U.S. Government works

ISBN-13: 978-0-415-68395-1 (hbk)
ISBN-13: 978-1-138-11254-4 (pbk)

Visit the Taylor & Francis Web site at
http://www.taylorandfrancis.com

and the CRC Press Web site at
http://www.crcpress.com

Computational Vision and Medical Image Processing – Tavares & Natal Jorge (eds)
© 2012 Taylor & Francis Group, London, 978-0-415-68395-1

Table of contents

Preface xi

Acknowledgements xiii

Invited lectures xv

Thematic sessions xvii

Scientific committee xix

Invited lecturers

Towards human-sequence evaluation 3
C. Fernandez, J. Gonzàlez & X. Roca

Finite-context models for image compression 9
A.J. Pinho

Learning classifier families for object detection and parameter estimation 15
S. Sclaroff, A. Thangali, Q. Yuan & V. Ablavsky

Contributed papers

Generation of planar radiographs from 3D anatomical models using the GPU 19
A.S. Cardoso, D.C. Moura & J.G. Barbosa

An on-line system for medical and biological image sharing 23
G.M. Porcides, L.A.P. Neves, L.C.M. de Aquino & G.A. Giraldi

Stapes replacement-different ways to replace its function 27
F. Gentil, C. Garbe, M. Parente, P. Martins, R.N. Jorge & J. Paço

Vision-based hand segmentation techniques for human-robot interaction
for real-time applications 31
P. Trigueiros, F. Ribeiro & G. Lopes

Database implementation for clinical and computer assisted diagnosis of dermoscopic images 37
B.S.R. Amorim, T. Mendonça, A.R.S. Marcal, J.S. Marques & J. Rozeira

The finite element analysis of skull deformation after correction of scaphocephaly 43
W. Wolański, M. Gzik, E. Kawlewska, D. Larysz & P. Larysz

Modeling and simulation of trigonocephaly correction with use of Finite Elements Method 47
M. Gzik, W. Wolański, E. Kawlewska, K. Kawlewski & D. Larysz

Computer-aided diagnosis of dementia using medical imaging processing
and artificial neural networks 51
G. Gavidia, R. López & E. Soudah

Automated extraction of the Femoral Shaft Axis and its distal entry point from full
and reduced 3D models 57
S. Van Cauter, M. De Beule, A. Van Haver, P. Verdonk & B. Verhegghe

Facial expression recognition using MPEG-4 FAP-based 3D MMM 63
H. Ujir & M. Spann

Using aerial photographs and characteristic points for automatic estimation of altitude
of the references points 69
M.A.P. Domiciano, E.H. Shiguemori, O.D. Zaloti Jr. & L.A.V. Dias

Simple and fast shape based image retrieval 73
J.F. Nunes, P.M. Moreira & J.M.R.S. Tavares

Bone registration using a robotic ultrasound probe 79
P.M.B. Torres, P.J.S. Gonçalves & J.M.M. Martins

The use of 3D mandibular movement simulation in total
denture construction 85
P. Fonseca, J. Reis-Campos, M.H. Figueiral, N. Viriato & M.A.P. Vaz

A practical and robust image processing method for evaluating the External
Apical Root Resorption 89
S. Alves, N.G. de Posada & M.A.G. López

Preliminary study of the clinical application of the Clinical Decision Support System ORAD II
in a university dental clinic 93
A.F. Simões, A. Correia, T. Marques & R. Figueiredo

Medicine application of laser holography and speckle interferometry 97
V.A. Antonov, M.H. Grosmann, A.I. Larkin, A.V. Osintsev & V.P. Schepinov

Image processing techniques in the analysis of the stresses exerted on the abutment tooth
for a Removable Partial Denture 101
M.J. Santos, M.H. Figueiral, A. Correia, J.M. Monteiro & M.A.P. Vaz

Current quality control procedures in Digital Radiography 107
S.D. Kordolaimi, A.-L.N. Salvara & M.E. Lyra

Image segmentation algorithms on female pelvic ultrasound images 111
P.F. Silva, Z. Ma & J.M.R.S. Tavares

Image segmentation algorithms and their use on doppler images 117
T.D.C.A. Silva, Z. Ma & J.M.R.S. Tavares

Morphometric and immunohistochemical image analysis in pre-pubertal lamb testes
after prenatal betamethasone treatment 123
G. Pedrana, E. Souza, M.H. Viotti, C. Trouche, D. Sloboda & G.B. Martin

Colourquantisation as a preprocessing step for image segmentation 131
H. Palus & M. Frąckiewicz

Reconstruction of a stratified flow inside a duct using X-ray transform for constant
by parts functions 137
A.R. Teixeira & N.C. Roberty

Parallelization environment of digital images processing for medical applications 143
C.A.B. Pariente & P.E. Ambrósio

Fovea and optic disc detection in retinal images 149
J. Pinão & C.M. Oliveira

Displacement measurements with block motion algorithms 155
G. Almeida, J. Fonseca & F. Melício

Automatic segmentation of the secondary austenite-phase island precipitates
in a superduplex stainless steel weld metal 161
V.H.C. Albuquerque, R.Y.M. Nakamura, J.P. Papa, C.C. Silva & J.M.R.S. Tavares

Discrete t-norms in noisy image edge detection 167
M. González-Hidalgo, S. Massanet & A. Mir

An object-based image analysis approach to spine detection in CT images 173
M. Schwier, T. Chitiboi, L. Bornemann & H.K. Hahn

Comparing different filtering and enhancement methods to evaluate the impact on the geometry reconstruction for medical images 179
A.J. João, A.M. Gambaruto & A. Sequeira

Fast identification of individuals based on iris characteristics for biometric systems 183
J.G. Rogeri, M.A. Pontes, A.S. Pereira, N. Marranghello, A.F. Araujo & J.M.R.S. Tavares

Monitoring feet temperature using thermography 189
D. Bento, F.C. Monteiro & A.I. Pereira

Identification of foliar diseases in cotton crop 193
A.A. Bernardes, J.G. Rogeri, N. Marranghello, A.S. Pereira, A.F. Araujo & J.M.R.S. Tavares

A local invariant features approach for classifying acrosome integrity in boar spermatozoa 199
L.F. Robles, V. González-Castro, O. García-Olalla, M.T. García-Ordás & E. Alegre

Analysis of mixing of a clothoid based passive micromixer: A numerical study 205
*F. Pennella, S. Ripandelli, L. Ridolfi, F. Mastrangelo, M.A. Deriu, F.M. Montevecchi,
U. Morbiducci, M. Rasponi, M. Rossi & C.J. Kähler*

Flow visualization of trace particles and Red Blood Cells in a microchannel with a diverging and converging bifurcation 209
V. Leble, C. Fernandes, R. Dias, R. Lima, T. Ishikawa, Y. Imai & T. Yamaguchi

Does fluid shear stress represent the degree of a Red Blood Cell deformation? 213
M. Nakamura & S. Wada

Flow of Red Blood Cells through a microfluidic extensional device: An image analysis assessment 217
T. Yaginuma, A.I. Pereira, P.J. Rodrigues, R. Lima, M.S.N. Oliveira, T. Ishikawa & T. Yamaguchi

An automatic method to track Red Blood Cells in microchannels 221
D. Pinho, F. Gayubo, A. Isabel & R. Lima

Speech articulation assessment using dynamic Magnetic Resonance Imaging techniques 225
S.R. Ventura, M.J.M. Vasconcelos, D.R. Freitas, I.M. Ramos & J.M.R.S. Tavares

The breast lesions characterization by *b* values variation in the DW-Magnetic Resonance Imaging 233
A.A. Fernandes, M.B. Ribeiro, J.C. Janardo, S.D. Jaguegivane & M.E. Pereira

Efficient lesion segmentation using Support Vector Machines 239
J.-B. Fiot, L.D. Cohen, P. Raniga & J. Fripp

Multimodality imaging population analysis using manifold learning 245
*J.-B. Fiot, L.D. Cohen, P. Bourgeat, P. Raniga, O. Acosta, V. Villemagne,
O. Salvado & J. Fripp*

2D MRI brain segmentation by using feasibility constraints 251
V. Pedoia, E. Binaghi, S. Balbi, A. De Benedictis, E. Monti & R. Minotto

Stochastic bone remodeling process: From isotropy to anisotropy 257
N. Mellouli & A. Ricordeau

Carotid artery atherosclerosis plaque analysis using CT and histology 261
F. Santos, A. Joutsen, J. Salenius & H. Eskola

Level set framework for detecting arterial lumen in ultrasound images 267
A.R. Abdel-Dayem

Micromovement measurements of endosseous dental implants with 3D Digital Image Correlation (DIC) method 273
A.T. Rodrigues, B.A. Neto & C.P. Nicolau

Monte Carlo simulation of PET images for injection dose optimization 279
J. Boldyš, J. Dvořák, O. Bělohlávek & M. Skopalová

The use of medical thermal imaging in obstetrics 285
R. Simões & C. Nogueira-Silva

Analysis system of sudomotor function using digital image processing 291
J.L. Quintero, E. Nava & M.S. Dawid

3D geometry reconstruction from gray and RGB medical images 297
P. Talaia, M. Parente, A. Fernandes & R.N. Jorge

The breast phantom construction for a research purpose 303
M. Ribeiro, J. O'Neill & J. Mauricio

Engineer methods of assistance of toraco-chirurgical operation 307
B. Gzik-Zroska, W. Wolański, M. Gzik & J. Dzielicki

Stress analysis of the tympanic membrane through image 311
C. Garbe, M. Parente, P. Martins, R.N. Jorge, F. Gentil & J. Paço

Simulation and modeling the thermal behaviour of textile structures 315
M.J. Geraldes, L. Hes & M. Araújo

Reaction force produced in the coccyx in different degrees of prolapse 319
T.H. Da Roza, R.N. Jorge, M. Parente, T. Mascarenhas, J. Loureiro & S. Duarte

Texture analysis and pattern recognition in X-band SAR images for urban forestry 323
S. Canale, A. De Santis, D. Iacoviello, F. Pirri & S. Sagratella

Cosmo-Skymed SAR data for urgency situations-study of a real case 329
R.L. Paes, E.H. Shiguemori, M. Habermann, A.M.R. Neto & R.M. Andrade

Using satellite imagery to develop a detailed and updated map of imperviousness to improve
flood risk management in the city of Lisbon
T. Santos, S. Freire, J.A. Tenedório & A. Fonseca 333

Feature extraction from satellite imagery and LiDAR to update exposure to tsunami
and improve risk assessment in dynamic urban areas
S. Freire, T. Santos & J.A. Tenedório 337

Situational awareness on Rio de Janeiro's terrain sliding using Cosmo-Skymed data-study
of a real case
R.L. Paes, O.D. Zaloti Jr., F.M. Barros & C.H.L. Ribeiro 343

Identification of wildfire precursor conditions: Linking satellite based fire and soil moisture data 347
C. Aubrecht, C.D. Elvidge, K.E. Baugh & S. Hahn

Development of an automated procedure for a patient specific segmentation of the human
femur body from CT scan images
D. Almeida, J. Folgado, P.R. Fernandes & R.B. Ruben 355

Pseudo Fuzzy colour calibration for sport video segmentation 361
C.B. Santiago, A. Sousa & L.P. Reis

Combining hierarchical watershed metrics and Normalized Cut for image segmentation 367
T.W. Pinto & M.A.G. de Carvalho

A comparison between segmentation algorithms for urinary bladder on T2-weighted MR images 371
Z. Ma, R.N. Jorge & J.M.R.S. Tavares

Computational algorithms for the segmentation of the human ear 377
E.M. Barroso, Z. Ma, J.M.R.S. Tavares & F. Gentil

Evaluation of wavelets in noise reduction of Electromyographic signals 383
F. Ballesteros & J. de Castro

Assessing the detection of embolic signals using continuous wavelet transform 387
I.B. Gonçalves, A. Leiria & M.M.M. Moura

Comparison between some time-frequency analysis methods on electromyography
(EMG) signal
*H.A. Weiderpass, C.G.F. Pachi, J.F. Yamamoto, I.C.N. Sacco, A. Hamamoto &
A.N. Onodera* 393

A new interface for manual segmentation of dermoscopic images   399
P.M. Ferreira, T. Mendonça, P. Rocha & J. Rozeira

InVesalius-An open-source imaging application   405
T.F. de Moraes, P.H.J. Amorim, F.S. Azevedo & J.V.L. da Silva

GPU acceleration of legendre moments as biomarkers of bone tissue   409
J.A. Lachiondo & M. Ujaldón

On the accurate classification of bone tissue images   415
J.E. Gil, J.P. Aranda, E. Mérida-Casermeiro & M. Ujaldón

Automated quantification of histone relocation in cell nuclei   423
T. Rieß, C. Dietz, M. Horn, O. Deussen, M. Leist, T. Waldmann & D. Merhof

An automated vehicle counting system from UAV images   429
A.M.R. Neto, E.H. Shiguemori & A.P.A. de Castro

Tracking rural and urban landmarks for UAV autonomous navigation   433
R.M. Andrade, E.H. Shiguemori & A.P.A. de Castro

Author index   439

Preface

This book contains invited lectures and full papers presented at VipIMAGE 2011 – III ECCOMAS Thematic Conference on Computational Vision and Medical Image Processing, which was held in Olhão, Algarve, Portugal, during the period 12–14 October 2011. The event had 6 invited lectures, and 79 contributed presentations originated from 16 countries: Austria, Belgium, Brazil, Canada, Czech Republic, France, Germany, Greece, Italy, Japan, Malaysia, Poland, Portugal, Russia, Spain and Uruguay.

Computational methodologies of signal processing and analyses, namely considering 2D, 3D and 4D images, have been commonly used in our society. For instances, full automatic or semi-automatic Computational Vision systems have been increasing used in surveillance tasks, traffic analysis, recognition process, inspection purposes, human-machine interfaces, 3D vision and deformation analysis.

One of the notable aspects of the Computational Vision domain is the inter- and multi-disciplinarily that are always presented. In fact, in this considerably recent field, methodologies of more traditional sciences, such as Informatics, Mathematics, Statistics, Psychology, Mechanics and Physics, are regularly embraced. Additionally, one of the key reasons that contributes for the continually effort done in this field of the human knowledge is the number of applications that can be found in Medicine. For instance, statistical or physical procedures can be used on medical images in order to model the represented structures, and then attain shape reconstruction, motion and deformation analysis, tissue characterization or computer-assisted diagnosis and therapy.

The main objective of these ECCOMAS Thematic Conferences on Computational Vision and Medical Image Processing, initiated in 2007, is to promote a comprehensive forum for discussion on the recent advances in the related fields trying to identify widespread areas of potential collaboration between researchers of different sciences. Henceforth, VipIMAGE 2011 brought together researchers representing fields related to Computational Vision, Computer Graphics, Computer Sciences, Computational Mechanics, Mathematics, Signal Processing, Statistics, Medical Imaging and Medicine.

The expertises spanned a broad range of techniques for Image Acquisition, Image Processing and Analysis, Signal Processing, Data Interpolation, Registration, Acquisition and Compression, Image Segmentation, Tracking and Analysis of Motion, 3D Vision, Simulation, Medical Imaging, Computer Aided Diagnosis, Surgery, Therapy, and Treatment, Computational Bioimaging and Visualization and Telemedicine, Virtual Reality, Software Development and Applications.

The Conference co-chairs would like to take this opportunity to express gratitude for the support given by The International European Community on Computational Methods in Applied Sciences and The Portuguese Association of Theoretical, Applied and Computational Mechanics, and thank to all sponsors, to all members of the Scientific Committee, to all Invited Lecturers, to all Session-Chairs and to all Authors for submitting and sharing their knowledge.

João Manuel R.S. Tavares
R.M. Natal Jorge
Conference co-chairs

Acknowledgements

The editors and the Conference co-chairs acknowledge the support towards the publication of the Book of Proceedings and the organization of the III ECCOMAS Thematic Conference VipIMAGE to the following organizations:

- Universidade do Porto (UP)
- Faculdade de Engenharia da Universidade do Porto (FEUP)
- Instituto de Engenharia Mecânica – Pólo FEUP (IDMEC-Polo FEUP)
- Instituto de Engenharia Mecânica e Gestão Industrial (INEGI)
- European Community on Computational Methods in Applied Sciences (ECCOMAS)
- International Association for Computational Mechanics (IACM)
- Fundação para a Ciência e a Tecnologia (FCT)
- Associação Portuguesa de Mecânica Teórica Aplicada e Computacional (APMTAC)

Computational Vision and Medical Image Processing – Tavares & Natal Jorge (eds)
© 2012 Taylor & Francis Group, London, 978-0-415-68395-1

Invited lectures

During VipIMAGE 2011, were presented Invited Lectures by 6 Expertises from 5 countries:

– Finite-context Models for Image Compression
  Armando J. Pinho – University of Aveiro, Portugal
– Deterministic vs DSMC Solvers for Boltzmann-Poisson Dynamics of Charged Transport in Nanostructures
  Irene M. Gamba – The University of Texas at Austin, USA
– 3D from Video for Static and Dynamic Scenes
  Marc Pollefeys – ETH Zurich, Switzerland
– Thoracic Image Processing for Nanoparticle Delivery
  Marc Thiriet – Universite Pierre et Marie Curie (Paris VI), France
– Towards Human-Sequence Evaluation
  Xavier Roca Marvà – Autonomous University of Barcelona, Spain
– Learning Classifier Families for Object Detection and Parameter Estimation
  Stan Sclaroff – Boston University, USA

Thematic sessions

Within VipIMAGE 2011 were organized 6 Thematic Sessions:

- Imaging Techniques Applied to Soft Tissue Biomechanics
  Organizers: Pedro A.L.S. Martins (IDMEC-Polo FEUP, Portugal), Patrick Dubois (University North of France, France)
- Simultaneous MR-PET Imaging
  Organizers: Pedro Almeida (University of Lisboa, Portugal), Liliana Caldeira (University of Lisboa, Portugal)
- Satellite Image Analysis for Environmental Risk Assessment
  Organizers: Alberto De Santis (Sapienza University of Rome, Italy), Daniela Iacoviello (Sapienza University of Rome, Italy)
- Dental Imaging and Processing Techniques
  Organizers: André Correia (University of Porto, Portugal), J.C. Reis Campos (University of Porto, Portugal), Mário Vaz (University of Porto, Portugal)
- Digital Mammography
  Organizers: Susana Branco Silva (Polytechnic Institute of Lisboa, Portugal), Nuno Machado (Polytechnic Institute of Lisboa, Portugal), Luis Freire (Polytechnic Institute of Lisboa, Portugal)
- Imaging of Biological Flows: Trends and Challenges
  Organizers: Alberto Gambaruto (Instituto Superior Técnico, Portugal), Mónica S.N. Oliveira (University of Porto, Portugal), Rui Lima (Polytechnic Institute of Bragança, Portugal)

Scientific committee

All works submitted to VipIMAGE 2011 were evaluated by an International Scientific Committee composed by 120 expert researchers from recognized institutions of 22 countries:

Adelino F. Leite-Moreira, Portugal
Ahmed El-Rafei, Germany
Ahmed Fadiel, USA
Alberto De Santis, Italy
Alberto Gambaruto, Portugal
Alejandro F. Frangi, Spain
Alexandre Cunha, USA
Amr R. Abdel-Dayem, Canada
Ana Mafalda Reis, Portugal
André Correia, Portugal
André R.S. Marçal, Portugal
André Vital Saúde, Brazil
Andrew D. Bagdanov, Spain
Antonio Vernet, Spain
Armando Sousa, Portugal
Arrate Muñoz Barrutia, Spain
Aubrecht Christoph, Austria
Bernard Gosselin, Belgium
Bhargab B. Bhattacharya, India
Bogdan Raducanu, Spain
Charles A. Taylor, USA
Christos Constantinou, USA
Christos Grecos, UK
Constantino Reyes-Aldasoro, UK
Daniela Iacoviello, Italy
David A. Steinman, Canada
Djemel Ziou, Canada
Durval C. Costa, Portugal
Eduardo Borges Pires, Portugal
Eduardo Soudah Prieto, Spain
Emmanuel A. Audenaert, Belgium
Enrique Alegre Gutiérrez, Spain
Eugenio Oñate, Spain
Fernão Abreu, Portugal
Filipa Sousa, Portugal
Fiorella Sgallari, Italy
George Bebis, USA
George Papaioannou, USA
Gerald Schaefer, UK
Gerhard A. Holzapfel, Sweden
Helcio R.B. Orlande, Brazil
Hélder Rodrigues, Portugal
Hemerson Pistori, Brazil
Henryk Palus, Poland
Hugo Proença, Portugal

Huiyu Zhou, UK
Isabel M.A.P. Ramos, Portugal
Ioannis Pitas, Greece
J. Paulo Vilas-Boas, Portugal
J. Tinsley Oden, USA
Jackie Shen, China
Jaime S. Cardoso, Portugal
Jan C de Munck, The Netherlands
Javier Melenchón, Spain
Jeffrey A. Weiss, USA
Jerome Darbon, France
J.C. Reis Campos, Portugal
Jimmy T. Efird, USA
João M.A. Rebello, Brazil
João Paulo Papa, Brazil
João Sanches, Portugal
Joaquim Jorge, Portugal
Joaquim Silva Gomes, Portugal
Jordi Gonzàlez, Spain
Jorge M.G. Barbosa, Portugal
Jorge S. Marques, Portugal
Jose M. García Aznar, Spain
Jun Zhao, China
Khan M. Iftekharuddin, USA
Kristian Sandberg, USA
Laurent Cohen, France
Liliana Caldeira, Portugal
Lionel Moisan, France
Lyuba Alboul, UK
Luís Amaral, Portugal
Luís Freire, Portugal
Luís Paulo Reis, Portugal
M. Emre Celebi, USA
Mahmoud El-Sakka, Canada
Manuel Filipe Costa, Portugal
Manuel González Hidalgo, Spain
Manuel Laranjeira, Portugal
Manuel Ujaldon, Spain
Manuele Bicego, Italy
Marcos Rodrigues, UK
Maria Petrou, UK
Mário Forjaz Secca, Portugal
Mário M. Freire, Portugal
Mário Vaz, Portugal
Masud Rahman, Australia

Invited lecturers

Computational Vision and Medical Image Processing – Tavares & Natal Jorge (eds)
© *2012 Taylor & Francis Group, London, ISBN 978-0-415-68395-1*

Towards human-sequence evaluation

Carles Fernandez, Jordi Gonzàlez & Xavier Roca

Department of Computer Science & Computer Vision Centre, Edifici O. Universitat Autonoma de Barcelona, Bellaterra, Spain

ABSTRACT: The increasing ubiquitousness of digital information in our daily lives has positioned video as a favored information vehicle, and given rise to an astonishing generation of social media and surveillance footage. This raises a series of technological demands for automatic video understanding and management, which together with the compromising attentional limitations of human operators, have motivated the research community to guide its steps towards a better attainment of such capabilities. As a result, current trends on cognitive vision promise to recognize complex events and self-adapt to different environments, while managing and integrating several types of knowledge. Future directions suggest to reinforce the multi-modal fusion of information sources and the communication with end-users.

1 INTRODUCTION

The revolution of information experienced by the world in the last century, especially emphasized by the household use of computers after the 1970s, has led to what is known today as the society of knowledge. Digital technologies have converted post-modern society into an entity in which networked communication and information management have become crucial for social, political, and economic practices. The major expansion in this sense has been rendered by the global effect of the Internet: since its birth, it has grown into a medium that is uniquely capable of integrating modes of communication and forms of content.

In this context, the assessment of interactive and broadcasting services has spread and generalized in the last decade—e.g., residential access to the Internet, video-on-demand technologies–, posing video as the privileged information vehicle of our time, and promising a wide variety of applications that aim at its effcient exploitation. Today, the automated analysis of video resources is not tomorrow's duty anymore. The world produces a massive amount of digital video files every passing minute, particularly in the fields of multimedia and surveillance, which open windows of opportunity for smart systems as vast archives of recordings constantly grow.

Automatic content-based video indexing has been requested for digital multimedia databases for the last two decades (Foresti, Marcenaro & Regazzoni 2002). This task consists of extracting high-level descriptors that help us to automatically annotate the semantic content in video sequences; the generation of reasonable semantic indexes makes it possible to create powerful engines to search and retrieve video content, which finds immediate applications in many areas: from the efficient access to digital libraries to the preservation and maintenance of digital heritage. Other usages in the multimedia domain would also include virtual commentators, which could describe, analyze, and summarize the development of sport events, for instance.

More recently, the same requirements have applied also to the field of video surveillance. Human operators have attentional limitations that discourage their involvement in a series of tasks that could compromise security or safety. In addition, surveillance systems have strong storage and computer power requirements, deal with continuous 24/7 monitoring, and manage a type of content that is susceptible to be highly compressed. Furthermore, the number of security cameras increases exponentially worldwide on a daily basis, producing huge amounts of video recordings that may require further supervision. The conjunction of these facts establishes a need to automatize the visual recognition of events and content-based forensic analysis on video footage.

We find a wide range of applications coming from the surveillance domain that point to real-life, daily problems: for example, a smart monitoring of elder or disabled people makes it possible to recognize alarming situations, and speed up reactions towards early assistance; road traffic surveillance can be useful to send alerts of congestion or automatically detect accidents or abnormal occurrences; similar usage can be directed to urban planning, optimization of resources for transportation allocations, or detection of abnormality in crowded locations —airports, lobbies, etc.–.

Such a vast spectrum of social, cultural, commercial, and technological demands have repeatedly motivated the research community to direct their steps towards a better attainment of video understanding capabilities.

1.1 Collaborative efforts on video event understanding

A notable amount of EU research projects have been recently devoted to the unsupervised analysis of video contents, in order to automatically extract events and behaviors of interest, and interpret them in selected contexts. These projects measure the pulse of the research in this field, demonstrate previous success on particular initiatives, and propose a series of interesting applications to such techniques. And, last but not least, they motivate the continuation of this line of work. Some of them are briefly described next, and shown in Figures 1–2.

ADVISOR (IST-11287, 2000–2002). It addresses the development of management systems for networks of metro operators. It uses CCTV for computer assisted automatic incident detection, content based annotation of video recordings, behavior pattern analysis of crowds and individuals, and ergonomic human computer interfaces.

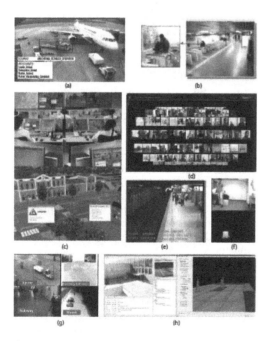

Figure 1. Snapshots of the referred projects. (a) AVITRACK, (b) ADVISOR, (c) BEWARE, (d) VIDI-Video, (e) CARETAKER, (f) ICONS, (g) ETISEO, (h) HERMES.

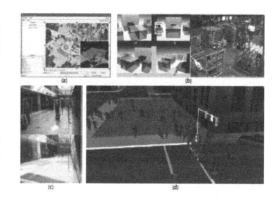

Figure 2. Some of the most recent projects in the field. (a) SHARE, (b) SCOVIS, (c) SAMURAI, (d) ViCoMo.

ICONS (DTI/EPSRC LINK, 2001–2003). Its aim is to advance towards (i) zero motion detection, detection of medium- to long-term visual changes in a scene—e.g., deployment of a parcel bomb, theft of a precious item—, and (ii) behavior recognition—characterize and detect undesirable behavior in video data, such as thefts or violence—only from the appearance of pixels.

AVITRACK (AST-CT-502818, 2004–2006). It develops a framework for automatically supervision of commercial aircraft servicing operations from the arrival to the departure on an airport's apron. A prototype for scene understanding and simulation of the apron's activity was going to be implemented during the project on Toulouse airport.

ETISEO (Techno-Vision, 2005–2007). It seeks to work out a new structure contributing to an increase in the evaluation of video scene understanding. ETISEO focuses on the treatment and interpretation of videos involving pedestrians and (or) vehicles, indoors or outdoors, obtained from fixed cameras.

CARETAKER 5 (IST-027231, 2006–2008). This project aims at studying, developing and assessing multimedia knowledge-based content analysis, knowledge extraction components, and metadata management sub-systems in the context of automated situation awareness, diagnosis and decision support.

SHARE 6 (IST-027694, 2006–2008). It offers an information and communication system to support emergency teams during large-scale rescue operations and disaster management, by exploiting multimodal data—audio, video, texts, graphics, location—. It incorporates domain dependent ontology modules, and allows for video/voice analysis, indexing/retrieval, and multimodal dialogues.

HERMES (IST-027110, 2006–2009). Extraction of descriptions of people's behavior from videos in restricted discourse domains, such as inter-city roads, train stations, or lobbies. The project studies human movements and behaviors at several scales —agent, body, face—, and the final communication of meaningful contents to end-users.

BEWARE (EP/E028594/1, 2007–2010). The project aims to analyze and combine data from alarm panels and systems, fence detectors, security cameras, public sources and even police files, to unravel patterns and signal anomalies, e.g., by making comparisons with historical data. BEWARE is self-learning and suggests improvements to optimize security.

VIDI-Video (IST-045547, 2007–2010). Implementation of an audio-visual semantic search engine to enhance access to video, by developing a 1000 element thesaurus to index video content. Several applications have been suggested in surveillance, conferencing, event reconstruction, diaries, and cultural heritage documentaries.

SAMURAI (IST-217899, 2008–2011). It develops an intelligent surveillance system for monitoring of critical public infrastructure sites. It is to fuse data from networked heterogeneous sensors rather than using CCTV alone; to develop real-adaptative behavior profiling and abnormality detection, instead of using predefined hard rules; and to take command input from human operators and mobile sensory input from patrols, for hybrid context-aware behavior recognition.

SCOVIS (IST-216465, 2007–2013). It aims at automatic behavior detection and visual learning of procedures, in manufacturing and public infrastructures. Its synergistic approach based on complex camera networks also achieves model adaptation and camera network coordination. User's interaction improves behavior detection and guides the modeling process, through high-level feedback mechanisms.

ViCoMo (ITEA2-08009, 2009–2012). This project concerns advanced video interpretation algorithms on video data that are typically acquired with multiple cameras. It is focusing on the construction of realistic context models to improve the decision making of complex vision systems and to produce a faithful and meaningful behavior.

As it can be seen, many efforts have been taken in the last decade, and are still increasing nowadays, in order to tackle the problem of video interpretation and intelligent video content management. It is clear from this selection that current trends on the field suggest a tendency to focus on the multi-modal fusion of different sources of information, and on more powerful communication with end-users. From the large amount of projects existing in the field we derive another conclusion: such a task is not trivial at all, and requires research efforts from many different areas to be joint into collaborative approaches, which success where individual efforts fail.

2 PAST, PRESENT, AND FUTURE OF VIDEO SURVEILLANCE

The field of video surveillance has experienced a remarkable evolution in the last decades, which can help us think of the future characteristics that would be desirable for it. In the traditional video surveillance scheme, the primary goal of the camera system was to present to human operators more and more visual information about monitored environments, see Figure 3. First-generation systems were completely passive, thus having this information entirely processed by human operators. Nevertheless, a saturation effect appears as the information availability increases, causing a decrease in the level of attention of the operator, who is ultimately in charge of deciding about the surveilled situations.

The following generation of video surveillance systems used digital computing and communications technologies to change the design of the original architecture, customizing it according to the requirements of the end-users. A series of technical advantages allowed them to better satisfy the demands from industry,

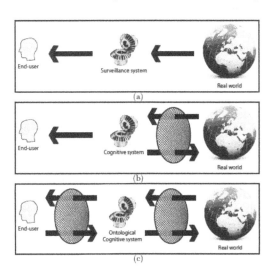

Figure 3. Evolution of video surveillance systems, since its initial passive architecture (a) to the reactive, bidirectional communication scheme offered by cognitive vision systems (b), which highlight relevant footage contents. By incorporating ontological and interactive capabilities to this framework (c), the system performs like a semantic filter also to the end-users, governing the interactions with them in order to adapt to their interests and maximize the efficiency of the communication.

i.e., higher-resolution cameras, longer retention of recorded video—DVRs replaced VCRs, video encoding standards appeared–, reduction of costs and size, remote monitoring capabilities provided by network cameras, or more built-in intelligence, among others (Nilsson 2009).

The continued increase of machine intelligence has derived into a new generation of smart surveillance systems lately. Recent trends on computer vision and artificial intelligence have deepened into the study of cognitive vision systems, which use visual information to facilitate a series of tasks on sensing, understanding, reaction, and communication, see Figure 3 (b). Such systems enable traditional surveillance applications to greatly enhance their functionalities by incorporating methods for:

i. Recognition and categorization of objects, structures, and events.
ii. Learning and adaptation to different environments.
iii. Representation, memorization, and fusion of various types of knowledge.
iv. Automatic control and attention.

As a consequence, the relation of the system with the world and the end-users is enriched by a series of sensors and actuators —e.g., distributions of static and active cameras, enhanced user interfaces—, thus establishing a bidirectional communication flow, and closing loops at a sensing and semantic level. The resulting systems provide a series of novel applications with respect to traditional systems, like automated video commentary and annotation, or image-based search engines. In the last years, European projects like CogVis or CogViSys have investigated these and other potential applications of cognitive vision systems, especially concerning video surveillance.

Recently, a paradigm has been specifically proposed for the design of cognitive vision systems aiming to analyze human developments recorded in image sequences. This is known as Human Sequence Evaluation (HSE) (Gonzàlez, Rowe, Varona & Roca 2009). An HSE system is built upon a linear multilevel architecture, in which each module tackles a specific abstraction level. Two consecutive modules hold a bidirectional communication scheme, in order to

i. generate higher-level descriptions based on lower-level analysis—bottom-up inference—, and
ii. support low-level processing with high-level guidance—top-down reactions—. HSE follows as well the aforementioned characteristics of cognitive vision systems.

Nonetheless, although cognitive vision systems conduct a large number of tasks and success in a wide range of applications, in most cases the resulting prototypes are tailored to specific needs or restricted to definite domains. Hence, current research aims to increase aspects like extensibility, personalization, adaptability, interactivity, and multi-purpose of these systems. In particular, it is becoming of especial importance to stress the paper of communication with end-users in the global picture, both for the fields of surveillance and multimedia: end-users should be allowed to automatize a series of tasks requiring content-mining, and should be presented the analyzed information in a suitable and efficient manner, see Figure 3(c).

As a result of these considerations, the list of objectives to be tackled and solved by a cognitive vision system has elaborated on the original approach, which aimed at the single—although still ambitious today—task of transducing images to semantics. Nowadays, the user itself has become a piece of the puzzle, and therefore has to be considered a part of the problem.

3 MIND THE GAPS

The search and extraction of meaningful information from video sequences is dominated by 5 major challenges, all of them defined by gaps (Smeulders, Worring, Santini, Gupta & Jain 2000). These gaps are disagreements between the real data and that one expected, intended, or retrieved by any computer-based process involved in the information flow conducted between the acquisition of data from the real world, and until its final presentation to the end-users. The 5 gaps are presented next, see Figure 4(a).

1. Sensory gap
   The gap between an object in the world and the information in an image recording of that scene. All these recordings will be different due to variations in viewpoint, lighting, and other circumstantial conditions.
2. Semantic gap
   The lack of coincidence between the information that one can extract from the sensory data and the interpretation that same data has for a user in a given situation. It can be understood as the difference between a visual concept and its linguistic representation.
3. Model gap
   The impossibility to theoretically account the amount of notions in the world, due to the limited capacity to learn them.
4. Query/context gap
   The gap between the specific need for information of an end-user and the possible retrieval solutions manageable by the system.

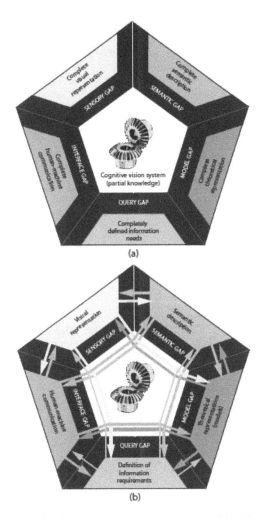
(a)

(b)

Figure 4. (a) The five gaps that need to be bridged for the successful analysis, extraction, search, retrieval, and presentation of video content. (b) In some cases, a collaborative and integrative use of different knowledge sources allows us to achieve or enrich the accomplishment of these tasks. Arrows stand for reusing ontological knowledge to enhance analyses in other areas.

5. Interface gap

The limited scope of information that a system interface offers compared to the amount of data actually intended to transmit.

Although each of these challenges becomes certainly difficult to overcome by its own, a proper centralization of information sources and the wise reutilization of knowledge derived from them facilitates the overwhelming task of bridging each of these gaps. There exist multiple examples of how the multiple resources of the system can be redirected to solve problems in a different domain, let us consider three of them:

– From semantic to sensory gap: tracking errors or occlusions at a visual level can be identified by high-level modules that imply semantics oriented to that end. This way, the system can be aware of where and when a target is occluded, and predict its reaparition.
– From sensory to interface gap: the reports or responses in user interfaces can become more expressive by adding selected, semantically relevant key-frames from the sensed data.
– From interface to query gap: in case of syntactic ambiguities in a query—e.g., "zoom in on any person in the group that is running"—, end-users can be asked about their real interests via a dialogue interface: "Did you mean 'the group that is running', or 'the person that is running'?".

Given the varied nature of types of knowledge involved in our intended system, an ontological framework becomes a sensible choice of design: such a framework integrates different sources of information by means of temporal and multimodal fusion—horizontal integration—, using bottom-up or top-down approaches—vertical integration—, and incorporating prior hierarchical knowledge by means of an extensible ontology.

We propose the use of ontologies to help us integrate, centralize, and relate the different knowledge representations—visual, semantic, linguistic, etc.— implied by the different modules of the cognitive system. By doing so, the relevant knowledge or capabilities in a specific area can be used to enhance the performance of the system in other distinct areas, as represented in Figure 4(b). Ontologies will enable us to formalize, account, and redirect the semantic assets of the system in a given situation, and exploit them to empower the aforementioned capabilities, especially targeting the possibilities of interaction with end-users.

4 CONCLUSIONS

Human Sequence Evaluation (HSE) concentrates on how to extract descriptions of human behaviour from videos in a restricted discourse domain, such as (i) pedestrians crossing inner-city roads where pedestrians appear approaching or waiting at stops of busses or trams, and (ii) humans in indoor worlds like an airport hall, a train station, or a lobby. These discourse domains allow exploring a coherent evaluation of human movements and facial expressions across a wide variation of scale. This general approach lends itself to various cognitive surveillance scenarios at varying degrees of resolution: from wide-field-of-view multiple-agent scenes, through to more specific inferences of emotional state that could be elicited from high resolution imagery of faces. The true challenge of the HERMES project will consist in the development of a system facility which starts with basic knowledge about pedestrian behaviour in the chosen discourse domain, but could cluster evaluation results into semantically meaningful subsets of behaviours. The envisaged system will comprise an internal logic-based representation which enables it to comment each individual subset, giving natural language explanations of why the system has created the subset in question.

Multiple issues will be contemplated to perform HSE, such as detection and localization; tracking; classification; prediction; concept formation and visualization; communication and expression, etc. And this is reflected in the literature: a huge number of papers confront some of the levels, but rarely all of them. Summarizing, agent motion will allow HSE to infer behavior descriptions. The term behaviour will refer to one or several actions, which acquire a meaning in a particular context.

Body motion will allow HSE to describe action descriptions. We define an action as a motion pattern, which represents the style of variation of a body posture during a predefined interval of time. Therefore, body motion will be used to recognize style parameters (such as age, gender, handicapped, identification, etc.).

Lastly, face motion will lead to emotion descriptions. The emotional characteristics of facial expressions will allow HSE to confront personality modeling, which would enable us to carry out multiple studies and researches on advanced human-computer interfaces.

So these issues will require, additionally, assessing how, and by which means, the knowledge of context and a plausible hypothesis about he internal state of the agent may influence and support the interpretation processes.

ACKNOWLEDGEMENT

The authors wish to acknowledge the support of the Spanish Research Programs Consolider-Ingenio 2010: MIPRCV (CSD200700018); Avanza I+D ViCoMo (TSI-020400-2009-133); along with the Spanish projects TIN2009-14501-C02-01 and TIN2009-14501-C02-02; MICIN the A.I. PT2009-0023.

REFERENCES

Foresti, G.L., Marcenaro, L. & Regazzoni, C.S. Automatic detection and indexing of video-event shots for surveillance applications. IEEE Transactions on Multimedia, 4(4):459–471, 2002. [Page 9].

Gonzàlez, J., Rowe, D., Varona, J. & Roca, X. Understanding dynamic scenes based on human sequence evaluation. Image and Vision Computing, 27(10):1433–1444, 2009. [Pages 16, 27, 32, 33, 63, 71 and 83].

Nilsson, F. Intelligent network video: understanding modern video surveillance systems. CRC Press, 2009. [Page 14].

Smeulders, A.W.M., Worring, M., Santini, S., Gupta, A. & Jain, R. Contentbased image retrieval at the end of the early years. IEEE Transactions on Pattern Analysis and Machine Intelligence, 22(12):1349–1380, 2000. [Pages 16 and 53].

Computational Vision and Medical Image Processing – Tavares & Natal Jorge (eds)
© 2012 Taylor & Francis Group, London, ISBN 978-0-415-68395-1

Finite-context models for image compression

Armando J. Pinho

Signal Processing Lab, IEETA/DETI, University of Aveiro, Aveiro, Portugal

ABSTRACT: Finite-context modeling has been applied to the problem of image compression with remarkable success. In this talk, we address this topic, showing examples with various types of images, including medical images of several modalities and DNA microarray images. We also show how finite-context modeling can be used for image complexity estimation and how this relates to image compression.

1 INTRODUCTION

Modeling plays a key role in data compression. With the invention of the first practical algorithm for arithmetic coding (Rissanen 1976), the problem of finding out an efficient representation for a certain information source could be restated as a data modeling problem. For our purposes, a model is a mathematical description of the information source, providing a probability estimate of the next outcome. The entropy of this model sets a lower bound on the compression performance of the arithmetic encoder. This bound is tight, meaning that it is possible to generate a bitstream with average entropy as close as desired to the entropy of the model, suggesting that the effort should be made in the direction of finding good models for the information sources.

For about ten years, we have been addressing the problem of data compression using arithmetic coding. Initially in the context of image coding (Pinho 2001b; Pinho 2001a; Neves and Pinho 2006b; Neves and Pinho 2006a; Pinho and Neves 2006; Pinho and Neves 2007; Neves and Pinho 2008; Pinho and Neves 2009; Neves and Pinho 2009) and, more recently, in the context of DNA sequence coding (Pinho et al., 2006; Pinho et al., 2011), we have been relying on finite-context models for describing the data in an efficient way. Finite-context models assume that the source has Markovian properties, i.e., that the probability of the next outcome of the information source depends only on some finite number of (recent) past outcomes. This past is normally referred to as the "context", hence the name "finite-context model".

In this talk, we will start by giving a brief overview of the main aspects associated with arithmetic coding. Then, we will present the principles of finite-context modeling, both in the case

of one and two-dimensional data. We proceed with a discussion of image compression applications, some of them proposed by us, such as lossy-to-lossless image coding approaches (Pinho and Neves 2006; Pinho and Neves 2007; Pinho and Neves 2009) and microarray image compression (Neves and Pinho 2009). In the remaining part of the talk, we will put forth some ideas that link finite-context modeling with the problem of estimating the complexity of data.

2 FINITE-CONTEXT MODELS

Consider an information source that generates symbols, s, from an alphabet $\mathcal{A}$, and denote by $x^n = x_1, x_2 \ldots, x_n$ the sequence of symbols generated by the source after n outcomes. A finite-context model of an information source (see Fig. 1

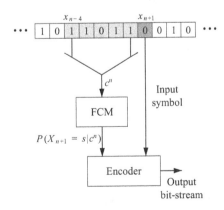

Figure 1. Example of a finite-context model for the binary alphabet, i.e., for $A = \{0,1\}$. The probability of the next outcome, X_{n+1}, is conditioned by the k last outcomes. In this example, $k = 5$.

for an example where $\mathcal{A} = \{0,1\}$) assigns probability estimates to the symbols of the alphabet, according to a conditioning context computed over a finite and fixed number k of past outcomes (order-k finite-context model) (Bell et al., 1990; Salomon 2007; Sayood 2006). At position n, we represent these conditioning outcomes by $c_n = x_{n-k+1} \cdots x_{n-1} x_n$. The number of conditioning states of the model is $|\mathcal{A}|^k$, determining the model complexity or cost.

In practice, the probability that the next outcome, X_{n+1}, is $s \in \mathcal{A}$, is obtained using the estimator

$$P(X_{n+1} = s \mid c^n) = \frac{N_s^n + \alpha}{\sum_{a \in \mathcal{A}} N_a^n + |\mathcal{A}|\alpha}, \qquad (1)$$

where N_s^n represents the number of times that, in the past, the information source generated symbol s having c^n as the conditioning context. The parameter α controls how much probability is assigned to unseen (but possible) events, and plays a key role in the case of high-order models. In fact, when k is large, the number of conditioning states, $|\mathcal{A}|^k$, is high, implying that statistics have to be estimated using only a few observations. The estimator defined in (1) reduces to Laplace's estimator for $\alpha = 1$ (Laplace 1814) and to the frequently used Krichevsky-Trofimov (Jeffreys 1946; Krichevsky and Trofimov 1981) estimator when $\alpha = 1/2$.

Initially, when all counters are zero, the symbols have probability $1/|\mathcal{A}|$, i.e., they are assumed equally probable. The counters are updated each time a symbol is encoded. Since the context is causal, the decoder is able to reproduce the same probability estimates without needing additional information.

The block denoted "Encoder" in Fig. 1 is an arithmetic encoder. It is well known that practical arithmetic coding generates output bitstreams with average bitrates almost identical to the entropy of the model (Bell et al., 1990; Salomon 2007; Sayood 2006). The theoretical bitrate average (entropy) of the finite-context model after encoding N symbols is given by

$$H_N = -\frac{1}{N} \sum_{n=0}^{N-1} \log_2 P(X_{n+1} = x_{n+1} \mid c^n) \text{ bps}, \qquad (2)$$

where "bps" stands for "bits per symbol".

3 IMAGE COMPRESSION USING FINITE-CONTEXT MODELS

JBIG, JPEG-LS and JPEG2000 are image coding standards that have been developed with different goals in mind. JBIG (ISO/IEC 1993; Sayood 2006;

Salomon 2007) is more focused on bi-level imagery, JPEG-LS (ISO/IEC 1999; Weinberger et al., 2000) is dedicated to the lossless compression of continuous-tone images and JPEG2000 (ISO/IEC 2000; Taub-man and Marcellin 2002) was designed with the aim of providing a wide range of functionalities. These three standard image encoders cover a great variety of coding approaches. Whereas JPEG2000 is transform based, JPEG-LS relies on predictive coding and JBIG relies on context-based arithmetic coding.

Usually, the compression techniques are classified according to their capability for recovering the original data. Lossy methods waive away that capability in exchange for increased compression, whereas loss-less techniques stick to the principle of exact recovery of the original data, even if that implies modest compression rates. Lossy methods are typically used in consumer products, such as photographic cameras. Lossless methods are generally required in applications where cost, legal issues or value play a decisive role, such as, for example, in remote and medical imaging or in long-term image archiving.

Therefore, the nature of the application is a key aspect when choosing between a lossy or a lossless representation. However, there are situations where different users may require different levels of reproduction quality, for example, because they might have reproduction equipments (displays, printers) with different capabilities. Users may have different downloading capacities and may want to trade quality for download time. Or, different users may be willing to pay different amounts for a given image and, therefore, may want to trade image quality for money. In conclusion, the image provider may be asked to deliver copies of the same image at an eventually large number of different qualities, including loss-less. Lossy-to-lossless technology is the answer to this need.

To provide lossy-to-lossless capabilities, we have to rely on embedded bitstream techniques, where a single bitstream is able to generate images with different quality. This is offered by the JPEG2000 image coding standard, but the rate-distortion can only be guaranteed in terms of the L_2 error norm. JBIG can also be used to achieve this goal, because it is able to handle multi-bit-plane images on a bit-plane by bit-plane basis. However, although JBIG might offer L_∞ error control, it is not prepared for exploiting inter-bit-plane dependencies, making it somewhat inefficient in this case.

Our work concerning lossy-to-lossless image coding has been focused in two approaches. One of them, is based on binary tree decomposition and arithmetic coding driven by size-adaptive finite-context models (Pinho and Neves 2006; Pinho and Neves 2007; Pinho and Neves 2009). These codecs

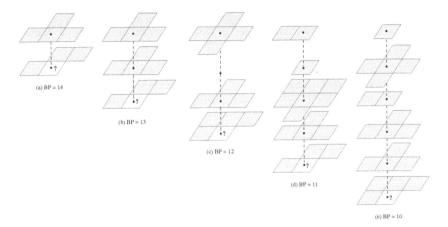

Figure 2. Example of image-dependent finite-context modeling. Each square represents a bit of a certain bit-plane of the image. For example, (a) indicates that the context for encoding the bit-plane number 14 is formed of four pixels of the upper bit-plane (number 15) and three more pixels of the current bit-plane. Bit-planes are processed from the most significant (bit-plane number 15) to the least significant bit-plane (number 0). The shape of the contexts depends on the image being encoded and is constructed on-the-fly using a greedy algorithm.

have shown better performances than the image coding standards both for mixed types of images (Pinho and Neves 2006; Pinho and Neves 2007) and for the special case of medical images (Pinho and Neves 2009). Moreover, they can provide both L_2 and L_∞ error control.

The other approach relies on bit-plane decomposition, sophisticated finite-context modeling, and bitrate monitoring and control. This technique is one of the best performing in terms of compression efficiency of microarray images (Neves and Pinho 2009). Microarrays generate pairs of 16 bits per pixel grayscale images, which may require several tens of megabytes in order to be stored or transmitted. The common approach for microarray compression has been based on image analysis for spot finding (griding followed by segmentation) with the aim of separating the microarray image data into different streams based on pixel similarities (Jörnsten et al., 2002; Hua et al., 2002; Jörnsten et al., 2003; Hua et al., 2003; Faramarzpour et al., 2003; Faramarzpour and Shirani 2004; Lonardi and Luo 2004; Zhang et al., 2005; Adjeroh et al., 2006). We have developed methods that do not require spot segmentation. This approach is based on arithmetic coding that is driven by image-dependent multi-bit-plane finite-context models (see Fig. 2 for an example).

4 ESTIMATING THE COMPLEXITY OF IMAGES

The works of researchers such as Solomonoff, Kolmogorov, Chaitin and others (Solomonoff 1964a; Solomonoff 1964b; Kolmogorov 1965; Chaitin 1966; Wallace and Boulton 1968; Rissanen 1978) related to the problem of defining a complexity measure of a string have been of paramount importance for several areas of knowledge. However, because it is not computable, the Kolmogorov complexity of a string A, $K(A)$, is usually approximated by some computable measure, such as Lempel-Ziv complexity measures (Lempel and Ziv 1976), linguistic complexity measures (Gordon 2003) or compression-based complexity measures (Dix et al., 2007).

One of the important problems that can be formulated using the Kolmogorov theory is the definition of similarity. Following this line, Li et al., (Li et al., 2004) proposed a similarity metric based on an information distance (Bennett et al., 1998), defined as the length of the shortest binary program that is needed to transform strings A and B into each other. This distance depends not only on the Kolmogorov complexity of A and B, respectively $K(A)$ and $K(B)$, but also on conditional complexities, for example $K(A|B)$, that indicates how complex string A is when string B is known. Because this distance is based on the Kolmogorov complexity (not computable), they proposed a practical analog based on standard compressors, which they call the normalized compression distance (Li et al., 2004).

According to Li et al., (Li et al., 2004), a compression method needs to be "normal" in order to be used in the normalized compression distance. One of the conditions for a compression method to be normal is that compressing string AA (the concatenation of A with A) should generate essentially the same number of bits as compressing A alone (Cilibrasi and Vitányi 2005). This characteristic holds, for example, in Lempel-Ziv based compressors, making them a frequent choice in this kind of applications.

Generally, Lempel-Ziv based compressors do not perform well on images. Moreover, most of the best performing image compression algorithms are not normal compressors. A normal compression algorithm accumulates knowledge of the data while compression is performed. It finds dependencies, collects statistics, i.e., it creates a model of the data. Most state-of-the-art image compressors, such as the JPEG2000 or JPEG-LS standards, start by decorre-lating the data using a transformation or a predictive method. Therefore, they assume an *a priori* data model that remains essentially static during compression. Moreover, this first step destroys most of the data dependencies, leaving to the entropy coding stage the mere task of encoding symbols from an (assumed) independent source.

The image coding methods that we have been developing work directly on the intensity data, i.e., they do not require a previous transformation or prediction step. These compression methods are normal and attain state-of-the-art or better than state-of-the-art compression performance, which makes them a potential choice for computing effective compression-based image complexity measures.

As an example to show the potential of the complexity measures, we consider the problem of finding unknown patterns that appear multiple times in a digital image. We want to find the number of repetitions and their positions in the image without constraining the nature and shape of the pattern in any way.

Fig. 3 displays the modified "Lena" image and the corresponding complexity surface. A complexity surface is an image ϕ, with the same geometry as the original image f, where each pixel $\phi_{i,j}$ contains the code length required to encode $f_{i,j}$ estimated by the finite-context model. For facilitating

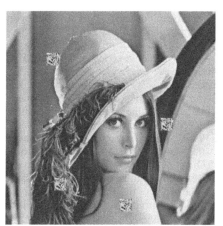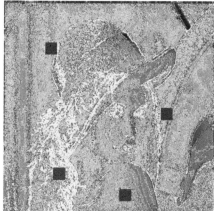

Figure 3. On the left, the "Lena" image changed by inserting the same small textured region into four different places. On the right, the logarithm of the complexity surface obtained with the method proposed in this paper, where it can be seen four darker regions corresponding to low complexity occurrences motivated by the repeating pattern.

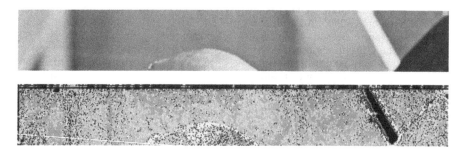

Figure 4. At the top, the first 70 rows of the "Lena" image. Below, the corresponding image of the logarithm of the complexity surface, showing a horizontal dark strip, indicating a repetitive pattern that might has been created during some previous manipulation of the image. The oblique strip is also marked as a low complexity region.

the observation of the details, we display the logarithm of the complexity surface scaled to the [0, 255] range (0 indicates the lowest complexity, whereas 255 corresponds to the highest complexity).

It is easy to find, in the complexity surface, the dark squares revealing the zones of low complexity that have been originated by the repetition of the pattern that we have inserted. In Fig. 4, we show in greater detail the first 70 rows of the "Lena" image and the corresponding complexity surface showing a horizontal dark strip. It is curious that we have only noticed the existence of a repeated pattern in the first few rows of the image after visualizing its complexity surface, demonstrating one of the potential uses of the technique.

REFERENCES

Adjeroh, D., Zhang, Y. and Parthe, R. (2006, February). On denoising and compression of DNA microarray images. *Pattern Recognition 39*, 2478–2493.

Bell, T.C., Cleary, J.G. and Witten, I.H. (1990). *Text compression*. Prentice Hall.

Bennett, C.H., Gács, P. Vitányi, M.L.P.M.B. and Zurek, W.H. (1998, July). Information distance. *IEEE Trans. on Information Theory 44*(4), 1407–1423.

Chaitin, G.J. (1966). On the length of programs for computing finite binary sequences. *Journal of the ACM 13*, 547–569.

Cilibrasi, R. and Vitányi, P.M.B. (2005, April). Clustering by compression. *IEEE Trans. on Information Theory 51*(4), 1523–1545.

Dix, T.I., Powell, D.R., Allison, L., Bernal, J., Jaeger, S. and Stern, L. (2007). Comparative analysis of long DNA sequences by per element information content using different contexts. *BMC Bioinformatics 8*(Suppl. 2), S10.

Faramarzpour, N. and Shirani, S. (2004, March). Lossless and lossy compression of DNA microarray images. In *Proc. of the Data Compression Conf., DCC-2004*, Snowbird, Utah, p. 538.

Faramarzpour, N., Shirani, S. and Bondy, J. (2003, November). Lossless DNA microarray image compression. In *Proc. of the 37th Asilomar Conf. on Signals, Systems, and Computers, 2003*, Volume 2, pp. 1501–1504.

Gordon, G. (2003). Multi-dimensional linguistic complexity. *Journal of Biomolecular Structure & Dynamics 20*(6), 747–750.

Hua, J., Liu, Z., Xiong, Z., Wu, Q. and Castleman, K. (2003, September). Microarray BASICA: background adjustment, segmentation, image compression and analysis of microarray images. In *Proc. of the IEEE Int. Conf. on Image Processing, ICIP-2003*, Volume 1, Barcelona, Spain, pp. 585–588.

Hua, J., Xiong, Z., Wu, Q. and Castleman, K. (2002, October). Fast segmentation and lossy-to-lossless compression of DNA microarray images. In *Proc. of the Workshop on Genomic Signal Processing and Statistics, GENSIPS2002*, Raleigh, NC.

ISO/IEC (1993, March). *Information technology—Coded representation of picture and audio information—progressive bi-level image compression.* International Standard ISO/IEC 11544 and ITU-T Recommendation T. 82.

ISO/IEC (1999). *Information technology—Lossless and near-lossless compression of continuous-tone still images.* ISO/IEC 14495-1 and ITU Recommendation T. 87.

ISO/IEC (2000). *Information technology—JPEG 2000 image coding system.* ISO/IEC International Standard 15444-1, ITU-T Recommendation T. 800.

Jeffreys, H. (1946). An invariant form for the prior probability in estimation problems. *Proc. of the Royal Society (London) A 186*, 453–461.

Jörnsten, R., Wang, W., Yu, B. and Ramchandran, K. (2003). Microarray image compression: SLOCO and the effect of information loss. *Signal Processing 83*, 859–869.

Jörnsten, R., Yu, B. Wang, W. and Ramchandran, K. (2002, September). Compression of cDNA and inkjet microarray images. In *Proc. of the IEEE Int. Conf. on Image Processing, ICIP-2002*, Volume 3, Rochester, NY, pp. 961–964.

Kolmogorov, A.N. (1965). Three approaches to the quantitative definition of information. *Problems of Information Transmission 1*(1), 1–7.

Krichevsky, R.E. and Trofimov, V.K. (1981, March). The performance of universal encoding. *IEEE Trans. on Information Theory 27*(2), 199–207.

Laplace, P.S. (1814). *Essai philosophique sur les probabilités (A philosophical essay on probabilities).* New York: John Wiley & Sons. Translated from the sixth French edition by F.W. Truscott and F.L. Emory, 1902.

Lempel, A. and Ziv, J. (1976, January). On the complexity of finite sequences. *IEEE Trans. on Information Theory 22*(1), 75–81.

Li, M., Chen, X., Li, X., Ma, B. and Vitányi P.M.B. (2004, December). The similarity metric. *IEEE Trans. on Information Theory 50*(12), 3250–3264.

Lonardi, S. and Luo, Y. (2004, August). Gridding and compression of microarray images. In *Proc. of the IEEE Computational Systems Bioinformatics Conference, CSB-2004*, Stanford, CA.

Neves, A.J.R. and Pinho, A.J. (2006a, May). A bit-plane approach for lossless compression of color-quantized images. In *Proc. of the IEEE Int. Conf. on Acoustics, Speech, and Signal Processing, ICASSP-2006*, Volume 2, Toulouse, France, pp. 429–432.

Neves, A.J.R. and Pinho, A.J. (2006b, October). Lossless compression of microarray images. In *Proc. of the IEEE Int. Conf. on Image Processing, ICIP-2006*, Atlanta, GA, pp. 2505–2508.

Neves, A.J.R. and Pinho, A.J. (2008, August). A bitplane based algorithm for lossless compression of DNA microarray images. In *Proc. of the 16th European Signal Processing Conf., EUSIPCO-2008*, Lausanne, Switzerland.

Neves, A.J.R. and Pinho, A.J. (2009, February). Lossless compression of microarray images using image-dependent finite-context models. *IEEE Trans. on Medical Imaging 28*(2), 194–201.

Pinho, A.J. (2001a, January). Adaptive context-based arithmetic coding of arbitrary contour maps. *IEEE Signal Processing Letters 8*(1), 4–6.

Pinho, A.J. (2001b, May). Region-based near-lossless image compression. In *Proc. of the IEEE Int. Conf. on Acoustics, Speech, and Signal Processing, ICASSP-2001*, Volume 3, Salt Lake City, UT, pp. 1761–1764.

Pinho, A.J., Ferreira, P.J.S.G., Neves, A.J.R. and Bastos, C.A.C. (2011). On the representability of complete genomes by multiple competing finite-context (Markov) models. *PLoS ONE in press*.

Pinho, A.J. and Neves, A.J.R. (2006, October). Lossy-to-lossless compression of images based on binary tree decomposition. In *Proc. of the IEEE Int. Conf. on Image Processing, ICIP2006*, Atlanta, GA, pp. 2257–2260.

Pinho, A.J. and Neves, A.J.R. (2007, November). L-infinity progressive image compression. In *Proc. of the Picture Coding Symposium, PCS 07*, Lisbon, Portugal.

Pinho, A.J. and Neves, A.J.R. (2009, April). Progressive lossless compression of medical images. In *Proc. of the IEEE Int. Conf. on Acoustics, Speech, and Signal Processing, ICASSP2009*, Taipei, Taiwan.

Pinho, A.J., Neves, A.J.R., Afreixo, V., Bastos, C.A.C. and Ferreira, P.J.S.G. (2006, November). A three-state model for DNA protein-coding regions. *IEEE Trans. on Biomedical Engineering 53*(11), 2148–2155.

Rissanen, J. (1976, May). Generalized Kraft inequality and arithmetic coding. *IBM J. Res. Develop. 20*(3), 198–203.

Rissanen, J. (1978). Modeling by shortest data description. *Automatica 14*, 465–471.

Salomon, D. (2007). *Data compression—The complete reference* (4th ed.). Springer.

Sayood, K. (2006). *Introduction to data compression* (3rd ed.). Morgan Kaufmann.

Solomonoff, R.J. (1964a, March). A formal theory of inductive inference. Part I. *Information and Control 7*(1), 1–22.

Solomonoff, R.J. (1964b, June). A formal theory of inductive inference. Part II. *Information and Control 7*(2), 224–254.

Taubman, D.S. and Marcellin, M.W. (2002). *JPEG2000: image compression fundamentals, standards and practice*. Kluwer Academic Publishers.

Wallace, C.S. and Boulton, D.M. (1968, August). An information measure for classification. *The Computer Journal 11*(2), 185–194.

Weinberger, M.J., Seroussi, G. and Sapiro, G. (2000, August). The LOCO-I lossless image compression algorithm: principles and standardization into JPEG-LS. *IEEE Trans. on Image Processing 9*(8), 1309–1324.

Zhang, Y., Parthe, R. and Adjeroh, D. (2005, August). Lossless compression of DNA microarray images. In *Proc. of the IEEE Computational Systems Bioinformatics Conference, CSB-2005*, Stanford, CA.

Computational Vision and Medical Image Processing – Tavares & Natal Jorge (eds)
© *2012 Taylor & Francis Group, London, ISBN 978-0-415-68395-1*

Learning classifier families for object detection and parameter estimation

Stan Sclaroff & Ashwin Thangali
Department of Computer Science, Boston University, Boston, MA, USA

Quan Yuan
US Research Center, Sony Electronics, San Jose, CA, USA

Vitaly Ablavsky
EPFL-I&C-CVLAB, Lausanne, Switzerland

ABSTRACT: We describe methods that can learn a single family of classifiers for detecting object classes that exhibit large within-class variation. One common solution is to use a divide-and-conquer strategy, where the space of possible within-class variations is partitioned, and different detectors are trained for different partitions. However, these discrete partitions tend to be arbitrary in continuous spaces, and the classifiers have limited power when there are too few training samples in each subclass. To address this shortcoming, explicit feature sharing has been proposed, but it also makes training more expensive. We show that foreground-background classification (detection) and within-class classification of the foreground class (pose estimation) can be jointly solved in a multiplicative form of two kernel functions. One kernel measures similarity for foreground-background classification. The other kernel accounts for latent factors that control within-class variation and implicitly enables feature sharing among foreground training samples. The multiplicative kernel formulation enables feature sharing implicitly; the solution for the optimal sharing is a byproduct of SVM learning. The resulting detector family is tuned to specific variations in the foreground. The effectiveness of this framework is demonstrated in experiments that involve detection, tracking, and pose estimation of human hands, faces, and vehicles in video.

1 OVERVIEW

A computer vision system for object recognition typically has two modules: a detection module and a foreground state estimation module. The detection module is often implemented as a scanning window process where each window location in an image is evaluated by a binary classifier, i.e., foreground class vs. background class. The invocation of the foreground state estimation module is conditioned on the detection of an instance of the foreground class; in other words, the second module is tuned to the variations within the foreground class. This second module can be implemented in numerous ways. For discrete state spaces—for example, face ID, hand shape class, or vehicle type—estimation can be framed as a multiclass classification problem. For continuous state spaces—for example, face age, hand joint angles, vehicle orientation—estimation can be formulated in terms of regression. Another common approach for foreground state estimation is to use nearest neighbor methods (Athitsos and Sclaroff 2003; Shakhnarovich et al., 2003).

In any case, when object classes exhibit large within-class variations, detection and foreground state estimation can be chicken-egg problems. Assuming the objects are detected and segmented from the background, foreground state estimation is relatively straightforward. Assuming specific variations of the foreground class, detection can be achieved as in (Ramanan et al., 2005). However, if neither the foreground state nor detection is given, then challenges arise. For example, it is difficult for a single detector to cope with all variations of the foreground class, while at the same time providing reliable discrimination between the foreground and background—especially in applications where there are widely varying, or even unconstrained backgrounds.

A common strategy in this setting is divide-and-conquer (Viola and Jones 2003; Wu and Nevatia 2007): divide the foreground class into subclasses by partitioning the space of within-class variations, and then train a separate detector for each partition. Thus, a set of detectors is trained, where each detector discriminates between the background class and its subset of the foreground class.

An additional advantage of such a strategy is that coarse estimation of the object pose can also be obtained during detection process. For example, in multi-pose face detection, the detector of the correct face pose tends to have a high response. However, in a divide-and-conquer strategy, the partitioning of a foreground class is oftentimes arbitrary. Moreover, to keep ample training examples in each subclass, the partitioning of the foreground class is usually coarse, which limits the ability of pose estimation.

We propose a different strategy that avoids explicit partitioning of the foreground class in this paper: learning a family of detectors, where the detectors themselves are parameterized over the space of within-class variations (Yuan et al., 2011). Our formulation utilizes a product of two kernel functions: a within-class kernel k_θ to handle foreground state variations and feature sharing, and a between-class kernel k_x to handle foreground-background classification. This kernel formulation is used in a Support Vector Machine (SVM) (Cortes and Vapnik 1995) training algorithm that outputs support vectors and their weights, which can be used to construct a family of detectors that are tuned to foreground variations. After SVM training, a sample set of detectors can be generated, where each detector is associated with a particular foreground state parameter value. All the samples from the detector family share the same support vectors, but the weights of these support vectors vary depending on the within-class state value. A useful side effect of this support vector sharing is that features are implicitly shared across the whole detector family.

The formulation is useful in solving detection, state estimation, and tracking problems. For detection using a scanning window process, an image window can be classified as foreground if at least one of the detectors in the family produces a score that is above a predefined threshold. For a given image window, the foreground state can be estimated simply by examining the state values associated with detectors that produce the highest responses for that input. For particle filter-based tracking methods, like CONDENSATION (Isard and Blake 1998), importance sampling from the detector family can be driven by a dynamical model at each frame, where the objects are allowed to undergo a range of state variations over time.

With proper nonparametric kernel functions, our formulation can be extended to nonparametric cases, when explicit parameter annotation of the foreground class examples is too expensive to obtain. A mode finding method is proposed that selects a representative subset of samples from the detector family in the nonparametric case. This generally reduces the number of detectors to be invoked, and thereby makes detection more efficient. If state estimation or tracking is desired, then the user can label the state for each sample in the representative subset. This alleviates the burden of assigning ground truth states for the complete training set, and instead focuses only on labelling the smaller representative subset.

The proposed framework is demonstrated in three application areas. The first involves hand detection, segmentation, and shape estimation for images taken from videos of Flemish and American Sign Language. There is a wide variation of hand shapes and orientations in these videos. The framework is also tested in estimating index finger angles. The second application involves detection, orientation estimation and tracking of vehicles driving on highways, and the more challenging case of race cars careening on dirt roads. The third application focuses on the problem of detecting and tracking multiple human faces, while simultaneously estimating the left-right rotation angles under illumination variations.

REFERENCES

Athitsos, V. and Sclaroff, S. (2003). Estimating 3D hand pose from a cluttered image. In *Proc. CVPR*.

Cortes, C. and Vapnik, V. (1995). Support vector networks. *Machine Learning 20*, 273–297.

Isard, M. and Blake, A. (1998). CONDENSATION: conditional density propagation for visual tracking. *International Journal of Computer Vision 29*(1), 5–28.

Ramanan, D., Forsyth, D.A. and Zisserman, A. (2005). Strike a pose: Tracking people by finding stylized poses. In *Proc. CVPR*.

Shakhnarovich, G., Viola, P. and Darrell, T. (2003). Fast pose estimation with parameter-sensitive hashing. In *Proc. ICCV*.

Viola, P. and Jones, M. (2003). Fast multi-view face detection. In *Proc. CVPR*.

Wu, B. and Nevatia, R. (2007). Cluster boosted tree classifier for multi-view multi-pose object detection. In *Proc. ICCV*.

Yuan, Q., Thangali, A. Ablavsky, V. and Sclaroff, S. (2011). Learning a family of detectors via multiplicative kernels. *IEEE Trans. on Pattern Analysis and Machine Intelligence 33*(3), 514–530.

Contributed papers

Computational Vision and Medical Image Processing – Tavares & Natal Jorge (eds)
© 2012 Taylor & Francis Group, London, ISBN 978-0-415-68395-1

Generation of planar radiographs from 3D anatomical models using the GPU

A.S. Cardoso
Faculdade de Engenharia, Universidade do Porto, Portugal

D.C. Moura & J.G. Barbosa
Departamento de Engenharia Informática, Laboratório de Inteligência Artificial e Ciência dos Computadores, Faculdade de Engenharia, Universidade do Porto, Portugal

ABSTRACT: This paper describes the development of parallel, high performance algorithms for generation of DRRs out of 3D vertebrae models, using the GPU. NVIDIA CUDA platform was chosen for the implementation of these algorithms because it provides flexible and fine-grain control over the hardware when compared with other platforms.

This research is motivated by recent work aiming to attain a process to recover the shape of the human spine of scoliosis patients using two planar radiographs. A DRR generation algorithm would allow for 2D/3D registration during the process, for best reconstruction accuracy. However, this requires generation of hundreds of DRRs per second, which is not compatible with a CPU implementation.

The top performance registered for the DRR generation of a lumbar vertebra was 828 FPS with an entry-level graphic card, showing that the GPU implementation achieves performances compatible with 2D/3D registration problems while keeping hardware requirements low.

1 INTRODUCTION

The generation of planar radiographs from anatomical models is, nowadays, an important research field because of the potential shown to solve many 2D/3D image registration problems. The use of digitally reconstructed radiographs (DRRs) has been reported on many medical procedures, such as computer aided surgery (CAS) (Knaan and Joskowicz 2003; Zollei et al., 2001; van de Kraats et al., 2004), radiotherapy (Mori et al., 2009) or surface recovery of human bone structures (Moura et al., 2009).

1.1 Motivation

Correct assessment of scoliosis patients' condition is only possible using three-dimensional reconstructions of the spine, from which clinical indexes such as the maximum plane of curvature can be quantified (Stokes 1994). Computer Tomography (CT) or Magnetic Resonance Imaging (MRI) are regarded as the gold standard on clinical 3D reconstruction techniques. However, they are not suitable for scoliosis patients because they require a lying down position, thus altering the spine configuration (Mitulescu et al., 2002). To deal with this issue, several methods were proposed which aim to recover the scoliotic spine (Mitulescu et al., 2001; Pomero et al., 2004; Mitton et al., 2006; Mitulescu et al., 2002). In particular, in (Moura et al., 2009; Moura et al., 2011), the authors proposed a semisupervised reconstruction method, which seeks to recover the spine shape using one posterior-anterior radiograph, and one lateral radiograph. This method requires only the identification of a spline on each radiograph, decreasing the amount of user input during the process.

The work herein described is in line with the former 3D reconstruction procedure: most of the reconstruction methods do not use image data and solely rely on the experience of the operator. Having a DRR generator would allow to perform 2D/3D registration of vertebrae models for recovering the vertebrae's shape. However, this would translate into an optimization process, requiring the computation of hundreds of DRRs per second, thus creating a computational bottleneck when considering this task on CPUs (Russakoff et al., 2003; Ruijters et al., 2008).

1.2 Objectives

In this paper, we propose the implementation of a parallel algorithm, based on a single-pass fragment capturing technique reported in (Liu et al., 2010), for DRR computation on the GPU. The algorithm is implemented under NVIDIA Compute Unified Device Architecture platform, a parallel computing platform that enables GPU programming and allows fine-grain control over the hardware when compared with other graphics APIs.

We believe that a GPU implementation can overcome the performance issues that the DRR computation procedures presents, by taking advantage of recent GPU technologies and the processing power they present. Also, the work is based on polygon mesh models, which is a much simpler representation compared to voxel-based volumes. This characteristic may allow us to achieve higher DRR generation performances.

2 DRR GENERATION CONCEPTS

DRRs try to mimic the physical process that takes place in planar radiography procedures. This process is explained by the attenuation law, which relates the absorption of electromagnetic radiation to the properties of the material traversed by the X-rays. This law can be described by Equation 1, in an integrated form, for a monochromatic X-ray beam:

$$N_{out}(E) = N_{in}(E) \times e^{-\int \mu(E, \rho(x), Z(x)) dx} \qquad (1)$$

where $N_{out}(E)$ is the number of photons that reach the image detector; N_{in} is the number of photons initially transmitted; and μ is the attenuation coefficient which dictates the interaction photons will have with the material.

For the purpose of the computation of a digital radiograph, one can emit rays from the X-ray source to each pixel of the final image, storing the path length of each ray—distance a ray traverses inside the object. Equation 2 (Vidal et al., 2009) shows the discrete approximation of the attenuation law, used to compute the intensity of each pixel on the DRR.

$$N_{out}(E) = N_{in}(E) \times exp\left(\sum_{i=0}^{i<objs} \mu(i) L_p(i) \right) \qquad (2)$$

where *objs* is the total number of objects; and $L_p(i)$ is the path length of the conceptual ray traversing the *ith* object, which is simply the distance a ray covers inside the object's volume.

3 PARALLEL DRR GENERATION

3.1 Overview

DRR generation algorithms need to compute the path length of a X-ray traversing an object

towards a pixel of the image detector. Intuitively, one can emit rays from the projection source to every pixel in the detector, and evaluate the intersections of each ray with the triangular mesh. These intersections could be further used to compute the path length of the ray, using the distance to the projection source. However, ray casting approaches rely on computationally expensive procedures, such as ray-triangle intersection tests and euclidean distances between two 3D points. In (Vidal et al., 2009) is reported an efficient GPU implementation—based on depth-peeling (Everitt 2001)—which uses OpenGL to peel away depth layers of the scene. Each peel allows the computation of the fragments' depths, which are stored in an off-screen buffer and used to calculate the path length of a ray, avoiding otherwise expensive arithmetic.

3.2 Method

Similarly to the approach followed in (Vidal et al., 2009), we propose a depth-peeling based algorithm for GPU implementation. It exploits CUDA atomic operations in order to store, without concurrency hazards, each fragments' depth on a *depth array*. The algorithm is implemented in two separate CUDA kernels:

- Capturing of each triangle fragment's depth;
- Final blending of each pixel *depth array*.

The first kernel launches one thread per triangle of the 3D model. Each thread determines all the pixels covered by the triangle projection by scanning the triangle row by row. This scanline procedure resorts to the Bresenham-line algorithm (Bresenham 1965) to calculate the minimum and maximum pixel positions of each row, thus avoiding floating-point arithmetic to determine the next pixel along the edge.

During this stage, the fragments' depths are interpolated in the integer domain using each triangle vertex depth value. Once the pixel position corresponding to the fragment is known, the interpolated depth is stored in the pixel *depth array*, using an approach reported in (Liu et al., 2010). The approach exploits the CUDA atomicInc() operation to provide concurrent threads with an unique index that can be used to access the pixel *depth array*, without concurrency hazards. Algorithm 1 shows the pseudo-code for this approach, where a shared integer value, previously initialized with zero, is incremented—using the atomicInc() atomic operation—by any thread that needs to write in the *depth array*.

It is common to assume a filling convention (or filling geometry) during polygon rasterization procedures, in order to avoid pixel overlapping by adjacent polygons of the model. Similarly, our DRR algorithm uses a *top-left* filling convention during the scanline procedure, avoiding the generation of artifacts in the DRR image. This demonstrates how the finegrain control provided by CUDA allows preventing the generation of artifacts, while previous OpenGL approaches (e.g., (Vidal et al., 2009)) that rely on the OpenGL pipeline require an additional post-processing step for removing artifacts.

Algorithm 1 Concurrent fragment depth insertion in *depth array*

1: *counter ← &(pixelCounters[pixel])*
2: *offset ← atomicInc(counter, INT_MAX)*
3: *index ← pixel + offset*
4: *depthArrays[index] ← fragmentDepth*

The first kernel processes all the triangles, capturing all the fragments' depths in submission order. The second kernel uses these values, captured in the *depth arrays*, blending them using Equation 2. Spanning one thread for each pixel, the kernel starts by ordering each *depth array*. Due to the small number of depth layers, a simple *bubble-sort* is used, running from 0 to *pixelCounters[pixel]*. This value is set in the previous kernel run, and corresponds to the number of fragments captured for one pixel. Once the ordering is done, the kernel continues with the blending stage, where each pair of consecutive values of the *depth arrays* are subtracted and the result accumulated. Finally, the result is multiplied by a suitable bone attenuation factor and stored as the final pixel value. This approach is shown in Algorithm 2.

Algorithm 2 Blending stage

1: *n ← depthCounters[pixel]*
2: *depthArray ← &(depthArrays[pixel])*
3: *bubbleSort(depthArray,n)*
4: **for** *i = 0 to n−1* **do**
5:    **if** *i % 2 != 0* **then**
6:       *acum ← ptr[i]−dec*
7:    **else**
8:       *dec ← ptr[i]*
9:    **end if**
10: **end for**
11: *drr_result[index] = exp(acum * μ)*

---

4 RESULTS AND DISCUSSION

The algorithms herein presented were developed under CUDA 3.1, and tested using a desktop equipped with a Intel Core 2 6400 and a NVIDIA GeForce GT 240 with 512 MB of RAM memory.

Figure 1 shows a DRR computed using the described algorithm.

For benchmarking the DRR generation process, 500,000 DRRs were generated and the processing time was recorded. The average number of DRRs generated per second were calculated (frames per second—FPS) for two anatomical models of different complexity: an human L3 vertebra with 1,552 triangles and a complete human spine with 21,792 triangles. DRRs were also generated for two different views: Posterio-anterior (PA) and Lateral (LAT). Since copying the DRR from GPU to CPU memmory can compromise performance and may not be required depending of the application, the benchmarking was performed both with and without copying the DRRs to CPU memory. Results are summarized in Table 1.

In (Vidal et al., 2009), a CPU implementation for DRR generation shows performances in the interval 10–100 FPS, when comparing similar object models and image dimensions. Those results assume a detector area coverage by the test object of only 21.5%. On the other hand, our benchmarks count with an average detector coverage of 47.0%, reaching a top performance of 828 FPS on the smaller object and 85 FPS on the bigger spine model. Moreover, our benchmarks encompass the dynamic region of interest (ROI) computation on each iteration, which is also done on GPU. Due to these differences, and due to non-negligeble differences in the graphics hardware, a comparison

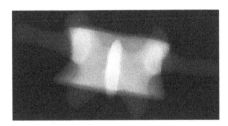

Figure 1. DRR for a L3 vertebra in the posterioanterior plane generated from a 3D mesh model.

Table 1. Benchmarking Results for the DRR generation algorithm, in frames per second (FPS). PA: posterior-anterior perspective; LAT: lateral view; Nomem: DRR was not transfered from GPU memory to CPU memory; Mem: DRR was transfered to CPU memory. Model Size is in triangle number units.

Model size	View	Pixel number	Performance no-mem	(FPS) mem
1,552*t*	PA	36,305	622.1	595.4
	LAT	26,664	828.2	722.4
21,792*t*	PA	396,526	84.6	74.5
	LAT	528,770	85.7	73.8

with the GPU implemention of (Vidal et al., 2009) is not possible.

5 CONCLUSIONS

This paper presents a single-pass DRR generation algorithm, implemented under NVIDIA CUDA, a GPU programming platform. The algorithm exploits CUDA atomic operations in order to capture fragment depths in submission order, while avoiding artifact generation during a carefully planned scanline rasterization stage. This shows an advantage over previous algorithms based on OpenGL that required a post-processing step for eliminating artifacts created by the DRR generation process.

Benchmark results for the generation of DRRs from 3D polygon mesh vertebrae models, show that the CUDA implementation delivers DRR generation rates compatible with 2D/3D registration procedures. Furthermore, it was shown that an entry level graphical card is already capable of delivering high performances.

The algorithm implementation proposed here follows a shared memory model and may be ported to other parallel hardware architectures. Future work will include incorporating the method proposed here in a 2D/3D registration framework and taking advantage of the GPU for calculating registration metrics, allowing to substantially decrease memory transfers from GPU memory to CPU memory.

REFERENCES

Bresenham, J.E. (1965). Algorithm for computer control of a digital plotter. *IBM Systems Journal 4*(1), 25–30.

Everitt, C. (2001). Interactive order-independent transparency. NVIDIA OpenGL SDK. http://developer. nvidia.com/object/Interactive_Order_Transparency. html.

Knaan, D. and Joskowicz, L. (2003). Effective intensity-based 2d/3d rigid registration between fluoroscopic x-ray and ct. In *Medical Image Computing and Computer-Assisted Interventio—MICCAI 2003*, Volume 2878 of *Lecture Notes in Computer Science*, pp. 351–358. Springer Berlin/Heidelberg.

Liu, F., Huang, M.-C., Liu, X.-H. and Wu, E.-H. (2010). Freepipe: a programmable parallel rendering architecture for efficient multi-fragment effects. In *I3D '10: Proceedings of the 2010 ACM SIGGRAPH symposium on Interactive 3D Graphics and Games*, New York, NY, USA, pp. 75–82.

Mitton, D., Landry, C., Vèron, S., Skalli, W., Lavaste, F. and Guise, J.A.D. (2006). 3d reconstruction method from biplanar radiography using non-stereocorresponding points and elastic deformable meshes. *Medical and Biological Engineering and Computing*, 133–139.

Mitulescu, A., Semaan, I., De Guise, J., Leborgne, P., Adamsbaum, C. and Skalli, W. (2001). Validation of the non-stereo corresponding points stereoradiographic 3d reconstruction technique. *Medical and Biological Engineering and Computing 39*, 152–158.

Mitulescu, A., Skalli, W., Mitton, D. and Guise, J.A.D. (2002). Three-dimensional surface rendering reconstruction of scoliotic vertebrae using a non stereo-corresponding points technique. *European Spine Journal*.

Mori, S., Kobayashi, M., Kumagai, M. and Minohara, S. (2009). Development of a gpu-based multithreaded software application to calculate digitally reconstructed radiographs for radiotherapy. *Radiological Physics and Technology*.

Moura, D.C., Boisvert, J., Barbosa, J.G., Labelle, H. and Tavares, J.M.R.S. (2011). Fast 3D reconstruction of the spine from biplanar radiographs using a deformable articulated model. *Medical Engineering & Physics (in press)*.

Moura, D.C., Boisvert, J. Barbosa, J.G. and Tavares, J.M. (2009). Fast 3d reconstruction of the spine using user-defined splines and a statistical articulated model. In *ISVC '09: Proceedings of the 5th International Symposium on Advances in Visual Computing*, Berlin, Heidelberg, pp. 586–595. Springer-Verlag.

Pomero, V., Mitton, D., Laporte, S., de Guise, J.A. and Skalli, W. (2004). Fast accurate stereoradiographic 3d-reconstruction of the spine using a combined geometric and statistic model. *Clinical biomechanics (Bristol, Avon) 19(3)*.

Ruijters, D., ter Haar-Romeny, B.M. and Suetens, P. (2008). Gpu-accelerated digitally reconstructed radiographs. In *BioMED '08: Proceedings of the Sixth IASTED International Conference on Biomedical Engineering*, Anaheim, CA, USA, pp. 431–435. ACTA Press.

Russakoff, D., Rohlfing, T., Rueckert, D., Shahidi, R., Kim, D., Kima, D. and Maurer, C.R. Jr. (2003). Fast calculation of digitally reconstructed radiographs using light fields. In M. Sonka and J.M. Fitzpatrick (Eds.), *Medical Imaging: Image Processing*.

Stokes, I.A. (1994). Three-dimensional terminology of spinal deformity. a report presented to the scoliosis research society by the scoliosis research society working group on 3-d terminology of spinal deformity. *Spine (Phila Pa 1976) 19(2)*, 236–48.

van de Kraats, E.B., Penney, G.P., Tomaževič, D.D., van Walsum, D. and Niessen, W.J. (2004). Standardized evaluation of 2d-3d registration. In *Medical Image Computing and Computer—Assisted Intervention*, Volume 3216 of *Lecture Notes in Computer Science*, pp. 574–581. Springer Berlin/Heidelberg.

Vidal, F.P., Garnier, M., Freud, N., Létang, J.M. and John, N. (2009). Simulation of x-ray attenuation on the gpu. In *Proceeding of TCPG'09—Theory and Practice of Computer Graphics*, pp. 25–32. Eurographics.

Zollei, L., Grimson, E., Norbash, A. and Wells, W. (2001). 2d-3d rigid registration of x-ray fluoroscopy and ct images using mutual information and sparsely sampled histogram estimators. In *Computer Vision and Pattern Recognition, 2001. CVPR 2001. Proceedings of the 2001 IEEE Computer Society Conference on*, Volume 2, pp. II-696–II-703 vol. 2.

Computational Vision and Medical Image Processing – Tavares & Natal Jorge (eds)
© *2012 Taylor & Francis Group, London, ISBN 978-0-415-68395-1*

An on-line system for medical and biological image sharing

Gustavo M. Porcides & Luiz A.P. Neves
Federal University of Paraná, Curitiba, Brazil

Luiz C.M. de Aquino & Gilson A. Giraldi
National Laboratory for Scientific Computing, Petrópolis, Brazil

ABSTRACT: This work presents an on-line tool for sharing and processing medical and biological images. Developed with PHP and Javascript using the DBMS PostgreSQL, this tool currently has several image processing algorithms, as well as marking and zooming tools. The system was validated using the Web Application test techniques proposed by Pressman (Pressman 1995).

1 INTRODUCTION

This project aims to create a web-based system that allows its users to store, share and process images. Though there are some on-line image processing systems, like Picnik (Picnik) and Pixlr (Pixlr), the proposed system has several advantages, like the possibility to store images and other functionalities that improve the communication among researchers and the analysis of images.

Therefore, the main objective of the SBIM (Shared Biological Image Manager) project is to offer to the researchers an easy to use system with several functionalities to ease the storage and manipulation of digital medical and biological images.

2 RELATED WORKS

To develop this system, several studies (Azevedo-Marques, Caritá, Benedicto, and Sanches 2005) (Azevedo-Marques, Trad, Júnior, and Santos 2001) (Pires, Medeiros, and Schiabel 2004) (Caritá, Seraphim, Honda, and Azevedo-Marques 2008) (d'Ornellas, Mussoi, and Dias 2004) (Santos and Furuie 2005) (Brito 1993) are being analysed. These studies propose methodologies, tools and functionalities that are useful to the proposed system. By analysing these works, we found many techniques that will improve this project, like CBIR algorithms (Content-Based Image Retrieval), keywords search, image processing algorithms and other functionalities related to the interface.

3 METHODOLOGY

The used methodology to develop this project is divided in three stages. During the first stage the system was modelled accordingly to the collected theoric referential. The second stage consisted of the development of the interface and the definition of how the data would be handled. In the last stage, the system is being implemented and the tests are being made.

4 ANALYSIS OF RESULTS

In this section we present the results obtained during the development of this system.

4.1 *Results of the data modelling*

One of the objectives of this project is to allow users to store and share images. For this purpose, a database composed of 15 tables was created.

The main table, called Image stores data about images, like format, compression, resolution and dimensions.

Other tables store data about the use history of the system, data about the users, messages and access levels. The data modelling of the system is shown in Porcides et al. (Porcides, Stein, Kamada, Neves, and Giraldi 2010), with minor modifications.

4.2 *Results of interface development*

During this stage, the main focus of the work was to develop an ease to use interface that would offer a friendly work environment.

Figure 1 shows the interface developed using techniques proposed by Reinhard (Oppermann 2010), who suggests methods for the development of clean interfaces and the use of colors to draw attention to the main areas of the website.

The central section of the website varies accordingly to the page that the user is currently visiting,

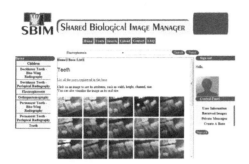

Figure 1. Image list of SBIM.

while the other sections remain static. Figure 1 show the list of images registered in a base.

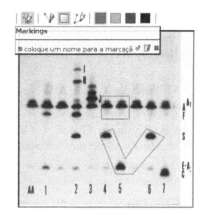

Figure 2. Marking tool.

4.3 Results of system implementation

Currently, the system is being developed using the programming languages PHP and Javascript and implementing HTML5 features. The Database Base Management System (DBMS) PostgreSQL is being used based on Porcides et al. (Porcides, Stein, Kamada, Neves, and Giraldi 2010).

The proposed system has several tools to improve the users experience in the system. These tools are:

- zoom;
- image marker;
- image processing algorithms;
- message system and
- automatic feature extractor.

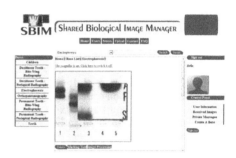

Figure 3. Zoom tool.

The marking tool was developed using Javascript and the HTML5 Canvas element. One interesting aspect of this tool is that the system does not need to create a copy of the image each time a line is drawn on it, because it stores the marking information,like color and coordinates, in a separate table, not in the actual image. The user must select the marking in a list in order to display it over the image as illustrated in Figure 2. Due to the fact that there are no copies of the images, it decreases largely the amount of computational resources used to store them. Also, users may attach text to the markings.

Another functionality of the proposed system is the tool that allows users to zoom in images as shown in Figure 3. Developed with Javascript, this tool is very interactive, because it allows the control of the size of the zoomed area as well as the zoom rate, that may be up to 1000%. This feature makes the image analysis more dynamic.

Moreover, the system has an automatic image feature extractor. The extracted features are resolution, format, compression, channel, height and width. These informations may be used to retrieve images using the advanced search engine, where users can search by format or set intervals of height and width.

The extraction process is imperceptible to the user, because it gets the information during the upload.

Another feature of the proposed system is the message module that allows the communication among researchers using a method similar to most e-mail systems. These messages are stored until the destinatary deletes them. Also, users can attach images to the messages, easing the sharing of information.

One of the main functionalities of this system is image processing tool, developed with the Javascript library Pixastic (Pixastic 2010). This tool has algorithms for color inversion, solarizing, emboss, sharpening, unsharpen mask, desaturation, grayscale and color histograms, rotation, noise removal, brightness, color and contrast control, saturation and three edge detection algorithms (Laplace, Robert and Sobel). Many of these algorithms accept several values, allowing usersto customize the tool accordingly to their needs. This tool also allows users to visualize the modified image side by

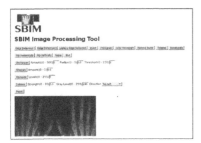

Figure 4. SBIM's image processing tool.

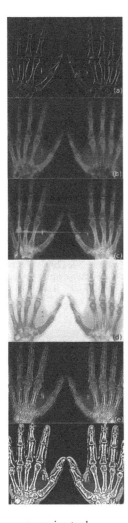

Figure 5. Image processing tool.

side with the original image. The Figure 4 shows the image processing tool of the SBIM system.

For example, the Figure 5 shows some features of Image Processing Tool such as: the edge detection using a 3×3 Laplacian mask (5-a), solarizing (5-b), color histogram (5-c), color inversion (5-d), sharpening (5-e) and unsharpen mask (5-f).

For the system security, there are three user classes with different access levels.

The first one, called *Researcher* can upload images and use all the features of the system. The second one, *Base Administrator*, can request the creation of a image database and control the access to it, inviting users to it or remove them from the base. Also, the Base Administrator can delete images from the base he administrates and disable some users from downloading images. The last class, *System Administrator*, can create and delete databases and also delete users, besides all the rights of the other classes. Non-registered users can see only a limited number of images and do not have access to all the features.

Therefore, the SBIM system offers tools that improve the image analysis and storage, for it puts together, in a single system, several features that could be spread among several softwares.

The proposed system can be seen at http://200.236.3.11/gustavo/sbim/.

5 TESTS

The tests were performed based on the Web Applications specific tests proposed by Pressman (Pressman 1995). In this stage, nine tests were performed, validating interface, features and system capacity.

Due to the fact that for several tests it is required the opinion of users, a group composed of 5 users was assembled, helping in several tests.

These tests aimed to validate functionalities, links, redirectings, Javascript, multiplatform test and processing, storage and network capacity.

For the tests related to the interface, 50 users answered a checklist, with questions about the ease of use and understanding, functionalities and predictability (how informative are the messages, and how easy it is to understand the static content of the system).

Most users, 55%, considered the system simple and 30% considered it easy to use. Only 15% rated it as hard to use.

This test also detected that 62.5% considered the interface clean, and 35% rated it as ambiguous and 2.5% as confusing. This happened due to the fact that the system is written in the English language and most of the testers are not English speakers.

By analyzing these answers, we concluded that 40% of the users rated the system as predictable and 50% as usually predictable. Though, 7.5% considered it usually unpredictable and 2.5% unpredictable.

The functionality test aimed to detect flaws in the functionalities. This test is is very useful, for it it performed by several testers in several computing environments. This test detected that the zoom tool does not on the Opera Web browser and the image processing tool doesn't work on Internet Explorer. Nevertheless, the majority of users, 77.5%, used all the features without problems and on 22.5% reported problems, all related tothe already mentioned tools.

Regarding the performance of the image processing tools, it was found out that it is well suited to run even on computers with low computational resources. For example, applying filters on a BMP image with the resolution of 1800 × 1800 took only 3 seconds on the worst case, sometimes being instantaneous.

By analyzing these results, it was found that the system is able to deal with many users at a time without great losses of performance.

6 CONCLUSIONS

Therefore, though there are systems with similar functionalities, the proposed system offers an interactive experience to the users, offering tools that improves the analysis of medical and biological images in an integrated environment.

This system achieves its objective, that is offer an way to share, store and process biological and medical images in a web-based system. At the moment, the system has over 100 images spread among 7 image databases.

For future projects, we intend to improve the tools that are already on-line and also implement new functionalities.

REFERENCES

Azevedo-Marques, P.M., Caritá, E.C. Benedicto, A.A. and Sanches, P.R. (2005). Implantação de um ris/pacs no hospital das clínicas de ribeirão preto: Uma solução baseada em web. *Radiol Bras 2005, São Paulo*, 37–43.

Azevedo-Marques, P.M., Trad, C.S. Júnior, J.E. and Santos, A.C. (2001). Implantação de um mini-pacs (sistema de arquivamento e distribuição de imagens) em hospital univer-sitário. *Radiol Bras 2001, São Paulo*, 221–224.

Brito, C.J. (1993). Gerencia de bases de imagens usando microisis.

Caritá, E.C., Seraphim, E. Honda, M.O. and Azevedo-Marques, P.M. (2008). Implementaçã e avaliação de um sistema de gerenciamento de imagens médicas com suporte á recuperação baseada em conteúdo. *Radiol Bras 2008, São Paulo*, 331–336.

d'Ornellas, M.C., Mussoi, S.R. and Dias, A.P. (2004). Avaliação e gerenciamento de qualidade de metadados de imagens médicas. *XVIII Congresso Brasileiro de Engenharia Biomédica Santa Maria*.

Oppermann, R. (2010). User-interface design.

Picnik. Available on http://www.picnik.com accessed on february 15th, 2011.

Pires, S.R., Medeiros, R.B. and Schiabel, H. (2004). Banco de imagens mamográficas para treinamento na interpretação de imagens. *Radiol Bras 2004, São Paulo*, 239–244.

Pixastic (2010). Available on http://www.pixastic.com accessed on february 13rd, 2011.

Pixlr. Available on http://www.pixlr.com. accessed on february 25th, 2011.

Porcides, G.M., Stein, L.H. Kamada, T. Neves, L.A.P. and Giraldi, G.A. (2010). An on-line medical imaging management for shared research in the web using pattern features. *Anais do VI Workshop da Visão Computacional 2010, WVC2010, Presidente Prudente, SP, Brasil*.

Pressman, R.S. (1995). *Engenharia de Softwar*. São Paulo: Pearson Makron Books.

Santos, M. and Furuie, S.S. (2005). Base de imagens para avaliação de algoritmos de processamento de imagens médicas. *IV SBQS—V Workshop de Informáatica Médica*.

Computational Vision and Medical Image Processing – Tavares & Natal Jorge (eds)
© 2012 Taylor & Francis Group, London, ISBN 978-0-415-68395-1

Stapes replacement-different ways to replace its function

Fernanda Gentil
IDMEC, FEUP, Clínica ORL-Dr. Eurico Almeida, Widex, ESTSP, Portugal

Carolina Garbe, Marco Parente, Pedro Martins & Renato Natal Jorge
IDMEC, Faculdade de Engenharia da Universidade do Porto, Portugal

João Paço
Hospital CUF, Faculdade de Medicina da Universidade de Lisboa, Portugal

ABSTRACT: The human ear is divided into three parts: outer, middle and inner ear. The middle ear is formed by ossicles (malleus, incus and stapes), ligaments, muscles and tendons, that transfer sound vibrations from the eardrum to the inner ear, linking with mastoid and Eustachian tube. The smaller bone of the human body, the stapes, can be replaced by a prosthesis when is damaged by exaggerated ossification. Different types of materials and morphology have been used, like stainless steel, teflon and titanium among others. In this work, a finite element modelling of the tympano-ossicular system of the middle ear was developed. The comparison between models with different prosthesis were compared with model representative of normal ear.

1 INTRODUCTION

The middle ear is a closed, air-filled chamber, separated from the external ear by the eardrum, and ventilated by the Eustachian tube. The stapes, the smallest bone in the human body, is the third in the tympano-ossicular chain of the middle ear (Fig. 1). The other two bones are the malleus and the incus (Fig. 2). It is through this bone which makes the connection between the middle ear and the inner ear by stapes footplate (Paço 2003). Mechanical energy already transformed from the sound energy at the eardrum is now transformed into hydraulic energy.

When the vibration of the stapes not renders correctly due to overgrowth of bone in this area, one may experience hearing loss (otosclerosis). This hearing loss can be corrected by hearing aids, but the most appropriate treatment is surgery which consists in the removal of the supra-structure of the stapes (stapedotomy) or entire stapes (stapedectomy), and its replacement by a prosthesis that make the link in the long crus of the incus. Initially the stapes replacement prosthesis was made directly by the surgeon, at the operating table. After removal of the stapes bone (which is not properly vibrating), a small window is made to the inner ear and

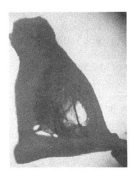

Figure 1. Stapes.

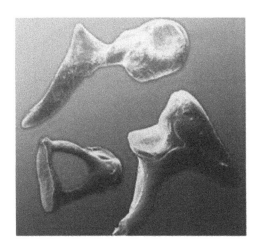

Figure 2. Middle ear ossicles.

was covered with a graft of vein, ear lobe adipose tissue or perichondrium. An artificial replacement made out of teflon and platinum or other material is then substituted for the non-functioning stapes bone. The artificial replacement (prosthesis) is very tiny, since the stapes bone, which it is replacing, is only about 3.5 mm in height and its weight is 2 mg. Was John Shea, in 1956, who introduced this technique, and in 1960, performed the first stapedotomy (Glasscock et al., 1995).

Initially a thin wire made of stainless steel (Fig. 3) was used for the wire loop. Among the different implants that have been used in stapes surgery, variations exist in size, shape, weight and mass. The first stapes prosthesis was carved of Teflon by Treace and used by Shea, and its size was similar to that of a normal human stapes (Treace 1994).

A number of different designs have been proposed and used for prosthesis attachment to the incus and also used to improve transmission of sound through the oval window to the inner ear. Currently available prosthesis are most commonly composed of different materials such as teflon-type polymer, titanium, stainless steel, gold or platinum (Tange et al., 2004). Teflon-metal wire prosthesis (Fig. 4) is often immersed directly into the perilymph without a vein graft.

Titanium prosthesis (Figs. 5, 6) represents the latest development in the field of all-metal prosthesis. It is known for its particularly good biocompatibility. Titanium and platinum assure MRI compatibility. The physical parameters that influence sound transmission include mass, elasticity and rigidity.

The main objective is always to improve and approximate as closely as possible the results obtained in the normal ear function.

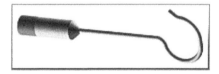

Figure 3. Stainless steel prosthesis.

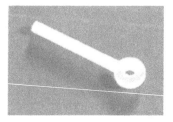

Figure 4. A teflon stapes prosthesis.

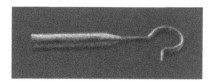

Figure 5. Titanium stapes prosthesis.

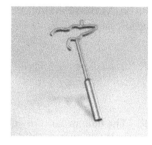

Figure 6. Titanium stapes prosthesis.

Different kind of titanium prosthesis are possible, like as shown in Figure 6, that has a safe fixation onto the long process of the incus, making the most efficient and effective solutions for stapedectomy.

2 MATERIALS AND METHODS

2.1 Model of tympano-ossicular chain

The first step of this work was the construction of the tympano-ossicular chain of the middle ear (eardrum and three ossicles, malleus, incus and stapes) including ligaments and muscles based on computerized tomography images (Gentil et al., 2009). The finite element method was applied using the ABAQUS software (ABAQUS 2007).

The eardrum is modeled by hexahedral (C3D8) elements. It was divided into *pars flaccida* (with only one layer) and *pars tensa* (with three layers). The elements of the ossicles are four tetrahedral nodes (C3D4). The ligaments and muscles are modeled using linear elements of type T3D2. The simulation of the cochlear fluid is modeled with fluid elements, of type F3D3, assuming an incompressibility condition.

Boundaries of the finite element model include the *pars tensa* of the eardrum periphery to simulate the tympanic annulus; the connection between the stapes footplate and the cochlea, in the oval window, to simulate the stapes annular ligament; the connection of suspensory ligaments to the temporal bone (the superior and the anterior of the malleus, the superior and the posterior of the incus) and muscles (the tensor tympani and the stapedius).

Table 1. Material properties for the prosthesis.

Material	Young's modulus (N/m²)	Poisson's ratio	Density (Kg/m³)
Steel	2.10E+11	0.30	7.80E+03
Teflon	6.00E+08	0.44	2.20E+03
Titanium	1.14E+11	0.34	4.43E+03

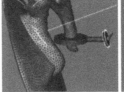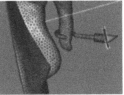

Figure 7. Teflon and stainless steel prosthesis.

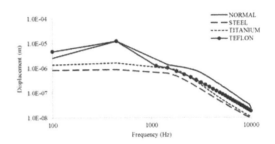

Figure 8. Stapes footplate displacement.

The connection between the malleus and the incus, simulating the incudomallear joint, is done using contact formulation. In this sense, the basic Coulomb friction model available in the ABAQUS software is used, being the friction rate equal to 0.7 (Gentil et al., 2007).

2.2 *Material properties*

The eardrum was divided into *pars flaccida*, and *pars tensa*. The *pars flaccida* was considered as isotropic, and the internal and external layers of the *pars tensa* were considered isotropic and the middle one, fibrous, was considered orthotropic (Garbe et al., 2009). The ossicles are assumed to have isotropic behavior, and with elastic properties obtained by literature (Prendergast 1999). Based on the Yeoh model (Yeoh 1990), the present work uses hyperelastic non-linear behavior for the ligaments (Gentil et al., 2006, Martins et al., 2006), being the Hill model used for the muscles (Martins et al., 1998). The constitutive model, for the middle ear muscles, is a modified form of the incompressible transversely isotropic hyperelastic model proposed by Martins et al. (1998), based on the work of Humphrey and Yin (1987).

In this work, the stapes was replaced by different kind of prosthesis (stainless steel, teflon and titanium) where respective material properties are shown in Table 1.

3 RESULTS AND CONCLUSIONS

Based on the original model of the tympano-ossicular chain of the middle ear, the stapes was replaced for three different kind of prosthesis and their results were compared.

In Figure 7 we can see two of these prosthesis (teflon and stainless steel).

For a sound pressure level of 130 dB SPL, applied in the eardrum, a dynamic study was made for a frequencial range between 100 Hz and 10 kHz. The displacements obtained from the central part of the stapes footplate (Fig. 8), were compared between the representative model of normal chain tympano-ossicular with the three distinct models.

When the stapes prosthesis is replaced by steel and titanium, the displacements have lower values along the entire frequencial range. The material which most closely approximates the normal model is teflon, especially at low frequencies.

Nowadays, although otosclerosis is considered to be one of the most known causes of hearing loss, it still remains a field of surgical improvements. The complete understanding of otosclerosis, remains a challenge for the scientific community. Despite the effort of introducing various other therapeutical options, otosclerosis management is undoubtedly surgical, with stapedotomy to be considered as the most scientifically accepted surgical option. The introduction of new materials in stapes prosthesis, has given the opportunity to the surgeon to eliminate the duration and technical difficulties of the surgery. Improvement of the stapes prosthesis can offer significant advantages in better audiological results, with absence of major postoperative complications.

As conclusions of this work, we can see that teflon can be a good option for replaced stapes, maybe for its small stiffness and density.

ACKNOWLEDGMENTS

The authors would like to thank the Ministério da Ciência, Tecnologia e Ensino Superior—Fundação para a Ciência e a Tecnologia in Portugal and by FEDER for the funding provide under the research project "Estudo bio-computacional do zumbido" with the reference PTDC/SAU-BEB/104992/2008.

REFERENCES

ABAQUS. 2007. Analyses User's Manual, Version 6.5.
Garbe, C. 2010. *Estudo biomecânico para reabilitação do ouvido médio humano*. Tese de Mestrado. Mestrado em Engenharia Biomédica. Faculdade de Engenharia da Universidade do Porto. Portugal.
Garbe, C., Gentil, F., Parente, M., Martins, P. & Natal Jorge, R. 2009. Aplicação Do Método Dos Elementos Finitos No Estudo Da Membrana Timpânica. *Audiologia Em Revista*. Volume II, (3): 99–106.
Gentil, F., Jorge, R.M.N., Ferreira, A.J.M., Parente, M.P.L., Martins, P.A.L.S. & Almeida, E. 2006. Biomechanical simulation of middle ear using hyperelastic models, *Journal of Biomechanics*. 39, Supplement 1: 388–389.
Gentil, F., Jorge, R.M.N., Ferreira, A.J.M., Parente, M.P.L., Moreira, M. & Almeida, E. 2007. Estudo do efeito do atrito no contacto entre os ossículos do ouvido médio, *Revista Internacional de Métodos Numéricos para Cálculo y Diseño en Ingeniería*. (23) 2: 177–187.
Gentil, F., Jorge, R.N., Parente, M.P.L., Martins, P.A.L.S. & Ferreira, A.J.M. 2009. Estudo biomecânico do ouvido médio, *Clínica e Investigação em Otorrinolaringologia*, 3 (1): 24–30.
Glasscock, M.E., Storper, I.S., Haynes, D.S. & Bohrer, P.S. 1995. Twenty-Five Years of Experience with Stapedectomy. *Laryngoscope*, 105: 899–904.

Humphrey, J.D. & Yin, F.C.P. 1987. On constitutive relations and finite deformations of passive cardic tissue: I. A pseudostrain-energy function, *ASME J. Biomech. Engrg.*, (109): 298–304.
Martins, P.A.L.S., Jorge, R.M.N. & Ferreira, A.J.M. 2006. A Comparative Study of Several Material Models for Prediction of Hyperelastic Properties: Application to Silicone-Rubber and Soft Tissues. *Strain*. (42): 135–147.
Martins, J.A.C., Pires, E.B., Salvado, R. & Dinis, P.B. 1998. A Numerical model of passive and active behavior of skeletal muscles. *Computer methods in applied mechanics and engineering*. (151): 419–433.
Paço, J. 2003. *Doenças do timpano*. Lisboa. Portugal: Lidel.
Prendergast, P.J., Ferris, P., Rice, H.J. & Blayney, A.W. 1999. Vibro-acoustic modelling of the outer and middle ear using the finite element method, *Audiol Neurootol*, (4): 185–191.
Tange, R.A., Grolman, W. & Dreschler, W.A. 2004. Gold and titanium in the oval window: a comparison of two metal stapes prostheses. *Otol Neurotol.*, 25(2): 102–5.
Treace, H.T. 1994. Biomaterials in ossiculoplasty and history of development of prostheses for ossiculoplasty. *Otolaryngol Clin North Am*, 2(4): 655–662.
Yeoh, O.H. 1990. Characterization of elastic properties of carbon-black-filled rubber vulcanizates, *Rubber Chemistry and Technology*, 63: 792–805.

Computational Vision and Medical Image Processing – Tavares & Natal Jorge (eds)
© 2012 Taylor & Francis Group, London, ISBN 978-0-415-68395-1

Vision-based hand segmentation techniques for human-robot interaction for real-time applications

Paulo Trigueiros
Instituto Superior de Contabilidade e Administração do Instituto Politécnico do Porto, Portugal

Fernando Ribeiro & Gil Lopes
Universidade do Minho, Portugal

ABSTRACT: One of the most important tasks in hand recognition applications for human-robot interaction is hand segmentation. This work presents a method that uses a Microsoft Kinect camera, for hand localization and segmentation. One important aspect for robot control besides hand localization is hand orientation, which is used in this work to control robot heading direction (left or right) and linear velocity. The system first calculates hand position, and then a kalman filter is used to estimate displacement and linear velocity in a smoother way. Experimental results show that the system is easy to use, and can be applied on several different human-computer interface applications.

Keywords: human-robot interaction, hand segmentation, hand control, kalman filter, kinect

1 INTRODUCTION

Recent applications in Human-Computer Interaction (HCI) and Computer Vision (CV) are raising a great opportunity to improve human life.

Nowadays, the keyboard, the mouse and remote controls are used as the main interfaces for transferring information and commands to computerized equipment (Hassanpour and Shahbahrami 2010). In some applications involving three-dimensional information, such as visualization, computer games and control of robots, other interfaces based on trackballs, joysticks and data gloves (Garg, Aggarwal et al., 2009) (Murthy and Jadon 2009) (Chen, Georganas et al., 2007) are being used. In our daily life, however, humans use vision and hearing as main sources of information in an environment. Therefore, one may ask to what extent it would be possible to develop computerized equipment able to communicate with humans in a similar way, by understanding visual input.

Main advantages of using visual input in this context are that visual information makes it possible to communicate with computerized equipment at a distance, without the need for physical contact with the equipment to be controlled.

The purpose of this project is to develop a user interface able of extracting user hands position and orientation on each frame, and use that information to communicate remotely with a robot.

Several human-computer applications use skin-color as one of the basic features to detect and analyze human hands for human-computer or human-robot interaction. These applications have different aims and different constraints under which the human hands must be analyzed. One crucial point, which is common to most of these applications, is the accuracy of hand segmentation. Due to this important fact, it was decided to use a Kinect camera, and take advantage of the depth camera module to acquire the hand blobs for further processing, eliminating this way, one constant problem faced in this kind of applications being the illumination variation. The blob centroid and hand orientation are calculated to take control of linear velocity and direction as well as the heading direction for the robot. The method has the advantage of being robust and easy to use.

This paper describes the method implemented to solve the problem of hand recognition in order to achieve remote robot control and presents the software developed to prove its feasibility.

The paper is organized as follows: state of the art on related work in section 2, this new approach describing hand segmentation and detection of orientation in section 3, experiments and results of this method are presented in section 4. The discussion of the proposed method is given in section 5, and conclusions are given in section 6.

2 RELATED WORK

Nowadays, human computer and human robot interaction using technology like Microsoft Kinect is giving its first steps. The solutions are starting to appear in many areas, and some examples of it are the work carried out at JAHIR—Joint-Action for Humans and Industrial Robots—in which a human co-worker is tracked using a Microsoft Kinect in a human-robot collaborative scenario (Robots).[1] The solution that uses a kinect with OpenNI[2], is able to track a human and automatically send this tracking data to an interface between the Kinect and an industrial robot so that it will dynamically avoid contact with that human being.

During Health and Wellness Innovation 2011, the Microsoft Kinect was also used by Jin Joo Lee (Personal Robots group at the MIT Media Lab) to advance her research in modelling the dynamics of social interaction. The goal is to better understand the subtle cues in human-human communication in order to improve human-robot interactions. This project applies machine learning and gesture recognition algorithms to the motion capture data from the Kinect in order to detect nonverbal cues including mimicry and synchronous movement.[3]

Another example of hand gesture detection using kinect is the work being done at the MIT Computer Science and Artificial Intelligence Lab (CSAIL) (MIT).[4] The project uses ROS (Robot Operating System), a set of tools that help software developers create robot applications, libfreenect driver and MIT developed gesture recognition.

Hand segmentation for gesture recognition is a difficult task to solve, mainly because of different lighting conditions that normal cameras have to adapt to.

In the proposed approach this kind of problem is not a concern, since the kinect depth sensor, that consists of an infrared laser projector combined with a monochrome CMOS sensor and which captures video data in 3D, is not dependent on light and therefore works under any light conditions.

Our focus in the proposed method is to segment the obtained depth image to extract the hand coordinates, and calculate movement and heading to remotely control a robot.

---

[1] http://www6.in.tum.de/Main/ResearchJahir
[2] OpenNI is available from http://www.openni.org/
[3] http://newmed.media.mit.edu/blog/jom/2011/03/29/modeling-dynamics-social-interactions-kinect-better-healthcare
[4] http://www.ros.org/wiki/mit-ros-pkg/KinectDemos/MinorityReport

3 OUR APPROACH

The proposed approach uses the kinect sensor system to gather depth information. The depth information will be used to detect and segment hands using two planes that define the minimum and maximum thresholds. These thresholds are calculated taking into account the closest point to the camera. The extracted hand centroid (relative position) is then used to control the robot movement as indicated in Figures 1 and 2.

Hand rotation is used to control robot heading as illustrated in Figure 3.

3.1 *Hand Segmentation*

In order to segment the hand region, the nearest point to the camera is calculated on each frame. For each time t, the closest point on the depth image I is calculated according to the formula:

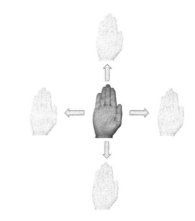

Figure 1. Hand movement used to control robot displacement.

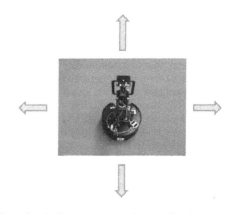

Figure 2. Robot movement relative to hand movement.

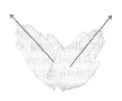 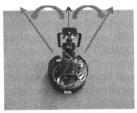

Figure 3.   Robot heading dependent on hand rotation.

$$distMin = \min\begin{Bmatrix} I(x,y): 0 \le x \le height(I) \\ and\, 0 \le y \le width(I) \end{Bmatrix} \quad (1)$$

Using this value, two parallel planes are defined to extract the hand binary mask and hand contours from the depth image.

Algorithm 1—Nearest Point

Given the frame depth array (depth) and the image that is going to store the resulting binary mask (thImage) calculate:

```
Initialize minDistance = depth[0];
Initialize nrPixels = imageWidth * imageHeight;
for i = 0, ..., nrPixels
  if minDistance = 0 and depth[i] > 0
    minDistance = depth[i]
  else if depth[i] > 0 and depth[i] < minDistance
    minDistance = depth[i]
  endif
end for

Initialize nearThreshold = minDistance −5
Initialize farThreshold = minDistance +5
for i = 0, ..., nrPixels
  if depth[i] > nearThreshold and
    depth[i] < farThreshold
    thImage[i] = 255
  else
    thImage[i] = 0
  endif
end for
```

The hand centroid (Equations 1 and 2) is then calculated, using the OpenCV method *findcontours*, being this value used for the relative hand position.

$$\bar{x} = \frac{1}{n}\sum x_i \quad (2)$$

$$\bar{y} = \frac{1}{n}\sum y_i \quad (3)$$

Using this centroid values $(\bar{x}, \bar{y})$, an estimated value for the new position is calculated using a kalman filter (Welch and Bishop 2001) (Press 1979), thereby enabling a smoother centroid movement,

and respectively a smoother robot movement. This smoother robot movement not only makes it more visibly attractive but also increases the life expectancy of the robot motors.

The robot direction of movement is calculated according to the hand vector angle related to the image centre as illustrated in Figure 4.

$$direction = \text{atan2}(dx, dy) \quad (4)$$

The vector length represented by the distance between the image centre and the hand centroid, is then used to calculate the robot linear velocity, which is proportional to that value according to Equation 5.

$$linearV = \sqrt{dx^2 + dy^2}\,/6 \quad (5)$$

where *linearV* is the linear velocity transmitted to the robot and the constant value 6 was learned from the experiments to avoid sudden accelerations.

These values used to control the robot are then sent to the robot via a wireless client-server application.

3.2   Orientation

Hand orientation (θ) is calculated taking into account two vectors: one formed between the hand centroid and the farthest point from it, and another, a vector parallel to a horizontal line that passes through the centre of the image (Figure 5). The angle θ is then obtained by using the dot product[5] between the two vectors according to equation 6.

$$\theta = \arccos\left(\frac{a \bullet b}{\|a\|\|b\|}\right) \quad (6)$$

being $a \bullet b$ the dot product between the two vectors and $\|a\|$ the norm of the vector.

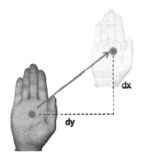

Figure 4.   Direction of movement.

---

[5] http://en.wikipedia.org/wiki/Dot_product

Computational Vision and Medical Image Processing – Tavares & Natal Jorge (eds)
© 2012 Taylor & Francis Group, London, ISBN 978-0-415-68395-1

The finite element analysis of skull deformation after correction of scaphocephaly

W. Wolański, M. Gzik & E. Kawlewska
Department of Applied Mechanics, Silesian University of Technology, Gliwice, Poland

D. Larysz & P. Larysz
Department of Neurosurgery, Medical University of Silesia, Katowice, Poland

ABSTRACT: Scaphocephaly is a type of non-syndromic craniosynostosis with premature fusion of sagittal suture. It is the most common type of craniosynostosis [5]. In the paper the technique of finite element analysis was used to analyze cranial deformation and changes in intracranial pressure, after surgical correction of scaphocephaly. With methods of finite element analysis, an intuitive prediction of surgical results is possible. It could give neurosurgeons possibility to improve surgical treatment in more accurate, safer and faster way.

Keywords: finite element method; preoperative planning; craniosynostosis; skull mechanics

1 INTRODUCTION

The main purpose of correction of craniosynostotic skull is to reopen cranial sutures with some bone slots in order to free the skull bones and allow proper brain development inside [8]. The intent of this paper is to analyze the relationships between various possibilities of bone osteotomies and skull rigidity.

Finite element analysis methods are used to obtain the deformation clouds of the different surgery schemes. Then the best option of cranial vault correction was chosen according to the simulation results of deformation distribution.

2 MATERIALS AND METHODS

We present a case of 5 months old boy with non-syndromic craniosynostosis—scaphocephaly (premature closure of sagittal suture). The case was selected to design the surgery plan according to virtual preoperative planning. Few plans of osteotomies was used for reconstruction to simulate the deformation distribution.

It was applied inverted modified π-squeeze procedure to perform the skull shape correction. In this method four incisions are made, along the frontal and parietal bones (Fig. 1). The separated bones can be repositioned to obtain the correct shape.

A three-dimensional model of skull was created with Mimics software from standard CT data. Planned correction of craniosynostotic skull is shown in Figure 1. Slots shown in Figure 2 were formed in the surgery procedure to reduce the rigidity in the parietal region. In order to get optimal cosmetic postoperative effects the parietal bones should allow proper brain expansion from inside.

For changes of the skull shape three schemes are designed by variation of osteotomies. Separated cranial bone models of scheme 1 to scheme 3 are made cranial bones remodeling and slots cutting off. At the scheme 1 there are intact parietal bones. Parietal boned were cut into two segments at the scheme 2. The scheme 3 are represented the

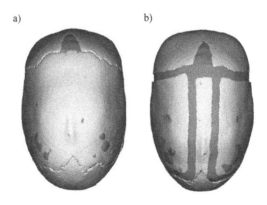

Figure 1. a) Original malformation, b) The "π" procedure for scaphocephaly.

scheme 1

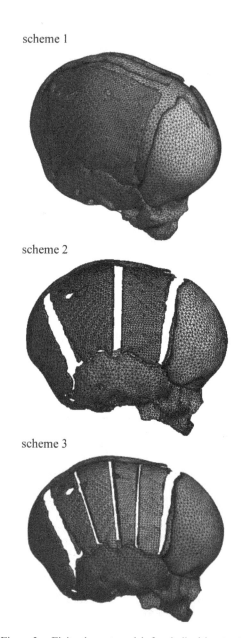

scheme 2

scheme 3

Figure 2. Finite element models for skull with osteotomies of parietal bone.

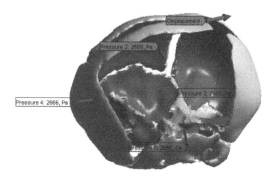

Figure 3. Boundary condition of the finite-element skull model.

Table 1. Material properties [9].

| Models | Materials properties | | |
	Young modulus (MPa)	Poisson's ratio	Density (kg/cm³)
Skull bones	2500	0.22	2.15
Brain	34.5	0.45	1.14

The whole model was supported on the lower surface of the skull base. 10 mm displacement was applied to the occipital bone to correct the scaphocephaly. Intracranial pressure was loaded through the inside surface of cranial bone models as a constant value of 2.66 kPa [10] (Fig. 3). Brain and skull bones were defined as the isotropic elastic material, and the viscoelastic material effects can be ignored. Material properties such as Young's modulus, Poisson's ratio and density of those models were presented in Table 1.

3 RESULTS

Firstly the basic dimensions before and after the virtual surgery were measured to check the value of cephalic index. Cephalic index is the relation between maximal skull width and length, multiplied by 100%. Proper cephalic index value for children is between 63,8 to 69,8. To obtain maximal skull length and width it was performed the basic craniometry. Four characteristic anatomical points were marked on the model: Euryon left (Eu.L), Euryon right (Eu.R), Lambda (L) and Glabella (G) (Fig. 4).

On the basis of these dimensions it was calculated the index value and the results were presented in Table 2. After the surgery the cephalic index increase, that is the positive result.

Finite element analysis was performed in ANSYS environment. It was applied boundary

parietal bones divided into four parts (refer as Figure 2).

Finite element mesh models were generated with application of Mimics software and were exported as data format for Ansys. When cranial bones and brain mesh models were imported into Ansys software, some tasks should be made to assemble the cranial bones and the brain meshes with contact relationship.

conditions and loads. Finite element analysis results of the scheme with intact parietal bone slot models were presented in Figure 5. Results of displacement clouds show that larger distortion appears at the posterior portion of brain and upper region of parietal bone. Maximum deformation was 5.859 mm at this scheme.

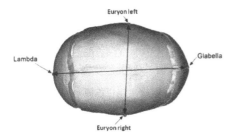

Figure 4. Marked anatomical points.

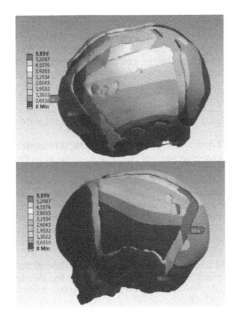

Figure 5. Displacement clouds for cranium without any slots.

Table 2. The craniometry results.

Dimension	Description	Before surgery	After surgery
Eu.R-Eu.L	Maximal skull width [mm]	90,75	91,75
G-L	Maximal skull length [mm]	148,79	142,67
Cephalic index	(Eu.R-Eu.L/ G-L)*100	60,99	64,31

a)

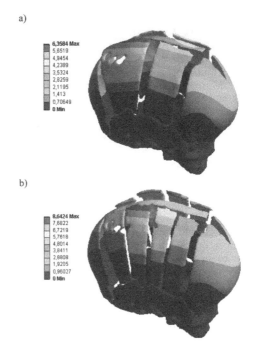

b)

Figure 6. The FEA results of: a) scheme 2, b) scheme 3.

From the analysis results we can assume that cranial bone rigidity is an important factor which has a great influence on postoperative results of correction congenital craniosynostosis. The lower bone rigidity, the better surgery results are possible to achieve. Figure 6 shows the displacement clouds for second and third scheme. From the figure we find out that the last scheme has high deformation level. The maximum displacement value of the scheme 3 was 8.642 mm, respectively are the best scheme.

At the Figure 2 we can see that the scheme 2 represented medium rigidity of cranial bones, because the maximum displacement was 6.358 mm. Therefore the primal cranial bone without any slots it's the worst type of surgery in all plans. So in the steps of making preoperative craniosynostosis treatment, effective measures should be taken such as the methods in scheme 3, for reasonable layout the rigidity of cranial bone.

4 DISCUSSION

The case exemplifies how biomechanical modeling can be used to support surgical procedures. Craniosynostosis surgery planning requires the sequence of bone osteotomies and repositioning. Virtual models could help better imagination of the skull shape and its crucial details such as sutures and foramina. The models play an important role during preoperative planning of neurosurgical cranial reconstruction especially in terms of ranges, angles and proper contours of osteotomies [1,2], [3,4]. Moreover, these bone segments are deformable and the surgery plan needs to choose which scheme of osteotomies will be better.

Modeling in biomechanics connected with modern visualization methods gives new possibilities of engineer support for medical procedures [6,7]. The clinical case presented in this paper, were successfully planned using the CAD-based planning procedure. The results unexpectedly revealed the important influence of age on correction results. By the time a child is five months old, the skull has stiffened to the point that a substantially larger number of osteotomies is needed to accommodate brain growth. Performing the operation at an early age reduces both the number of osteotomies needed and the invasiveness of the operation.

5 CONCLUSIONS

The results of deformation distribution of cranial bones under the intracranial pressure after surgical correction of craniosynostosis can be obtained by the finite element method. These results reflect the ability of the cranial bone expanding with the brain tissues growth. With finite element method, surgical prediction can be made to guide surgeons to make the decision of improving surgical treatment.

Pre-operative planning enable to choose the optimal method of treatment for individual patients. The use of the planning procedure led to significant surgery time reduction—with blood loss and infection risk reduction as a consequence—compared to previous surgical experiences.

Also the evaluation of results and preventing complications is possible. The three-dimensional visualization of results are helpful for the neurosurgeons and the comparison of models before and after the surgery enable the qualitative and quantitative evaluation of treatment.

ACKNOWLEDGMENTS

The researches are supported by Polish Ministry of Science and Higher Education, as the project No. 03006306, in years 2009–2012.

REFERENCES

[1] Altobelli, et al., 1993. Computer-assisted three-dimensional planning in craniofacial surgery. *Plastic and Reconstructive Surgery*, 92, pp. 576–587.
[2] Bohner et al., 1997, Operation planning in craniomaxillofacial surgery. *Computer Aided Surgery*, 2, pp. 153–161.
[3] Cutting, et al., 1986. Three-dimensional computer-assisted design of craniofacial surgical procedures: optimization and interaction with cephalometric and CT-based models. *Plastic and Reconstructive Surgery*, 77, pp. 877–887.
[4] Girod, et al., 2001. Computer-aided 3-D simulation and prediction of craniofacial surgery: a new approach. *Journal of Maxillofacial Surgery*, 29(3), pp. 156–158.
[5] Gzik, M., Wolański, W., Tejszerska, D., Gzik-Zroska, B., Koźlak, M. & Larysz D. 2009. Interdisciplinary researches supporting neurosurgical correction of children head deformation. *In Modeling and Optimization of Physical Systems*, No. 8, 49–54.
[6] Jans, et al., 1999. Computer-aided craniofacial surgical planning implemented in CAD software. *Computer Aided Surgery*, 4, pp. 117–128.
[7] Lo, et al., 1994. Craniofacial computer-assisted surgical planning and simulation. *Clinics in Plastic Surgery*, 21, pp. 501–516.
[8] Mommaerts, et al., 2001. On the assets of CAD planning for craniosynostosis surgery. *Journal of Craniofacial Surgery*, 12, pp. 547–554.
[9] Roth, S., Raul, J.S. & Willinger, R. 2008. Biofidelic child head FE model to simulate real world trauma, *Computer methods and programs in biomedicine*, vol. 90, 262–274.
[10] Yu, P.L. & Yang, Y.J. 1999. Hydrocephalus and encephalic high pressure of children, *Beijing People's Medical Publishing House*, 1st ed., vol. 14., 183–185.

Computational Vision and Medical Image Processing – Tavares & Natal Jorge (eds)
© *2012 Taylor & Francis Group, London, ISBN 978-0-415-68395-1*

Modeling and simulation of trigonocephaly correction with use of Finite Elements Method

M. Gzik, W. Wolański, E. Kawlewska & K. Kawlewski
Department of Applied Mechanics, Silesian University of Technology, Gliwice, Poland

D. Larysz
Department of Neurosurgery, Medical University of Silesia, Katowice, Poland

ABSTRACT: In this paper the trigonocephaly, that is one of the type of craniosynostosis was described. It was presented the virtual planning of the surgical treatment and the simulation of skull shape after the correction. Also the main strain, that occur during the surgery were calculated. To obtain the 3-dimensional geometry from CT scans it was used the Mimics v14 software and to obtain the results of biomechanical analysis it was used the Ansys software.

1 INTRODUCTION

Craniosynostosis is the children's disease, that results in incorrect head shape from premature fusion of one or more sutures [2]. Because the brain cannot expand in the direction of the fused suture, it is forced to grow in the direction of the open sutures, often resulting in an abnormal head shape and facial features. Some cases of craniosynostosis may result in increased pressure on the brain and developmental delays. It is estimated that cranio-synostosis affects 1 in 2000 live births [1, 3]. It can be the result of an inherited syndrome or sporadic. In sporadic cases, the cause is unknown.

There are a few types of craniosynostosis, depending on which suture has fused prematurely. The trigonocephaly occurs when the metopic suture (on the forehead) was fused. The triangular shape of forehead is characteristic for this malformation. Also there are complications in neuropsychological development and the problems with seeing and ocular hypotelorism can occur [8]. In trigonocephaly it is necessary to rebuild the whole forehead, that's why

the surgery is relatively complicated [6, 9]. In these cases the engineering support is helpful, because there is a possibility to plan the incisions virtually and to simulate the results of treatment [5].

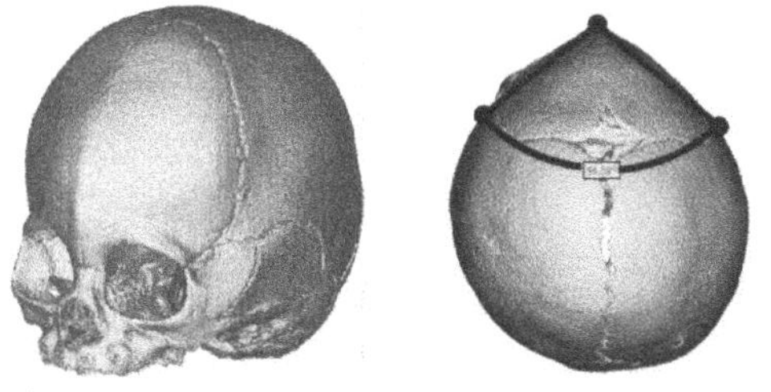

2 MATERIALS AND METHODS

The correction of complicated skull deformations must be planned individually for each patient. In this paper 3-months old boy with diagnosis of trigonocephaly was considered (Fig. 1).

Three-dimensional model of skull geometry obtained on the basis of standard CT scanning that was carried out to establish the diagnosis. With the using of *Mimics v14* software it was possible to separate the bone tissue (based on Hounsfield scale) from the images and perform the simulations of incisions and repositions (Fig. 2).

At the beginning it was also performed the analysis of bone thickness, to evaluate if it is possible

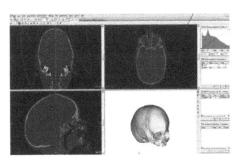

Figure 1.   Model of skull with trigonocephaly.

Figure 2.   Screen of the Mimics software window.

to perform the endoscopic surgery instead of open, more invasive treatment. It was calculated that the thickest elements of skull are 6 mm and they are located on the forehead (Fig. 3).

2.1 Virtual surgery

The "virtual surgery" was performed step by step, with the strictly cooperation of the neurosurgeon. The main procedure of planning was presented on the schema below (Fig. 4).

The simulation of surgery was carried out in two variants, in which it was applied three and five incisions respectively.

In variant "1" (Fig. 5) at the beginning the forehead was separated from the skull. It was possible by performing two incisions: above the orbital and along the coronal sutures. Then another incision was performed along the metopic (frontal) suture, that was prematurely fused [7]. After that the separated bones were parted in the transverse plane to obtain the optimal, more spherical skull shape. The parts of bones were stabilized by the biodegradable plates.

In variant "2" assumed to perform three incisions like in the variant "1" and two additional incisions, in the middle of each half of frontal bone (Fig. 6).

The separated elements were moved to obtain the correct skull shape. All the incisions and repositions of skull bones were consulted with the neurosurgeon. The virtual surgery gave him the possibility to choose the optimal variant of treatment that should be performed in real operation.

2.2 Modeling of correction

In Mimics it was marked the desired bone fragments displacements. Subsequently it was measured the dimensions between the original and reshaped skull, to find the values of boundary conditions that were put into the Ansys. It was found that the tilt of the bones of 12 mm ensures improved shape of the skull (Fig. 7).

Three-dimensional geometrical models were exported to *.stl files and next imported to Ansys

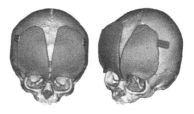

Figure 5.   Model of planned incisions in variant "1".

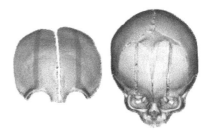

Figure 6.   The simulation of variant "2" with five incisions.

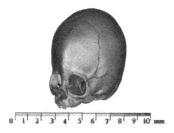

Figure 3.   Results of the skull bone thickness analysis.

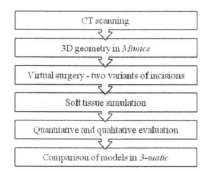

Figure 4.   Schema of procedure in the preoperative planning of surgical treatment in craniosynostosis [4].

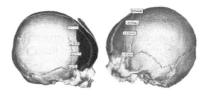

Figure 7.   The measurements of displacements of separated bones in Mimics.

Table 1.   Material properties of model [4].

	Young modulus MPa	Poisson's ratio	Density kg/cm³
Skull bones	380,0	0,22	2,15

48

environment, to perform the biomechanical analysis. On the basis of own experimental researches it was entered the material properties, presented in Table 1.

3 RESULTS

The biomechanical analysis enable to obtain the color map of stress and deformation (Fig. 8 & Fig. 10), that occurs during the correction. It was used the Huber—von Misses yield criterion to calculate the reduced stress (Fig. 9 & Fig. 11). The results of bio-mechanical analysis were presented in Table 2.

Subsequently the generated models, that present the real deformation were imported back to Mimics environment. It was possible to compare the assumed correctness, that was performed manually in Mimics with the neurosurgeon support and the automatic reposition, that occurred in Ansys during the analysis, when the displacement equals 12 mm was imposed (Fig. 12).

FEM model of frontal bone was also com-pares before and after the surgery in two variants (Fig. 13 & Fig. 14). It was possible to evaluate the forehead shape after the treatment.

With the use of 3-matic module it was performed the soft tissue simulation and also the comparison of results. The skin tissue was calculated, on the basis of the Hounsfield scale of the CT images and then it was imposed on the corrected bone tissue. This simulation enabled the qualitative evaluation of the surgery effects.

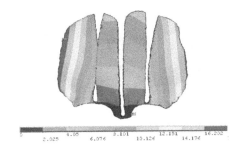

Figure 10. The colour map of deformation for variant "2".

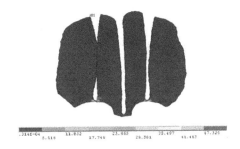

Figure 11. The map of reduced stress for variant "2".

Table 2. Results of biomechanical analysis.

	Maximal stress [MPa]	Maximal deformation [mm]
Variant "1"	40,56	19,26
Variant "2"	53,25	18,23

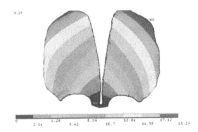

Figure 8. The colour map of deformation for variant "1".

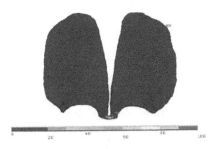

Figure 9. The colour map of reduced stress for variant "1".

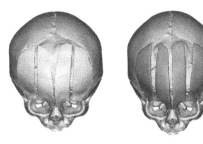

Figure 12. The forehead bone after the correction a) the assumed reposition obtained manually in Mimics, b) reposition obtained automatically in Ansys.

As results it was obtained the deformation of skull after the performed procedure of correction. The angle of forehead was increased from 96.58° before the surgery to 125.65° after the surgery (Fig. 15).

The shape of head before and after the correction of trigonocephaly was presented below (Fig. 16). The planned improvement of shape is sufficient.

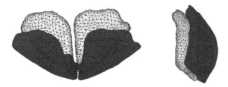

Figure 13. The forehead bone before and after the correction—variant "1" (light and dark model respectively).

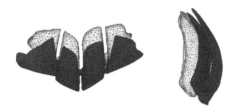

Figure 14. The forehead bone before and after the correction—variant "2" (light and dark model respectively).

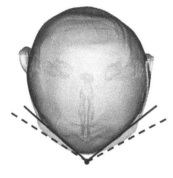

Figure 15. The effect of correction—the angle of forehead before (solid line) and after the surgery (dashed line).

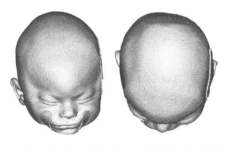

Figure 16. Final result—the model of patient's head after the correction (front and top view).

4 CONCLUSIONS

Preoperative planning enables the neurosurgeon to predict the effects of the treatment. Applied qualitative and quantitative evaluation enable to choose the kind of osteotomies of forehead bone in trigonocephaly.

In this individual case the virtual surgery allowed to qualification the patient to the endoscopic surgery.

The numeric analysis enable to ensure that the optimal solution was variant "1", because there were only three incisions and the maximal stress were lower than in variant "2". Also the final effect of the surgery was acceptable. Hypotelorism that occurred in this individual patient was decreased during the correction.

Virtual planning of the treatment was helpful for the neurosurgeon, because he could "practice" the incisions before the real surgery. It is especially important in the endoscopic method.

The individual planning for each patient increases the quality of treatment and the safety during the operation. The time of surgery decreases so the blood loss is also less.

ACKNOWLEDGMENTS

The researches are supported by Polish Ministry of Science and Higher Education, as the project No. NN501 157038, in 2010–2012.

REFERENCES

[1] Aldridge, K., Marsh, J.L., Govier, D. & Richtsmeier, J.T.: Central nervous system phenotypes in craniosynostosis, Journal of Anatomy (2002), nr 202, str. 31–39.
[2] Erlanger Health System Tennessee Craniofacial Center (1997), No. 1(800), pp. 418–3223.
[3] Gaskill, S. & Marlin, A.E.: Neurologia i neurochirurgia dziecięca, Wyd. I, TA. WPN UNIVERSITAS. Kraków, 2000.
[4] Gzik, M., Tejszerska, D., Wolański, W., Gzik-Zroska, B., Larysz, D. & Mandera, M. 2009. Komputerowe wspomaganie planowania zabiegu korekcji trigonocefalii u dzieci. In Modelowanie Inżynierskie, No. 7(38), 51–56, Gliwice.
[5] Gzik, M., Wolański, W., Tejszerska, D., Gzik-Zroska, B., Koźlak, M. & Larysz, D. 2009. Interdisciplinary researches supporting neurosurgical correction of children head deformation. In Modeling and Optimization of Physical Systems, No. 8, 49–54. Gliwice, Poland.
[6] Hayward, R., Jones, B., Dunaway, D. & Evans, R. 2004. The clinical management of craniosynostosis. London: Mac Keith Press.
[7] Marchac, D. & Renier, D.: Craniofacial Surgery for Craniosynostosis, Little, Brown and Company, Boston, 1982.
[8] Marieb, E.N. & Hoehn, K.: Human Anatomy and Physiology, Seventh Edition, 2007.
[9] Neurochirurgia, w zarysie. Red. M. Pawlina, Wyd. I. PZWL. Warszawa, 1999.

Computer-aided diagnosis of dementia using medical imaging processing and artificial neural networks

G. Gavidia, R. López & E. Soudah

International Center for Numerical Methods in Engineering, Polytechnical University of Catalonia, Barcelona, Spain

ABSTRACT: The Alzheimer's Disease (AD) is a disorder neurodegenerative, which is one of the most common causes of dementia in the older people, it constitutes one of the diseases with great social impact in Europe and America. The progress of medical diagnosis using Magnetic Resonance Imaging (MRI) is widely used for the treatment of neurological diseases; it allows obtaining, increasingly, more functional and anatomical information from the brain of the patients, with a great precision in time and space. However, this big amount of data and images are impossible to analyze directly, is necessary to develop methodologies of calculus for quantified the parameters more relevant in the MRI.

This work proposes a methodology for the diagnosis of dementia based on Alzheimer's disease combining imaging processing and artificial intelligence techniques. We created an Artificial Neural Network (ANN) of classification based on architecture Multilayer Perceptron. In order to construct a complete dataset for training and testing of the network, initial inputs-target variables were obtained from the database OASIS (Open Access Series of imaging studies) with a total of instances equal to 235. The variables were classified into 3 groups: demographic, clinical and morphometric data. Task of training and testing were applied on initial data, obtained a 48% of confusion of the diagnosis. For minimize this percentages of error, image processing and Voxel Based Morphometry (VBM) techniques were implemented to obtain new morphometric variables of three areas of the brain: White Matter (WM), Gray Matter (GM) and fluid (CSF) cerebro-espinal. In this way, we reduced the percentage of confusion to 17%. The results obtained with the ANN, demonstrated that the demographic and clinical information from patients, combined with morphometric information of areas of the brain, are input variables useful to train an ANN of diagnosis of dementia with 83% of reliability, and in this way, help to the early diagnosis of AD.

Keywords: Medical imaging processing, segmentation, neural network (ANN), Magnetic resonance imaging (MRI), tissues of brain, Alzheimer's disease (AD), Voxel based morphometry (VBM), Multilayer Perceptron

1 INTRODUCTION

AD is a disorder neurodegenerative, which is one of the causes of most common dementia in the elderly, also constitutes one of the diseases with great social impact in Europe and America.

Although AD is not a normal success of old age population, the risk of developing this disease increases in elderly persons. For the past 2005, in Europe were diagnosed 3600,000 patients affected by AD (source: Frost & Sullivan) and in recent research carried by *Alzheimer Europe*, was estimated that 7.3 million people have dementia.

Normally, the diagnosis of AD is done after the exclusion of other forms of dementia, but the definitive diagnosis requires not only the presence of large cognitive deficits in patients, also require the confirmation in the autopsy, which consist in a study of brain tissue.

Under these circumstances, the early diagnosis of dementia establishes new goals in clinical research of AD (Morris, Storandt, et al., 2001) (Mueller, Weiner, et al., 2005b). Numerous studies based on magnetic resonance imaging (MRI) are used to describe the differences of the brain structure between demented patients and healthy subjects (Jack, et al., 1997) (Killiany, et al., 2002) (Morra, et al., 2008), being the main objective to find degree of relation between brain abnormalities and development of the disease.

In this paper, we describe a methodology to combine medical images processing, VBM and ANN techniques for the diagnosis of dementia based on AD, making the task of diagnosis as a problem of classification using the Clinical Dementia Rating (CDR) (Morris 1993) as output of the network. The inputs- targets variables for the training and testing of the ANN were obtained from

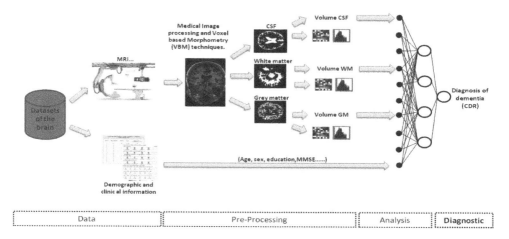

Figure 1. Flowchart of stages implicated in the building of artificial neural network of AD diagnostic.

a free database of MRI aimed at research of AD. In order to improve the results of diagnosis, techniques of image processing and VBM were applied into MRI datasets to extract numerical information of affected brain tissues.

The Figure 1 shows the stages implicated in the development of diagnostic ANN of AD, from obtaining initial datasets until building the ANN.

2 MATERIALS AND METHODS

2.1 Obtaining the initial dataset and inputs-target variables from OASIS database

Obtain successful results in the training and testing of the network depends of the proper choice of variables and a sufficient sample of instances. In order to obtain these, we used the datasets of brain MRI with clinical and demographic data of subject provided by OASIS (Marcus, et al., 2010), which is a project aimed at making MRI datasets of the brain freely available to the neurology researches. This dataset included 235 cross-sectional collections of 416 subjects aged 18 to 96 years (where 100 the included subjects older than 60 years have been clinically diagnosed with very mild to moderate AD).

In the first stage, all variables of OASIS database were used to integrate three groups of data: a) demographic data integrated by sex (1), age (2), Handedness (3), education (4), socio-economic status (SES) (5); b) Clinic data integrated by Mini-Mental State Examination (MMSE) (6) and Clinical Dementia Rating (CDR) (7); and c) morphologic data conformed with eTIV (*Estimated total intracranial volume*) (Buckner, et al., 2004) (8), (Fotenos, et al., 2005); nWBV (*Normalized whole brain volume*, nWBV) (Fotenos, et al., 2005) (9),

y (3) ASF (*Atlas Scaling Factor*) (Fotenos, et al., 2005) (10), which is a factor of increase or decrease of the volume of the brain to be registered to an atlas-template supplied by Talairach and Tournoux (Talairach and Tournoux 1988).

The CDR factor constituted the target variable of ANN, it was developed at the Memory and Aging Project at Washington University School of Medicine in 1979 and it is used in both research and clinical settings to characterize the level of cognitive and functional performance in patients at risk for or suspected of having AD or another dementing disorder In clinic diagnosis, the CDR score is calculated by standard algorithm and its possible values are: CDR = 0: no impairment; CDR = 0.5: very mild; CDR = 1: mild; CDR = 2: moderate; and CDR = 3: severe dementia. However, as the database used only had two instances with CDR = 2 and zero instances with CDR = 3, in this work was used the dataset with CDR = 0, 0.5, 1 y 2.

– Additional brain morphological parameters obtained using image processing techniques

Research in neurology have shown that the volume of the brain and the zones involved in memory have a significant degree of atrophy in patients with mild *cognitive impairment* (MCI) and early stages of AD (Jack, et al., 1997), (Killiany, et al., 2002), (Fotenos, et al., 2005), (Morra, et al., 2008). Based on this, we decided complemented the morfometric group obtaining the total volume of important brain tissues: white matter (WM), gray matter (GM) and cerebrospinal fluid (CSF).

The brain tissues are characterized by a varied, complex and often overlapping morphology, for these reasons, the task of obtain precise volumes for statistical and morphometric studies is not an easy and trivial task. In order to obtain them, we applied techniques of image processing, which were implemented in four stages: (a) reading and three-dimensional reconstruction of each cross-section of MRI; (b) Preprocessing, to remove artifacts and improve the quality of the images; (c) Segmentation of three tissues of interest and (d) quantification of the volumes segmented, using techniques of *Voxel Based Morphometry* (VBM). The workflow of algorithms used for obtain the volumes is based in the methodology presented in (Gavidia, et al., 2011).

After obtain the three volumes, were calculated the total number of voxels of WM (*voxels_WM*), the total number of voxels of GM (*voxels_GM*) and the total number voxels of CSF (*voxels_CSF*). Then, were calculated the percentage of tissue for each one relative to the sum of three amounts referred above total volumes (total_voxels), see ec. 1. On this way, were obtained three new inputs-variables: %WM, %GM and %CSF, which were included into morphometric group.

$$\%WM = 1/(voxels\_WM / total\_voxel)$$
$$\%GM = 1/(voxels\_GM / total\_voxels) \quad (1)$$
$$\%CSF = 1/(voxels\_CSF / total\_voxels)$$

– Analysis of the input-target variables

In the previous sections, we described how were obtained 12 initial variables (9 inputs and 1 target) from OASIS database. The current stage consisted in calculate the correlation between the inputs variables and target variable, analyzing their values and determine their dependence. This process showed that Handedness, Education and SES variables have not a correlation clearly defined with the rest of variables. Also, the analysis showed that nWBV and ASF variables could be eliminated because not provided relevant information to the training. The first one is implicit in the sum of %_WM and %_GM variables and the second one is equal to 1755 divided by eTIV variable (Buckner, et al., 2004). Thus, this stage allowed us to establish that nine of twelve initial variables could be more suitable for training and testing of the ANN, however, the definitive exclusion of these variables only will be confirm in the phase of training and testing by compare the confusion percentage de la ANN using different groups of variables.

2.2 Artificial neural network training

At this stage, we determined the characteristics and functionalities would be applied in the training of the ANN.

– Selection of the rule of learning and training algorithm

First, was necessary to determine the type of rule of learning and the training most appropriate to solve our problem of diagnosis. Given that the same occurrence of the set of *inputs* always will be associated to a specific *target*, that is, the occurrence of certain values in each one of the 12 inputs should correspond to a same diagnosis CDR (*target*), we decided establish the problem of diagnosis as a problem of classification. Likewise, based in the nature of the problem, we decided use the Multilayer Perceptron, which is a type of supervised learning network and as task of learning was selected the Pattern Recognition technique, widely used in the solution of problems of classification. In the practice, pattern recognition approach compared the obtained outputs with the correct target, by adjusting the weights (W) and biases (b) of the network and ensures that the outputs were closer to the target. Figure 2 shows a general scheme of the ANN architecture implemented in this research.

– Training of the network

The main tasks were:

a. *The dataset pre-processing.* All inputs-targets were normalized in the interval [–1 1];
b. *Division of the data.* The dataset was divided in two groups, the first one was used in the training with 80% of total sample and the second one was used in the testing with 20% remaining. This division of data was done randomly.
c. *Determine the architecture of ANN most effective,* by setting the number of entry layers and hidden layers.
d. *Training and testing of the network,* these processes were repeated until to find the *weights and biases* more adequate for minimize the percentage of confusion between *targets* and obtained outputs.

Likewise, this step allowed us establishes definitely which combinations of inputs variables were more suitable for diagnosis of dementia.

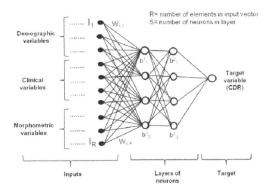

Figure 2. General scheme of the ANN architecture.

e. *Post-processing of the outputs*, the continuous values obtained as output were post processed to locate into any of the four classes of CDR target.

3 RESULTS

In the testing process applied to three different groups of inputs, the results confirmed the assertions done in the previous section about the correlation between variables and the importance of considering information about the size of affected brain tissues in patients with AD:

a. *Group of original nine inputs from OASIS database* (Sex, handedness, age, education, SES, MMSE, eTIV, nWBV, ASF) was obtained 48% of confusion error, that is, only 122 of 235 diagnostics were correct;
b. *Group of 6 inputs without additional morphometric data* (Sex, age, MMSE, eTIV, nWBV, ASF), gave a 25% of confusion error, that is, only 122 of 235 diagnostics were correct.
c. *Group of 7 inputs variables including additional morphometric inputs* (Sex, age, MMSE, eTIV, %_WM, %_GM(13), %CSF), gave a 17% confusion error.

The Figure 3 shows the regression plot of the results obtained in the testing of ANN showing normalized values to CDR: CDR = 0→−1, CDR = 0.5→−0.5, CDR = 1→0, CDR = 2→1. The dashed line in each axis represents the perfect result, the solid line represents the best fit linear regression line between outputs and targets. The R value is an indication of the relationship between the outputs and targets. If the training were perfect, the network outputs and the targets would be exactly equal, that is R = 1, but the relationship is rarely perfect in practice. For this research, using the third group of variables, the testing data indicated R value that greater than 0.8, which is a good result. The plot showed that certain data points have poor fits, for example, there are data points in whose output values are close to −0.5 (CDR = 0.5: very mild), while the corresponding target values are about −1 (CDR = 0: no impairment); in another case, there are data points in whose output values are close to 0.5 (CDR = 1: mild dementia), while the corresponding target values are about 1 (CDR = 2: moderate dementia). A possible reason to this confusion could be the extrapolation of some instances outside of the training dataset, which is comprehensible given the small number of instances to CDR = 2.

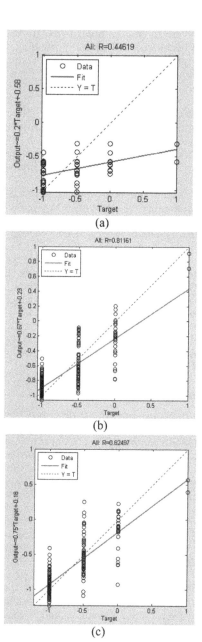

(a)

(b)

(c)

Figure 3. Regression plot of the results obtained in the testing of ANN. (a) 48% confusion (122/235) obtained in testing applied to 235 instances with nine original input variables (Sex, handedness, age, education, SES, MMSE, eTIV, nWBV, ASF). (b) 25% confusion (178/235) obtained in testing applied to 235 instances with six input variables (Sex, age, MMSE, eTIV, nWBV, ASF). (c) 17% confusion (195/235) obtained in testing applied to 235 instances with seven input variables (Sex, age, MMSE, eTIV, %_WM, %_GM, %CSF). (Plots obtained using Neural Network Toolbox of MATLAB) (R2009b 2011).

4 CONCLUSIONS

Through this research was demonstrated that the combination of appropriate demographic, clinical and morphometric brain data of a patient obtained with medical imaging processing and VBM techniques are *inputs* suitable to build a successful ANN of diagnosis of AD.

The ANN learned from MRI data in 235 cases. In the general testing, the percentage of confusion was 17%, this error indicates that only 195 of 235 cases were incorrectly diagnosed. However, the existence of small error rate reflects that always is necessary the continuous monitoring of the ANN diagnosis by an expert in neurology.

This research has some limitations. The experimental data sample is small and maybe the number of variables is limited. In order to improve the results of diagnosis of CDR, it is necessary to collect more samples from other brain database, for example, include datasets from Alzheimer's Disease Neuroimaging Initiative (ADNI) (Mueller, Weiner, et al., 2005a), (Mueller, Weiner, et al., 2005b). Also, studies dedicated to investigate atrophied brain by AD, make reference to another areas affected by this disease as the ventricles, the hypothalamus and the sea-horses (Morra, et al., 2008). Thus, it is possible to obtain better results in the diagnosis of dementia including new morphometric inputs. Additionally, could be considered statistical descriptors (entropy, correlation, standard deviation, etc., calculated) from segmented volumes of the brain.

Finally, we believe that the methodology applied to build the ANN with the monitoring by medical personal, could be applied to another type of pathological diagnosis.

REFERENCES

Buckner, R.L. et al. "A unified approach for morphometric and functional data analysis in young, old, and demented adults using automated atlas-based head size normalization: reliability and validation against manual measurement of total intracranial volume." *Neuroimage* 23 (2004): 724–738.

Fotenos, A.F., Snyder, A.Z., Girton, L.E., Morris, J.C. and Buckner, R.L. "Normative estimates of cross-sectional and longitudinal brain volume decline in aging and AD." *Neurology* 64 (2005): 1032–1039.

Gavidia, Giovana, Eduardo Soudah, Miguel Cerrolaza, and Miguel Landrove. "Generación de modelos discretos de tejidos del ser humano a través del pre procesamiento y segmentación de imágenes médicas." *Revista Internacional de Métodos Numéricos en Ingeniería*, 2011.

Jack, Clifford, R. et al. "Medial temporal atrophy on MRI in normal aging and very mild Alzheimer's disease." *Neurology* 49, no. 3 (1997): 786–794.

Killiany, R.J. et al. "MRI measures of entorhinal cortex vs hippocampus in preclinical AD." *Neurology* 58, no. 8 (2002): 1188–1196.

Marcus, Daniel, Anthony, F Fotenos, John G Csernansky, John C Morris, and Randy L Buckner. "Open Access Series of Imaging Studies (OASIS): Longitudinal MRI Data in Nondemented and Demented Older Adults." *Journal of Cognitive Neuroscience* 22, no. 12 (2010): 2677–2684.

Morra, J.H. et al. "Automated mapping of hippocampal atrophy in 1-year repeat MRI data from 490 subjects with Alzheimer's disease, mild cognitive impairment, and elderly controls." *Neuroimage* 43, no. 1 (2008): 59–68.

Morris, J.C. "The Clinical Dementia Rating (CDR): current version and scoring rules." *Neurology* 43 (1993): 2412–2414.

Morris, J.C. et al. "Mild cognitive impairment represents early-stage Alzheimer." *Archives of Neurology* 58 (2001): 397–405.

Mueller, S.G. et al. "The Alzheimer's disease neuroimaging initiative." *Neuroimaging Clin. North*, 2005a: 869–877.

Mueller, S.G, et al. "Ways toward an early diagnosis in Alzheimer's disease: The Alzheimer's Disease Neuroimaging." *Alzheimers Dement*, 2005b: 55–66.

R2009b, MATLAB. "Neural Network Toolbox™ User's Guide." *R2009b documentation, Neural Network Toolbox*. 2011. http://www.mathworks.com/help/toolbox/nnet/

Talairach, J. and Tournoux, P. *Co-Planar Stereotaxic Atlas of the Human Brain*. New York: Thieme, 1988.

Automated extraction of the Femoral Shaft Axis and its distal entry point from full and reduced 3D models

S. Van Cauter & M. De Beule
IBiTech-bioMMeda, Ghent University, Ghent, Belgium

A. Van Haver
Engineering Department, Ghent University College, Ghent, Belgium
Department of Mechanical Construction and Production, Ghent University, Ghent, Belgium

P. Verdonk
Department of Orthopaedic Surgery, Ghent University Hospital, Ghent, Belgium

B. Verhegghe
IBiTech-bioMMeda, Ghent University, Ghent, Belgium

ABSTRACT: During conventional total knee arthroplasty, the shaft or medial axis of the femur (FSA) is referenced by inserting an intramedullary rod (FIR), which is then used to position the femoral prosthesis. In this study, an automated technique, based on geometrical entity fitting, is presented for extracting the FSA and FIR from a 3D triangular surface mesh. The algorithms are tested using computed tomography scans of 50 cadaveric femurs. Furthermore, reduced models are processed and compared to the full models to study the feasibility of partially scanning the thigh. The mean deviations for two outer parts of 25% and a central part of 5% of the femoral length are smaller than 1 mm for the FSA and 0.3° and 0.5 mm for the orientation and entry point of a 150 mm long FIR. The automated methods could offer a valuable assistance to the surgeon for preoperative planning of FIR insertion.

Keywords: automated landmark extraction, femoral shaft axis, computed tomography, total knee arthroplasty

1 INTRODUCTION

The identification of anatomical reference parameters or landmarks, which are defined as prominent features of the body, is a well-established technique in orthopaedic surgery. A variety of morphological measurements and joint coordinate systems have been defined using such anatomical features. Landmarks are typically obtained by manual palpation of the subject or by virtual localization on a medical image. Manual analyses are, however, time-consuming and prone to observer variability and, consequently, an increasing amount of techniques for automated landmark extraction are being presented.

The femoral shaft (or anatomical) axis (FSA) is defined as the medial axis of the shaft (or diaphysis) of the femur and is usually straight in the frontal plane but curved in the sagittal plane. It is used as a reference parameter for positioning the femoral prosthesis in conventional total knee arthroplasty (TKA). The distal part of the axis is determined by manually inserting a metal rod into the medullary canal of the femur. The distal femur is then resected at a certain angle with respect to the intramedullary rod (FIR), aiming to put the femoral prosthesis orthogonally to the mechanical axis. As it has been shown that the entry point location of the rod has an important influence on the alignment of the prosthesis (Reed 1997, Mihalko 2005), preoperatively determining this entry point could improve the alignment accuracy of TKA. In addition, the preoperative planning of the insertion of the FIR could be used to obtain a patient-specific distal femoral resection angle.

Different methods have been presented to automatically determine the FSA on 3D virtual femurs generated from computed tomography (CT) scans, such as distance-controlled thinning (Subburaj 2010), circle fitting (Mahaisavariya 2002) and cylinder fitting (Cerveri 2010). However, because of the radiation exposure involved in CT scanning, obtaining full femur scans is not feasible in patient treatment. A new method for computing the FSA, based on geometrical entity fitting, is therefore proposed, which can be applied to full and reduced models of the femur. Moreover, the orientation and entry point of a FIR with a length of 150 mm are computed from the distal part of the FSA. The femur is reduced in different ways and the analyses are compared to those of the full femur to determine the effect of the scanning reduction on the computed FSA and FIR.

2 MATERIALS & METHODS

To develop and test the algorithms, 50 CT scans of cadaveric femurs, with 0.79×0.79 mm pixel size and 0.63 mm slice increment, are processed. The bones are segmented and 3D triangular surface meshes are created using Mimics (Materialise NV, Leuven, Belgium). All further processing is performed automatically in pyFormex (http://pyformex.org), an open-source program under development at IBiTech-bioMMeda, providing a wide range of operations on surface meshes.

2.1 Preprocessing

Some preprocessing algorithms are applied to simplify the 3D mesh and to remove undesirable noise. First, the edge reduction algorithm of the GNU Triangulated Surface Library is applied, resulting in 66668 triangles for the full femur. The edge reduction is run with equal weights for volume, boundary and shape optimization (Lindstrom 1998). Next, the 3D model is smoothed with a volume-preserving low-pass filter (Taubin 1995), by applying 20 smoothing iterations with a scale factor of 0.5.

2.2 Standardised coordinate system

The femur, which is positioned randomly during CT scanning, is then oriented in a standardised way. The centre of gravity (C) and principal axes of inertia of the surface are calculated. These axes serve as a coarse approximation of the antero-posterior (AP), right-left (RL) and disto-proximal (DP) directions. Then, the RL axis is rotated parallel to the posterior condylar line (PCL) in the axial plane (Fig. 1). The PCL is calculated as the line connecting the most posterior points of the medial and lateral condyles. As the PCL depends on the AP direction, the coordinate system is iteratively rotated until the RL and PCL axes are parallel.

2.3 Reference parameters

The following step is to extract the femoral middle shaft axis (FMSA), which is defined as the straight

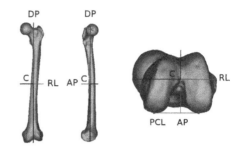

Figure 1. Standardised coordinate system: centre of gravity C and principal axes of inertia (RL, AP, DP) with RL rotated parallel to the posterior condylar line (PCL).

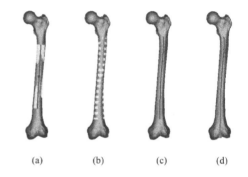

Figure 2. Reference parameters in the frontal plane: (a) femoral middle shaft cylinder and axis (FMSA); (b) femoral shaft hyperboloids; (c) femoral shaft axis (FSA); (d) femoral intramedullary rod (FIR).

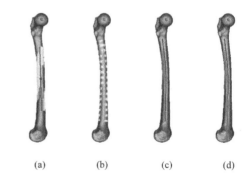

Figure 3. Reference parameters in the sagittal plane: (a) femoral middle shaft cylinder and axis (FMSA); (b) femoral shaft hyperboloids; (c) femoral shaft axis (FSA); (d) femoral intramedullary rod (FIR).

medial axis of the middle diaphysis. This axis will be used to reduce the full models and thus simulate a partial scanning of the thigh. The FMSA is calculated by fitting an elliptic cylinder to a set of points that lies symmetrically around C and has a height that is equal to half of the femoral length along DP (Figs. 2–3 (a)). The axes of the standardised coordinate system are used as a starting estimate for the principal axes of the cylinder. The FMSA is defined by the longitudinal axis of the fitted cylinder.

The optimal position and sizes of the cylinder are computed by minimizing the sum of squares of the distances of the points to the cylinder. This minimization is done with the nonlinear Levenberg-Marquardt least-squares optimization routine of the SciPy library. For a general quadric, calculating the orthogonal Euclidean distance requires solving the following set of equations, which states that the line connecting the point x_p and its closest point x_c on the quadric $Q(x)$ should be orthogonal to $Q(x)$ in x_c:

$$\begin{cases} Q(x_c) = x_c A x_c^T + b x_c^T + c = 0 \\ x_p - x_c = t \nabla Q(x_c) = t(2 x_c A + b) \end{cases} \quad (1)$$

The closest point x_c can be written as

$$x_c = (x_p - tb)(I + 2tA)^{-1} \quad (2)$$

Eliminating x_c from Equation 1 results in

$$\begin{aligned} &(x_p - tb)(I + 2tA)^{-1} A (I + 2tA)^{-1} (x_p - tb)^T \\ &+ b(I + 2tA)^{-1}(x_p - tb)^T + c = 0 \end{aligned} \quad (3)$$

Calculating the orthogonal distances thus involves finding the roots of a (at most) sixth degree polynomial for every point. Moreover, these distances need to be computed for each iteration of the minimization algorithm. An approximate geometrical distance is therefore calculated for every point x_p by intersecting the quadric with the normal vector n of the surface mesh at x_p. This problem is described by Equation 4 and involves solving a second degree polynomial, as shown in Equation 5.

$$\begin{cases} Q(x_c) = x_c A x_c^T + b x_c^T + c = 0 \\ x_p - x_c = tn \end{cases} \quad (4)$$

$$(x_p - tn)A(x_p - tn)^T + b(x_p - tn)^T + c = 0 \quad (5)$$

To determine the FSA, which is defined as the curved medial axis of the diaphysis, a series of elliptic hyperboloids of one sheet are fitted to the shaft (Figs. 2–3 (b)). The axes of the standardised coordinate system are used as an initial guess for the principal axes of the first (central) hyperboloid and each following hyperboloid is initialized by the principal axes of the previous one. All hyperboloids have a height between 5 and 10 mm, to provide enough surface points for the fitting procedure,

while allowing to capture the curvedness of the shaft. The FSA is then represented by a cubic Bezier curve that is computed from the longitudinal axes of the fitted hyperboloids (Figs. 2–3 (c)). To find the distal and proximal endpoints of the curve, a stop criterion is implemented, stating that the radius change along the FSA should not be larger than 10%.

Finally, the orientation and entry point of a FIR with a length of 150 mm are computed by fitting a line to the distal part of the FSA and intersecting it with the distal surface of the femur (Figs. 2–3 (d)). An iterative process is used to fit the line to the part of the FSA lying 150 mm above the entry point.

2.4 Comparison of full and reduced femur models

To simulate the effect of obtaining a partial scan of the patient's thigh, the femur model is reduced along its FMSA. Three reduction methods (distal, central and proximal part; distal and proximal part; distal part), two reduction amounts for the distal and proximal parts (30% and 25% of the femoral length) and two reduction amounts for the central part (10% and 5% of the femoral length) are studied. Figure 4 shows the different types of reductions with distal and proximal parts of 30% and a central part of 10% of the length. For the models consisting of more than one part, the FSA is interpolated to estimate the medial axis in the non-scanned regions.

The FSA and FIR computed from the full and reduced models are compared using the following values: maximum orthogonal distance between the FSA (FSA-max); 3D distances between the distal/proximal endpoints of the FSA (FSA-DP/FSA-PP); absolute 3D angle between the axes of

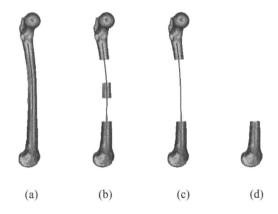

(a)   (b)   (c)   (d)

Figure 4. FSA computed on different types of models: (a) full model; (b) reduced model with distal, central and proximal part; (c) reduced model with distal and proximal part; (d) reduced model with distal part.

the FIR (FIR-A); 3D distance between the entry points of the FIR (FIR-EP).

3 RESULTS AND DISCUSSION

Figure 5 shows the mean values and standard deviations for the 50 femur models for distal and proximal parts of 30% of the femoral length. The orthogonal distance between the FSA varies between 0.10 ± 0.07 and 2.21 ± 0.50 mm (FSA-max). It should be noticed that the smallest value is obtained for the reduction to one distal part, because no interpolation can be used here to estimate the FSA in the non-scanned regions. The largest value is found for the reduction to a distal and proximal part. The FSA of these models has a highly larger deviation from the FSA of the full model compared to the first two cases. Removing the central part forces the curve to interpolate directly between the outer parts, thereby misestimating the curvature of the bone. The 3D distances between the endpoints (FSA-DP and FSA-PP) are rather similar for the different cases and have a maximum value of 0.40 ± 0.36 mm. The values for the FIR orientation and entry point are between 0.14 ± 0.09 and 0.94 ± 0.45° (FIR-A) and between 0.23 ± 0.16 and 1.43 ± 0.65 mm (FIR-EP). The best results are obtained for the models with a central part of 10%, while a large increase is shown for the models without central part. Overall, the models with central parts of 10% and 5% have similar mean values and standard deviations.

The results for distal and proximal parts of 25% of the femoral length are displayed in Figure 6. The same observations as in Figure 5 can be made between the different reduction cases. Compared to the outer parts of 30%, larger values are shown. Good results for all parameters are obtained for the central part of 5%, with mean deviations from the full models smaller than 1 mm (FSA-max), 0.5 mm (FSA-DP and FSA-PP), 0.3° (FIR-A) and 0.5 mm

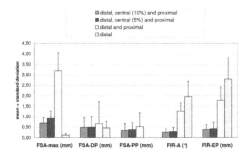

Figure 6. Comparison of the analyses of the full and reduced femur models for distal and proximal parts of 25% of the length.

(FIR-EP). The maximum values are smaller than 2 mm, 3.1 mm, 1.3° and 2.1 mm.

It was found that reducing the outer parts to 20% results in too few hyperboloids in these regions and incorrect endpoints for the FSA.

The results of this study indicate that scanning 55% of the thigh gives precise values for the FSA and a 150 mm long FIR. To correctly capture the curvedness of the shaft (and thus of the FSA), it is recommended to scan a distal, central and proximal part of the thigh. It is also shown that the orientation of the FIR largely depends on the curvedness of the FSA, as considerably higher deviations from the full model are obtained when the central part is omitted.

The automated extraction of the FIR orientation and entry point may contribute to a faster and more objective planning of TKA. However, some limitations of the current study should be mentioned. Mesh simplification and smoothing was applied on the 3D models, but the effect of various parameters for these preprocessing operations should be investigated. Also, the insertion of intramedullary rods with different lengths should be studied. In particular, larger rods may inhibit a complete insertion because the medullary canal is curved, and it might thus be important to take into account the canal width. Further work is being carried out to evaluate the computed values by comparison with a set of manually identified parameters and to extract the mechanical axis of the femur to find a patient-specific distal resection angle for TKA procedures. The proposed methods could then allow for automatic planning of FIR insertion and distal femoral resection preoperatively, offering a valuable assistance to the surgeon.

4 CONCLUSIONS

An automated method for computing the FSA was developed and tested on 50 femur models.

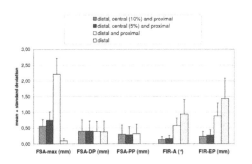

Figure 5. Comparison of the analyses of the full and reduced femur models for distal and proximal parts of 30% of the length.

The orientation and entry point of a FIR used for TKA alignment was derived from the distal part of the FSA. It was shown that the FSA and FIR can be determined with high precision by scanning two outer parts and a central part of the thigh. The automated method could offer a valuable assistance to the surgeon for TKA procedures by preoperatively planning FIR insertion.

ACKNOWLEDGEMENT

The authors gratefully acknowledge Dr. Emmanuel Audenaert (Department of Orthopaedic Surgery, Ghent University Hospital) and the Department of Experimental Anatomy of the Vrije Universiteit Brussel for providing the CT scans.

REFERENCES

Cerveri P., Marchente, M., Bartels, W., Corten, K., Simon, J.P. & Manzotti, A. 2010. Automated method for computing the morphological and clinical parameters of the proximal femur using heuristic modeling techniques. Ann Biomed Eng 38(5): 1752–1766.

Lindstrom, P. & Turk, G. 1998. Fast and memory efficient polygonal simplification. Proceedings of IEEE Visualization '98. Research Triangle Park, North Carolina, 18–23 October, pp. 279–286.

Mahaisavariya, B., Sitthiseripratip, K., Tongdee, T., Bohez, E.L., Vander Sloten, J. & Oris, P. 2002. Morphological study of the proximal femur: a new method of geometrical assessment using 3-dimensional reverse engineering. Med Eng Phys 24(9): 617–622.

Mihalko, W.M., Boyle, J., Clark, L.D. & Krackow, K.A. 2005. The variability of intramedullary alignment of the femoral component during total knee arthroplasty. J Arthroplasty 20(1): 25–28.

Reed, S.C. & Gollish, J. 1997. The accuracy of femoral intramedullary guides in total knee arthroplasty. J Arthroplasty 12(6): 677–682.

Subburaj, K., Ravi, B. & Agarwal, M. 2010. Computer-aided methods for assessing lower limb deformities in orthopaedic surgery planning. Comput Med Imaging Graph 34(4): 277–288.

Taubin, G. 1995. A signal processing approach to fair surface design. Paper presented at: SIGGRAPH '95. Proceedings of the 22nd Annual Conference on Computer Graphics. Los Angeles, CA, USA, 6–11 August, pp. 351–358.

Computational Vision and Medical Image Processing – Tavares & Natal Jorge (eds)
© 2012 Taylor & Francis Group, London, ISBN 978-0-415-68395-1

Facial expression recognition using MPEG-4 FAP-based 3D MMM

Hamimah Ujir
Universiti Malaysia Sarawak, Malaysia

Michael Spann
University of Birmingham, UK

ABSTRACT: A 3D Modular Morphable Model (3DMMM) is introduced to deal with facial expression recognition. The 3D Morphable Model (3DMM) contains 3D shape and 2D texture information of faces extracted using conventional Principal Component Analysis (PCA). I this work, Modular PCA approach is used. A face is divided into several components according to different facial features which are categorized based on Facial Animation Parameters (FAP). FAP is the measurement of muscular action relevant to the Action Units and it provides temporal information that is needed in order to have a realistic facial expression effect. Each region will be treated separately in the PCA analysis. Our work is about recognizing the six basic emotions, provided that the properties of an emotion are satisfied.

Keywords: Modular PCA, 3D Morphable Model, Facial Expression Recognition

1 INTRODUCTION

Facial expression recognition deals with the application of facial motion and facial feature deformation into abstract classes that are purely based on visual information (Fasel & Luettin, 2003). Facial expression studies are beneficial to various applications. Among the applications are physiological studies, face image compression, synthetic face animation, robotics as well as virtual reality.

In this paper, we propose a novel approach for facial expression recognition called 3D Modular Morphable Model (3DMMM) that combines three advances in the face processing field: 3D Morphable Model (3DMM), Modular Principle Component Analysis (MPCA) and Facial Animation Parameters (FAP).

There have been numerous works in this area. However, our work has the following differences with others: (1) the fitting of 3D shape and texture (face appearance) is done according to the components and therefore each component has their own eigenvalues and eigenvectors; and (2) each component are given priority in the fitting process which depends on its importance in recognizing facial expression.

The outline of the paper is as follows: In the second section, the motivation of the work is described. In the third section, the three separate advances are discussed. The framework of this work can be found in the fourth section. In the fifth section is about the database description. The experiment as well as its analysis is presented in sixth section. Finally, we give the conclusion.

2 MOTIVATION

PCA algorithms produce a set of values of uncorrelated variables called principal component (PC). All PCs are then ordered so that the first few retain most of the variation in all of original variables while the rest of the components contain the remaining original variables after all correlation with the preceding PCs has been subtracted out. The number of PCs is normally chosen to explain at least 90% of the variation in the training set. The fitting process of a new image to the model involved projecting the 2D image onto the face space and then finding the minimum of the distance all of the faces stored in the database and the closest matching one is recognised. With the number of subjects involved, as well as large variation of expressions, poses and illumination in the training set, the number of principal components to be considered is rather high. Logically, the fitting processing time is increased proportionally with the number of PCs.

Different combination of facial features produces different type of facial expressions. For instance, how to differentiate between the true smile and polite smile since both types of smile share the same action unit (AU) deformation which is the lip corner puller. In this case, the cheek raiser AU needs to be checked; if it's in action, the true smile is performed and vice versa. Most work in face processing is based on linear combination approach. Employing PCA on one whole face is like learning a face as one big component. In other word, the local features and its holistic information are not being taken full advantage of.

Since the facial expression really depends on the deformation of facial features and muscles, a face is divided into several components. In this work, a Modular PCA (MPCA) is implemented where each face component is treated separately in the PCA process. The face components are decided based on the facial features which are categorized according to the Facial Animation Parameters (FAP). Basic related concepts of FAP are described in Lavagetto and Pockaj (1999).

One major prominent feature of MPCA is it yields new modules to recognize different facial expressions which could be the new addition to the existing facial expression in the training set. The new modules here are the combination of different components. Besides that, with MPCA, a smaller error is generated compared to conventional PCA as it pays more attention to the local structure (King and Xu, 1997).

Since a different PC is calculated for each region the number of PCs for each region is less than when a face is treated as a whole. Priority in the fitting process goes to the components with intransient facial features which are facial features that are always present in the face and may be deformed due to the facial expressions such as the eyebrows and mouth.

3 APPROACHES

3.1 Modular PCA

Using PCA, a face is represented by a linear combination of physical face geometries, S_{model} and texture images, T_{model} and both models are within a few standard deviations from their means. PCA is indeed a promising approach in for face analysis. It is fast, reliable and able to produce good results. However, according to Mao et al. (2009), PCA does not cope well with variations of expression, facial hair, and occlusion. Thus, we chose a slightly different PCA version which is MPCA.

Zhao et al. (2003) state that face recognition using eigenmodules (i.e.: mouth, nose and eyes) showed improvement in facial recognition compared to using only eigenfaces. Other work using MPCA showed a significant result especially when there are large variations in facial expression and illumination is by Gottumukkal and Asari (2004). As mentioned in the last section, MPCA generates a smaller error as it pays more attention to the local structure (King and Xu, 1997).

However, according to Gottumukkal and Asari (2004), MPCA is known as not giving a significant advancement in pose and orientation problem. It also requires the location of each facial feature to be identified initially.

King and Xu (1997) divided a face into 4 components; centre-of-the-left-eye, centre-of-the-right-eye, tip-of-the-nose and centre-of-the mouth feature points. Chiang et al. (2009) used 5 components which include the left eye, the right eye, the nose, the mouth, and the bare face with each facial component identified by a landmark at the component centre. In this work, a face is divided into several components according to different facial features which are categorized based on the Facial Animation Parameters (FAPs). The computational part of MPCA is further discussed in section 3.3.

3.2 Facial animation parameters

FAPs are a set of parameters, used in animating MPEG-4 models that define the reproduction emotions, expressions and speech pronunciation. It gives the measurement of muscular action relevant to the AU and it provides temporal information that is needed in order to have a life-like facial expression effect (Zhang et al, 2008). Figure 2 shows FAP and feature points on a neutral face and both define FAPU.

FAPs represent a complete set of basic facial actions, such as stretch nose, open or close eyelids, and therefore allow the representation of most natural facial expressions, as shown in Figure 1. In this work, six FAP-based components are used to represent a whole face, see Table 1. Each component contains the facial features that correspond to the FAP in that component. For example, in group 1, stretch_l_nose and stretch_r_nose, refer to horizontal displacement of both side of nose. Therefore, all facial features that belong to the red box in Figure 2 are set in component group

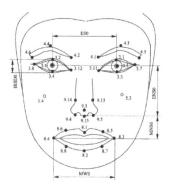

Figure 1. A neutral face with FAPs and feature points to define FAPU (Zhang et al., 2008).

Table 1. Face components represented in FAP group (Zhang et al., 2008).

Group	Facial Animation Parameters (FAP)
1	stretch_l_nose, stretch_r_nose,
2	open_jaw, raise_b_midlip, stretch_r_cornerlip, raise_l_cornerlip, raise_r_cornerlip, push_b_lip, stretch_l_cornerlip, depress_chin
3	raise_r_i_eyebrow, raise_r_i_eyebrow, squeeze_r_eyebrow., raise_l_i_eyebrow, raise_l_o_eyebrow, squeeze_l_ eyebrow,
4	raise_b_midlip_o, stretch_r_cornerlip_o, raise_l_cornerlip_o, raise_r_cornerlip_o, stretch_l_cornerlip_o
5 & 6	lift_l_cheek (group 5), lift_r_cheek (group 6)

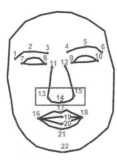

Figure 2. Three facial features in one of the face components corresponding to FAP.

1 which is also the group with highest priority. In group one, the two FAPs is only exist in disgust expression and when there is a change for these two parameters, it means the subject is showing the disgust or anger expression.

3.3 FAPs-Based 3D MMM

3D MM is based on a series of example 3D scans represented in an object centred system and registered to a single reference (Romdhani et al., 2005). It will be used for MPCA-based representation of faces; this combination of algorithms will then be named as the 3D Modular Morphable Model (3D MMM).

The training of MPCA is similar to conventional PCA with the algorithm applied to each of the seven groups in Table 1. For convenience, six disjoint sets of facial features are denotes as $P \in$ {$lower, rbrow, lbrow, cheek, nose, mouth$}.

The training examples are stored in terms of x, y z-coordinates of all vertices in the same components of a 3D mesh. The following is the example of the nose component:

$$S_{nose} = \{x_1, y_1, z_1, x_2, y_2, z_2, \ldots, x_n, y_n, z_n\} \quad (1)$$

Accordingly, the texture vectors are formed from the red, green and blue of all vertices.

$$T_{nose} = \{r_1, g_1, b_1, r_2, g_2, b_2, \ldots, r_n, g_n, b_n\} \quad (2)$$

The linear space of face geometries and texture are denoted in Equations 3 and 4 and both assume a uniform distribution of the shapes and the textures. a_{nose} and b_{nose} are the coefficients that determine the variation between 3D nose components for all faces in the training set.

$$S_{nose} = \bar{S}_{nose} + \sum_{i=1}^{n} a_i s_i \quad (3)$$

$$T_{nose} = \bar{T}_{nose} + \sum_{i=1}^{n} b_i t_i \quad (4)$$

4 OUR FRAMEWORK

Given a 2D image of a subject with facial expression, a matched 3D model for the image is found by fitting them to our 3D MMM. Figure 3 describes our 3D Modular Morphable Model Framework. As mentioned before, the fitting is done according to the components, not for the whole face and it will be in order of the importance in facial expressions recognition.

After all matched components are found, they are combined and rendered; finally a new 3D face model is generated. Since the input could involve any type of facial deformations; the only way to define the facial expressions shown by the input image is by comparison with the mean face which is set to be a neutral face. The deformation of each facial feature that corresponds to a FAP is measured. This measurement is done according to the priority order of the component set. The next step is to check the symmetry of facial features. Therefore, a second step to recognize the deformed facial features is by checking the face symmetry. An asymmetric facial feature means there is difference between the left and right side, for example the left eyebrow is in raise state while the right eyebrow is neutral. Those asymmetric facial features are also labelled as the deformed facial features.

The collections of deformations by all facial features tell us the type of facial expression shown by the model. However, if the collection of deformed facial features does not describe the properties of any six basic emotions, then it will be stated as unrecognized; instead, and all deformed facial features involved are listed. In the case where no deformed facial features, the face is noted as a neutral face.

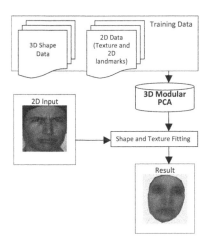

Figure 3. 3D Modular morphable model framework.

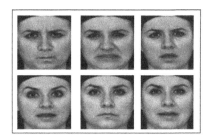

Figure 4. Six different emotions of a subject. Top row: anger, disgust, fear. Bottom row: surprise, neutral and few combinations of deformation.

5 DATABASE DESCRIPTION

A multi–attribute database developed by Savran et al. (2008) from Bogazici University, Turkey called The Bosphorus Database is used. The data is acquired using Inspeck Mega Capturor II 3D which is a commercial structured-light based 3D digitizer device. The Bosphorus Database contains 24 facial landmark points; provided that they are visible in the given scan (i.e., the right and left ear lobe cannot be seen from frontal pose). It provides a rich set of expressions, systematic variation of poses and different types of realistic occlusions. Each scan is intended to cover one pose and/or one expression type. Thirty-four facial expressions are composed of a wisely chosen subset of Facial Action Units (FAU) as well as the six basic emotions. Besides the facial expression data, this database contains different occlusion and head poses data.

In this work, our 3DMMM is derived from statistics computed on 30 subjects with 6 different expressions. One of the expressions must be a neutral face and the remaining five expressions could be among the six basic emotions or simply a deformation of any facial features. Figure 4 shows a subject with six different facial expression.

We are dealing with two type of information, 2D and 3D data, and both data need to go under a few processes before they are ready to be used in modular PCA computation as well the fitting procedure. The 3D points of every faces are aligned to each other and 97 3D points and 174 meshes are used to represent one whole face. The aligned 3D points are then divided into six facial components. For each component, the eigenvalues and its corresponding eigenvectors as well as the weight parameters are computed. Out of certain amount of eigenvalues, only 97% of the eigenvalues of the whole training data are kept and used in the next step which is fitting.

In two dimensional data, two important data are needed: (1) 2D-points that mark the facial features on a texture and (2) a texture (RGB values). The 2D points are warped using Thin Plate Spline (TPS) algorithm to ensure the colour profiles are obtained cross a free shape patch. On the other hand, all training texture are also normalized using affine transformation, this way all training texture have the same brightness and contrast. The RGB values of the texture are extracted from the normalized texture and eigenvalues and its corresponding eigenvectors are computed.

We can recognize the facial expression by measuring the similarity (mean square error) between input image and the reconstructed 3D face model with 2D face appearance. Given a 2D image input, a 3D model is generated and the new texture is reconstructed by fitting the model to the new input. Following Blanz et al. (2007) work's, rigid transformation and perspective projective are implemented in the fitting process. A further discussion of fitting a new 2D image can be found in Blanz et al. (2007).

6 RESULTS

To assess the viability of this approach, we have performed the experiments to recognize the six facial expressions. In the training set, there are 3 subjects and each subject shown the 6 facial expressions. Figure 5 shows a test image with anger expression and the generated 3D model.

The challenging part in this experiment is to fit a component with other components that would define an identifiable facial expression. As mentioned, the first priority is set to be the nose area since it will assist in differentiating anger and disgust expression from others, i.e: a stretch nose only happens in anger and disgust expression.

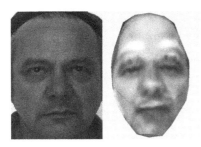

Figure 5. Left: Input image with anger expression. Right: 3D model with anger appearance.

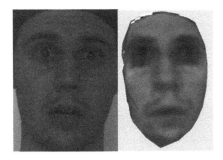

Figure 6. Left: Input image with fear expression. Right: 3D model with fear appearance.

The following component, the eyes area, needs to comply with the first component properties and this is repeated by the other components according to the priority list. Wrong matched components will result a face with unrecognized facial emotion or even worse, an odd looking face.

Another noticeable outcome from the experiment is the wrinkle and dimple feature. In real life, these two features are two keys that help in identifying people and it also become one of the important feature that project certain facial expression. For example, in Figure 6, lines of wrinkles on the forehead and a line from inner eyes to the outer cheek are part of the fear expression. However, this cannot be seen in the 3D model generated.

7 CONCLUSION

This paper explores the potential of facial expression recognition using modular approach. A face is divided into six components and each component will have their own eigenvalues as well as eigenvector. A test image is divided into the six components and the fitting is done component by component. A facial expression is considered as identified when the changes of facial expression parameters are detected and the result of the

experiment is a 3D model with facial expression. The system developed also yields various facial expressions even though that certain expression is not in the training set.

Our future work will emphasize in efficiently classifying facial expression where it will identify any facial deformation instead of only six facial emotions. In order to have an effective classification system, the fitting process needs to be improved and number of test image will be added. We will pursue these three aspects in the future.

REFERENCES

Blanz, V., Scherbaum, K. & Seidel, H. 2007. "Fitting a Morphable Model to 3D Scans of Faces", *Computer Vision, IEEE International Conference on*, vol. 0, pp. 1–8.

Chiang, C.-C., Chen, Z.-W. and Yang, C.-N., 2009. "A Component-based Face Synthesizing Method", *APSIPA Annual Summit and Conference*, pp. 24.

Fasel, B. & Luettin, J. 2003, "Automatic Facial Expression Analysis: A Survey", *Pattern Recognition*, vol. 36, no. 1, pp. 259–275.

Gottumukkal, R. & Asari, V.K. 2004. "An improved face recognition technique based on modular PCA approach", *Pattern Recogniton .Letter.*, vol. 25, no. 4, pp. 429–436.

King, I. & Xu, L. 1997. "Localized Principal Component Analysis Learning for Face Feature Extraction and Recognition", *Proc. Workshop 3D Computer Vision*, p. 124.

Lavagetto, F. & Pockaj, R. 1999. "The Facial Animation Engine: towards a high-level interface for the design of MPEG-4 compliant animated faces", *IEEE Trans. on Circuits and Systems for Video Technology*, Vol. 9, no. 2, pp. 277–289.

Mao, X., Xue, Y., Li, Z., Huang, K. & Lv, S. 2009. "Robust Facial Expression Recognition based on RPCA and AdaBoost", *10th Workshop on Image Analysis for Multimedia Interactive Services*.

Romdhani, S., Pierrard, J.-S & Vetter, T. 2005. "3D Morphable Face Model, a Unified Approach for Analysis and Synthesis of Images" in *Face Processing: Advanced Modeling and Methods*, ed. R.C. Wenyi Zhao, Elsevier.

Savran, A., Alyüz, N., Dibeklioğlu, H., Çeliktutan, O., Gökberk, B., Sankur, B. & Akarun, L. 2008. "Biometrics and Identity Management" in *Bosphorus Database for 3D Face Analysis*, eds. B. Schouten, N.C. Juul, A. Drygajlo & M. Tistarelli, Springer-Verlag, Berlin, Heidelberg, pp. 47–56.

Zhang, Y., Ji, Q., Zhu, Z. & Yi, B. 2008. "Dynamic Facial Expression Analysis and Synthesis With MPEG-4 Facial Animation Parameters", *IEEE Trans. Circuits System.Video Technology*, vol. 18, no. 10, pp. 1383–1396.

Zhao, W., Chellappa, R., Phillips, P.J. & Rosenfeld, A. 2003. "Face recognition: A literature survey", *ACM Computing Survey.*, vol. 35, no. 4, pp. 399–458.

Computational Vision and Medical Image Processing – Tavares & Natal Jorge (eds)
© 2012 Taylor & Francis Group, London, ISBN 978-0-415-68395-1

Using aerial photographs and characteristic points for automatic estimation of altitude of the references points

M.A.P. Domiciano, E.H. Shiguemori & O.D. Zaloti Jr.
Institute for Advanced Studies, São José dos Campos, SP, Brazil

L.A.V. Dias
Brazilian Aeronautics Institute of Technology, São José dos Campos, SP, Brazil

ABSTRACT: This work aims to present a study, which employs aerial photography keypoints to altitude estimation from coincident points in images. It has been employed an algorithm to automatic images characteristic estimation. From flying and camera information, the elevation of the keypoints is estimated. This information is important and can be employed in UAV's autonomous navigation.

1 INTRODUCTION

Using images in applications that require real-time execution has grown in recent years, mainly due to computational and technological development. Among these applications stand out the autonomous aerial navigation based on images.

This work aims to present an approach for provide position information to an unmanned aerial vehicle (UAV) based on images (Canhoto et al., 2009), (Domiciano et al., 2008).

2 PROBLEM

According to (Simons 2011) the first operational UAV was A.M. Low's "aerial target" of 1916. The Hewitt-Sperry Automatic Airplane developed on Sept. 12, 1916 and controlled by Elmer Sperry gyroscope demonstrated the feasibility of unmanned assault aircraft. The scientist Hugo Gernsback already saw the advantages of a pilotless via radio control and a television link, in 1924; although the current technology was inadequate for such a device.

The V-1 (introduced in 1944) was the first weapon to use the classic cruise missile layout of a bomb-like fuselage with short wings and a dorsally mounted engine, along with a simple inertial guidance system (Ekütekin 2007).

According to (Kane 2007) the UAVs have been often utilized on missions that are too "dull, dirty, or dangerous" for manned aircraft.

For autonomous navigation, it is important to extract accurate navigation parameters of an aircraft such as position and velocity. Using them,

one can adjust a velocity or direction to the desired destination (Sim & Park 2002).

One possibility to obtain the position of the aircraft in a given time is based on construction, real-time and embedded, of a digital elevation model of references (DEM-R) from the images obtained during the flight of a UAV and compare it with a model pre-existing (Domiciano et al., 2008), (Lowe 2004), (Schultz 1995).

3 METHODOLOGY

The methodology consisted of the following steps: to find characteristic points in images with the application of the SIFT algorithm (Lowe 2004), make the correspondence between the centers of the images in order to find the misalignment between them.

After that it is necessary to find the starting point of search. Then, it is applied the Zernike moments from this starting point in parts of the images, windows search, find corresponding points, and finally the altitude is estimated.

In order to achieve this, it's necessary to identify corresponding points in two sequential images. Thus, this study used the SIFT algorithm (Lowe 2004), which provided punctual previous information necessary for the calculation.

After that, the Zernike Moments (Khotanzad & Hong 1990), (Chen & Sun 2010) were used to identify correspondents points in two images and then builds a DEM-R in a regular grid.

Then the altitude of each point identified in relation to a datum specified has been obtained using the following equation used in photogrammetry (Wolf 1983), (Domiciano et al., 2008):

$$h_a = H - \frac{B \cdot f}{x_a - x'_a} \qquad (1)$$

where H is the altitude of flight in relation to a datum, B the air baseline, f the focal distance, x_a the distance from the point "A" to the center of the first image and x'_a the distance from the point "A" to the center point of the second image.

4 RESULTS

For preliminary results obtained in the study, it has been employed two aerial photos of the city of Sao Jose dos Campos, Brazil, with overlap of approximately 60%. These images were provided by (1°/6° Grupo de Aviação 1999). The methodology applied in these images obtained altitudes close to the real terrain, indicating that it can be applied in the estimation of position of the UAV through the DEM-R.

The next step is to compare the obtained DEM-R with the pre-existing reference model to estimate the error of the algorithm.

In order to compare the obtained altitudes with the reference ones, it was selected a part of the image that contains the runway of the city.

The criteria for choosing this area were:

- The area is approximately flat;
- To have the DEM of the area;
- The area has a slope;
- Ease of access, and
- Easily identifiable in the image.

Figure 1 shows some Sao Jose dos Campos images used in this work.

Figure 2 shows the digital elevation model obtained with the points returned after use of Zernike Moments in the images shown by Figure 1.

Figure 3 shows the Triangulated Irregular Network (TIN) obtained with the points returned after use of Zernike Moments in the images shown by Figure 1.

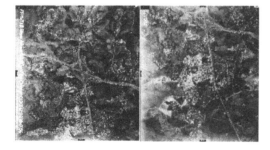

Figure 1. Sao Jose dos Campos images.

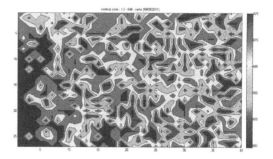

Figure 2. Sao Jose dos Campos DEM-R.

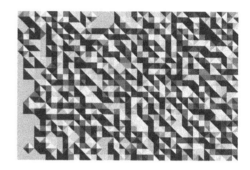

Figure 3. Sao Jose dos Campos—Triangulated Irregular Network (TIN).

Figure 4 shows the area of the runway utilized in tests.

It was applied Zernike moments on the area corresponding to the runway and performed a subsequent search to locate the corresponding points between two images of the runway by applying the Zernike Moments. After that, it was calculated the altitudes of these points as shown in Figure 5.

The results obtained are similar to the altitude of the reference DEM-R, as can be seen in Figure 5.

The resolution of the reference DEM-R is approximately 5 m while the resolution of the images used is approximately 2.56 m, because the resolutions are not equal or proportional and using two pixels in an image to one in the DEM-R, each 98 pixels in the image correspond to 50 pixels in the DEM-R and not 49, thus there may be a mismatch of altitudes with the corresponding removal of one of the points.

The spatial resolution along with the fact that the area is flat with a slight slope, contributes to small displacements of points, providing similar altitudes in the range analyzed.

Comparing the reference DEM-R with calculated DEM-R it was obtained for the maximum altitude 649.9990 m for the reference DEM-R and 649.9906 m for the calculated DEM-R.

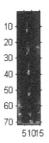

Figure 4. Part of the runway of Sao Jose dos Campos.

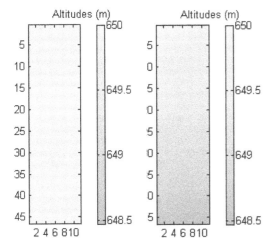

Figure 5. Calculated DEM-R and reference DEM-R.

As far as maximum difference from the reference DEM-R to the calculated DEM-R it was obtained 1.5187 m.

The minimum difference for altitudes on the calculated DEM-R was zero, and for the reference DEM-R was 1.5271 m.

The average absolute difference among the altitudes on reference and the calculated DEM-R was 0.7617 m, been this result is equivalent to an average error of 0.1173%.

The imprecision of the measurements of height, the median plane, flight altitude, and air baseline are sources of error for automatic determination of altitudes.

5 CONCLUSION

This paper presented a methodology for obtaining elevations of terrain points using aerial photographs and their characteristics. The results are promising, however, work is still under way and different methodologies and case studies will be dis-cussed with the aim of application in autonomous UAV navigation.

REFERENCES

1°/6° Grupo de Aviação (1999). Fotografias Aéreas de São José dos Campos. Recife, Brazil, Brazilian Air Force.

Canhoto, A., Shiguemori, E.H. & Domiciano, M.A.P. (2009). Image Sequence Processing Applied to Autonomous Aerial Navigation. *IEEE International Conference on Signal and Image Processing Applications (ICSIPA)*. Kuala Lumpur, IEEE. **1**.

Chen, Z. & Sun, S.-K. (2010). "A Zernike Moment Phase-Based Descriptor for Local Image Representation and Matching." *IEEE TRANSACTIONS ON IMAGE PROCESSING* **19**(1): 15.

Domiciano, M.A.P., Vitalli, R.A.P. Shiguemori, E.H. et al., (2008). Estudo da Influência do Tamanho Real do CCD para o Cálculo do DEM. *Encontro de Usuários de Sensoriamento Remoto das Forças Armadas—SERFA*.I.d.E. Avançados. Instituto de Estudos Avançados—São José dos Campos—São Paulo—Brasil, Instituto de Estudos Avançados.

Ekütekin, V. (2007). Navigation and Control Studies on Cruise Missiles. *Mechanical Engineering*. Ankara—Turquia, Middle Easr Technical University. **Doutorado:** 330.

Kane, M. (2007). Autonomous Systems and Future Capability, Bae Systems.

Khotanzad, A. & Hong, Y.H. (1990). "Invariant Image Recognition by Zernike Moments." **IEEE Transactions on Pattern Analysis and Machine Intelligence 12** (05): 09.

Lowe, D.G. (2004). "Distintive image features from scale-invariant keypoints" International Journal of Computer Vision **60** (2): 91–110.

Schultz, H. (1995). *Reconstruction from Widely Separated Images*. Proc. SPIE.

Sim, D.-G. & Park, R.-H. (2002). "**Localization Based on DEM Matching Using Multiple Aerial Image Pairs.**" *IEEE Transactions on Image Processing* **11**(1): 52–55.

Simons, G. (2011). Drone Diplomacy. *The Link*. Nova Iorque, Americans for Middle East Understanding, Inc. **44:** 16.

Wolf, P.R. (1983). Elements of Photogrammetry, McGraw-Hill. **único:** 628.

Computational Vision and Medical Image Processing – Tavares & Natal Jorge (eds)
© *2012 Taylor & Francis Group, London, ISBN 978-0-415-68395-1*

Simple and fast shape based image retrieval

João Ferreira Nunes
Escola Superior de Tecnologia e Gestão, Instituto Politécnico de Viana do Castelo, Portugal
Departamento de Engenharia Informática, Faculdade de Engenharia Universidade do Porto, Portugal

Pedro Miguel Moreira
Escola Superior de Tecnologia e Gestão, Instituto Politécnico de Viana do Castelo, Portugal
Laboratório de Inteligência Artificial e Ciências de Computadores, Universidade do Porto, Portugal

João Manuel R.S. Tavares
Faculdade de Engenharia Universidade do Porto, Portugal

ABSTRACT: Content Based Image Retrieval (CBIR) is a challenging and active topic of research. This paper focuses on the shape of the represented objects as the main criterion in respect to evaluate the relevance of the retrieval results. There are several shape descriptors described in the literature, which are reported to achieve good results. However some of them are not obvious to implement or are computationally demanding. In this paper we propose a simple and fast to compute set of features to achieve shape based image retrieval. We conducted retrieval experiments on the MPEG-7 Core Experiment CE-Shape-1 test set and the results obtained demonstrate usefulness and competiveness against reported results from other more elaborated descriptors. Results demonstrate that our approach is also valuable when objects represented in the images share similar shapes, although being conceptually different. Another interesting result is that users tend to be very stringent when a good result set is presented (very similar shapes) whilst they are more permissive when the result set does not present a very high level of similarity between the shapes.

1 INTRODUCTION

The "democratization" of technology increased the access to digital devices and consequently amplified the amount of multimedia contents produced, raising significantly the size of the multimedia repositories. Simultaneously several applications in entertainment, art and commerce arise, needing to accurately access the unstructured data stored on those repositories. For example, for a distinctive trademark registry application (Eakins et al., 2007), one might need to ensure that a new registered trademark is sufficiently unique from the existing marks by searching the database.

To accomplish this need for managing and searching within multimedia collections we can find several tools. On one hand the tools based on textual information (keywords) describing the multimedia content. These tools require humans to label all the content stored. This task turns out to be very subjective since it depends on the interpretation of the person that catalogs and also impractical in circumstances where the amount of information is enormous, as in situations where the contents are generated automatically, like a surveillance cameras system. On the other hand the tools that comprise extracting the hidden useful knowledge embedded on the multimedia content, and then attempt to discover relationships between them, to classify them based on their content and to extract data patterns. Having regard only to images, this last approach is the basis of a Content Based Image Retrieval system (CBIR), which builds on the image analysis to extract information that is used to retrieve the images.

Most researches on CBIR have contributed to color/texture based indexing and retrieval. Comparatively, little work has been done on image retrieval using shape. In fact, among all the visual features, shape is the most valuable feature to identify or describe objects represented in images since it is easier for users to describe in the query, either by example or by sketch rather than sketch a colored or a textured image as query. In some circumstances shape contains more intrinsic information about the represented object than color, texture or any other feature.

This paper focuses on presenting a reduced set of image features simple and fast to extract and that can be used to describe 2D shapes in images.

To validate our approach we conducted experiments on image retrieval. The reported experiments were conducted with the well-known MPEG-7 Core Experiment CE-Shape-1 test set and the results obtained demonstrate usefulness and competiveness against existing descriptors.

The paper is organized into six sections: after this introduction, on Section 2 we present related work in respect to shape descriptors and CBIR. On the third section we describe the proposed set of features as well as the experiments conducted to assess and validate our approach. Results and conclusions are presented in section four and five, respectively.

2 RELATED WORK

2.1 *Shape descriptors*

Image description consists in one of the key elements of multimedia information description. In the Multimedia Content Description Interface (MPEG-7) images are described by their contents featured by color, texture and shape. The shape descriptor aims to measure geometric attributes of an object to be used for classifying, matching, and recognizing objects. There are available several techniques for shape representation that are summarized in (Mehtre et al., 1997), such as Fourier descriptors (Zhang & Lu 2002; El-ghazal et al., 2009), Wavelet descriptors, grid-based, Delaunay triangulation (Shahabi & Safar 2006), among others. The study in (Mehtre et al., 1997) classifies the shape description techniques into boundary based and region based methods. Boundary based methods use only the contour of the objects' shape, while the region based methods use the internal details in addition to the contour.

2.2 *Image retrieval*

Many works have been done in the field of image retrieval, known as Content Based Image Retrieval (CBIR), see e.g., (Lew et al., 2006; Wong et al., 2007). The key to a successful retrieval system is to choose the right features that represent the images as accurately and uniquely as possible. We can find different implementations of CBIR with various types of user queries: some fed with queries by example, where users draw a rough approximation of the image they are looking for (Chatzichristofis et al., 2010; Langreiter 2011), or they provide a pre-existing image; in other implementations the query is made by direct specification of image features; and in others the query is done by image region (rather than the entire image); or by multiple example images; or even using multimodal queries.

3 METHOD

With this work we intended to define a set of image features that are simple and fast to extract involving very light math operations, and yet robust enough to distinguish 2D shapes in images. To validate our proposal set we conducted some experiments on image retrieval using the Part B of the MPEG-7 Core Experiment CE-Shape-1 dataset. To measure the performance of those experiments we used the metric known as Bulls Eye Percentage (BEP). As we also intended to evaluate how our proposed methods perform in respect to the users' subjective relevance of retrieved shapes, we have developed a web-based tool to support these experiments.

3.1 *The MPEG-7 dataset*

The MPEG-7 Core Experiment CE-Shape-1 was created by the Moving Picture Experts Group to evaluate the performance of 2D shape descriptors under the change of a viewpoint with respect to objects, non-rigid object motion (e.g., people walking or horse running) and noise resulted from digitization and/or segmentation (Latecki & Lakamper 2000).

The dataset consists of 1400 shapes grouped into 70 classes, each class containing 20 similar objects. Some of the shapes have experienced a number of transformations, such as scales, cuts and rotations and also some of them have holes. Finally, the image resolution is not constant among them. The next figure (Fig. 1) illustrates a representative shape image of each one of the 70 classes.

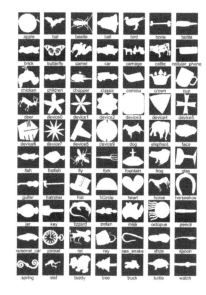

Figure 1. The MPEG-7 Core Experiment CE-Shape-1 dataset.

This dataset offers the possibility for experimental comparison of the existing approaches evaluated based on the retrieval rate. In (Veltkamp & Latecki 2006) we can find a wide-ranging comparison of shape descriptor methods that were tested against the MPEG-7 dataset, also used by us to compare our results.

3.2 Image features

Since the images in the MPEG-7 dataset were inconsistent in terms of resolution, scalability and rotation we had to apply some preprocessing operations in order to produce a feature set as generic as possible. Thus, using some Matlab functions we cropped the images by their bounding box. We also applied a morphological close filter smoothing boundaries, reducing small inward bumps and filling small holes caused by noise.

We also developed a procedure that computed several geometric features and to guarantee that all of them were weight balanced, we had to assure that they were normalized (between 0 and 1). After a correlation study between all the features, our initial extensive set of image features was reduced into the following:

f1. Solidity—it is the ratio between the image area (number of pixels in the foreground region) and its convex-hull area (number of pixels of the area of the smallest convex polygon that can contain the same region).

f2. Perimeter-Area Ratio—results from the ratio between the image perimeter and the image area.

f3. Eccentricity—specifies the eccentricity of the ellipse that encloses the shape having the same second-moments as the shape. It finds how much the conic section deviates from being circular. An ellipse whose eccentricity is zero is actually a circle, while an ellipse whose eccentricity is one it is a line segment.

f4. Extent—it is the result from the ratio between the number of pixels in the foreground region of the shape with the number of pixels in the bounding-box area.

f5. Area vs. Contour—this feature intends to distinguish shapes in respect to their ratio of the occupied area in respect to the contour, normalized by the area and perimeter of the minimal axis aligned bounding box (AABB) enclosing the shape image.

f6. Compactness—the compactness of a shape represents the degree to which a shape is compact. It is computed by the ratio of the shape's area to the area of a circle (the most compact shape) having the same perimeter.

f7. This feature intends to capture the relation between the elongatedness and the complexity

of the contour in respect to the minimal bounds given by the enclosing circumference and bounding box.

The features f1, f2, f4, f5, f6 and f7 according to the taxonomy reported in (Zhang & Lu 2003) are classified as a region-based techniques while f3 is classified as a conventional contour-based technique.

In Figure 2 we can see the seven extracted features in the form of radar plots of each shape image that was illustrated in Figure 1.

3.3 Retrieval experiments

To measure the performance of our proposed features applied on a shape based image retrieval system we used the Bulls Eye test. This is an automatic and frequently used test in shape retrieval, which enables the comparison of our approach against other performing shape retrieval techniques.

This test is to present each of the images of the dataset as the query image and through a Euclidean-distance, based on the nearest neighbor approach, the top 40 matches are retrieved. The number of relevant images (images that are labeled within the same class as the query image) is summed and then divided by the highest number of relevant images. The resulting Bulls Eye Percentage (BEP) is then the total number of relevant retrieved images divided by 20 (number of instances per class) × 1400.

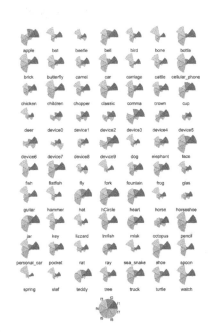

Figure 2. Radar plots of the average feature values.

3.4 *User study*

In some related research projects that also work with the MPEG-7 dataset, like the one reported in (Chen & Huang 2008) the authors claim that a possible reason of their proposed scheme performs poorly in some shapes is because the categorization of those shapes is not consistent with the human perception. In fact, after a visual examination of the dataset we also noticed that some shapes categorized in different classes are graphically similar. Some of the disputed categories are the *guitar*, the *spoon* and the *key*, where their images have a great resemblance in shape as well as in their features' values, here represented in form of radar plots in Figure 3.

This fact motivated us to conduct a study to confirm if there are images of the MPEG-7 dataset that are categorized in different classes, but nevertheless that they could be considered valid in a resulting set of an image retrieval experiment.

Thus we developed a web-based tool that uses a methodology quite similar to the one we used on the automatic retrieval experiments: for each image picked from the dataset and presented as the query image, the tool presents the top forty matches using the same metric—the Euclidean distance, based on the nearest neighbor approach. The main difference between both methodologies

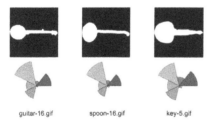

guitar-16.gif   spoon-16.gif   key-5.gif

Figure 3. Sample images from the *guitar*, *spoon* and *key* classes (top) and the corresponding extracted features (bottom).

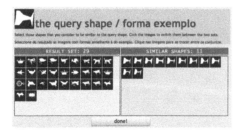

Figure 4. Sample screen interface of the developed web-based tool. Initially, all the images are placed at the left container. Users have to select relevant shapes (right container) by clicking over the images to switch their container.

lies in selecting the relevant images. While in this method the selection is made by the users' judgment, in the automatic method the relevant images are automatically selected according to the a priori known classification of each represented object.

Once developed, our tool was made available at (Nunes et al., 2011), we invited via email a significant number of volunteers to perform the retrieval experiments. For each experiment the users were asked to distinguish the images that they considered to be shape similar to the reference image (the relevant images) from those that they considered to be shape dissimilar (Figure 4). Both resulting sets of every experiment containing the similar and dissimilar shapes were stored on a database for further analysis.

4 EVALUATION AND RESULTS

The achieved result of our automatic retrieval experiments was a BEP of 59%. We reinforce the fact that our shape description is short, and easy to extract and to implement.

A comprehensive comparison of shape descriptor methods is reported by Veltkamp & Latecki (2006) where distinct shape descriptors were compared, re-implemented and tested against the same dataset we used. This comparison is partially reproduced in Table 1.

As the authors observe, there are some important differences between the reimplementation and the reported performances. This can be due

Table 1. BEP performance (reported and re-implemented) for several shape similarity measures using the MPEG-7 Part B dataset (adapted from (Veltkamp & Latecki 2006)).

Method	BEP reported	BEP reimp.
Shape context	76.51	
Image edge orientation histogram		41
Hausdorff region		56
Hausdorff contour		53
Grid Descriptor		61
Distance set correspondence	78.38	
Fourier descriptor		46
Delaunay triangulation angles		47
Deformation effort	78.18	
Curvature scale space	81.12	52
Convex parts correspondence	76.45	76
Contour-to-centroid triangulation	84.33	79
Contour edge orientation histogram		41
Chaincode nonlinear elastic matching		56
Angular radial transform		53
Our method	**59**	

to several issues such as: lack of information to devise a proper implementation, some methods are inherently complex and some fine tuning in respect to the datasets for which the performance values were reported. We notice that our proposed approach ranks in fourth place with respect to the re-implemented performances. Another possible reason for this result derives from the fact that we consider the dataset has some images that despite being associated with a particular class, they could also be classified within other classes and therefore being valid in a retrieval experience.

We used a total of 1535 individual experiments via our web-based tool. The overall result was similar to that obtained automatically of 58%. Although, it is clear that in some classes the retrieval rate increased significantly (e.g., class device 2) leading to the conclusion that for these classes the resulting set of the top forty relevant images contains images from different classes but considered by users to be shape similar. Both retrieval results are illustrated in Figure 5. As it can be observed there are noticeable differences. The retrieval performances for the BEP range from 14% to 100% while for the user tests range from 18% to 97%. Since we used the same criteria in both methods to get the forty more relevant images, it would not be expected retrieval rates from the user tests above the retrieval rates

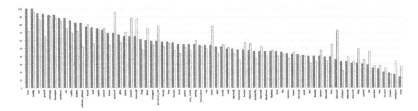

Figure 5. BEP per class for the automatic retrieval (dark grey) and for the retrieval rate for the user experiment (light gray). The classes are ranked left to right in decreasing order in respect to the achieved BEP for the automatic retrieval.

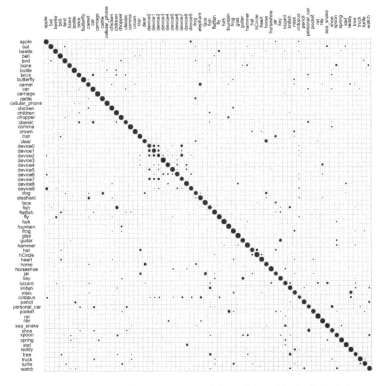

Figure 6. Detailed relevance results assigned by users. For each line of the grid, the dark circles, are correlated to the number of shapes from each class that were considered relevant (shape similar) in respect to the example image (class).

achieved with the BEP, unless the resulted set of relevant images has images from disputed classes sharing similar shapes. This has turned out to be more clearly when a good result set is presented, as for instance, the *face* class (leftmost), for which users tend to be more rigorous (100% of retrieval rate for the BEP against 72% for the user tests). However, users are more permissive when the result set does not present a very high level of similarity between the shapes, like in the *tree* class (the rightmost) where the retrieval rate for the Bulls Eye test is 14% and the twice for the user tests (28%).

The confusion matrix in Figure 6 presents the detailed, per class, relevant results assigned by users. For each line of the grid, the dark circles, are correlated to the number of shapes from each class that were considered relevant (similar) in respect to the example image. A first conclusion that can be drawn is that the results, although not strictly symmetrical, present a high degree of symmetry. For instance, there are a comparable number of *guitar* shapes considered relevant when the retrieval is based on a *key*, in respect to the number of *key* shapes when the retrieval is based on a *guitar* shape. As it was expected, there are classes that are considered by users to exhibit shape similarity. As a consequence shapes belonging to objects from these classes are considered relevant by users when asked to separate the images from the retrieved result set. For instance, it can be observed that shapes from *deer* class are considered to be similar to those from the *horse* class. A high level of subjective similarity is also present amid the *device* classes of objects.

5 CONCLUSIONS AND FUTURE WORK

We have presented a simple method supported by few set of simple geometric image features to describe shapes that are simple and fast to compute.

We conducted our experiments on the MPEG-7 Core Experiment CE-Shape-1 and the achieved results demonstrate usefulness and competiveness against other reported approaches. We also developed a web-based tool to conduct user experiments in order to investigate subjective relevance of the retrieved shapes. Results indicate that users tend to be very stringent when a good result set is presented (very similar shapes) whilst they are more permissive when the result set does not present a very high level of similarity between the shapes. We intend to further investigate this behavior by conducting more experiments using, for example, a set of identical images with different rotations or scales.

There are several avenues for future work. A first one is to learn feature weights using, as for instance, evolutionary algorithms (e.g., genetic algorithms) to properly tune the used similarity distance metric. Another improvement is to make use of relevance feedback from the users.

REFERENCES

Chatzichristofis, S.A., Boutalis, Y., Papamarkos N. & Zagoris, K. 2010. Accurate Image Retrieval Based On Compact Composite Descriptors And Relevance Feedback Information. *Int. J. Patt. Recog. Art. Intel.* 24: 207.

Chen, C. & Huang P. 2008. A New Method for Image Retrieval Based on Shape Decomposition *In 2008 Congress on Image and Signal Processing IEEE*, pp. 439–444.

Eakins, J.P., Boardman J.M. & Shields K. 2007. Retrieval of Trade Mark Images By Shape Feature.

El-ghazal, A., Basir, O. & Belkasim, S. 2009. Farthest point distance: A new shape signature for Fourier descriptors. *Signal Processing: Image Communication* 24: 572–586.

Langreiter, 2011. Available at: http://labs.systemone.at/retrievr [Accessed June 2011].

Latecki, L.J. & Lakamper, R. 2000. Shape Similarity Measure Based on Correspondence of Visual Parts. *IEEE Transactions On Pattern Analysis And Machine Intelligence 22*: 1–6.

Lew M.S., Sebe, N., Djeraba, C. & Jain, R. 2006. Content-based Multimedia Information Retrieval—State of the Art and Challenges. *ACM Transactions on Multimedia Computing, Communications, and Applications*: 1–26.

Mehtre, B.M., Kankanhalli, M.S. & Lee, W.F. 1997. Shape Measures for Content Based Image Retrieval. *Information Processing & Management*: 1–19.

Nunes, J.F., Moreira, P.M. & Tavares, J.M.R.S. 2011. Fast and Simple Shape Based Image Retrieval—Web Based Tool. Available at: http://shapes.estg.ipvc.pt

Shahabi, C. & Safar, M. 2006. An experimental study of alternative shape-based image retrieval techniques. *Multimedia Tools Appl 32*: 29–48.

Veltkamp, R.C. & Latecki, L.J. 2006. Properties and Performance of Shape Similarity Measures *In 10th IFCS Conf. Data Science and Classification Slovenia*, pp. 1–9.

Wong, W., Shih, F.Y. & Liu, J. 2007. Shape-based image retrieval using support vector machines, Fourier descriptors and self-organizing maps. *Information Sciences 177*: 1878–1891.

Zhang, D. & Lu, G. 2002. An Integrated Approach to Shape Based Image Retrieval *In ACCV2002: The 5th Asian Conference on Computer Vision*, pp. 1–6.

Zhang, D. & Lu, G. 2003. Evaluation of MPEG-7 shape descriptors against other shape descriptors. *Multimedia Systems 9*: 15–30.

Computational Vision and Medical Image Processing – Tavares & Natal Jorge (eds)
© 2012 Taylor & Francis Group, London, ISBN 978-0-415-68395-1

Bone registration using a robotic ultrasound probe

Pedro M.B. Torres
Polytechnic Institute of Castelo Branco, School of Technology, Av. Empresário, Castelo Branco, Portugal

Paulo J.S. Gonçalves
Polytechnic Institute of Castelo Branco, School of Technology, Av. Empresário, Castelo Branco, Portugal
Technical University of Lisbon, IDMEC/IST, Av. Rovisco Pais, Lisboa, Portugal

Jorge M.M. Martins
Technical University of Lisbon, IDMEC/IST, Av. Rovisco Pais, Lisboa, Portugal

ABSTRACT: This paper reports two important pieces of work: automatic positioning of the ultrasound (US) probe through an anthropomorphic robot, and point set registration of ultrasound images with Computerized Tomography (CT) images of a femur bone. The US probe was placed in the end effector of the *Eurobtec IR52C* robot, responsible for scanning the femur and extract the US images, at constant speed. Registration between the two sets of points, US and CT, is performed by two different methods, to compare results and draw appropriate conclusions. The first method used is the Iterative Closest Point (ICP) method, based on an iterative approach between two rows of points in order to achieve the closest relationship between them. The second method, Coherent Point Drift (CPD), recently proposed, is based on the probabilistic concept to relate two data sets. Throughout the paper are described the following steps, need to achieve the ultimate goal: acquisition and processing of CT and US images; 3D reconstruction of surfaces and registration between the two surfaces, using ICP and CPD methods. Although computationally heavy, CPD is the method that presents better results for the bone registration, in terms of mean squared error.

Keywords: image-guided surgery, surface-based registration

1 INTRODUCTION

Multimodal image registration is an important task in many application areas, particularly in surgical navigation. Registration of medical images allow to relate a group of images obtained in a preoperative scenario, with images obtained in the intra operative scenario, assisting the surgeon in surgical navigation (Dang et al., 2010). Minimally invasive surgical interventions performed using computer-assisted surgery (CAS) (Sugano 2003) systems require reliable registration methods for pre-operatively acquired patient anatomy representations that are compatible with the minimally invasive paradigm. At the moment, minimally invasive surgery is a topic with great focus and contribution to this has been the increasing development of robots that cooperate with surgeon in surgical procedures, as example the famous DaVinci robot or ZEUS Robotic Surgical System. Robot-assisted surgery was developed to overcome limitations of minimally invasive surgery, among other factors include tremor filters and increase the precision of surgery. Orthopedic surgery also did not stayed

behind this technological developments, and in recent years robotic systems with applications in orthopedic surgery have emerged, e.g., ROBODOC or ACROBOT. Robots need navigation systems to perform accurately in the operating room. Surgical navigation systems allow the surgeon to perform surgical actions in real time using information conveyed through a virtual world, which consist of computer-generated models of surgical instruments and the virtual representations of the anatomy being operated. Virtual representations can be generated from data obtained through Computer Tomography scans, ultrasound images, amongst others. Fiducial markers placed through incisions in the bone is a common practice in actual surgical navigation systems, to know the position and orientation of bone during an orthopedic surgery. Studies on the patients reported persistent severe pain at the site of pin implantation, after surgery, caused by the injuries to the nerves, caused by fiducial markers (Nogler et al., 2001). One of the important steps that is tackled in the paper is to avoid the use of fiducial markers, (Amiot and Poulin 2004), (Nabeyama et al., 2004) in orthopedic surgery, using minimal invasive methods such as ultrasound navigation of a surgical robot. The HIPROB project avoids fiducial markers in the development an robotic system for Hip Resurfacing surgery, with navigation based on ultrasound images. The orientation of the robot is based on the registration of ultrasound images acquired in the intra-operative scenario, with the CT images of the femur obtained pre-operatively. This paper is organized as follows. Section 2 describe the theoretical concepts of 3D point set registration, Iterative Closest Point and Coherent Point Drift methods. Sections 3 and 4 describes the experimental setup and presents the obtained results. Finally, conclusions and future work are presented.

2 3D POINT SET REGISTRATION

Registration is an essential task in computer-assisted surgery (CAS) systems. It consists of finding a transformation that aligns common features from two modality data sets taken at different times (Maintz and Viergever 1998). 3D multi-modal point set Registration of anatomical structures, such as bone, is complex because the datasets arrive from different scans. Adequate feature extraction algorithms are essential to accurately align the two datasets. In recent years several algorithms have been developed for the registration of 3D point clouds, mainly based on the ICP method (Granger et al., 2010), (Salvi et al., 2006).

2.1 Iterative closest point method

The ICP method, presented by (Besl and Mckay 1992) is the standard method used to perform registration between two sets (clouds) of 3D points. It transforms two sets of points to a common coordinate frame. If the exact correspondences of the two data sets could be known, then the exact translation t and rotation R can be found. The main issue of the method is to find the corresponding points between the two data sets, $Y = (y_1, ..., y_M)^T$ and $X = (x_1, ..., x_N)^T$.

To obtain the closest point of Y to a point in X, the Euclidean distance is applied. When all points of the data set Y are associated to the point in X the transformation is estimated by minimizing a mean square cost function:

$$E_{ICP} = \sum_i \| R \cdot x_i + t - y_i \|^2 \qquad (1)$$

2.2 Coherent Point Drift method

Coherent Point Drift (CPD) is a probabilistic method for point set registration, described in (Myronenko and Song 2010). Given two n-dimensional point sets, where a given point set is expressed as $Y = (y_1, ..., y_M)^T$ and should be aligned with the reference point set $X = (x_1, ..., x_N)^T$. Points in Y are considered the centroids of the Gaussian Mixture Model, and fit it to the data points X by maximizing a likelihood function. Bayes theorem is used to find the parameters Y by maximizing the posteriori probability, or minimizing the energy function:

$$E_{CPD}(Y) = -\sum_{n=1}^{N} log \sum_{m=1}^{M} e^{-\frac{1}{2}\|\frac{x_n - y_m}{\sigma}\|^2} + \frac{\lambda}{2}\phi(Y) \qquad (2)$$

where E is the negative log-likelihood function, $\phi(Y)$ is a regularization term, and λ is a trade-off parameter.

3 EXPERIMENTAL SETUP

A cow femur was used in the experiments to validate the ICP and CPD methods. For obtaining the CT images, a *Siemens* commercial machine was used with 0.75 mm between slices. The experimental apparatus, illustrated in Figure 1, used to acquire US images, consists of an IR52C robot manipulator, an *ALOKA prosound* 2 echograph with a 5 MHz probe and a computer with a standard video card for image acquisition. With this system, it is possible to acquire images with 0.55 mm spacing, keeping the probe, always with the same orientation relative to the bone. The relation between the base of the robot and its end-effector, obtained by the robot kinematics (T1), the relation between the end-effector and the probe support (T2) and the relation between the probe support and the probe (T3) are needed to calibrate the system (Figure 2) and obtain the relationship from a

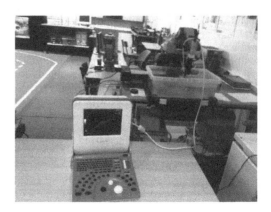

Figure 1. Experimental setup.

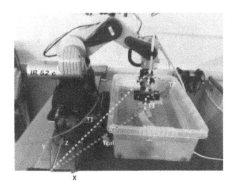

Figure 2. Overview of the robotic system and transformations.

2D US pixel image, (u, v), and its 3D coordinates, i.e., the transformation T_{cal}.

$$T_{cal} = T_1 T_2 T_3 P(u, v) \qquad (3)$$

where,

$$P_x = \begin{bmatrix} S_x u \\ S_y v \\ 0 \\ 1 \end{bmatrix}$$

S_x and S_y are the scale factors for the (u, v) pixel coordinates.

3.1 Image processing and surface extraction

Processing of CT images was quite simple, since such images are not affected by large amounts of noise. The objective of the paper is the registration between CT images, and US images. Knowing that the bone is a rigid anatomical structure, and that the ultrasound signals are all reflected in the bone, is only possible see the upper surface of the bone, in the US image. Accordingly, only the top surface of the bone was considered as the region of interest in CT images. Figure 3 shows a CT image of the bone and the corresponding result of its skeletonization. The next step is to extract the coordinates of the skeleton of the 360 CT images captured in the experiment. With these 3D coordinates and the spacial resolution, i.e., the gap between slices, a surface reconstruction of the surface can be obtained, presented in Figure 5.

To acquire the ultrasound images of the cow bone, it was necessary to place the bone into a tub of water (Figure 2) to achieve a good coupling of the probe to the bone and acquire images with minimal noise. Although the bone being immersed

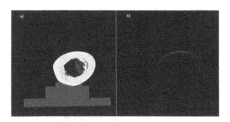

Figure 3. a) A CT Bone image with the support, b) Skeletonization result of the region of interest.

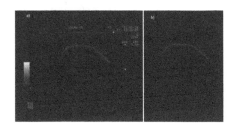

Figure 4. a) A US Bone image, b) Skeletonization result of the region of interest.

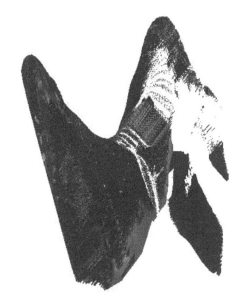

Figure 5. CT Surface, seen in MeshLab.

in water and the coupling is the best possible, ultrasound images have noise. To clean and smooth the images, an *Denoising* algorithm described in (Sanches et al., 2008), was used. The image resulting is a blurred image and it was necessary extract its skeleton, using a similar procedure as for the CT images. The most important point in the processing of ultrasound images is the segmentation of the region of interest, to obtain the skeleton of the

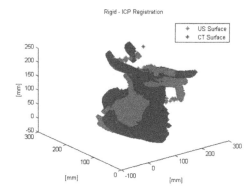

Figure 7.   ICP rigid registration.

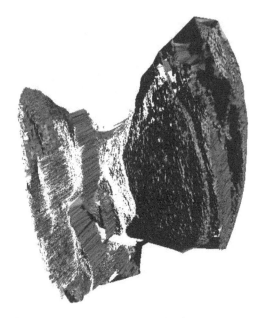

Figure 6.   US Surface, seen in MeshLab.

bone structure. Figure 4 shows an US image of the central bone area and the result of the corresponding skeletonization. When the images after segmentation presented gaps, interpolation was used to obtain a regular skeleton. The 3D reconstruction of the surface, shown in Figure 6, is constructed through the coordinates extracted from 489 ultrasound images processed. The reconstruction of surfaces present in Figures 5 and 6, was made in *MATLAB*, but their representation was made with the aid of *MeshLab* software.

4   REGISTRATION RESULTS

The registration methodology can be classified into two main physical categories: rigid and non-rigid registration, or mathematical categories: linear and nonlinear registration, or complexity categories: parametric and non-parametric registration (NOPPADOL and KE 2009).

Rigid registration involves a linear rigid-body transformation, consisting of rotation and translation. Affine transformation is composed of linear transformations (rotation, scaling or shear) and a translation (or "shift"). Affine and Rigid registration of CT and US surfaces were performed in this work through the ICP and CPD algorithms.

The results of the registration between the two surfaces are depicted in Figures 7, 8 and 9. Table 1 shows the results of root mean square error (RMSE), according to Equation 4, and the time consumed for each simulation.

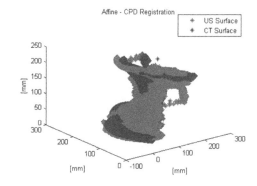

Figure 8.   CPD affine registration.

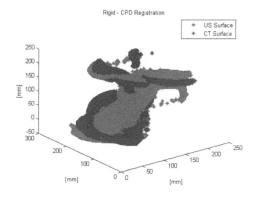

Figure 9.   CPD rigid registration.

Table 1.   Errors results.

	Reg. errors [mm]			
	Before	After	iter.	time
CPD affine	51.8662	44.1493	40	17 m:22 s
CPD rigid		47.4229	26	11 m:40 s
ICP rigid		47.7152	27	10 m:86 s

Algorithms were tested in *MATLAB*, with an Intel Core 2 Duo, 2.27 GHz computer, with 4 GB RAM. Better results, were presented by affine registration performed by the CPD method, although it takes longer to converge. ICP Affine method, was also implemented and tested, but failed to obtain an adequate registration, and the simulations lasted one full day, it was decided to exclude this method, because its contribution was not valid for this study.

The errors obtained are quite high, however at this stage of the work was intended to apply the methods to register the bone and understand the difficulties that must be overcome.

$$RMSE = \sqrt{\frac{1}{n}\sum(\hat{y}_i - y_i)^2} \qquad (4)$$

5 CONCLUSIONS

This paper presents the work developed to register 3D surfaces, with data from ultrasound and CT images. The well known ICP and the recent CPD methods were tested to register the points of US and CT images of a cow femur bone. The results obtained validate the approach for the femur application. CPD algorithm presents better results although with high computational cost. The affine transformation, as seen in Figure 8 achieves a better approximation between the points of two surfaces, resulting in a lower value of mean square error (Table 1). For the bone registration procedure and when attaching the ultrasound probe to the robot end-effector, the results obtained are more precise than the ones obtained using a free-hand ultrasound system (Gonçalves and Torres 2010). However these results still show high error values. To improve the presented results, the contour segmentation procedure must be improved. Bone segmentation in ultrasound images is a complex task, so the study of active contours have been a hypothesis to segment the region of the bone with precision. The results of the error does not exclude the approaches studied for registration, because the surfaces are very irregular and with different spatial resolutions, i.e., there are few similarities between the points of two surfaces.

6 FUTURE WORK

As future work is expected to test the algorithms with images of human femurs. Apply more precise methods, like active contours, for extracting features and use the POLARIS system, as spacial localizer, in order to increase the precision in image acquisition and 3D surface reconstruction.

ACKNOWLEDGEMENTS

The authors would like to thank: the Portuguese Science Foundation, FCT, for the funding to IDMEC through LAETA; the FCT project: PTDC/EME-CRO/099333/2008. Pedro Torres would like to thank FCT for the funding of its PROTEC program.

REFERENCES

Amiot, L. and Poulin, F. (2004). Computed tomography-based navigation for hip, knee, and spine surgery. *Clin. Orthop. Relat. Res. 421*, 77–86.

Besl, P.J. and McKay, N.D. (1992). A method for registration of 3-d shapes. *Pattern Analysis and Machine Intelligence 14(2)*, 239–256.

Dang, H., Gu, L., Zhuang, X. and Luo, Z. (2010). Hierarchical normal vector information based registration for surgical navigation by using saliency information. pp. 137–142.

Gonçalves, P. and Torres, P. (2010). Registration of Bone Ultrasound Images to CT based 3D Bone Models. In *6th International Conference on Technology and Medical Sciences, Porto, Portugal*, pp. 21–23.

Granger, S., Pennec, X. and Roche, A. (2010). Rigid point-surface registration using an EM variant of ICP for computer guided oral im-plantology. In *Medical Image Computing and Computer-Assisted Intervention-MICCAI 2001*, pp. 752–761. Springer.

Maintz, J.B.A. and Viergever, M.A. (1998). A Survey of Medical Image Registration. *Image (Rochester, N.Y.) 2*(1), 1–37.

Myronenko, A. and Song, X. (2010). Point set registration: Coherent point drift. *IEEE Transactions on Pattern Analysis and Machine Intelligence 99* (PrePrints).

Nabeyama, R., Matsuda, S. Miura, H. Mawatarim, T. Kawano, T. and Iwamoto, Y. (2004). The accuracy of image-guided knee replacement based on computed tomography. *J. Bone Joint Surg. 86-B*, 366–371.

Nogler, M., Maurer, H., Wimmer, C., Gegenhuber, C., Bach, C. and Krismer, M. (2001, October). Knee pain caused by a fiducial marker in the medial femoral condyle: a clinical and anatomic study of 20 cases. *Acta orthopaedica Scandinavica 72*(5), 477–80.

NOPPADOL, C. and KE, C. (2009). A robust affine image registration method. *6*(2), 311–334.

Salvi, J., Matabosch, C., Fofi, D. and Forest, J. (2006). A review of recent range image registration methods with accuracy evaluation. *Image and Vision Computing*.

Sanches, J.M., Nascimento, J.C. and Marques, J.S. (2008). Medical image noise reduction using the sylvesterlyapunov equation. *IEEE Trans. Image Process 17*, 1522–1539.

Sugano, N. (2003). Computer-assisted orthopedic surgery. *Computer-Aided Design*, 442–448.

Computational Vision and Medical Image Processing – Tavares & Natal Jorge (eds)
© 2012 Taylor & Francis Group, London, ISBN 978-0-415-68395-1

The use of 3D mandibular movement simulation in total denture construction

P. Fonseca, J. Reis-Campos & M.H. Figueiral
FMDUP, Porto, Portugal

N. Viriato & M.A.P. Vaz
FEUP—INEGI, Porto, Portugal

ABSTRACT: Total denture manufacture still remains a very demanding work to the clinician and to the technician. The aim of this research is to test the utility of 3D mandibular movement simulation in the construction of total dentures with bilateral balanced occlusion. By an optical scanning process and computer simulation, the authors demonstrate that articulator's individualization is important to the construction of a total denture with a balanced occlusion in equilibrium with the physiology of the temporomandibular joint.

1 INTRODUCTION

Over the last few years, it is possible to combine engineering techniques and computer-aided-design systems (CAD) applied to dental medicine.

3D optical scanning proved to be useful in oral rehabilitation, predominantly in implant surgery (Frisard et al., 2011, Valente et al., 2009). However some economical, aesthetical or functional limitations made sometimes the conventional complete denture the only way for edentulous patients' rehabilitation.

We can determinate in such patients the adapted centric relation, the value of bilateral condylar guidance and Bennett angles. When the subject's casts are mounted in a semi adjustable articulator by use of a facebow and intraoral or extraoral records to adjust the posterior determinants of occlusion, a close approximation of the patient's mandibular movements and oclusal relationships can be obtained (Santos et al., 2003).

The main aim of this study is to test the ability to simulate the three-dimensional mandibular movement for the construction of total dentures with bilateral balanced occlusion.

2 MATERIALS AND METHODS

2.1 Scanning process

The casts of a bi-maxillary total prosthesis were mounted in a semi adjustable articulator (Bioart®) with standard posterior determinants and with balanced occlusion. The scanning process used to determinate the geometry of the manually fabricate plaster models was a 3Shape D250 3D dental scanner from Materialise®. This machine provides an accurate, reliable and fast optical scanning of dental full casts. The object moves on 3 axes (rotation, translation and tilting) and permit that high resolution digital cameras capture images of the laser plànes projected onto the cast. The point cloud generated by the software of the scanning unit, is inserted in a CAD software, SolidWorks®, and then processed to have the final geometry of the plaster models (Figures 1 and 2).

2.2 Mandibular movement simulation

Bilateral condylar guidances, Bennett angles, intercondylar distance and condylar axis of rotation were determinate in patient and then transferred to the computer. This way the solids were ori-

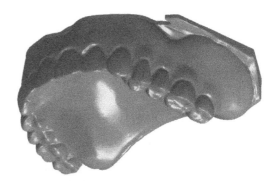

Figure 1. Geometry of maxilar plaster model.

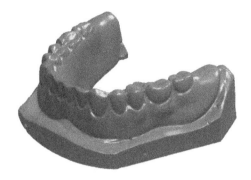

Figure 2.   Geometry of mandibular plaster model.

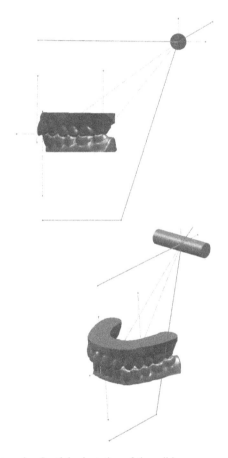

Figure 3.   Spatial orientation of the solids.

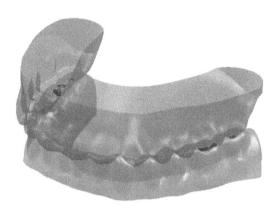

Figure 4.   Premature contacts during clench.

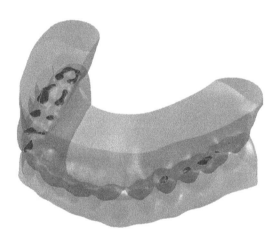

Figure 5.   Contacts evaluation during left lateral movement.

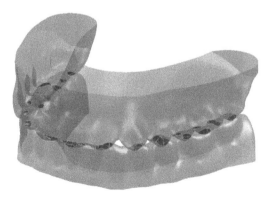

Figure 6.   Contacts evaluation during protrusive movement.

ented in space with the reference of oclusal plane (Figure 3).

Using a software that simulates the real patient's mandibular movement, enables the clinician/technician to see more clearly the premature contacts (Figure 4) and interferences generated during physiologic movements (Figures 5 and 6).

3 RESULTS

With the computer simulation of the mandibular movement it is possible to determinate the dental interferences during mandibular function and failure of the bilateral balanced occlusion when posterior determinants are individualized.

4 DISCUSSION AND CONCLUSIONS

The use of a 3D optical scanner and computer simulation of the mandibular movement can help the clinician to choose the most indicate teeth to use in the fabrication of complete dentures. This way it is possible to promote better functional mandibular movements according to the posterior determinants of occlusion in order to obtain bilateral balanced contacts. All temporomandibular movements are more physiological and contribute to a better longevity and successful of the oral rehabilitation with conventional total prosthesis.

This is only the beginning of a research that the authors hope to prove the importance of clinical articulator individualization and to facilitate the construction of a complete denture with bilateral balanced occlusion.

REFERENCES

Drago, C.F. & Peterson, T. 2007. Treatment of an edentulous patient with CAD/CAM technology: a clinical report. *J Prosthodont* 16(3): 200–8.

Frisardi, G., Chessa, G., Barone, S., Paoli, A., Razionale, A. & Frisardi, F. 2011. Integration of 3D anatomical data obtained by CT imaging and 3D optical scanning for computer aided implant surgery. *BMC Medical Image* 11: 5.

Neto, A.F., Junior, W.M. & Carreiro, A.F.P. 2010. Masticatory efficiency in denture wearers with bilateral balanced occlusion and canine guidance. *Braz Dent J* 21(2): 165–9.

Santos, J., Nelson, S. & Nowlin, T. 2003. Comparison of condylar guidance setting *g: A pilot study. *J Prosthet Dent* 89: 54–9.

Valente, F., Schiroli, G. & Sbrenna, A. 2009. Accuracy of computer-aided oral implant surgery: a clinical and radiographic study. *Int J Oral Maxillofac Implants* 24(2): 234–42.

Computational Vision and Medical Image Processing – Tavares & Natal Jorge (eds)
© 2012 Taylor & Francis Group, London, ISBN 978-0-415-68395-1

A practical and robust image processing method for evaluating the External Apical Root Resorption

Sónia Alves
Faculty of Medicine, University of Coimbra, Coimbra, Portugal

Naimy Gonzalez de Posada & Miguel A. Guevara López
INEGI-FEUP Institute of Mechanical Engineering and Industrial Management, Faculty of Engineering, University of Porto, Porto, Portugal

ABSTRACT: This work presents a practical and robust image processing method to identify the proportion of External Apical Root Resorption (EARR) allowing a standardized EARR classification metric of severity, based on crown and root length ratio in the panoramic radiographs. The proposed algorithm combine suitably digital image processing techniques that includes image denoising, image enhancing, deformable models and feature extraction techniques, allowing computing in a precise and reproducible way the crown/root (length and area) ratios using as input a cross constructed for each particular teeth. The proposed method was tested experimentally in a representative database with 200 anonymous patient's cases from orthodontic historical archives (complying with current privacy regulations as they are also used to teach regular and postgraduate students) supplied by the Faculty of Medicine at Coimbra University, Portugal.

1 INTRODUCTION

External apical root resorption (EARR) is an undesirable sequel of orthodontic treatment that results in permanent loss of the dental structure of the root apex and can affect the dentition longevity (Al-Qawasmi, Hartsfield et al., 2003). This is a frequent iatrogenic result associated with orthodontic treatment, especially reported for the maxillary incisors, followed by the mandibular incisors (Brezniak and Wasserstein 1993). The etiologic factors are complex and multifactorial, but it seems that EARR results from a combination of the effect of mechanical factors, individual biological variability and genetic predisposition.

The prevalence of EARR associated with orthodontic treatment greatly varies in the literature, depending on the methods used to determine it in the studies. Histological studies show high prevalence, whereas clinical studies, using diagnostic radiographic techniques, show lower and variable prevalence rates (HARRY and SIMS 1982).

With panoramic radiographs, EARR is usually less than 2.5 millimeters (mm) (Linge and Linge 1983), or varying from 6% to 13% for different teeth (Blake, Woodside et al., 1995). By using graded scales, EARR in frequently classified as minor or moderate in most orthodontic patients (Brin, Tulloch et al., 2003). Severe resorption, is defined as exceeding 4 mm, or a third part of the original root length.

In clinical orthodontics, panoramic radiograph is always included as a complementary diagnostic method, so it's important to have a feasible method to measure crown and root length in this dental radiograph.

Digital radiography is used frequently in dental clinics because of its speed of use and easier storage and images interpretation. Recent studies are demonstrating that the combination of digital image processing, pattern recognition and artificial intelligence techniques can support the development of new and more precise computer-aided dental x-ray analysis methods and systems.

In this work was developed a practical and robust method to identify the proportion of EARR in the most usually affected teeth that allows establish a standardized EARR classification metric of severity, based on crown and root length ratio in the panoramic radiographs. The proposed algorithm combine suitably digital image processing techniques that includes image denoising, image enhancing, deformable models and feature extraction techniques (Chenyang and Prince 1998; Guevara, Silva et al., 2003; Paragios, Mellina-Gottardo et al., 2004; Pastorinho, Guevara et al., 2005). This allows computing in a precise an reproducible way the crown and root length and area ratios using as input a cross constructed for each particular tooth.

This method was tested experimentally in a representative database formed with 200 anonymous patient's cases from orthodontic historical archives (complying with current privacy regulations) supplied by the Faculty of Medicine at Coimbra University, Portugal.

2 MATERIALS AND METHODS

2.1 *Database preparation*

With the approbation of the Research Ethics Commission (Faculty of Medicine at Coimbra University in Portugal), two hundred anonymous patients selected from the historical archives of the Orthodontic Service were invited to participate in this research study. All patients received comprehensive orthodontic treatment (straight-wire technique). Multibonded appliances with 0.018×0.025-inch bracket slots were used in all cases. With this, was formed a ground true database (200 patients cases), including digital content (panoramic radiographs) and associated metadata (clinical patient's information). As the etiology of root resorption during orthodontic treatment is complex, for each patient were analyzed several risk factors, such as patient's age, duration of treatment, type of orthodontic appliance, dental vulnerability, oral habits, gender etc.

The panoramic radiographs includes in this study were digitalized (with a resolution of 150 dpi and 256 gray levels) before (T-1) and after (T-2) orthodontic treatment using a scanner (scanner model Epson Expression 1680 Pro) and saved in tagged image file format (tiff).

2.2 *Proposed method*

The proposed method includes the following four steps: (1) image preprocessing, (2) cross selection, (3) segmentation and (4) feature extraction.

Image preprocessing: To increase the potential for teeth's area discrimination first is selected a rectangular image part: the region of interest (ROI) including maxillary central and lateral incisors, maxillary canines and mandibular incisors.

Then image preprocessing step is based on applying first a median filter with a mask of size 5×5 (see Fig. 1b) to the created image ROI and hereafter are combined morphological operations (top hat and bottom hat) and histogram based techniques (adjust image intensity values, contrast-limited adaptive histogram equalization, etc.) to obtain an enhanced ROI image.

Cross selection: This step allow selecting (manually) four points, which are used to produce a

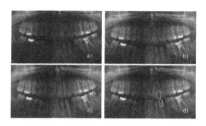

Figure 1. a) Original image; b) Enhanced image; c) Selected cross ends points and d) Segmented root and crown.

"cross". (see Fig. 1c). This cross is constructed for maxillary central and lateral incisors, maxillary canines and mandibular incisors. For each tooth we selected the mesial and distal dento-enamel junction and the apex and incisal edge.

Segmentation: the selected four "cross ends points" are used to create (applying an spline function) an initial approximated teeth contour (the initial snake), which is then deformed with an adjusted variant of gradient vector flow snake (Chenyang and Prince 1998) producing in an automatically way the final and more precise teeth contour segmentation (final snake). To follow final snake is divide to produce the root and crown final contours based on the selected horizontal cross ends points (see Figure 1d).

Feature Extraction: Taking as input the selected cross ends points and the final snake, root and crown length and area are computed respectively. However to simplify the process, direct metric analysis of the panoramic radiographs are not indicated due to their lack of reproducibility. So the basis of this study was the percentage (proportion) of fixed final root/initial root, calculated using the selected cross (ends points), constructed for each tooth.

With this approach, two segments of lines are created: (1) connecting the incisal edge to the apex and (2) connecting the mesial and distal dento-enamel junction (see Fig. 1c). Finally, we used the rule "of three" of Brezniak and Wasserstein (Brezniak and Wasserstein 1993) to compute the fixed final root (*FFR*) which represents the real root length after treatment.

Mathematical formulation of the main features computed is the following:

$$FFR = FR * IC / FC$$

where *FFR* represents the fixed final root, *FR* is the final root, *IC* is the initial crown and *FC* is the final crown.

$$ratio = FFR / IR$$

where *FFR* is the fixed final root and *IR* is the initial root.

$$\%EARR = 1 - ratio$$

where *%EARR* represents the percentage of *EARR*.

3 RESULTS

We implemented in MATLAB a system prototype to test the new proposed method. Then we measured in maxillary central and lateral incisors, maxillary canines and mandibular incisors (ten teeth) the changes in root and crown length in both radiographs (T-1 and T-2 pre and post treatment respectively). As it is accepted that during orthodontic treatment the crown length does not change (unless it was fractured), the ratio between the initial crown length and the final crown length is used to determine the enlargement factor of the radiographs to adjust the final root length. When no changes occurred in the root length during treatment, the ratio initial root (IR)/final root (FR) should be equal to the initial crown(IC)/final crown ratio (FC). Then, the rule "of three" of (Brezniak and Wasserstein 1993), as mentioned, was used to calculate the change in root length after treatment (FFR) and it was also added the ratio between the initial root and FFR area. However in this study we only consider the IR/FFR ratio.

Figure 2. shows the application of the proposed algorithm, in which two patients were evaluated: one witness in different times a) initial and b) after and the other one with orthodontic treatment c) T-1 and d) T-2.

In the witness case all teeth (maxillary central and lateral incisors, maxillary canines and mandibular incisors) were measured (see results in Table 1) and in the case of the patient with orthodontic treatment only teeth with treatment were considered (see results in Table 2).

Table 1 shows the results achieved on the witness patient, where it can be observed that the percentage of external root resorption (%EARR) is zero or near zero in all measured teeth. Only on teeth 41 and 31 the percentage of EARR presents a value of 0.02, which can be assumed due to differences in the mandibular tooth position, patient exposure to the x-ray beam, etc. of the teeth in the two panoramic radiographs—initial and after.

In Table 2 can be observed that IC/FC is uniform for all mandibular incisors as the reduction of their root length after treatment. We also consider of great value IC/FC to correct FR, in

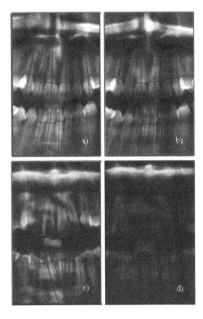

Figure 2. A witness patient measured in different times: a) initial and b) after. Patient with orthodontic treatment measured: c) before, T-1 and d) after, T-2.

Table 1. Results archived with the witness patient.

Teeth	IC	IR	FC	FR	IC/FC	FFR	FFR/IR	%EARR	IC/IR	FC/FR	IR-FFR
13	145,53	220,84	132,37	200,03	1,10	219,91	1,00	0,00	0,66	0,66	0,93
12	106,10	222,40	103,41	215,27	1,03	220,88	0,99	0,01	0,48	0,48	1,52
11	133,06	247,16	127,04	233,08	1,05	244,14	0,99	0,01	0,54	0,55	3,03
21	138,01	242,02	143,22	250,36	0,96	241,26	1,00	0,00	0,57	0,57	0,76
22	122,20	189,26	116,28	179,45	1,05	188,59	1,00	0,00	0,65	0,65	0,67
23	148,57	202,80	139,61	188,86	1,06	200,99	0,99	0,01	0,73	0,74	1,82
42	89,82	198,29	90,09	198,73	1,00	198,13	1,00	0,00	0,45	0,45	0,15
41	93,21	200,57	98,73	208,63	0,94	196,97	0,98	0,02	0,46	0,47	3,60
31	88,02	207,12	97,13	223,27	0,91	202,33	0,98	0,02	0,42	0,44	4,78
32	97,05	227,11	99,25	229,61	0,98	224,52	0,99	0,01	0,43	0,43	2,59

Table 2. Results archived in patient with treatment.

Teeth	IC	IR	FC	FR	IC/FC	FFR	FFR/IR	%EARR	IC/IR	FC/FFR	IR-FFR
42	121	280,6	102	205	1,18	242,3	0,86	0,14	0,43	0,42	38,35
41	116	206,8	103	164	1,12	184,1	0,89	0,11	0,56	0,56	22,73
31	114	203,8	101	158	1,12	177	0,86	0,14	0,56	0,57	44,49
32	117	240,2	100	185	1,17	216,7	0,9	0,1	0,49	0,46	23,51

order to eliminate all the external factors affecting the radiograph measurements. The %RRAE shows a consistent presence of external root resorption on all mandibular incisors.

Summarizing, the proposed method demonstrated the following advantages: (1) it allows enhanced (improved) ROI details in the panoramic radiographs, facilitating the visual analysis of the teeth under study; (2) it is invariant to changes in image rotation and scale due to the correction factor determined and (3) facilitate a metric to measure in a fast and reproducible way the external apical root resorption.

4 CONCLUSIONS

Here is presented a simple, practical and robust image processing method to identify the proportion of external apical root resorption (EARR), which allows a standardized EARR classification metric of severity in the panoramic radiographs. This semiautomatic algorithm permits computing in a precise way the crown/root length and area ratios using as input crosses ends points constructed for each particular teeth. The proposed approach appears to be efficient to study qualitatively and quantitatively the EARR evolution in orthodontic treatments.

Compared with traditional methods, our method facilitated EARR measurements, assessing a higher number of teeth in a semiautomatic, fastest and reproducible way and minimizing the typical manual measurement errors.

Future work will be focused to construct an EARR prediction model. With this model, we intend to evaluate the expected EARR, exploring the influence of relative value of each risk factor, which is of great value in clinical practice. It is very interesting to apply this prediction model before beginning the treatment, once the patient can be involved on the decision of realizing or not his orthodontic treatment. Finally, it is also very advisable and convenient to have a panoramic radiograph and an EARR evaluation, every 12 months after beginning the treatment. Extreme EARR cases can then be identified and it will be possible to stop the treatment in order to preserve the integrity teeth.

ACKNOWLEDGEMENTS

Prof. Guevara acknowledges POPH—QREN-Tipologia 4.2—Promotion of scientific employment funded by the ESF and MCTES, Portugal.

REFERENCES

Al-Qawasmi, R.A., Hartsfield, J.K. et al., (2003). "Genetic predisposition to external apical root resorption." *American Journal of Orthodontics and Dentofacial Orthopedics* **123**(3): 242–252.

Blake, M., Woodside, D.G. et al., (1995). "A radiographic comparison of apical root resorption after orthodontic treatment with the edgewise and Speed appliances." *American Journal of Orthodontics and Dentofacial Orthopedics* **108**(1): 76–84.

Brezniak, N. and Wasserstein, A. (1993). "Root resorption after orthodontic treatment: Part 1. Literature review." *American Journal of Orthodontics and Dentofacial Orthopedics* **103**(1): 62–66.

Brin, I., Tulloch, J.F.C. et al., (2003). "External apical root resorption in Class II malocclusion: a retrospective review of 1- versus 2-phase treatment." *American Journal of Orthodontics and Dentofacial Orthopedics* **124**(2): 151–156.

Chenyang, X. and Prince, J.L. (1998). "Snakes, shapes, and gradient vector flow." *Image Processing, IEEE Transactions on* **7**(3): 359–369.

Guevara, M.A., Silva, A. et al., (2003). Segmentation and Morphometry of Histological Sections Using Deformable Models: A New Tool for Evaluating Testicular Histopathology. *Progress in Pattern Recognition, Speech and Image Analysis*, Springer Berlin/Heidelberg. **2905**: 282–290.

Harry, M.R. and Sims, M.R. (1982). "Root Resorption in Bicuspid Intrusion." *The Angle Orthodontist* **52**(3): 235–258.

Linge, B.O. and Linge, L. (1983). "Apical root resorption in upper anterior teeth." *The European Journal of Orthodontics* **5**(3): 173–183.

Paragios, N., Mellina-Gottardo, O. et al., (2004). "Gradient vector flow fast geometric active contours." *Pattern Analysis and Machine Intelligence, IEEE Transactions on* **26**(3): 402–407.

Pastorinho, M., Guevara, M. et al., (2005). Development of a New Index to Evaluate Zooplanktons' Gonads: An Approach Based on a Suitable Combination of Deformable Models. *Progress in Pattern Recognition, Image Analysis and Applications*. A. Sanfeliu and M. Cortés, Springer Berlin/Heidelberg. **3773**: 498–505.

Computational Vision and Medical Image Processing – Tavares & Natal Jorge (eds)
© *2012 Taylor & Francis Group, London, ISBN 978-0-415-68395-1*

Preliminary study of the clinical application of the Clinical Decision Support System ORAD II in a university dental clinic

A.F. Simões, A. Correia & T. Marques
Portuguese Catholic University, Viseu, Portugal

R. Figueiredo
Faculty of Odontology of the University of Barcelona, Spain

ABSTRACT: Clinical decision support systems (CDSS) are computer programs developed to give a specialized support to health providers in the clinical decision making process. In Dental Medicine, radiographic images are the primary auxiliary support for a correct diagnosis. ORAD II was developed to evaluate clinical and radiographic characteristics of intra-bone lesions. The aim of this research is to evaluate the reliability of this clinical decision support system in patients observed in a university dental clinic. Two Professors and two students analyzed radiographic images of oral pathologies of nine patients, and its parameters were introduced in the clinical decision support system ORAD II. Within the limitations of our study, we conclude that the software ORAD II is useful in assisting the differential diagnosis of oral pathologies, but should always be used only as a complement in the decision-making process.

Keywords: differential diagnosis; ORAD; CDSS; intra-bone lesions

1 INTRODUCTION

Clinical decision support systems (CDSSs) are computer programs designed to provide specialized support to health professionals in the clinical decision process related to prevention, diagnosis or treatment of a particular pathology. The use of computers and clinical decision support systems by health professionals has been studied since the middle of the 20th century. The first studies were focused on the development of diagnostic systems. According to Mendonça (2004), Ledley and Lusted in 1959 were the first to create such a system, using punched cards to indicate relationships between diseases and symptoms. However, problems associated with the limitations of the scientific foundation and the resistance by practitioners to accept a system that was not integrated into their daily practice prevented the evolution of the same. In 1972, Leaper applied the Bayesian probability theory to develop the system "The Leeds abdominal pain system". The system used sensitivity, specificity and disease prevalence in relation to signs, symptoms and test results to calculate the probability of seven causes of abdominal pain. MYCIN, was a CDSS developed in the mid-70s, that had treatment recommendations based on certainty factors and it was tested in cases of bacteremia and meningitis. The exponential development of the capabilities of these systems has played an important role in dentistry. Today, computers and specialized software are an integral part of dental office, and the biggest challenge is to incorporate evidence-based practice, clinical information needs of the dentist, and its integration in the complex clinic workflow. There has been research and development of CDSSs in dentistry for over two decades, using different types of knowledge representation and its application in various areas. Computer technology has brought many changes in clinical practice of Dentistry.

Within the scope of this article, ORAD—Oral Radiographic Differential Diagnosis—is a CDSS related to Oral Pathology. Originally created by White in 1989, it is a computer program developed to evaluate clinical and radiographic features of patients with intra-bony lesions, in order to assist in their identification, using the Bayes' theorem. Works with 16 variables, based on statistical information from over 150 of the most common lesions manifested in the mandible or maxilla. Including the features of the lesion in question, the program generates results by providing a list of possible diseases that may be associated with the described condition.

Although further development of CDSS in the field of dentistry is needed, the implementation of the basic conclusions of each software and their interaction with professionals is crucial for them to be accepted. The use and evaluation of such systems should be an integral part of medical and dental training. Students must acquire basic knowledge in computer technology applied to also enhance the levels of self-learning and continuing education. The use of information technologies and communication is a challenge to tailor training to the current reality and future needs.

2 MATERIAL AND METHODS

We used the computer program available online—ORAD II—Oral Radiographic Differential Diagnosis (http://www.orad.org/)

Lesions were submitted through the cases selected on the basis of available clinical data from the UCP, during the school year of 2009–2010 with confirmation by histological evaluation by biopsy.

The ORAD II includes 16 questions that, after responding to each of them allow us to obtain a differential diagnosis of the lesion. Answers to questions were made by two students of the course units of Oral Pathology and Dental Medical Informatics and two faculty members teaching in the University Clinic. None of them knew previously the biopsy diagnosis.

3 RESULTS

Table 1. ORAD Vs Biopsy Results (0 = Non coincident; 1 = Coincident; 2 = ORAD 2nd option; 3 = ORAD 3rd option).

Pat.	Lesion biopsy diagnosis	Prof_ 1	prof_ 2	stud_ 1	stud_ 2
1-L.C.R.	Inflammatory cyst	3	1	0	1
2-D.L.D.	Fibro-osseous lesions	1	1	1	1
3-L.A.M	Stafne bone cavity	1	1	1	1
4-F.G.Q.	Odontogenic cyst	0	0	0	0
5-R.F.C.S	Cemento-ossifying fibroma	3	0	0	0
6-R.F.C.S	Complex odontoma	3	0	0	0
7-I.S	Juvenile ossifying fibroma	0	0	0	0
8-L.B.	Periodontal cyst	1	2	1	2
9-S.S.	Radicular cyst	2	1	0	0

4 DISCUSSION

Analyzing Table 1, we can confirm that only in two cases, all differential diagnoses generated by ORAD II, with higher probability, correspond to the histopathological diagnosis obtained in laboratory (case n° 2 and 3). It is important to note that in case number three, "Stafne bone cavity", biopsy is unusual for its diagnosis. It is only possible to diagnose by radiograph image (see figure n° 2).

In this study, 67% of the ORAD´s submissions do not match with the biopsy results. Note that in cases n° 4 and 7 (see Table and Figure n°1), none of the hypotheses generated by the support system are in accordance with the definitive diagnosis obtained by biopsy.

In cases 1, 5, 6 8 and 9 the program provides probabilistic outcomes related definitive diagnosis by histopathology. However, it appears that these cases definitive diagnosis is not made by ORAD II as the first option, i.e. most likely to occur, but as the 2nd and 3rd option.

Since this system is based on statistical probabilities related to 16 variables, we can put the hypothesis that the relative probabilities of the

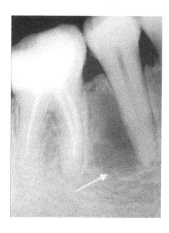

Figure 1. Periapical radiograph for case n° 7 (non coincident).

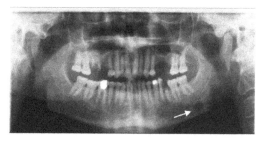

Figure 2. Orthopantomography for case n° 3—Stafne bone cavity.

necessary conditions in question may not be on the probabilistic database system, or may have been an error in the responses given by observers.

In this regard it should be noted the study by Lang (1996), which argues that the expansion and updating of the database software ORAD can increase the likelihood of correct diagnosis of the lesion. This author obtained more accurate diagnoses when the program was used by experienced radiologists, in contrast to student's results.

Zanet (2009), in a validation of interpretation of maxillo-mandibular bone changes with Delphi software concluded that the level of knowledge between specialists and general practitioners did not affect the end result of using this software.

Even after development of many modern imaging modalities, radiography still remains the most important mode of investigation for the evaluation of jaw lesions. ORAD II presents itself as a clinical decision support system for differential diagnosis in the field of radiology in dentistry. According to Mendonça (2004), decisions are made through use of a logical deductive system based on Bayes' theorem. These kind of logical systems are not useful if they are not adjusted to the rarity or prevalence of specific diseases. The application in the field of dentistry needs further improvement and development.

Results may be biased by errors in the preparation of the clinical history or introduction of the analysis parameters in ORAD II. The evolution of such systems should always pass through the sharing of clinical information between professionals in the areas involved. In a systematic review prepared by Mileman (2009), he claims a key factor for successful use of such systems, with regard to practice and knowledge of the software and specific disease by users.

5 CONCLUSION

Within the limitations of our study, especially with regard to the limited sample size, it was not possible to draw conclusions that demonstrate the reliability of the system ORAD II. Consequently, there was a discrepancy between the histopathological results and those provided by ORAD II.

No conclusions can be established with regard to diagnoses generated by lecturer/assistant professor and students.

Although it is a useful system, allowing the aid in the differential diagnosis, this clinical decision support system should be used as a complement in the decision-making and not as a definitive diagnosis. Prior knowledge in the field of oral pathology by the health professional is still a need and priority.

REFERENCES

Andrade, P.J. Specialized computer support systems for medical diagnosis. Relationship with the Bayes' theorem and with logi-cal diagnostic thinking. Arq Bras Cardiol. 1999 Dec. 73(6): 537–52.

Benn, D.K., Bidgood, W.D., Jr. & Pettigrew, JC, Jr. An imaging standard for dentistry. Extension of the radiology DICOM standard. Oral Surg Oral Med Oral Pathol. 1993 Sep;76(3): 262–5.

Borra, R.C., Andrade, P.M., Correa, L. & Novelli, M.D. Development of an open case-based decision-support system for diagnosis in oral pathology. Eur J Dent Educ. 2007 May;11(2): 87–92.

Brickley, M.R., Shepherd, J.P. & Armstrong, R.A. Neural networks: a new technique for development of decision support systems in dentistry. Journal of Dentistry. [doi: DOI: 10.1016/S0300-5712(97)00027-4]. 1998;26(4): 305–9.

Correia, A.R.M., Matos, C.R.Cd., Pinto, A.L.M., Filipe, M.J.M. & Costa, P.M.F.V. Dental Informatics: An emerging discipline. Rev odon-to ciênc. [Review]. 2008;23(4): 397–402.

Heithersay, G.S., Cohn, S.A. & Parkins, D.J. Central giant cell granu-loma. Aust Endod J. 2002 Apr;28(1):18–23.

Hochadel, M. How publishers are developing clinical decision support. J Evid Based Dent Pract. 2008 Sep;8(3): 206–8.

Lang, W.P. & Brooks, S.L. Use and Evaluation of an Expert System for Interpretation of Oral Radiographic Lesions. Proc AMIA Annu Fall Symp. 1996: 874.

Mendonca, E.A. Clinical decision support systems: perspectives in dentistry. J Dent Educ. 2004 Jun;68(6): 589–97.

Mileman, P.A. & van den Hout, W.B. Improving treatment decisions from radiographs: effect of a decision aid. Int J Comput Assist Radiol Surg. 2009 Jun;4(4): 367–73.

Newman, M.G. Clinical decision support complements evidence-based decision making in dental practice. J Evid Based Dent Pract. 2007 Mar;7(1): 1–5.

Neyaz, Z., Gadodia, A., Gamanagatti, S. & Mukhopadhyay, S. Radi-ographical approach to jaw lesions. Singapore Med J. 2008 Feb;49(2):165–76; quiz 77.

Schleyer, T., Mattsson, U., Ni Riordain, R., Brailo, V., Glick, M., Zain, R.B. et al. Advancing oral medicine through informatics and information technology: a proposed framework and strategy. Oral Dis. 2011 Apr;17 Suppl 1: 85–94.

Shortliffe, E.H., Davis, R., Axline, S.G., Buchanan, B.G., Green, C.C. & Cohen, S.N. Computer-based consultations in clinical therapeu-tics: explanation and rule acquisition capabilities of the MY-CIN system. Comput Biomed Res. 1975 Aug; 8(4): 303–20.

Song, M., Spallek, H., Polk, D., Schleyer, T. & Wali, T. How information systems should support the information needs of general dentists in clinical settings: suggestions from a qualitative study. BMC Med Inform Decis Mak. 2010;10: 7.

Umar, H. Capabilities of computerized clinical decision support systems: the implications for the practicing dental professional. J Contemp Dent Pract. 2002 Feb 15;3(1): 27–42.

Umar, H. Clinical decision-making using computers: opportunities and limitations. Dent Clin North Am. 2002 Jul;46(3): 521–38, vi.

Vikram, K. & Karjodkar, F.R. Decision Support Systems in Dental Decision Making: An Introduction. Journal of Evidence Based Dental Practice. [doi: DOI: 10.1016/j.jebdp.2009.03.003]. 2009;9(2): 73–6.

White, S. ORAD II Oral radiographic differential diagnosis. ORAD for the web- ORAD version 2.0. 1995 [updated July 9, 2005; cited 2010 May 26, 2010]; Available from: http://www.orad.org

White, S.C. Computer-aided differential diagnosis of oral radio-graphic lesions. Dentomaxillofac Radiol. 1989 May;18(2): 53–9.

White, S.C. Decision-support systems in dentistry. J Dent Educ. 1996 Jan;60(1): 47–63.

White, S.C. & Pharoah, M.J. The Evolution and Application of Dental Maxillofacial Imaging Modalities. Dental Clinics of North America. [doi: DOI: 10.1016/j.cden.2008.05.006]. 2008;52(4): 689–705.

White, B.A. & Maupome, G. Making clinical decisions for dental care: concepts to consider. Spec Care Dentist. 2003 Sep-Oct;23(5): 168–72.

Zanet, T. Sistema de apoio à decisão diagnóstica baseado em caracteristicas radiográficas. Sao Paulo: Universidade de São Paulo; 2009.

Computational Vision and Medical Image Processing – Tavares & Natal Jorge (eds)
© 2012 Taylor & Francis Group, London, ISBN 978-0-415-68395-1

Medicine application of laser holography and speckle interferometry

V.A. Antonov, M.H. Grosmann, A.I. Larkin, A.V. Osintsev & V.P. Schepinov
National Research Nuclear University MEPhI, Russia

ABSTRACT: Holography is highly suitable for classification of system's states because it offers unique possibilities of parallel processing two-dimensional data arrays, realizing the correlation algorithm in a simple way, handling information rapidly, and providing large memory density and capacity. Holographic and speckle interferometry important and actual for experimental prosthetic dentistry—investigation of bone stock, denture deformations and teeth displacements.

1   INTRODUCTION

The high coherent laser radiation is used effectively in different kinds of medical diagnostics such as: multiparametric analysis, optical coherence tomography, research of blood, skin and teeth states, etc. Holography is highly suitable for classification of system's states because it offers unique possibilities of parallel processing two-dimensional data arrays, realizing the correlation algorithm in a simple way, handling information rapidly, and providing large memory density and capacity.

Operative optics analysis of multiparametric states confirms that coherent optics and holography holds much promise for biomedical research and clinical examinations. The holographic methods are suitable for diagnose in the general case of no constraints imposed on the statistical function of system states and permits analyze information represented in multiparametric form. Investigation carried out with a optics diagnosing systems confirm that coherent optics and holography holds much promise for biomedical research and clinical examinations, in particular, for morphology of blood elements. The discussed holographic methods are suitable for diagnosing in the general case of no constraints imposed on the statistical function of system states. In distinction of the optical methods dealing with images in the natural form, holographic diagnostics can analyze information represented in multiparametric form, thereby offering a qualitatively new way of data processing. Accurate separation of diagnostic ranges in the space of characters may be achieved in two ways: by thoroughly selecting the most informative parameters of the system, or by increasing the space dimensionally.

At present time several methods have been used to solve the problems of experimental prosthetic dentistry—investigation of bone stock and denture deformations, teeth displacements. The limitations of method are: necessity for attaching of strain gages to the surface of investigated object and laboriousness of denture modeling. That's why recently the methods of coherent optics—holographic and speckle interferometry have been started to use. These methods allow non-contact measurements with accuracy up to laser wavelength and allow the creation of automated system for recording of displacement fields with computer data processing. Moreover, the measurements can be carried out on diffuse reflecting surface. Laser photonics experimental methods are very important and actual for medicine application. Particularly in prosthetic dentistry they give unique information leading to correct process of medical treatment and as a result many patients health safety.

2   MULTYPARAMETRIC DIAGNOSTICS

The last years marked the transition from the investigation and construction of simple pattern recognizing devices to the development of complex pattern recognition systems [1]. In holography this process is characterized by the extension of the range of investigation from the recognition of pattern of natural two-dimensional form to the multi-parameter pattern recognition as well as the problem of medical and technical diagnosis [2].

The procedure of making out a diagnosis with the aid holography involves the following stages:

– Data preparation and formalization. -Initial data coding and recording on optical transparencies to form a holographic memory file.
– Coding of the examination records on an optical transparency (data input).

– Comparison of tire patient's examination records with the stored statistical material and final decision making.

The first two stages are preparatory. It is expedient that they be carried out in leading public health institutions and then only once if the storage is not expected to be replenished with new data.

Diagnosing of a multiparametric system involves conversion of tulle initial naultidimensional space of characters and, at a first stage, requires its development into a one-dimensional sequence. Holography offers an advantage already at this stage enabling the source information to be represented in two dimensions, then the characters no longer need to he tried one by one as they can be processed simultaneously. In combination with spatial-matched filtering, this feature offers tulle possibility of conspiring in one operation the pattern on the input transparency with the entire holographic memory.

The principles of holographic data processing [2, 3], as used for signals, graphics or for diagnosing of multiparametric states, are applicable for biomedical research and clinical examinations where they proved convenient and economical, and where they open up new possibilities for diagnosing. In taking up electrophysiological records. a need arises to process simultaneously several waveforms incoming from a few interrelated points of the system. The analysis of electrophysiological signals involves the following operations:

– Averaging of several wave forms.
– Correlation analysis of wave trains, performed hy synchronizing and cross-correlating waveforms taken from various electrophysiological pickups.
– Spectral analysis of signals.

The holographic methods are suitable for diagnosing in the general case of no constraints imposed on the statistical function of system states and permits analyze information represented in multiparametric form.

Accurate separation of diagnostic ranges in the space of characters may be achieved in two ways: by thoroughly selecting the most informative parameters of the system, or by increasing the space dimensionally.

The first approach permits an exquisite solution. However, the search for most informative characters is an insolvable problem not only in the general case but also for most of specific situations. Besides, the weight of characters proves different and depends on the final diagnosis.

The simplest diagnostic algorithm is the search for a precedent. This is the only algorithm in which the data being processed virtually equals the storage capacity. Its number of possible states ranges into q^m, where q is the number of possible definite values of a certain parameter, and m is the number of parameters. Such an algorithm does not call for preliminary processing of the initial data, but imposes stringent requirements on the memory capacity. Moreover, the speed in exhaustive search proves the slowest of all. The diagnostic machine then turns out to be a spacious retrieval system rather than a system that implements a decision making algorithm. Therefore, machine diagnostics fairly often uses a deterministic method which establishes an explicit connection between definite parameters and diagnostic results, i.e., approximates the actual distribution by an (m+1)—dimensional parallelepiped. If an analyzable system does not fit by one of the parameters it is immediately discarded of those corresponding to a definite diagnosis. But this can result in gross mistakes, particularly where the intelligence weight of individual parameters is not known beforehand.

A more reliable diagnostic procedure seems to be the one using metric, methods in a pattern recognition algorithm. These methods employ a certain metric as a diagnostic measure.

Probabilistic algorithms, exploiting statistical distributions, play the highest flexibility. These rely on the Bayes theorem, according to which the information contained in a character S_i (or in the system of characters, S) on the condition that disease B_j takes place is equal to the information contained in diagnosis B_j provided that character S_i (or the system of characters, S) takes place. The posterior probability of the j-th diagnosis on condition that the system of characters—S is $P(B_j | S)$. The probabilities $P(S_j | B_j)$ are readily determinable from available medical statistics. The required storage capacity will be defined by the product qm rather than by the power q^m.

In implementing the "probabilistic diagnostics" on a computer, it is common to assume statistical independence of the parameters. This constraint can be avoided if we take advantage of the "correspondence diagnostics". In essence it is as follows. The initial distribution of $P(B_j|S)$ is approximated by a set of (m+1)-dimensional parallelepipeds whose number is determined by the shape of distribution and the desired accuracy is stating the diagnosis probability. With such an approach, the independent classes of diseases result from the value sets of the parameters, which correspond to a definite diagnosis subject to a given probability of the result. The requirements placed on the storage capacity become less stringent than in search for a precedent, but more stringent than for the deterministic method. Besides, the correspondence diagnostics calls for complete initial statistics which has to be processed for store.

The above diagnostic methods reduce in one way or another to comparison of a pattern formed by the set of symptoms with the pattern in the store. At a sufficiently large number of the parameters represented in an appropriate manner, such a comparison can be made, by correlation analysis. Diagnosing can then be thought of as a classification or even as identification, i.e., as a pattern recognition procedure. In holographic systems [2] the evaluation of the correlation function and the attendant pattern recognition procedure take little time and rely on comparatively simple means.

In the general case, a statistical processing of multiparametric information can yield a multivariate distribution. In the simplest case we need to decide on whether a situation pending to a definite set of characters belongs to a given class or extends beyond its limits (the problem of validity testing diagnosis or prognosis of a state).

We tried our diagnostic system on diagnosing liver using the data collected by Byhovski and Vishnevski. In the preliminary stage, we processed the data on a computer and selected 34 independent characters out of 150 available. We verified computationally 10^4 codes and determined their modification thresholds, which made it possible to construct a matrix for 16 possible disease in the analysis with 34 parameters. A check on a sample of 200 actual case histories revealed that the prognosis for these statistical data is over 80 percent accurate.

3 PROSTHETIC DENTISTRY

At present time several methods have been used to solve the problems of experimental prosthetic dentistry—investigation of bone stock and denture deformations and teeth displacements. These methods are: strain measurement method, photoelasticity method, method of photostress coating etc. The limitations of methods connected with necessity for attaching of strain gages to the surface of investigated object in strain measurement method, laboriousness of denture modeling in photoelasticity method. That's why recently the methods of coherent optics—holographic and speckle interferometry have been started to use. These methods allow non-contact measurements with accuracy up to parts of laser wavelength. Moreover, the measurements can be carried out on diffuse reflecting surface.

The major factors influencing resolution of interference fringe patterns in methods of holographic and digital speckle interferometry and essentially limiting opportunity of automation of measurements are considered below. Interference fringes in holographic and digital speckle interferometry are modulated by speckle noise.

For holographic interferograms registration at study of the bone deformation processes fabrics to mandible was used optical scheme shown on Fig. 1. The particularity of this scheme is using of two holders photoplate and two supporting bunches that allowed to research the mandible with two sides.

The beam of the coherent radiation from laser (LTN-402, 0,53 MKM) falls on mirror, changing its direction. The reflected by mirrow laser beam enlarges by microobjective. The flat wave, formed by lens, illuminates the under investigation object. The light wave, reflected from right sides of the object, falls on photoplate. From left sides of the object are reflected light wave and forms the subject wave for other photoplate. A part of flat wave front, reflected from mirror, moves on photoplate, the other part is reflected from mirror and forms the reference wave.

The optical scheme of the interferometer with use two registerring photoplates, installed on plug-in return parts device, allows to realize the simultaneous registration of the deformation process under investigation object as well as investigate the processes of relaxations deformation at time.

The interference strips picture on each step of the installation mini-implantat possible define the magnitudes a deformation for each step of its installation. Total picture bone deformation is received as a result of summations local deformations.

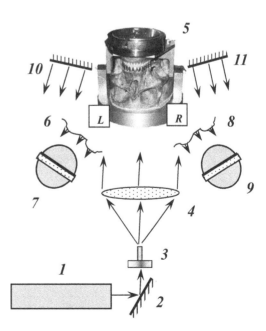

Figure 1.   The optical scheme of two-plates holographic interferometer.

The holographic interferogram with increase on which the speckle structure of the image of the body is well visible given in the Fig. 2. This phenomenon is especially typical in digital speckle interferometry as this method is based on subtraction of fields speckle reflected from a body surface before and after its deformation.

The typical holographic interferograms got at zone of the installation mini-implant are brought on Fig. 3a,b. The picture of the strips on Fig. 3a is received when installing mini-implant since the fourth on fifth turn, on Fig. 3b—since seventh on eighth turn. On brought interferograms is well seen that on all stage of the installation mini-implantat maximum deformation exists in the field of tops of the body to mandible and spreads over surface of the jaws. Herewith on initial stage of the installation—Fig 3a deformation small—exists one strip, but consequent increase—ten strips on Fig. 3b.

When installing cylindrical mini-implantats deformation bone arise only upon the first turn. When installing cone-shaped mini-implants deformation bone arise on top of alveolar and act on the whole process of the submersion that can bring about fission bone fabrics and, as complication, towards rift or fracture to bones.

4 CONCLUSIONS

Laser photonics experimental methods are very important and actual for medicine application. Particularly in prosthetic dentistry they give unique information leading to correct process of medical treatment. The discussed holographic methods are suitable for diagnosing in the general case of no constraints imposed on the statistical function of system states. In distinction from the optical methods dealing with images in the natural form, holographic diagnostics can analyze information represented in multiparametric form, thereby offering a qualitatively new way of data processing. A check on a sample of 200 actual cases revealed that prognosis for these statistical data in over 80 per cent accurate.

REFERENCES

[1] Antonov, V.A. et al. 1984. *Lasers and Holographic Data Processing.* Moscow: MIR,
[2] Grosmann, M.H. & Larkin, A.I. 2008. Fundamental connection between coherent optics and radiophysics *Les 6emes Journees d'Optique et de Traitement de l'Information,* Mohammedia, Maroc.
[3] Larkin, A.I. & Volkov, L.V. 1994. Capability of Quasi-Stationary Partially Coherent Radiation in Optical Systems of Recording and Information Processing. *Optical Review,* 1 (1) 12.

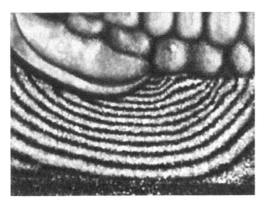

Figure 2. Typical interferograms of bone micro-deformation.

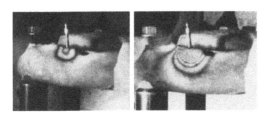

Figure 3. Typical interferograms at mini-implantat installation (a) fourth on fifth turn, (b) seventh on eighth turn.

Computational Vision and Medical Image Processing – Tavares & Natal Jorge (eds)
© 2012 Taylor & Francis Group, London, ISBN 978-0-415-68395-1

Image processing techniques in the analysis of the stresses exerted on the abutment tooth for a Removable Partial Denture

M.J. Santos, M.H. Figueiral & A. Correia
FMDUP, Porto, Portugal

J.M. Monteiro & M.A.P. Vaz
FEUP, Porto, Portugal

ABSTRACT: The stability of a Removable Partial Denture during its use is influenced by biological support structures and by the prosthesis design. The aim of this research is to study the stresses exerted on the abutments of a Removable Partial Denture Metal Framework by means of Digital Image Correlation and Holographic Interferometry techniques.

1 INTRODUCTION

According to the Glossary of Prosthodontic Terms (GTP), a Dental Prosthesis is an artificially made device that allows replacing, in whole or in part, of missing or damaged teeth and contiguous structures, with the goal of restoring function and aesthetics. [1]

There are several types of dental prostheses like: inlays/onlays, crowns, bridges, implants, partial and complete dentures and removable partial dentures (RPD), being these last the subject of this study. These are formed by major and minor connectors, teeth, saddles, clasps and occlusal support [2]. Prostheses can be dental supported (the support is given by virtually all abutment teeth) or supported by mucosa and teeth (support is also given by the mucosa of the alveolar ridge). In the case of RPD with dental support must be taken into consideration, among other factors, the number of remaining teeth, their distribution in the arch, its relationship with the antagonist teeth, as well as their health status. It is particularly important to evaluate the state of the periodontium, because it is responsible for anchoring the support teeth to the bone. Furthermore, the periodontal ligament assists in the dissipation of forces applied to bone during functional tooth contact, and even considered a natural buffer forces. For RPD with mucosal and teeth support there must also consider the quality and quantity of cortical bone, resilient and adhered sub mucosa and keratinized mucosa.

In Dentistry, it is extremely important to know the biomechanics of mandible movements and its influence on the success of the Oral Rehabilitation. The structures that support the Removable Partial Denture are biological structures that are subject to different forces, particularly during chewing. Therefore, the Dentist must consider the direction, duration, frequency and magnitude of the forces applied in order to preserve the health of these structures [3]. Sometimes, the forces transmitted through the prosthesis to the abutment teeth are larger than this can tolerate, which may result in mobility or fracture of the teeth and, ultimately, in its loss. [4]

As so, it is important to study the forces, stresses and strains exerted over the teeth, related structures and dental materials, by using engineering techniques like those related to Experimental Mechanics. With these techniques is possible to assess stresses in structural components when they are subjected to loads and they can be used in laboratory for *in vitro* stability evaluation of a RPD.

2 OBJECTIVES

The purpose of this study is the characterization of the stresses exerted on the abutment tooth for a removable partial denture, namely in the clasps design. The first step of the investigation is use to define and evaluate the methodology used and validate it according to the objective of this study.

3 MATERIAL AND METHODS

For this study was selected a plaster model of a mandible with acrylic teeth as abutments (teeth 35 and 45) simulating a Kennedy Class I clinical situation (Fig. 1).

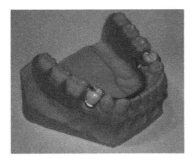

Figure 1. Plaster model with a removable partial denture.

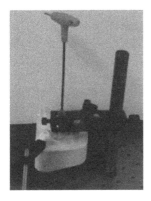

Figure 2. Experimental load rig.

The displacement fields were assessed with two non contact full field optical techniques, digital image correlation (DIC) and electronic speckle pattern interferometry (ESPI). With DIC the displacement is computed from the optical correlation established between two images of the object surface, which were recorded for two moments of different load. For this, the surface of object is first encoded, either by its natural texture, either by painting with an intensity pattern similar to a speckle field, see Figs. 4 and 5. The final resolution depends on the speckle size and can range from a few tenths to several hundredths of mm. 3D displacements can be obtained if two cameras are used to record de images.

To perform this measurement the denture was painted with the appropriate texture, and placed on a loading rig (Fig. 2). In this case the loading was obtained by applying a vertical displacement resulting by a screw tightening (screw thread— 0.25 mm). The loads were applied on prosthetic tooth 3.6 and 4.6. A single camera set-up was used to obtain the in-plane displacements.

ESPI was used with the same loading system (Fig. 3). In this technique the resolution is about

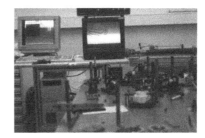

Figure 3. Optical setup for ESPI.

two orders of magnitude lower, 0,1 μm, therefore the load applied was significantly lower, about ¼ of a turn of the screw. Two different setups were used, one with out-of-plane sensitivity and the other one with dual illumination for in-plane displacement assessment.

This technique allows measuring displacements in a global and non-contact way, and with a resolution which can go down to 0.1×10^{-6}, corresponding to half of the laser wavelength used for illumination. Therefore both techniques are suitable for analyzing how the structure behaves under different loading conditions.

4 RESULTS

The follow images were obtained by Digital Image Correlation, dedicated software was used in this technique that divides in a cell matrix the selected area. After the division the software identifies the center of the initial image (Fig. 3) and the center of the final image (Fig. 4) and calculate the displacements and deformations (derivative of displacement) of the Dental Prosthesis. In Fig. 6 the digital processed mask that defines the measurement area.

In the following images the displacement in the X (horizontal) and Y (Figs. 7 and 8) axis directions and the respective deformation (Figs. 9 and 10) are presented. The interpretation of this images is made observing the color scale in the right side of each image. All the results presented in (Figs. 7 and 8) result from a correlation between pairs of images.

In the images above it was observed only movement in the clasps of the denture for high displacement amplitudes. In the first recordings obtained for reduced loads no displacement of the abutment tooth was detected.

In this direction of measurement it was observed the effect previously referred, no displacement occours for low loading amplitudes. However, when the load increases the deformation of the

Mandible left side

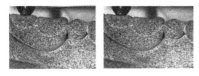

Figure 4. DIC Images recorded before and after loading.

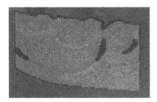

Figure 5. Digital mask for definition of the area of measurement.

Displacement in OX

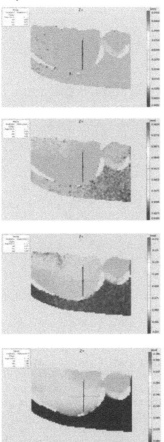

Figure 6. Displacement field in horizontal direction measured with DIC.

Displacement in OY

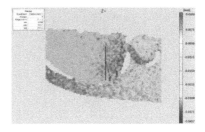

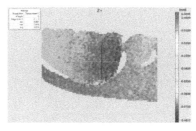

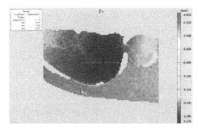

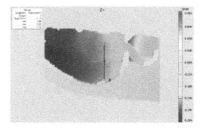

Figure 7. Displacement field in vertical direction measured with DIC.

RPD is transmited to the abutement. Acoording to the color scale a rotation of the RPD is detected because the denture undergoes a vertical displacement top to bottom and, on the other hand, the abutement (right side) has a vertical displacement upwords.

From the displacement fields obtained it is possible to extract the deformatins by numerical differentiation. With this calculation the deformed regions, with displacement gradients, become evident.

In this case, the deformation was observed only in the clasps as can be seen in the images above.

Deformation in OX　　　　　　　　　　　**Deformation in OY**

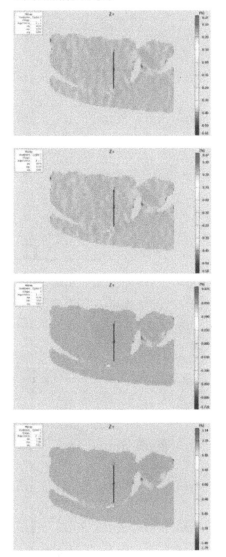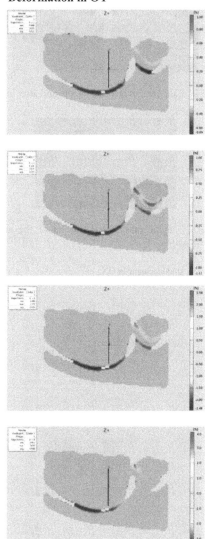

Figure 8. Deformation field in horizontal direction measure with DIC.

Figure 9. Deformation field in vertical direction measure with DIC.

Please note that the abutment tooth undergoes a rigid body movement and only the clasps reveal localized deformations.

In this case was also observed a deformation in the clasps of the denture. Furthermore it is evident a deformation on the saddle of the RPD, identified by a strong color between the RPD and the plaster model.

From the previous DIC measurements it becomes clear that the RPD support was well designed and only with arge loads it starts to move. To obtain

a better perspective of the behavior of the model with reduced loads the same measurements were performed with ESPI. The following images were obtained by ESPI with a set-up oriented to obtain the displacements through a direction perpendicular to the surface.

The ESPI technique relays on the interference between two coherent recordings of the surface image when it is illuminated with laser light. In this case the surface displacement is converted on an interference fringe pattern where each fringe

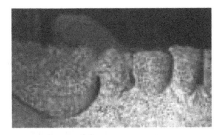

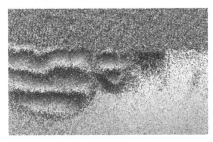

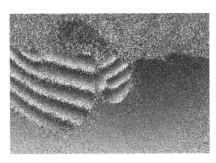

Figure 10. Initial image and the deformation phase map with displacements obtained by ESPI.

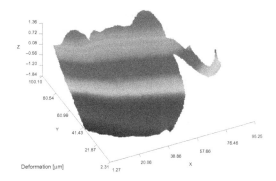

Figure 11. 3D representation of the out-of-plane displacement obtained with ESPI.

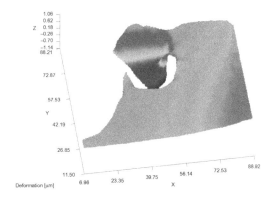

Figure 12. Detail of the 3D representation of the out-of-plane displacement showing the behavior of abutment tooth.

represents points undergoing the same displacement. Using phase modulation techniques it is possible to obtain the phase distribution corresponding to the object displacement, (Fig. 10).

In Fig. 10 it is shown an image of the area selected for displacement assessement and tow phase maps obtained with an out-of-plane ESPI set-up. The two measurements were carried out with the sensitivity vector oriented in a direction close to the normal to the surface.

The phase maps shown in (Fig. 10) present 2π discontinuities resulting from the phase calculation with an arctang function [5]. To obtain the continuous displacement field the phase discontinuities can be removed by unwrapping algorithms which can be combined with information about the sensitivity vector and laser wavelegth to obtain the 0,1 μm resolution displacement of each point [6].

After the displacement calculation it is possible to present the final results on a pseudo 3D presentation wich can be seen in (Figs. 11 and 12).

In the previous figure it is evident that the main displacement of the RPD is a rotation in a horizontal axis. Please note that the dimensions in the X and Y directions are in mm while displacements, in Z axis, are two orders of magnitude lower and codified in colors for better image interpretation.

The results shown in Fig. 12 were extracted from the last image of (Fig. 10). In this image is presented a detailed view of the abutment tooth showing an out-of-plane rotation which induces displacements through OZ direction. According to the experimental data the maximum displacement is about 1,4 mm in the direction to the recording camera.

5   DISCUSSION AND CONCLUSION

With these results is possible to conclude that both measurement techniques prove to be appropriate to the objectives of work and allows the global measurement, without contact, of the relative displacements of the removable partial denture during its in vitro experimental loading.

Digital image correlation, having a resolution close to 0,01 mm, still allowing access to the displacements and deformations of the prosthesis without detection of large motion in the abutment teeth.

However, the techniques of holographic interferometry seem more appropriate to study displacements of the abutment teeth. Due to its lower resolution it was possible to detect movement in the abutment teeth as shown in the images. However, the measured movements are due to the rotation and did not exceed about 2 μm for lower load levels.

REFERENCES

1. "The glossary of Prosthodontics Terms" The Journal of Prosthetic Dentistry, Vol. 94, n° 1, 55–56, 2005.
2. R.D. Phoenix, *et al.*, *Stewart's Clinical Removable Partial Prosthodontics*, Quintessence, Chicago, US, 3rd Ed., 2003.
3. J.D. Browning *et al.,* "Movement of three removable partial denture clasp assemblies under occlusal loading", The Journal of Prosthetic Dentistry, Vol. 55, n° 1, 69–74, 1986.
4. Carr, A.B. *et al.*, McCracken—*Prótesis Parcial Removable*, Elsevier Mosby, Madrid, Espanha, 11 Ed. 2006.
5. Katherine Creath, "Phase-shifting speckle interferometry", Applied Optics, Vol. 24, Issue 18, pp. 3053–3058 (1985).
6. Peter Ettl and Katherine Creath, "Comparison of phase-unwrapping algorithms by using gradient of first failure" Applied Optics, Vol. 35, Issue 25, pp. 5108–5114 (1996).

Computational Vision and Medical Image Processing – Tavares & Natal Jorge (eds)
© 2012 Taylor & Francis Group, London, ISBN 978-0-415-68395-1

Current quality control procedures in Digital Radiography

Sofia D. Kordolaimi, Aikaterini-Lampro N. Salvara & Maria E. Lyra
A' Department of Radiology, University of Athens, Athens, Greece

ABSTRACT: In the last decades, Computed Radiography (CR) and Direct Digital Radiography (DDR) are becoming more popular in relation to traditional film screen radiography. This derives mostly from the fact that digital image is prone to post-processing analysis and it can also be stored for future use. Various organizations worldwide have published protocols, in which guidelines concerning quality assurance and acceptance tests for digital systems are referred. In this review, apart from the Quality Control (QC) aspects that are also met in conventional mammography (e.g., kVp performance, accuracy, linearity, uniformity, resolution etc.), diverse methods for quality assurance of digital mammography are presented as well, based on current published protocols. These methods concern the display units, the detector's efficiency, the image quality (Contrast to Noise Ratio-CNR, Signal to Noise Ratio-SNR) and the erasure thoroughness of the cassette (for CR systems). Moreover, presentative phantoms utilised in clinical practice for QC of digital systems are also displayed.

Keywords: Direct Digital Radiography (DDR), Computed Radiography (CR), Quality Control, Signal to Noise Ratio (SNR), Contrast to Noise Ratio (CNR), Image Noise, Ghosting Erase, Test Patents, CR reader, Photostimulated Storage Phosphor (PSP), Detective Quantum Efficiency (DQE) Curve, Automatic Exposure Control (AEC)

1 INTRODUCTION

Digital Radiography (DR) gains ground toward conventional radiography, as it presents more benefits concerning the display, the post-processing and the storage of the images. Moreover, lower doses have been noticed in order to achieve same image quality. Digital radiographic systems are divided into direct and indirect DRs.

In direct digital sytems (DDR) the detection of the signal is one-step procedure. The x-ray beam passes through the object of interest and impinges upon a detector, which converts the radiation into electric signal. The detector could be either a Flat Panel Detector (FPD), or a High Density Line Scan Solid State detector.

In indirect digital sytems (CR) the detection is a two step procedure. For exposure, a storage phosphor plate (a photo-stimulable plate, or PSP) is placed in an x-ray cassette, instead of an X-ray film sheet. When exposed to x-rays, cassettes have the special property of storing the x-ray energy in a latent image, which is "developed" in a CR reader, when the phosphor plate is scanned by a light beam, such as a laser beam.

In this review, various quality control procedures for DR systems, implemented worldwide, as well as the suitable equipment for these measurements are presented.

2 QUALITY CONTROL PROCEDURES

2.1 Typical controls for both conventional and digital radiography

2.1.1 Entrance Surface Dose (ESD) or Entrance Surface Air Kerma (ESAK)

The entrance surface dose (ESD) is the absorbed dose on the phantom surface at a given location and it includes the backscattered radiation. While ESAK is defined as the incidence air kerma impinges upon the phantom surface. The calculation of these indices can be accomplished with several methods. Some of them are the calculation of the incident dose rate by using a copper phantom, which can be related to dose area product. ESD estimations can be also done by using an ionization chamber placed on the surface of a tissue equivalent phantom in order to measure the in-air exposure at several x-ray tube kilovoltages covering all the clinical range. Another well known method to measure the ESD, while reducing the patient dose, is to measure the radiation of the whole beam and then multiply the result with the backscattered factor of the material of the phantom (Goldman 2007, Martin 1995, Omrane et al., 2003, Marshall 2009).

2.1.2 *Reproducibility*

Reproducibility should be checked for kVp performance, timer and radiation output. These measurements can be achieved by keeping the potential and the current constant and repeating the measurements several times. Then, a coefficient of variation is estimated (McLean et al., 2009, Walsh et al., 2008, Fitzgerald et al., 1999):

$$CV = \frac{S}{\bar{X}} = \frac{1}{\bar{X}} \left[\frac{\sum\limits_{i=1}^{n}(X_i - \bar{X})^x}{n-1} \right]^{1/x}$$

where,

    CV: is the coefficient of variation,
    S: is the estimated standard deviation,
    X_i: is the value of the ith measurement,
    $\bar{X}$: is the mean value of the measurements,
    n: is the number of measurements.

2.1.3 *Accuracy*

The purpose of this measurement is to ensure that the kVp does not differ from the nominal value. This is accomplished by conducting measurements for the whole range of potential and current values in clinical use. This control should be performed every six months and the measured kVp should be within ±5% (McLean et al., 2009, IAEA 15.1).

2.1.4 *Image contrast*

Using various phantoms, high contrast and low contrast resolution can be measured. Low contrast resolution characterizes the minimum discernible contrast and is also known as Threshold Contrast Detail Detectability (TCDD). High contrast resolution is the special resolution defined as the number of line pairs per mm. This procedure is described analytically in various protocols worldwide (AAPM, ACPSEM, KCARE). Some of the protocols quantify this contrast (e.g., Image Quality Factor- IQF) while others simply based on visual inspection of the phantoms in display screen (Cowen et al., 1993, Wagner et al., 1991).

2.2 *Specific controls for digital radiographic systems*

2.2.1 *Image quality*

A variety of indices, that aim to assess the performance of the system, are available in literature.

Some of them are: Modulation Transfer Function (MTF), Noise Power Spectrum (NPS), Signal to Noise ratio (SNR), Contrast to Noise ratio (CNR) and uniformity.

The MTF of an imaging system is defined as the absolute value of its optical transfer function, normalized to unity at spatial frequency zero. It is recognised as the best indicator of equipment system resolution under the condition that the appropriate software does exist. One of the established methods to determine the MTF is based on the use of a sharp edge that is imaged to produce an edge spread function (ESF). The ESF is then differentiated to obtain the line spread function (LSF), from which the MTF is calculated by a Fourier transform. An edge test device with a well-defined edge is usually realized by carefully machining a thin piece of metal, (e.g., lead, tungsten, or platinum). Material thicknesses of 0.1 to 0.25 mm are often used to allow easy manufacturing and handling as well as accurate alignment of the edge in the x-ray beam. Depending on the actual thickness of the material and on the beam quality used for imaging, the metal sheet may be either (almost) fully absorbing or semitransparent. Every manufacturer usually has specific instructions for the acquisition of the MTF (Walsh et al., 2004, Beckett & Kotre 2000).

NPS can be determined by imaging a standard test block and by using appropriate software. The typical technique for estimating the NPS for real images is based on averaging the power of the Fourier transform of noisy image samples taken from several images, or more routinely from a single noise image. Despite the difficulties of estimating NPS, it is possible to achieve results with absolute normalization that agree between different laboratories (Blackman & Tukey 1958, Rabbani & Shaw 1987, Cunningham 2000).

SNR is the quotient of mean value of the linearized signal intensity and SD of the noise (intensity distribution) at this signal intensity. It depends on the dose (exposure time and conditions) at the detector, the radiographic system properties and it is also affected by the selection of the acquisition protocol. The European protocol recommends a tolerance limit of ≤15% of the baseline (Alexia 2004, Dimov & Vassileva 2008, Vano et al., 2005, Gennaro et al., 2009, Birch et al., 2006).

Even if the image has a high SNR, it is not useful unless there is a high enough contrast to noise ratio (CNR) to be able to distinguish among different tissues and tissue types, and in particular between healthy and pathological tissue. CNR is a measure for assessing the ability of imaging a procedure to generate clinically useful image contrast. CNR is calculated by the equation:

$$CNR = \frac{MPV_{ph} - MPV_A}{\sqrt{[(SD_{ph}^{x} + SD_{A}^{x})/2]}}$$

where,

MPV_{ph}: is the ROI (~0.25 cm²) located in a uniform part of the phantom,

MPV_{Al}: is the area where the Al foil is located,

SD_{ph}: is the Standard Deviation of MPV_{ph},

SD_{Al}: is the Standard Deviation of MPV_{Al}.

The European provisional specification requires that the CNR be at least 1.1 times and 0.9 times the CNR with 4 cm PMMA for 2 cm and 6 cm of PMMA, respectively [Neitzel et al., 2004].

As far as uniformity is concerned (also referred as "Homogeneity"), there are some differences as to the methodology. The most common method is to calculate the Mean Pixel Value (MPV) in some Regions of Interest (ROIs) throughout the image and compare them. However, if the software of the system does not support ROI processing, the uniformity of the detector can be assessed directly by visual inspection (McLean et al., 2009, KCARE 2009, Morgun 2003).

2.2.2 Automatic Exposure Control (AEC)

A well-designed AEC should be capable of modifying required detector exposures based on exposure conditions (typically selected kVP and mA) to compensate for energy dependence and exposure rate. Some indices that can quantify AEC performance are SNR or CNR, divided by the Average Glandular Dose (AGD). AGD is defined as the mean dose received by the radiation sensitive tissue contained within the breast phantom (Alexia 2004, Neitzel et al., 2004, Doyle & Martin 2006, Doyle et al., 2005, KCARE 2005, Samei et al., 2001).

2.2.3 Detector's performance control

The most commonly used parameter for the characterization of the dose efficiency of a DR detector is the Detective Quantum Efficiency (DQE). It can be determined experimentally (though it is quite difficult to make experimental measurements), and provides information about the additional noise added to the signal at all stages of the signal conversion. Thus, DQE makes it possible to compare on a quantitative basis different systems for X-ray imaging (Gagne et al., 2003, IEC 2003, IEC 2005, Illers et al., 2005, KCARE 2005, Rampado et al., 2006). The DQE for the spatial frequency (u) along the horizontal or vertical direction (along the lines or rows of the pixel matrix of the detector) is determined using the following defining equation:

$$DQE(u) = MTF^2(u) - \frac{W_{in}(u)}{W_{out}(u)}$$

where,

$DQE(u)$: is reported at frequency multiples of 0.5 mm⁻¹ up to the Nyquist frequency,

$MTF(u)$: the modulation transfer function of the detector,

$W_{in}(u)$: the noise power spectra of the input X radiation,

$W_{out}(u)$: the noise power spectra of the linearised detector output signal.

In CR systems where the detector is a phosphor cassette, additional quality controls should be conducted. Erasure thoroughness of the system should be checked in order to avoid ghost artefacts when re-exposing the cassette (Morgun et al., 2003).

2.2.4 Monitor display

A very useful and necessary control of a DR system is to test the quality of the image presentation on monitors and printers. These tests are made by using test patterns on each of the monitors used for reporting clinical images. The system must be able to differentiate all the lines, from thick to narrow and both horizontally and vertically.

In order to check the optimal function of the printers and the quality of the image presentation on them, test patterns are used to test geometrical distortion, contrast visibility, printer artefacts, density response and uniformity. The test patterns are print-out and they are checked for changes in geometric distortion, contrast visibility, resolution, optical density range and artefacts (McLean et al., 2009, KCARE 2003, DICOM 2003, Krupinski et al., 2007, Gray 1992, Jacobs et al., 2006, 20. Lu et al., 1999).

3 CONCLUSION

Currently, various protocols exist for quality control of the physical and technical aspects of digital mammography with regard to image quality and radiation dose. Each protocol has specific advantages and disadvantages that must be taken into account in reporting the results. Although, there are some individual efforts for creating quality assurance protocols in digital radiography, it is imperative to increase harmonisation as far as quality assurance and constancy checking is concerned, so as to compare the arising results among various systems. It is of outmost importance that the same parameters are measured using the same protocols, worldwide.

REFERENCES

Alexia L. 2004. Digital radiography in equine practice. *Clinical Techniques in Equine Practice* 3: 352–360.

Beckett J.R. & Kotre C.J. 2000. Estimation of Mean Glandular Dose for Mammography of Augmented Breasts. *Phys. Med. Biol.* 45: 3241–3252.

Birch I.P., Kotre C.J. & Padgett R. 2006. Trends in Image Quality in High Magnification Digital Specimen Cabinet Radiography. *Brit. J. Rad.* 79: 239–243.

Blackman R.B. & Tukey J.W. 1958. The measurement of power spectra. New York: Dover.

Cowen A.R., Workman A. & Price J.S. 1993. Physical Aspects of Photostimulable Phosphor Computed Radiography. *Brit. J. Rad.* 66: 332–345.

Cunningham I.A. 2000. Applied linear-systems theory. In: Beutel J., Kundel H.L., Van Metter R.L., eds. Handbook of medical imaging. Bellingham, WA: SPIE Press: 79–159.

DICOM: Digital Imaging and Communications in Medicine, grayscale standard display function. National Electrical Manufacturers Association. 2003; Part 14.

Dimov A. & Vassileva J. 2008. Assesment of performance of a new digital image intensifier fluoroscopy system. *Radiat. Prot. Dosim.* 129: 123–126.

Doyle P. & Martin C.J. 2006. Calibrating Automatic Exposure Control Devices for Digital Radiography. *Phys. Med. Biol.* 51: 5475–5485.

Doyle P., Gentle D. & Martin C.J. 2005. Optimising Automatic Exposure Control in Computed Radiography and the Impact on Patient Dose. *Rad. Prot. Dos.* 114: 236–239.

Fitzgerald M. *et al.* 1999. The European Protocol for the Quality Control of the Physical and Technical Aspects of Mammography Screening. Third Edition.

Gagne R.M., Boswell J.S & Myers K.J. 2003. Signal detectability in digital radiography: spatial domain figures of merit. *Med. Phys.* 30: 2180–2193.

Gennaro G., Golinelli P., Bellan E. *et al* 2009. In: Automatic Exposure Control in Digital Mammography: Contrast-to-Noise Ratio versus Average Glandular Dose. Springer Berlin/Heidelberg. 711–715.

Goldman L.W. 2007. Principles of CT: Radiation Dose and Image Quality. *J. Nucl. Med. Tech.* 35: 213–225.

Gray J.E. 1992. Use of the SMPTE Test Pattern in Picture Archiving and Communication Systems. *J. Digit. Imaging* 5: 54–58.

IAEA: International Atomic Energy Agency. Radiation Protection in Diagnostic and International Radiology. Training Material on Radiation Protection in Diagnostic and Interventional Radiology; Part 15.1.

IEC: International Electrotechnical Commission 2003. Medical Electrical Equipment—Characteristics of digital X-ray imaging devices—Part 1: Determination of the detective quantum efficiency. IEC 62220-1. First edition.

IEC: International Electrotechnical Commission 2005. Medical diagnostic Xray equipment—radiation conditions for use in the determination of characteristics. IEC 61267. Second Edition.

Illers H., Buhr E. & Hoeschen C. 2005. Measurement of the Detective Quantum Efficiency (DQE) of Digital X-ray Detectors According to the Novel Standard IEC 62220-1. *Rad. Prot. Dos.* 114: 39–44.

Jacobs J., Deprez T., Marchal G. & Bosmans H. 2006. In: Digital Mammography, Initial Results of the Daily Quality Control of Medical Screen Devices Using a Dynamic Pattern in a Digital Mammography Environment. Springer Berlin/Heidelberg. 416–423.

KCARE: King's Centre for the Assessment of Radiological Equipment Protocol for the QA of computed radiography systems, 2003; Draft 4.0.

KCARE: King's Centre for the Assessment of Radiological Equipment, Protocol for the QA of computed radiography systems, 2004; Draft 7.0.

KCARE: King's Centre for the Assessment of Radiological Equipment, Protocol for the QA of computed radiography systems, 2005; Draft 8.0.

Krupinski E.A., Williams M.B., Andriole K. *et al.* 2007. Digital Radiography Image Quality: Image Processing and Display. *J. Am. Coll. Radiol.* 4: 389–400.

Lu Z.F., Nickoloff E.L. & Terilli T. 1999. DryView Laser Imager: One Year Experience on Five Imation Units. *Med. Phys.* 26: 1817–1821.

Marshall N.W. 2009. An Examination of Automatic Exposure Control Regimes for Two Digital Radiography Systems. *Phys. Med. Biol.* 54: 4645–4670.

Martin C.J. 1995. Measurement of Patient Entrance Surface Dose Rates for Fluoroscopic X-ray Units. *Phys. Med. Biol.* 40: 823–834.

McLean I.D., Heggie J.C.P., Herley J., Thomson F.J. & Grewal R.K. 2009. Recommendations for a Digital Mammography Quality Assurance Program. *Austr. Phys. Eng. Sc. Med.* 2.

Morgun O.N., Nemchenko K.E. & Rogov Yu V. 2003. Detective Quantum Efficiency as a Quality Parameter of Imaging *Equipment. Biomed. Eng.* 37: 258–261.

Neitzel U., Buhr E., Hilgers G. & Granfors P.R. 2004. Determination of the Modulation Transfer Function Using the Edge Method: Influence of Scattered Radiation. *Med. Phys.* 31: 3485–91.

Omrane B.L. *et al.* 2003. An Investigation of Entrance Surface Dose Calculations for Diagnostic Radiology Using Monte Carlo Simulations and Radiotherapy Dosimetry Formalisms. *Phys. Med. Biol.* 48: 1809–1824.

Rabbani M., Shaw R. & Van Metter R. 1987. Detective quantum efficiency of imaging systems with amplifying and scattering mechanisms. *J Opt Soc Am A* 4: 895–901.

Rampado O., Isoardi P. & Ropolo R. 2006. Quantitative Assessment of Computed Radiography Quality Control Parameters. *Phys. in Med. Biol.* 51: 1577–1593.

Samei E., Seibert J.A., Willis C.E., Flynn M.J., Mah E. & Junck K.L. 2001. Performance Evaluation of Computed Radiography Systems. *Med. Phys.* 28: 361–371.

Vano E., Geiger B., Schreiner A., Back C. & Beissel J. 2005. Dynamic flat panel detector versus image intensifier in cardiac imaging: dose and image quality. *Phys. Med. Biol.* 50: 5731–5742.

Wagner A.J., Barnes G.T. & Wu X.Z. 1991. Assessing Fluoroscopic Contrast Resolution: A Practical and Quantitative Test Tool. *Med. Phys.* 18: 894–899.

Walsh C., Gorman D., Byrne P., Larkin A., Dowling A. & Malone J.F. 2008. Quality Assurance of Computed and Digital Radiography Systems. *Radiation Protection Dosimetry*, 1–5.

Walsh C., Larkin A., Dennan S. & Reilly G. 2004. Exposure Variations Under Error Conditions in Automatic Exposure Controlled Film–Screen Projection Radiography. *Brit. J. Rad.* 77: 931–933.

Computational Vision and Medical Image Processing – Tavares & Natal Jorge (eds)
© 2012 Taylor & Francis Group, London, ISBN 978-0-415-68395-1

Image segmentation algorithms on female pelvic ultrasound images

Patrícia F. Silva, Zhen Ma & João Manuel R.S. Tavares
Faculdade de Engenharia da Universidade do Porto (FEUP)/Instituto de Engenharia Mecânica e Gestão Industrial (INEGI), Porto, Portugal

ABSTRACT: The processing and analysis of structures presented in images has been one of the areas of Computational Vision with greater potential and applicability. The main goal of the researchers of this area has been the development of new computational methodologies to study the behaviour of structures in images. The mentioned image-based analysis is very important in many domains. For example, in Medicine, the information obtained by the proposed automatic analysis is crucial to understand the functioning and the behaviour of organs, and thus to assist medical doctors. A faithful simulation of organs is extremely important to improve the accuracy of medical virtual systems, as of the human body and of computational surgical simulators and robotic surgery. In this work, several algorithms of image segmentation are evaluated on ultrasound images acquired from female pelvic cavity.

1 INTRODUCTION

The pelvic floor constitutes the caudal border of the human's visceral cavity. It is characterized by a very complex morphology, mainly because different functional systems join in this region (Goldman & Vasavada 2007). A clear understanding of the pelvic anatomy is crucial for the diagnosis of female pelvic diseases, for female pelvic surgery as well as for fundamental mechanisms of urogenital dysfunction and treatment. Once knowing the more frequent pathologies, the analysis will be possible if an element does not match the "standard ones".

Pelvic floor disorders are highly prevalent diseases that affect women of different ages. Urinary incontinence is the most well-known of these dysfunctions. Stress urinary incontinence (SUI) affects 6 to 33% of the female population and, although not life-threatening, can severely compromise quality of life as well as impose a financial burden on the health care system (Rahmanian et al., 2008). Modern imaging techniques have been used in the diagnosis of pelvic floor disorders, as well as in determining the extent of pelvic diseases or the staging of pelvic tumors.

Diagnostic imaging is an invaluable tool in medicine. Magnetic resonance imaging (MRI), computed tomography (CT), Ultrasonography, digital mammography, and other imaging modalities provide effective means for noninvasively mapping the anatomy of a subject. These technologies have greatly increased knowledge of normal and diseased anatomy for medical research and are a critical component in diagnosis and treatment planning, allowing the medical research and the society to evolve.

In Computational Vision, segmentation refers to the process of partitioning a digital image into multiple sets of pixels, with respect to some characteristics such as intensity or texture. The goal of segmentation is to simplify and/or change the representation of an image into a form that is more meaningful and easier to analyze. Image segmentation is typically used to locate objects or structures (i.e., lines, curves, regions, etc.) in images.

The continuous growing size and number of medical images have triggered an increased need to use computers to ease processing and analysis. In particular, computational algorithms for the delineation of anatomical structures and other regions of interest are becoming increasingly important. In medical imaging, the segmentation process is the separation between anatomical regions or the classification between pathological and non-pathological sets of locations (Suri et al., 2005). These image segmentation algorithms play an essential role in numerous biomedical-imaging applications, such as the quantification of tissue volumes, identification of pathologies, assisting medical diagnosis, treatment planning and computer-integrated surgery.

In this paper, a review on image segmentation algorithms is presented. Hence, the algorithms are classified based on their principal features into three types: 1) threshold-based, 2) clustering-based and 3) deformable models-based (Bankman 2000; Ma et al., 2010). Additionally, the common features of each class are emphasized, discussed and summarized, including their advantages and disadvantages, and their employment on ultrasound images from the female pelvic cavity.

2 SEGMENTATION ALGORITHMS

2.1 *Threshold algorithms*

Global thresholding is simple and computationally fast. It is based on the assumption that the image has a bimodal histogram and, consequently, the structure of interest can be extracted from the background by a simple operation that compares image values with a threshold value T. Let suppose that there is an image $f(x, y)$ with a histogram containing two groups with different intensities, separated by T The threshold image g(x, y) is defined as:

$$g(x, y) = \begin{cases} 1 & if \ (x, y) > T \\ 0 & if \ (x, y) \leq T \end{cases} \qquad (1)$$

As a result, a binary image is obtained, with white pixels representing the structure and black pixels corresponding to the scene background (Figure 1).

There are many ways to select the value used in the global threshold process. However, frequently,

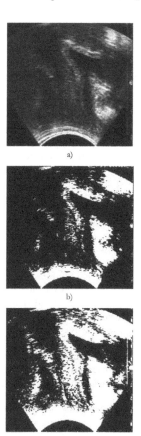

a)

b)

c)

Figure 1. Pelvic ultrasound image a); Result after applying a threshold value of 0.32 b); Result after applying a threshold value of 0.17 c).

a suitable value cannot be found from the histogram, or a single threshold value cannot give good segmentation results over an entire image. For example, when the intensity distribution of the background is not homogeneous and its contrast with the structures varies across the image, a case that often happens on medical images. In those cases, threshold may work well in some parts of the image, but not in other areas. A solution is to apply local thresholding, which can be determined by splitting an image into sub-images and calculating global thresholds for each one of those sub-images. Another approach to determine the local threshold values is by examining the image intensities of the neighboring pixels and selecting a threshold as the mean value of the local intensity distribution (or other statistics, such as mean plus standard deviation, mean of the maximum and minimum values or others based on local intensity gradient magnitude) (Bankman 2000).

Based on the information used to define the local threshold values, the segmentation algorithms can be classified as: region-based, edge-based or hybrid.

2.1.1 *Region-based algorithms*

The idea of region-based algorithms comes from the observation that quantifiable features inside a structure tend to be homogeneous. For example, a simple approach can be to choose a pixel, or group of pixels (called seeds) and merge their neighbor pixels whose intensities are within the threshold values until all the intensities of the surrounded pixels are outside the pre-defined ranges (Bankman 2000). If two adjacent pixels are similar, merge them into a single region. If two neighboring regions are collectively alike enough, merge them, likewise. This collective similarity is usually based on the comparisons between the statistics of the regions.

The selection of similarity criteria depends not only on the problem under consideration, but also on the type of image data available, for example, if the image is in grayscale or color (Gonzalez et al., 2003). Eventually, this method will converge when no further merging are possible (Suri et al., 2005).

The advantage of region growing-based approaches is the ability to correctly segmenting regions that have the equivalent properties and are spatially separated, generating connected regions (Bankman 2000). On the other hand, the primary disadvantage is that manual interaction to obtain the seed point is usually required. Thus, for each region that needs to be extracted, a seed must be defined, and different initial seeds can generate dissimilar segmentations on the same image (Suri et al., 2005).

An application of this type of approach to segment magnetic resonance images from the pelvic cavity can be seen in (Pasquier et al., 2007).

2.1.2 Edge-based algorithms

An edge (or contour) is the border between two regions with distinct properties in an image. Its detection is made by determining the points where the pixel intensity abruptly varies, since sudden changes in images usually reflect important events on the scene (like the transition between object/ background or changes on material properties). As such, an edge is defined by the local pixel intensity gradient, which is an approximation of the first-order derivative of the image function. For a given image $f(x, y)$, the magnitude of the gradient can be obtained as:

$$|G| = \sqrt{[Gx^2 + Gy^2]} = \sqrt{\left[\left(\frac{\partial f}{\partial x}\right)^2 + \left(\frac{\partial f}{\partial y}\right)^2\right]}, \qquad (2)$$

and the direction of the gradient as:

$$D = \tan^{-1}\left(\frac{G_y}{G_x}\right), \qquad (3)$$

where Gx and Gy denote the gradient in the directions x and y, respectively. Some of the most well-known algorithms of this type include the Sobel, Laplacian (Davis 1975) and Canny's edge detectors (Canny 1986), Figure 2.

An advantage of these methods is the fact that they are computationally fast and do not require priori information about the image. On the other hand, edge detection methods are very sensitive to noise and usually cannot correctly segment the entire image, causing discontinuous lines (Bankman 2000). For this reason, other image processing techniques are needed after the edges detection (Ma et al., 2010).

2.1.3 Hybrid algorithms

Hybrid segmentation algorithms combine different image clues to perform the segmentation. Typical examples are the watershed algorithms (Beucher & Lantuéjoul 1979), (Vincent & Soille 2001; Hamarneh & Li 2009), which combine edge-based with region-based approaches. There are several watershed algorithms, but they all use the same basic concept: A grey-level image is "seen" as a topographic relief, where the grey level of a pixel is interpreted as its altitude in the relief. A drop of water falling on a topographic relief flows along a path to finally reach a local minimum. Intuitively, the watershed of a relief corresponds to the limits of the adjacent catchment basins of the drops of water.

In image processing, different watershed lines may be computed. In graphs, some may be defined on the nodes, on the edges, or hybrid lines on both nodes and edges (Körbes & Lotufo 2010).

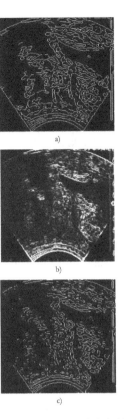

a)

b)

c)

Figure 2. Results of the Canny a), Sobel b) and Laplacian c) edge detectors applied on the image of Figure 1a.

These algorithms can present very good results, since they combine different information of the original image. However, the result of the watershed transform is degraded by the background noise and often produces over-segmentations. (Ma et al., 2010).

2.2 Algorithms based on clustering techniques

As structures in medical images can be treated as patterns, techniques from pattern recognition fields can be used to perform the segmentation. Two main types of these techniques are: supervised classification algorithms and unsupervised classification algorithms. These can be supervised if samples of each area to be classified are provided, so that the system "knows" a priori what the regions are, or unsupervised, if we allow the system to try to find which are the different kind of areas by itself (Suri et al., 2005).

Examples of supervised classification techniques include k-nearest neighbour (kNN) classifiers (Vrooman et al., 2006), maximum likelihood (ML) algorithms (Sarti et al., 2005), supervised artificial neural networks (ANN) (James 1985), support vector machines (SVM) (Cortes et al., 1995), active shape models (ASM) (Cootes et al., 1992), and active appearance models (AAM) (Cootes et al., 1992). A training set is needed to extract structure information and its definition is different among distinct algorithms.

Unsupervised clustering techniques include the *fuzzy K-means* (FKM) (Jacobs et al., 2000), the ISODATA (Ball et al., 1967) and the *unsupervised neural networks* (Bankman 2000).

Algorithms based on clustering techniques can be applied to segment the *levator ani* muscles (Ma et al., 2010).

2.3 Algorithms based on deformable models

Image segmentation (2D, 3D or 4D) based on deformable models has been considered one of the main successes in Computational Vision, over the last decades, mainly on the medical imaging field (Silva et al., 2004).

Compared with the two classes previously described, the ones based on deformable models are more flexible and can be used for more complex segmentations (Ma et al., 2010). These algorithms treat the structure boundary as the final status of the initial chosen contours.

Deformable models are geometrically or parametrically defined curves or surfaces that move under the influence of forces, which have two components: internal and external forces (Suri et al., 2005). Hence, these algorithms can be viewed as the deformation of an initial contour as a curve evolution that moves towards the boundaries of the structures (Silva et al., 2004).

The mathematical fundaments of this type of models can be found, for example, in (Bankman 2000) and (Xu et al., 1999).

2.3.1 Parametrical deformable models

Parametric deformable models, or active contours (being the most well-known the snake model), are a special case of a more general formulation that tries to adjust a deformable model to a contour in an image by using an energy minimizing formulation. Typically, the user initializes the snake near the wanted contour, and then it is driven towards an appropriate result (Silva et al., 2004).

The original mathematical formulation of the snakes can be found in (Kass et al., 1988). The segmentation process is defined as the evolution of the modeled curves that flow under the influence of internal forces, which keeps the model smooth during the deformation, and external forces that force the moving contours towards the borders.

A snake can be defined parametrically as $v(i) = [x(i), y(i)$, where $x(i)$ and $y(i)$ are the coordinates

x, y along the contour. The energy function to minimize can be described as (Suri et al., 2005):

$$E_{snake} = \sum_{i=1}^{N} [E_{int}(i) + E_{ext}(i)], \qquad (4)$$

where E_{int} and E_{ext} represent the internal and the external energies, and N is the total number of points of the snake.

The internal energy can be defined as:

$$E_{int}(i) = \propto_i \| v_i - v_{i-1} \|^2 + \beta_i \| v_{i-1} - 2v_i + v_{i+1} \|^2, \qquad (5)$$

where α_i and β_i specify the stiffness and the flexibility of the snake. These models are called "active" due to its dynamic (Kass et al., 1988), allowing not only the detection of boundaries but also the tracking of its movement, which can be extremely helpful to study the pelvic cavity (Rahmanian et al., 2008). A disadvantage of this method is its weak application to structures with great bends. There are several snake algorithms, like the one proposed in (Jr. et al., 1999). An example of its application to pelvic cavity ultrasound images can be seen in Figure 3.

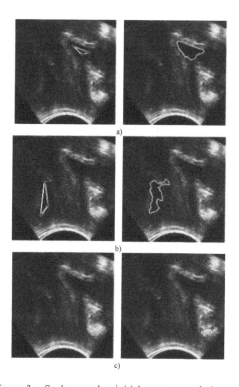

Figure 3. Snakes results: initial contour and the segmented bladder a); Initial contour and the segmented anal-rectal junction b); Initial contour and the segmented symphysis pubis c).

2.3.2 *Geometrical deformable models*

Geometric deformable models provide a solution to address the primary limitations of parametric deformable models. These models are based on the level set method (Osher & Sethian 1988) that was initially proposed to handle topological changes during the curve evolution. The main idea of the level set method is to implicitly embed the moving contour into a higher dimensional level set function and view the contour as its zero level set. Then, instead of tracking the discrete contour points, one can track the zero level set of the level set function (Ma et al., 2010). Examples can be found, for example, in (Malladi et al., 1993; Chan & Vese 2001).

The proficiency of adaptation to changes in the topology can be useful in many applications. However, sometimes it can lead to undesirable results, producing segmentations not consistent with the structure to be segmented. The level set methods have been commonly applied on medical images (Jayadevappa et al., 2009), (Schmid & Magnenat-Thalmann 2008), (Ma et al., 2011). An example can be seen in Figure 4, where the Chan-Vese's model was used to segment several organs in ultrasound images from the pelvic cavity.

3 CONCLUSIONS

The growing significance of medical imaging to diagnose and treat health problems or diseases has brought along a set of challenges to accurately segment anatomical structures from medical images. Segmentation on medical images is affected by many factors, like the size of the data involved, the complexity and variability of the structures to segment, and others, inherent to limitations from the information used.

There are a great number of image segmentation algorithms, and many of them have some kind of application to the medical field. However, the deformable models, namely the snakes and the level set methods, are the more complete ones, and the ones that usually provide best segmentation results.

The study in this area continues, looking for algorithms that are more robust to the influence of noise and initialization conditions, and can offer an entirely automatic segmentation, without manual intervention, particularly designed for the structures of the pelvic cavity in ultrasound images.

ACKNOWLEDGEMENTS

This work was partially done in the scope of the projects "Methodologies to Analyze Organs from Complex Medical Images—Applications to Female Pelvic Cavity", "Aberrant Crypt Foci and Human Colorectal Polyps: mathematical modeling and endoscopic image processing" and "Cardiovascular Imaging Modeling and Simulation—SIMCARD", with references PTDC/EEA-CRO/103320/2008, UTAustin/MAT/0009/2008 and UTAustin/CA/0047/2008, respectively, financially supported by Fundação para a Ciência e a Tecnologia (FCT), in Portugal.

The second author would like to thank FCT for his PhD grant with reference SFRH/BD/43768/2008.

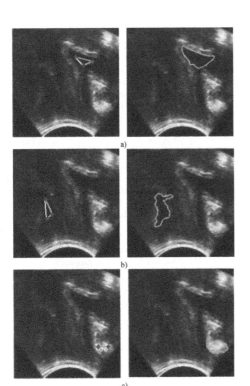

a)

b)

c)

Figure 4. Results of the Chan-Vese's model: Initial contour and the segmented bladder a); Initial contour and the segmented anal-rectal junction b); Initial contour and the segmented *symphysis* pubis c).

REFERENCES

Ball, G.H. & Hall, D.J. 1967. A clustering technique for summarizing multi-variate data. *Behavioral Science* 12 (2):153–155.
Bankman, I.N. ed. 2000. *Handbook Medical Imaging Processing Analysis.* San Diego/London: Academic Press.

Beucher, S. & Lantuéjoul, C. 1979. Use of watersheds in contour detection. *International Workshop on Image Processing, Real-Time Edge and Motion Detection/ Estimation*, at Renne.

Canny, J. 1986. A computational approach to edge detection. *IEEE Trans Pattern Anal Mach Intell* 8 (6):679–698.

Chan, T.F. & Vese, L.A. 2001. Active contour without edges. *IEEE Trans Image Process* 10:266–277.

Cootes, T.F., Taylor, C.J., Cooper, D.H. & Graham, J. 1992. Training models of shape from sets of examples. *British Machine Vision Conference*.

Cortes, C. & Vapnik, V. 1995. Support-vector networks. *Machine Learning* 20 (3):273–297.

Davis, L.S. 1975. A survey of edge detection techniques. *Computer Graphics and Image Processing* 4 (3):248–270.

Goldman, H.B. & Vasavada, S.P. 2007. *Female Urology— A practical clinical guide*. New Jersey: Human Press.

Gonzalez, R.C., Woods, R.E. & Eddins, S.L. 2003. *Digital Image Processing Using MATLAB*. New Jersey: Prentice-Hall.

Hamarneh, G. & Li, X.X. 2009. Watershed segmentation using prior shape and appearance knowledge. *Image Vis Comput* 27 (1):59–68.

Jacobs, M.A., RA, R.A.K., Soltanian-Zadeh, H., ZG, Z.G.Z., Goussev, A.V., Peck, D.J., Windham, J.P. & Chopp, M. 2000. Unsupervised segmentation of multiparameter MRI in experimental cerebral ischemia with comparison to T2, diffusion, and ADC MRI parameters and histopathological validation. *JMRI* 11 (4):425–437.

James, M. 1985. *Classification algorithms*. NY: Wiley-Interscience.

Jayadevappa, D., Kumar, S.S. & Murty, D.S. 2009. A New Deformable Model Based on Level Sets for Medical Image Segmentation. *IAENG International Journal of Computer Science* 36 (3).

Jr., A.Y., Andy, A. & Willsky, A. 1999. Seventh IEEE International Conference on Computer Vision.

Kass, M., Witkin, A. & Terzopoulos, D. 1988. Snakes: Active Contour Models. *International Journal of Computer Vision*:321–331.

Körbes, A. & Lotufo, R.A. 2010. Análise de Algoritmos da Transformada Watershed. *17th International Conference on Systems, Signals and Image Processing*.

Ma, Z., Jorge, R.N., Mascarenhas, T. & Tavares, J.M.R.S. 2010. A review of algorithms for medical image segmentation and their applications to the female pelvic cavity. *Computer Methods in Biomechanics and Biomedical Engineering* 13 (2):235–246.

Ma, Z., Jorge, R.N., Mascarenhas, T. & Tavares, J.M.R.S. 2011. Using Deformable Models to Segment Bladder Wall in Magnetic Resonance Images. *Annals of Biomedical Engineering* 39 (8):2287–2297.

Malladi, R., Sethian, J.A. & Vemuri, B. 1993. A topology independent shape modeling scheme. *SPIE—Conference on Geometric Methods in Computer Vision*.

Osher, S. & Sethian, J.A. 1988. Fronts Propagation with Curvature Dependent Speed: Algorithms Based on Hamilton-Jacobi Formulations. *Journal of Computational Physics* 79:12–49.

Pasquier, D., Lacorniere, T., Vermandel, M., Rousseau, J., Lartigau, E. & Betrouni, N. 2007. Automatic Segmentation of Pelvic Structures from Magnetic Ressonance Images for Prostate Cancer Radiotherapy. *International Journal of Radiation Oncology Biol. Phys* 68 (2):592–600.

Rahmanian, S., Jones, R., Peng, Q. & Constantinou, C.E. 2008. Visualization of Biomechanical Properties of Female Pelvic Floor Function Using Video Motion Tracking of Ultrasound Imaging. *Studies in Health Technology and Informatics*:132:390–395.

Sarti, A., Corsi, C., Mazzini, E. & Lamberti, C. 2005. Maximum likehood segmentation of ultrasound images with Rayleigh distribution. *IEEE Trans Ultrasoun Ferroelect Freq Control* 52 (6):947–960.

Schmid, J. & Magnenat-Thalmann, N. 2008. MRI Bone Segmentation Using Deformable Models and Shape Priors. *Medical Image Computing and computer-assisted intervention: MICCAI*, at New York.

Silva, J.S., Santos, B.S., Silva, A. & Madeira, J. 2004. Modelos Deformáveis na Segmentação de Imagens Médicas: uma introdução. *Revista do DETUA* 4 (3).

Suri, J., Wilson, D.L. & Laxminarayan, S., eds. 2005. *Handbook of Biomedical Image Analysis*. Vol. 2. New York: Kluwer Academic/ Plenum Publishers.

Vincent, L. & Soille, P. 2001. Watersheds in digital spaces: an efficient algorithm based on immersion simulations. *IEEE Trans Pattern Anal Mach Intell* 13 (6):583–598.

Vrooman, H.A., CA, C.A.C., Stokking, R., Arfan, I.M., Vemooij, M.W., Breteler, M.M. & Niessen, W.J. 2006. kNN-based multi-spectral MRI brain tissue classification: manual training versus automated atlas-based training. *SPIE Medical Imaging*.

Xu, C., Pham, D.L. & Prince, J.L. 1999. Image Segmentation Using Deformable Models. *SPIE: The International Society for Optical Engineering*.

116

Computational Vision and Medical Image Processing – Tavares & Natal Jorge (eds)
© 2012 Taylor & Francis Group, London, ISBN 978-0-415-68395-1

Image segmentation algorithms and their use on doppler images

Tatiana D.C.A. Silva, Zhen Ma & João Manuel R.S. Tavares
Faculdade de Engenharia da Universidade do Porto (FEUP)/Instituto de Engenharia Mecânica e Gestão Industrial (INEGI), Porto, Portugal

ABSTRACT: This paper aims to make a review on current segmentation algorithms used for medical images. Image segmentation algorithms can be classified according to their methodologies, namely the ones based on thresholds, clustering, and deformable models. Each type of algorithms is discussed as well as their main application fields identified; additionally, the advantages and disadvantages of each type are pointed out. Experiments that apply the algorithms to segment Doppler images are presented to further evaluate their behaviour.

1 INTRODUCTION

The main goal of this paper is to present and discuss methods for image segmentation suitable for the construction of geometric models of cardiovascular structures from medical images, appropriate for biomechanical studies.

Detection, localization, diagnostic, staging and monitoring treatment responses are the most important aspects and crucial procedures in diagnostic medicine and clinical oncology (Suri et al., 2005). In the last decades, there were significant advances in medical imaging and computer-aided medical image analysis. Both recent multidimensional medical imaging modalities and computing power have opened new insights in medical research and clinical diagnosis.

In the majority of the developed countries, cardiovascular diseases such as heart attack and cerebral infarction are the most common death causes. Cardiac imaging is an established approach to diagnose cardiovascular disease and plays an important role in its interventional treatment (Bankman 2000; Suri et al., 2005). While cardiac imaging capabilities are developing rapidly, the images are mostly analyzed qualitatively. The ability to quantitatively analyze the acquired image data is still not satisfactorily available in routine clinical care (Himeno 2003; Quarteroni et al., 2000; Taylor et al., 1996). A large part of the acquired data is not totally used because of the tedious and time-consuming characteristics of manual analysis (Mitchell et al., 2002).

Thanks to the new technologies of medical imaging data acquisition, such as computed tomography (CT), angiography, magnetic resonance imaging (MRI) and ultrasound (Doppler), it has become possible the construction of three dimensional models of blood vessels. However, these models still need manual interventions to attain high-quality models (Unal et al., 2008; Guerrero et al., 2007).

Image processing techniques can improve and enhance the information contained in the original images. Additionally, image analysis techniques, such as image segmentation, have a crucial role in extracting high-level information from the processed images. Regarding image segmentation, it plays an essential part in the extraction of useful information and attributes from medical images. Hence, it is a key task for understanding, analyses and interpretation of the image represented structures.

Non-invasive ultrasound imaging of human arteries is a widely used form of medical diagnosis of arterial diseases, like atherosclerosis (a disease of blood vessels caused by the formation of plaques inside the arteries). The diagnosis of atherosclerosis is one of the most important medical examinations for the prevention of cardiovascular events, like myocardial infarction and stroke. Since the carotid is a superficial artery, it is suited for medical ultrasound. B-mode images are user dependent and have poor quality due to some degrading factors such as: speckle, echo shadows, attenuation, low contrast and movement artifacts. However, this technique has lower cost and smaller risks to the patient, when compared to the other alternatives already mentioned. Due to the variability of the carotid shape and the possible existence of extensive occlusions, most of the known model-based segmentation techniques are inadequate (Rocha et al., 2010). This was one motivation for the search of segmentation algorithms.

The main goal of segmentation is to divide the original image into homogeneous regions (or classes) according to one or more characteristics (Ma et al., 2010; Withey et al., 2007). Each of the regions can be separately processed for information extraction. The most obvious application of this technique in medical imaging is anatomical localization, or in generic terms, region of interest delineation, whose main aim is to outline anatomic structures and regions of interest (Suri et al., 2005).

There are a large number of segmentation techniques that have been proposed, but there is still no gold standard approach that satisfies all of the segmentation criteria. In general, image segmentation techniques can be divided into three main classes: Thresholding-based, Clustering and Deformable Models (Withey & Koles 2007; Ma et al., 2010). These techniques are commonly employed in two-dimensional image segmentation. A review of each of these techniques will be presented in this paper as well as the discussions on their advantages and disadvantages when applied on Doppler images.

2 SEGMENTATION ALGORITHMS

2.1 *Algorithms based on thresholding*

Thresholding is a common segmentation technique because of its simplicity in implementation and intuitive properties. In this technique, predefined values (thresholds) are selected, and an image is divided into groups of pixels having values within the ranges defined by the thresholds and groups of pixels with values beyond such range.

There are several threshold algorithms. The most intuitive approach is the global thresholding, which is best suited for bimodal image. When only one threshold value is selected for the entire image, based on the image histogram, the thresholding is called global. If the threshold depends on local image properties, for example, the local average gray value, the thresholding is called local. If the thresholds are selected independently for each pixel or groups of pixels, then the thresholding is called dynamic or adaptive.

Global thresholding is based on the assumption that the image has a bimodal histogram; therefore, the structure can be extracted from the background by a simple operation that compares image values with a threshold value T. Suppose an image $f(x, y)$ with the histogram with two groups of intensities separated by T. The thresholded image $g(x, y)$ is defined as:

$$g(x,y) = \begin{cases} 1 & if \quad f(x,y) \geq T \\ 0 & if \quad f(x,y) \leq T. \end{cases} \quad (1)$$

As such, the result of thresholding is a binary image, where pixels with intensity value of 1 (one) correspond to structures, while pixels with value 0 (zero) correspond to the scene background. Otsu's method (Otsu 1979) obtains the threshold values automatically by choosing the ones that can minimize the intra-class variance, based on the image histogram, Figure 1.

Global thresholding is simple and computationally fast. It performs well if the intensity contrast between the structures and the background is high. However, it may fail when two or more structures have overlapping intensity levels and it may not lead by itself fully automatic. The accuracy of the resulting structures is also not guaranteed as they are separated from the image based on a single threshold value. Threshold selection becomes more difficult with the increasing number of regions or noise, or when the contrast of the image is low.

When the image background is not constant and the contrast of structures varies on the image, global thresholding may not work well in some areas. If the background variations can be described by a known function of position in the image, one could attempt to correct it by using gray level correction techniques, after which a single threshold should work for the entire image. Another

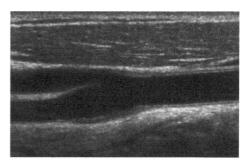

(a)

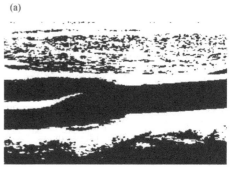

(b)

Figure 1. Image of carotid bifurcation obtained by Doppler (a) and the result of Otsu's method on such image (b).

solution is to apply local thresholding that can be determined by:

1. Splitting the input image into sub-images and calculating thresholds for each sub-image; or
2. Examining the image intensities in the neighborhood of each pixel.

In the first method, an image is divided into rectangular overlapping sub-images and the histograms are calculated for each of them. The sub-images used should be large enough to include both structures and background pixels. If the sub-image has a bimodal histogram, the local threshold should be the minimum between the histogram peaks. If the histogram is unimodal, then the threshold should be calculated by interpolation from the local thresholds found for nearby sub-images. In the end, a second interpolation is used to find the correct thresholds at each pixel. In the second method, the threshold is selected using the mean value of the local intensity distribution.

Local thresholding is computationally more expensive than global thresholding. It is very useful for segmenting structures from a varying background, and for extraction of regions that are very small and sparse.

According to the information used to define the threshold values, algorithms can be further classified as edge-based, region-based and hybrid ones.

2.1.1 *Edge-base segmentation*

An edge can be briefly described as a collection of connected pixels that lie on the boundary between two homogeneous regions having different intensities; i.e., edges can be defined as abrupt changes in pixel intensity that can be reflected by the gradient information. A gradient is an approximation of the first-order derivative of the image function. For a given image $f(x,y)$, it is possible to calculate the magnitude of the gradient as:

$$|G| = \sqrt{G_x^2 + G_y^2} = \sqrt{\left[\left(\frac{\partial f}{\partial x}\right)^2 + \left(\frac{\partial f}{\partial y}\right)^2\right]}, \qquad (2)$$

and the direction of the gradient as:

$$D = \tan^{-1}\left(\frac{G_y}{G_x}\right), \qquad (3)$$

where G_x and G_y are gradients in directions x and y, respectively.

Some know algorithms of this class are gradient operators, like Sobel, Laplacian and Canny operators (Ma et al., 2010). Laplacian edge detector uses the second derivation information of the image intensity, and both Canny and Sobel edge

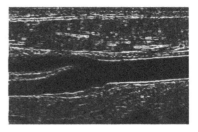

(a)

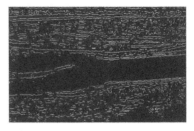

(b)

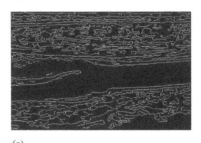

(c)

Figure 2. Results of Sobel (a), Canny (b) and Laplacian (c) edges detectors applied on the image of Figure 1a.

detectors use the gradient magnitude to find the potential edge pixels and suppresses them through non-maximal suppression and hysteresis thresholding.

Edge-based techniques are computationally fast and do not require a *priori* information about the image contents. A usual problem of these techniques is that often the edges do not enclose the structures completely. To avoid this problem, a postprocessing step of linking or grouping the detected edges that correspond to the structures' boundaries is needed. However, in general, edge linking is computationally expensive and not very reliable.

Results of Sobel, Canny and Laplacian edges detectors can be seen in Figure 2.

2.2 *Region based segmentation*

Region-based segmentation approaches examine pixels in an image and build disjoint regions by merging neighborhood pixels with homogeneous properties based on a predefined similarity criterion.

The simplest region-based segmentation technique is called *region growing*, and it is used to extract a connected region of similar pixels from an image. This technique starts with a pixel or group of pixels called *seed(s)*, which belongs to the structure of interest. Seeds can be chosen by the operator or determined by an automatic seed finding algorithm. Then, the neighboring pixels of each seed are inspected and the ones with properties similar enough to the seed are added to the region that the seed belongs to, and thus, the region is growing and its shape is also changing. The procedure continues until no more pixels can be added. It is possible that some image pixels may remain unlabeled when the growing process stops.

The results of region growing depend strongly on the selection of the homogeneity criterion. If it is not properly chosen, the regions leak out into adjoining areas and merge with regions that do not belong to the structure of interest. Another problem of region growing is that different starting points, i.e., seeds, may not grow into identical regions.

The advantage of region growing is that it enables the correct segmentation of regions that have the similar properties and are spatially separated, and also the building of connected regions.

The resultant segmentation of an image of carotid bifurcation by using a region growing algorithm can be seen in Figure 3

2.2.1 *Hybrid algorithms*
Hybrid segmentation algorithms combine different image properties to achieve the segmentation. Watershed is a region based technique that uses image morphology (Bankman 2000), and it has been a powerful tool for image segmentation. The basic concept of watershed is that a grey-level image may be seen as a topographic relief, where the grey level of a pixel is interpreted as its altitude in the relief. A drop of water falling on a topographic relief flows along a path to finally reach a local minimum. Intuitively, the watershed of a relief corresponds to the limits of the adjacent catchment basins of the drops of water.

The common watershed algorithm needs at least one marker ("seed" point) interior to each structure of the image, including the background as a separate structure. The operator is responsible by the manual selection of the markers or it can also be selected by an automatic seed finding algorithm. The neighboring pixels of each seed are inspected and the ones with properties similar enough to the seed are added to the corresponding region where the seed is, and therefore, the region is growing and its shape is also changing. The growing process is repeated until no pixel can be added to any region.

Due to the combination of diverse image clues, watershed algorithms can achieve satisfied results and always produce a complete segmentation of an image. However, watershed algorithms tend to present over-segmentation problems, especially when the images are noisy or the desired structures have low signal-to-noise ratio appearances.

2.3 *Clustering algorithms*

Clustering is the process of grouping similar image structures into a single cluster, while structures with dissimilar features are grouped into different clusters based on some similarity criteria. The similarity is quantified in terms of an appropriate distance measure.

Clustering techniques can be divided into two main classes: supervised and unsupervised.

Supervised clustering techniques need a training set to be efficient. They need predefined images with the structures of interest already segmented. With this training, there is an adaptation and these predefined images will be a prototype image. Afterwards, the prototype is overlapped to the image to be segmented. These techniques include k-nearest neighbor (kNN) (Vrooman et al., 2006), maximum likelihood (ML) algorithms (Sarti et al., 2005), supervised artificial neural networks (ANN) (James 1985), support vector machines (SVM) (Cortes et al., 1995), active shape models (ASM) (Cootes et al., 1992) and active appearance models (AAM) (Cootes et al., 1992).

Unsupervised classification techniques are also called clustering algorithms and, with these techniques, the structure features are extracted from the classified points. The system finds by himself the different structures to be segmented. Unsupervised classification includes fuzzy C-means algorithms (FCM) (Jacobs et al., 2000), iterative self-organizing data analysis technique algorithms (ISODATA) (Ball et al., 1967) and unsupervised neural networks (Bankman 2000).

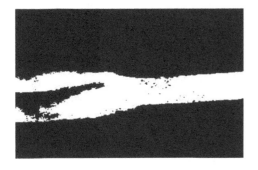

Figure 3.   Result of a region growing algorithm on the image of carotid bifurcation shown in Figure 1a.

2.4 Algorithms based on deformable models

Deformable models are segmentation techniques that are able to represent the complex shape and broad shape variability of anatomical structures. Deformable models overcome many of the limitations of traditional low-level image techniques, by providing compact and analytical representations of structures, by incorporating anatomical knowledge and by providing interactive capabilities.

Deformable models can be parametrically or geometrically defined, according to the way used to track the moving contours.

2.4.1 Parametrical deformable models

Parametric deformable models, or active contours, try to adjust a deformable model to an image by using an energy minimizing formulation. The snakes are the most well-known method in this category. The user starts the snake near the border of the structure of interest and it is driven to an appropriate result. However, the snake can get stuck in a place of local minimal solutions caused, for example, by noise or a wrong starting solution (Bankman 2000). After incorporating the deformable curve to an energy function, the optimization of the energy functional segmentation process is needed, led by an energy minimization of the contour, which makes the deformable curve evolve gradually from the initial contour to the desired limit of the structure. The energy function contains two parts: internal energy E_{int} and external energy E_{ext}.

Generally, the internal energy E_{int} only imposes restrictions on the smoothness of the curve, such as the behaviour of the elasticity and curvature, while the external energy E_{ext} is responsible for "pulling" the curve of the Snake in the direction of the boundaries of the structure to be segmented (Xu et al., 1999). These two energies are usually added to form an energy functional, which can be minimized by deforming the contour in an optimization process:

$$E_{Snake} = \sum_{i=1}^{N} \left[E_{int}(i) + E_{ext}(i) \right], \qquad (4)$$

$$E_{int}(i) = \alpha i \parallel v_i - v_{i-1} \parallel^2 + \beta i \parallel v_{i-1} - 2v_i + v_{i+1} \parallel^2, \qquad (5)$$

where α_i and β_i specify the stiffness and the flexibility of the snake, and N is the number of points.

A segmentation example obtained using a snake algorithm can be seen in Figure 4.

2.4.2 Geometrical deformable models

Geometric deformable models are based on the level set method, which was proposed to handle topological changes during the curve evolution. The main idea of the level set method is

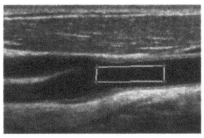

(a)

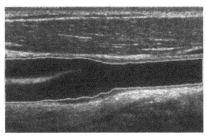
(b)

Figure 4. Initial contour used (a) with Yessi's algorithm (Snake) applied on an image of a carotid bifurcation (b).

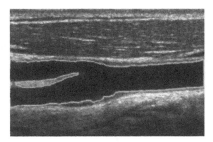

Figure 5. Result of the Chan-Vese's model on the image of a carotid bifurcation, with an initial contour similar to the one shown in Figure 4(a).

to implicitly embed the moving contour into a higher-dimensional level set function and view the contour as its zero level set (Osher et al., 1988). Then, instead of tracking the discrete contour points, one can track the zero level set of the level set function. The proficiency of adaptation to changes in the topology can be useful in many applications. A segmentation example can be seen in Figure 5, where the Chan-Vese's model was used to segment the carotid bifurcation in a Doppler image.

3 CONCLUSIONS

Most segmentation algorithms combine several techniques of image processing to improve their performances. For this reason, there is no universal classification on segmentation algorithm. In this paper, segmentation algorithms were classified into three categories, and their main characteristics were reviewed. Deformable models, namely the snakes and the level set methods, are the more complete ones, and the ones that provided better segmentation results in the Doppler images used.

Computerized segmentation methods have demonstrated their useful applications in medical image analysis and used for better understanding, diagnosis and treatment of disorders.

Research in this area remains active, while pursuing segmentation algorithms that are more robust to noise and initialization problems, as well as other factors that may prevent a successful segmentation.

Future research on the segmentation of medical images will be targeted to improve the accuracy, precision and computational speed of segmentation methods, as well as reduce the amount of the manual interaction required.

ACKNOWLEDGEMENTS

This work was partially done in the scope of the projects "Methodologies to Analyze Organs from Complex Medical Images—Applications to Female Pelvic Cavity", "Aberrant Crypt Foci and Human Colorectal Polyps: mathematical modeling and endoscopic image processing", "Cardiovascular Imaging Modeling and Simulation—SIMCARD" and "Blood flow simulation in arterial networks towards application at hospital", with references PTDC/EEA-CRO/103320/2008, TAustin/MAT/0009/2008, TAustin/CA/0047/2008 and PTDC/SAU-BEB/102547/2008, respectively, financially supported by Fundação para a Ciência e a Tecnologia (FCT), in Portugal.

The second author would like to thank FCT for his PhD grant with reference SFRH/BD/43768/2008.

REFERENCES

Ball, G.H. & Hall, D.J. 1967. A clustering technique for summarizing multi-variate data. *Behavioral Science* 12 (2):153–155.

Bankman, I.N. 2000. *Handbook of Medical Imaging*. Vol. II. San Diego/ London: Academic Press.

Cootes, T.F., Taylor, C.J., Cooper, D.H. & Graham, J. 1992. Training models of shape from sets of examples. Paper read at British Machine Vision Conference.

Cortes, C. & Vapnik, V. 1995. Support-vector networks. *Machine Learning* 20 (3):273–297.

Guerrero, J., Salcudea, S.E., McEwen, J.A., Masri, B.A. & Nicolaou, S. 2007. Real-Time Vessel Segmentation and Tracking for Ultrasound Imaging Applications. *IEEE Transactions on Medical Imaging* 26 (8):1079–1090.

Himeno, R. 2003. Blood Flow Simulation toward Actual Application at Hospital. *The 5th Asian Computational Fluid Dynamics*.

Jacobs, M.A., RA, R.A.K., Soltanian-Zadeh, H., ZG, Z.G.Z., Goussev, A.V., Peck, D.J., Windham, J.P. & Chopp, M. 2000. Unsupervised segmentation of multiparameter MRI in experimental cerebral ischemia with comparison to T2, diffusion, and ADC MRI parameters and histopathological validation. *JMRI* 11 (4):425–437.

James, M. 1985. *Classification algorithms*. NY: Wiley-Interscience.

Ma, Z., Tavares, J., Jorge, R. & Mascarenhas, T. 2010. A review of algorithms for medical image segmentation and their applications to the female pelvic cavity. *Computer Methods in Biomechanics and Biomedical Engineering* 13 (2):235–246.

Mitchell, S., Bosch, J.G., Lelieveldt, B.P.F., Geest, R.J.v.d., Reiber, J.H.C. & Sonka, M. 2002. 3-D Active Appearance Models: Segmentation of Cardiac MR and Ultrasound Images. *IEEE Transactions on Medical Imaging* 21.

Osher, S. & Sethian, J. 1988. Fronts propagating with curvaturedependent speed: algorithms based on Hamilton-Jacobi formulations. *Journal of Computational Physics* 79 (1):12–49.

Otsu, N. 1979. A threshold selection method from gray-level histrograms. *IEEE Transactions on Systems, Man, and Cybernetics* 9 (1):62–66.

Quarteroni, A. & Veneziani, M. 2000. Computational Vascular Fluid dynamics: problems, models and methods. *Computer and Visualization in Science*.

Rocha, R., Campilho, A., Silva, J., Azevedo, E. & Santos, R. 2010. Segmentation of ultrasound images of the carotid using RANSAC and cubic splines. *Computer Methods and Programs in Biomedicine* 101 (1):94–106.

Sarti, A., Corsi, C., Mazzini, E. & Lamberti, C. 2005. Maximum likehood segmentation of ultrasound images with Rayleigh distribution. *IEEE Trans Ultrasoun Ferroelect Freq Control* 52 (6):947–960.

Suri, J.S., Wilson, D.L. & Laxminarayan, S., eds. 2005. *Handbook of Biomedical Image Analysis*. Vol. 2. New York: Kluwer Academic/ Plenum Publishers.

Taylor, C., Hughes, C. & Zarins, T. 1996. Computational Investigations in Vascular Disease. *Computers Physics* 10 (3):224–232.

Unal, G., Bucher, S., Carlier, S., Slabaugh, G., Fang, T. & Tanaka, K. 2008. Shape-Driven Segmentation of the Arterial Wall in Intravascular Ultrasound Images. *IEEE Transactions on Information Technology in Biomedicine* 3 (12):335–347.

Vrooman, H.A., Cocosco, C.A., Stokking, R., Arfan, I.M., Vemooij, M.W., Breteler, M.M. & Niessen, W.J. 2006. kNN-based multi-spectral MRI brain tissue classification: manual training versus automated atlas-based training. *SPIE Medical Imaging*.

Withey, D.J. & Koles, Z.J. 2007. Medical Image Segmentation: Methods and Software. *International Conference on Functional Biomedical Imaging*:140–143.

Xu, C., Pham, D.L. & Prince, J.L. 1999. Image Segmentation Using Deformable Models (cap. III). *SPIE: The International Society for Optical Engineering*.

Computational Vision and Medical Image Processing – Tavares & Natal Jorge (eds)
© 2012 Taylor & Francis Group, London, ISBN 978-0-415-68395-1

Morphometric and immunohistochemical image analysis in pre-pubertal lamb testes after prenatal betamethasone treatment

G. Pedrana, E. Souza & M.H. Viotti
Facultad de Veterinaria, Montevideo, Uruguay

C. Trouche
Ecole Nationale Vétérinaire de Toulouse, Toulouse, Francia

D. Sloboda
University of Auckland, and the National Research Centre for Growth and Development, Auckland, New Zealand

G.B. Martin
UWA Institute of Agriculture, University of Western Australia, Crawley, Australia

ABSTRACT: Stereological evaluation provides information about morphometric changes that can occur in a tissue of interest. In the present study, we used image analysis to determine the effect of prenatal exposure to betamethasone during the third trimester of gestation on testicular tissue. Apoptotic enzyme immunoexpression and morphometric parameters were quantified in pre-pubertal lamb testes. Image analysis programs were used to calculate% of immunostained area and morphometric parameters. Sex cord diameter (betamethasone $42.0 \pm 0.4\,\mu$m *versus* saline $50.0 \pm 0.4\,\mu$m; $p = 0.001$) and volume density (betamethasone $46.0 \pm 0.9\%$ *versus* saline $49.1 \pm 0.8\%$; $p = 0.01$) were reduced in the betamethasone group. In addition, active caspase-3 immunoexpression also decreased in betamethasone group ($24.2 \pm 0.2\%$ *versus* $23.3 \pm 0.3\%$; $p = 0.01$). The morphometric testicular changes suggest that prenatal betamethasone treatment might influence postnatal development. Decreases in caspase-3 immunoexpression can lead to a reduction in the normal apoptotic process with negative consequences for future spermatogenesis.

1 INTRODUCTION

During fetal life, adverse events can lead to modifications in organ development, perhaps programming disruptions that persist during post-natal life (Rhind, 2004). Glucocorticoids are known to have long-term effects in the offspring (Ward & Weisz, 1980). Synthetic glucocorticoids such as betamethasone are commonly administered to pregnant woman at risk of preterm delivery. This prenatal therapy has positive effects on pulmonary development, improving fetal lung maturation (Liggins & Howie, 1972) and significantly reducing neonatal morbidity and mortality (Ikegami *et al.*, 1997; Alcalde-Herrero, 2006). However, many animal studies have reported short and long term deleterious effects of prenatal glucocorticoid therapy, including growth restriction and a predisposition to cardiovascular and metabolic diseases in postnatal life (Bishop, 1981; Seckl, 2004; Squires, 2006; Nyirenda *et al.*, 1998). Whether long term effects persist in humans, however, is still contentious (Dalziel *et al.*, 2005; De Vries *et al.*, 2008).

In sheep, excessive exposure to prenatal glucocorticoids produces hypertension in the offspring (Dodic *et al.*, 2002; Jensen *et al.*, 2002; Tangalakis *et al.*, 1992) and increased glucocorticoid receptor (GR) mRNA levels in *pars distalis* of the 146-day fetal pituitary gland (Sloboda *et al.*, 2000; 2002). In male rats prenatal administration of corticosterone analogues and ACTH have been shown to reduce testosterone production by Leydig cells (Lalau *et al.*, 1990; Sapolsky, 1985; Page *et al.*, 2001). In addition prenatal betamethasone treatment was associated with decreases in the fetal sex cords length and proliferation of Leydig cells (Pedrana *et al.*, 2008a). In adult rats, dexamethasone administration induces apoptosis in germinal (Yazawa *et al.*, 2000) and Leydig cells (Gao *et al.*, 2002). Apoptosis is a key regulatory process during normal spermatogenesis (Furuchi *et al.*, 1996). It is regulated by the activation of an enzymatic cascade by cysteinyl-aspartate-specific proteases called caspases that causes cellular death (Cooper, 2002; Said *et al.*, 2010). The activation of caspase-3 has been shown to be critical in apoptosis (Kim *et al.*, 2001).

We have previously reported that *in utero* betamethasone exposure increased the levels of key apoptosis-signaling proteins in fetal sheep testis (Pedrana *et al.*, 2008b). In the present study, we investigated long-term effects of *in utero* betamethasone exposure in morphometry and active caspase-3 immunoexpression in Merino lamb testes.

2 MATERIALS AND METHODS

2.1 Animals and prenatal treatments

Experimental procedures were approved by the Animal Experimentation Ethics Committee of the Department of Agriculture of Western Australia. Pregnant Merino ewes bearing singleton male fetus of known gestational age were allocated randomly to receive maternal injections of betamethasone (Celestone Cronodose ®, Schering Plough, Baulkham Hills, NSW, Australia), dose 0.5 mg/kg, n = 6) at 104, 111 and 118 days of gestation (dG) or 5 ml saline (n = 6). All animals were injected intramuscularly with 150 mg medroxyprogesterone acetate (Depo Provera; Upjohn, Rydalmere, NSW, Australia) at 100 dG to reduce pregnancy losses because of subsequent glucocorticoid treatment (Sloboda *et al.*, 2002). After spontaneous delivery male lambs were kept under optimal conditions with ewes until the time of sacrifice. At 90 days old lambs were sedated with ketamine (15 mg/kg) and xylazine (0.1 mg/kg, Troy Laboratories, Smithfield, NSW, Australia) and then killed by decapitation.

2.2 Tissue collection

Testicular tissues were dissected, weighed, fixed in Bouin's solution for 12 hours, dehydrated in increasing concentrations of ethanol (70, 96 and 100%), chloroform, and embedded in paraffin wax. Sections (5 μm) were cut in Leica Reichert Jung Biocut 2030, Wetzlar, Alemania) and mounted on slides.

2.3 Morphological measurements and stereological studies

Stereological studies were performed on haematoxylin and eosin sections and digital images were retrieved with a digital camera (Dino-Eyepiece, AM-423X) connected to a light microscope (Premiere Professional binocular, Model MRP-5000, Manassas, USA). Gonocytes, Leydig and Sertoli cells, sex cords diameter, sex cords and interstitial are were measured using Image J 1.43 m, Wayne Rasband, National Institutes of Health, USA (http://rsb.info.nih.gov/ij). Volume densities (Vv) were determined by using the image area

occupied by sex cords or interstitial tissue with Equation 1:

$$Vv = (An/At)100 \qquad (1)$$

where An = area overlying the tissue component of interest (sex cords or interstitial tissue) and At = is the total image area. Absolute volumes (Av) were estimated using Equation 2:

$$Av = Vv \times \text{testes volume} \qquad (2)$$

where Vv = volume density (of sex cords or interstitial tissue). For morphometric calculations, the specific gravity of testicular tissue (density) was considered to be 1.0 (Russell & Peterson, 1984; Bielli *et al.*, 1999; Franca *et al.*, 2000). Sex cords were assumed to be cylindrical and their lengths were estimated with Equation 3:

$$L = Av/An \qquad (3)$$

where Av = sex cords absolute volume; An = area overlying the sex cords. The total numbers of gonocytes, Leydig and Sertoli cells per testis were estimated using the number of cells counted in 50 transverse cord cross-sections for each animal. Cells were counted when the nucleus was observed in transverse cross-section. The total number of Sertoli cells per testis (TnSc) was calculated using Equation 4:

$$TnSc = Ns \times (L/\text{section thickness}) \qquad (4)$$

where Ns = mean number of Sertoli cells per transverse section of sex cord; L = sex cord length.

2.4 Immunohistochemistry

Sections were deparaffinised (60°C, 15 min and immersion in xilol); rehydrated in ethanol (100, 95, 70%) and immersed in phosphate buffered saline (PBS; pH 7.4). Antigen retrieval was performed in 0.01M citrate buffer (pH 6.0), heated in microwave (100%, 3 min and 40%, 5 min and cooling 20 min). Tissue-specific endogenous peroxidases were inactivated (3% hydrogen peroxide—H_2O_2, 30 min). Slides were washed in PBS and non-specific binding was blocked (10% normal bovine serum, 15 min). Slides were incubated with primary rabbit polyclonal IgG human/mouse anti-active caspase-3 (concentrated, volume 1 ml, dilution 1:100, catalog N° RP096, Diagnostic BioSystem, Pleasanton, USA) in a humidified chamber (18 h at 4°C). After washing with PBS, slides were incubated with secondary biotin-labeled antibody (30 min) followed by conjugated streptavidin horseradish peroxidase (30 min) both at room temperature (concentrated, volume 10 ml, Secondary goat polyclonal biotinylated-anti-mouse and anti-rabbit IgG, and S-HRP Conjugate, Universal HRP Immunostaining Kit, cat. # KP50D, Diagnostic Biosystems, Pleasanton, USA). Chromogen solution containing Diamino-benzidine (DAB) and H_2O_2 (substrate) 3% was previously prepared (volume 10 tabs, DAB Chromogen Universal HRP Immunostaining kit, cat. # KP50D Diagnostic BioSystems, Pleasanton, USA). Sections were counterstained with Mayer's haematoxylin, dehydrated and mounted. Specificity was verified by substitution of primary antibody with PBS. Digital images were retrieved as described above for morphometric evaluation.

2.5 Quantitative and semi-quantitative immunohistochemistry analyses

The percentage (%) of immunostained area (brown reaction) observed for active caspase-3 in testicular parenchyma was measured at 400 magnification using image analysis software (Image Pro-Plus 6.1®, Media Cybernetics, Silver Spring, MA, USA). Testicular images were evaluated in 30 fields with colour segmentation analysis by extracting brown stain objects and measuring % of immunostained area (Ortega *et al.*, 2007). Semi-quantitative analysis for gonocytes, Leydig and Sertoli cells staining intensity (Si) was score as: 0 absence of brown colour; 1 weak (pale brown); 2 moderate (brown); 3 intense (dark brown) (Boos *et al.*, 1996). Sections were analyzed with the observer blinded to treatment.

2.6 Statistical analyses

Morphometric and immunohistochemical data were expressed as mean ± standard error of the mean. Group means were compared using analysis of variance (ANOVA) with Statgraphics Plus ®5.1 (Statistical Graphic Corp, Rockville, Maryland, USA, 1994–2000). Post hoc differences between groups were assessed with Tukey's tests. In all cases, the level of statistical significance was taken to be P < 0.05.

3 RESULTS

At 90 days of age, the testicular parenchyma comprised testicular interstitial tissue and solid sex cords that did not have a lumen. Sertoli cells were localised in the periphery of the sex cords and showed a basophilic nucleus and irregular eosinophil cytoplasm. Gonocytes were found in small numbers, 2 or 3 per transverse cross-section of the sex cords. Leydig cells were found in interstitial tissue with round eosinophil cytoplasm and a round nucleus.

Control and betamethasone-treated lambs showed no differences in body weight (P = 0.49) or testicular weight (P = 0.24). There was a strong correlation between body weight and the testicular weight in both the controls (r = 0.82) and the treated offspring (r = 0.76). There was a very strong correlation (r = 1.0) between sex cord length and testicular weight in both groups. The correlation between transverse sex cord diameter and testicular weight was also strong for both the control (r = 0.72) and the treated offspring (r = 0.63).

Sex cord diameter was greatly reduced in offspring of mothers treated with betamethasone compared with the control group (P = 0.001; Table 1; Figure 1).

In the saline-exposed group, the area occupied by interstitial tissue was considerably less than that in the betamethasone-treated group. There was also a reduction in the volume density of the sex cords in the betamethasone-exposed offspring compared with the control (P = 0.013; Table 1). By contrast, the volume density of the interstitial tissue was higher in the exposed offspring than in the controls (P = 0.013). The number of Sertoli cells per transverse sex cord cross-section was higher in betamethasone-exposed (P = 0.04) compared to

Table 1. Body weight and testicular variables (mean ± SEM) in lambs at 90 days of age, after treatment *in utero* with betamethasone or saline vehicle.

| Variable | Prenatal treatment | |
	Saline	Betamethasone
Body weight (kg)	18.7 ± 0.8	17.8 ± 0.9
Testes mass (g)	8.7 ± 1.1	6.6 ± 1.2
Sex cords		
Diameter (µm)	50 ± 0.4[a]	42 ± 0.4[b]
Volume density (%)	49.1 ± 0.8[a]	46.0 ± 0.9[b]
Absolute volume (µm³)	$4.3 \times 10^8 \pm 1.3$[a]	$3.1 \times 10^8 \pm 1.5$[b]
Total length (m)	31.7 ± 9.8	22.0 ± 4.3
Gonocytes per cross section	2.7 ± 0.2	2.5 ± 0.2
Total gonocytes	13030 ± 1950	11040 ± 2130
Sertoli cells per cross section	45.1 ± 1.1[b]	48.6 ± 1.3[a]
Total Sertoli cells	265800 ± 370	217200 ± 410
Interstitial tissue		
Volume density (%)	50.9 ± 0.8[b]	54.0 ± 0.9[a]
Absolute volume (µm³)	$4.3 \times 10^8 \pm 0.9$[a]	$3.5 \times 10^8 \pm 1.0$[b]
Leydig cells per image	1.7 ± 0.1	2.0 ± 0.1
Total Leydig cells	$1.4 \times 10^7 \pm 0.2$	$1.4 \times 10^7 \pm 0.2$

Values in the same row with different superscripts: P < 0.05.

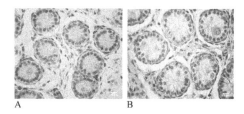

Figure 1. Haematoxylin-eosin-stained images of testicular parenchyma from Merino lambs at 90 days of age after treatment *in utero* with betamethasone (A) or saline vehicle (B). Betamethasone treatment showed smaller sex cord diameter and area compared with saline.

Table 2. Cellular distribution (Cytoplasmic: C, perinuclear: PN, nuclear: N) and immunoexpression levels of active caspase-3 in Sertoli cells, Leydig cells and gonocytes in testes from the betamethasone and saline groups. (0) Absence of brown color, (1) Weak (pale brown), (2) Moderate brown, (3) Intense (dark brown).

Testicular cells	Saline			Betamethasone		
	C	PN	N	C	PN	N
Sertoli	2	2	1	1	1	0
Gonocytes	2	3	1	1	2	0
Leydig	2	2	1	1	1	1

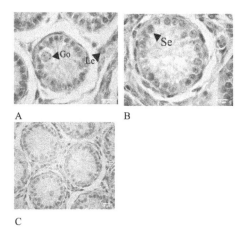

Figure 2. Immunohistochemical localization of active caspase-3 in lamb testis parenchyma after treatment *in utero* with betamethasone (A) or saline (B). Negative control (C) for immunohitochemistry without incubation of the primary antibody. Le = Leydig cell, Se = Sertoli cell, Go = gonocyte. Scale bar = 10 μm.

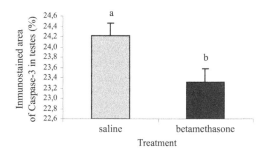

Figure 3. Immunopositive area (%; mean ± pooled SE) for active caspase-3 in lamb testis parenchyma after treatment in utero with betamethasone or saline vehicle. Bars with different letters are significantly different ($P < 0.05$).

The area immunostained for active caspase-3 decreased ($P = 0.01$) from 23% in betamethasone-treated animals to 24% the controls (Figure 3).

control lambs, but no differences were detected for gonocytes numbers or for sex cord length.

3.1 *Immunohistochemistry results*

Immunoreactive active caspase-3 was localised to germ cells, Sertoli cells and Leydig cells in testes of lambs at 90 days of age, in both the saline- and betamethasone treated groups (Figure 2).

In the saline-exposed offspring, the gonocytes showed the highest levels of immunoexpression in the perinuclear region whereas, in Sertoli and Leydig cells, active caspase-3 was localised in the cytoplasmic, perinuclear and nuclear regions However, in betamethasone-exposed offspring, active caspase-3 was evident in Sertoli, Leydig cells and gonocytes in the perinuclear region and the cytoplasmic and nuclear levels were low (Table 2).

4 DISCUSSION

The present study showed that *in utero* administration of synthetic glucocorticoids affects the testicular morphology of pre-pubertal lambs. Normally, the pre-pubertal lamb testis comprises mostly interstitial tissue and testicular sex cords that are solid and without a central lumen. The testicular parenchyma retains this composition until puberty when the solid sex cords become seminiferous tubules with a central lumen (Kerr *et al.*, 2006). In the present study, solid sex cords were observed in pre-pubertal testes from betamethasone-exposed offspring, but the lumen had started to appear in the middle of sex cords in saline-exposed offspring (Figure 2). In testes from betamethasone-treated animals, there was also a reduction in active caspase-3 immunoexpression, accompanied by a decrease in sex cord diameter and volume density.

Importantly, prenatal betamethasone exposure did not affect sex cord length but did decrease sex cord diameter in 90-day-old lambs. Previously, in the fetus, we observed the same outcome for sex cord length after betamethasone treatment, but no differences in sex cord diameter (Pedrana et al., 2008). During fetal life, an increase in sex cord size is mainly a consequence of increased cord length, not diameter. So, it is possible that, in betamethasone-exposed males, sex cord length increases to reach saline-exposed males, in order to compensate the reduction in sex cord diameter. In postnatal life, the process continues and becomes gonadotrophin-dependent, with sex cords lengthening 8-fold (Hochereau-de Reviers et al., 1995). This process leads to the onset of spermatogenesis and the formation of spermatozoa. Thus, adequate development of the sex cords and interstitial tissue is necessary for future spermatogenesis and adult fertility. In rams, sexual differentiation and postnatal testicular growth are separated by at least six months (Hochereau-de Reviers et al., 1995). The results of the present study suggest that prenatal administration of glucocorticoid may alter sex cord growth and, in doing so, postpone the onset of spermatogenesis.

Sertoli cells proliferate during the period between sexual differentiation in the embryo and fetus and the onset of puberty. When Sertoli cells differentiate into adult functional cells, they lose their capacity to proliferate (Herrera-Alarcón et al., 2007). In the fetal ovine testis, Sertoli cells undergo at least eight mitotic divisions, six of them before Day 110 of gestation and the remainder during the postnatal period leading to puberty (Hochereau-de Reviers et al., 1995). Variation in the number of Sertoli cells in the testis is strongly correlated with the number of germinal cells (Hochereau-de Reviers & Courot, 1978; Jahnukainen et al., 2004). Therefore, the number of Sertoli cells per testis is correlated with the number of spermatogonia necessary for appropriate development of spermatogenesis, and thus fertility (Hochereau-de Reviers & Courot, 1978). In our study, prenatal glucocorticoid exposure did not affect the total number of either gonocytes or Sertoli cells. Consistent with this, mitotic activity in ovine Leydig cells involves at least seven mitotic divisions before birth, but six are completed by Day 110 of gestation (Hochereau-de Reviers et al., 1995). It is therefore expected that glucocorticoid treatment on Days 104–118 did not affect the total number of Leydig cells in postnatal offspring.

In this study, we have demonstrated that in utero betamethasone exposure decreases the expression of the apoptotic protein, active caspase-3, in 90-day pre-pubertal lambs. However, this was not accompanied by any decrease in total number of Sertoli cells or gonocytes. It is possible that caspase-3 was expressed before the apoptosis was identified. Although we expected an increase in active caspase-3 apoptotic enzyme in lambs, as we had observed in the fetal testis (Pedrana et al., 2008), our postnatal data suggests the chance of a delay in the first apoptotic wave (Hafez, 2000).

Apoptosis contributes to the modulation of cell number on the pre-pubertal testis and determines potential fertility in adulthood (Berensztein et al., 2002). Spermatogenesis begins with an apoptotic germ cell wave that limits their number during the first cycle in most mammals, ensuring a balance between numbers of spermatogonia and Sertoli cells (Rodriguez et al., 2010). The development of normal spermatogenesis depends on a balance between testicular cells, which involves the process of apoptosis (Boulogne et al., 1999; Furuchi et al., 1996, Kimura et al., 2003). Sertoli cells can support a limited number of germ cells being one of the most important factors that regulate germ cell death (Pentikäinen et al., 1999). Once the activation of caspase-3 begins, it decides the destiny of the cell, a process that cannot be reversed (Said et al., 2010). Our data are consistent with this hypothesis because testes from control offspring showed an increase in the immunoexpression of active caspase-3.

The inhibition of an early apoptotic wave has been associated with the accumulation of spermatogonia and infertility in later life (Jahnukainen et al., 2004, Rodriguez et al., 1997). The reduction in active caspase-3 immunoexpression observed in the present study suggests alterations in the first pre-pubertal apoptotic wave in the testis that could have long-term effects on future spermatogenesis.

5 CONCLUSIONS

Prenatal treatment with synthetic glucocorticoids during the final third of ovine pregnancy affects the development of male testicular sex cords and protein caspase-3 expression in testicular cells in pre-pubertal 90 day-old lambs. This suggests changes in the beginning of the spermatogenesis process. Notably, studies are needed to determine whether antenatal glucocorticoid administration is associated with reproductive diseases in humans, given the frequent use of glucocorticoid therapy in pregnant women at risk of preterm delivery. Studies are also needed in the ovine model to determine whether the expression of caspases is permanently altered in the adult and to assess the differential impact of glucocorticoids on Sertoli cells, Leydig cells and gonocytes because changes in apoptosis regulatory enzymes may determine fertility.

REFERENCES

Alcalde-Herrero, A.I. 2006. Efectos sobre el comportamiento, salud y bienestar animal. In E.J. Squires, Endocrinología animal aplicada. Editorial Acribia, Zaragoza, España pp. 211–251.

Berensztein, E., Sciara, M., Rivarola, M., and Belgorosky, A. 2002. Apoptosis and proliferation of human testicular somatic and germ cells during prepuberty: high rate of testicular growth in newborns mediated by decreased apoptosis. The Journal of Clinical Endocrinology and Metabolism 87: 5113–5118.

Bielli, A., Perez, R., Pedrana, G., Milton, J.T.B., Lopez, A., Blackberry, M.A. Duncombe, G., Rodriguez-Martinez, H. and Martin, G.B. 2002: Low maternal nutrition during pregnancy reduces the numbers of Sertoli cells in the newborn lamb. Reprod. Fertil. Dev. 14, 333–337.

Bishop, E. 1981. Acceleration of fetal pulmonary maturity. Obstetrics and Gynecology 58: 48–51.

Boos, A., Meyer, W., Schwarz, R. and Grunert, E. 1996. Immunohistochemical assessment of oestrogen receptor and progesterone receptor distribution in biopsy samples of the bovine endometrium collected throughout the oestrous cycle. Animal Reproduction Science 44: 11–21.

Boulogne, B., Olaso, R., Levacher, C., Durant, P. and Habert, R. 1999. Apoptosis and mitosis in gonocytes of the rat testis during foetal and neonatal development. International Journal of Andrology 22: 356–365.

Cooper, B. 2002. Disease at the Cellular Level. In: D. Slauson & B. Cooper Mechanisms of disease a textbook of comparative general pathology. 3rd. ed. St. Louis, Mosby.

Dalziel, S.R., Lim, V.K., Lambert, A., McCarthy, D., Parag, V., Rodgers, A. and Harding, J.E. Antenatal exposure to betamethasone: psychological functioning and health related quality of life 31 years after inclusion in randomised controlled trial. British Medical Journal, doi:10.1136/bmj.38576.494363.

De Vries, W.B., Karemaker, R., Mooy, N.F., Strengers, J.L.M., Kemperman, H., Baerts, W., Veen, S., Visser G.H.A., Heijnen, C.J. and van Bel, F. 2008. Cardiovascular Follow-up at School Age After Perinatal Glucocorticoid Exposure in Prematurely Born Children. Perinatal Glucocorticoid Therapy and Cardiovascular Follow-up. Archive of Pediatrics and Adolescent Medicine 162(8): 738–744.

Dodic, M., Abouantoun, T., O'Connor, A., Marelyn, E., Karen, W. and Moritz, M. 2002. Programming effects of short prenatal exposure to dexamethasone in sheep. Journal of the American Heart Association 40: 729–734.

Franca, L.R., Silva, V.A., Chiarini-Garcia, J.R.H., García, S.K. and Debeljuk, L. 2000. Cell proliferation and hormonal changes during postnatal development of the testes in the pig. Biology of Reproduction 63: 1629–1636.

Furuchi, T., Masuko, K., Nishimune, Y., Obinata, M. and Matsui, Y. 1996. Inhibition of testicular germ cell apoptosis and differentiation in mice misexpressing Bcl-2 in spermatogonia. Development 122: 1703–1709.

Gao, H., Ming-Han, T., Yan-Qiang, H., Qing-Su, G., Renshan, G. and Matthew, P.H. 2002. Glucocorticoids induces apoptosis in rat Leydig cells. Endocrinology 143: 130–138.

Hafez, E.S.E. and Hafez, B. 2000. Reproducción e inseminación artificial en animales. 7a. ed. México DF, Mc Graw Hill.

Herrera-Alarcón, J., Villagómez-Amezcua, E., González-Padilla, E. and Jiménez-Severiano, H. 2007. Stereological study of postnatal testicular development in Blackbelly sheep. Theriogenology 68: 582–591.

Hochereau-de Reviers, M.T. & Courot, M. 1978. Sertoli cells and development of seminiferous epithelium. Annales de Biologie Animale, Biochimie, Biophysique 18: 573–583.

Hochereau-de Reviers, M.T., Perreau, C., Pisselet, C., Locatelli, A. and Bosc, M. 1995. Ontogenesis of somatic and germ cells in sheep fetal testis. Journal of Reproduction and Fertility 103: 41–46.

Ikegami, M., Jobe, A.H., Newnham, J., Polk, D.H., Willet, K.E. and Sly, P. 1997. Repetitive Prenatal Glucocorticoids Improve Lung Function and Decrease Growth in Preterm Lambs. American Journal of Respiratory and Critical Care Medicine 156: 178–184.

Jahnukainen, K., Chrysis, D., Hou, M., Parvinen, M., Eksborg, S. and Söder, O. 2004. Increased Apoptosis Occurring During the First Wave of Spermatogenesis Is Stage-Specific And Primarily Affects Midpachytene Spermatocytes in the Rat Testis. Biology of Reproduction. 70: 290–296.

Jensen, E.C., Gallaher, B.W., Breier, B.H. and Harding, J.E. 2002. The effect of a chronic maternal cortisol infusion on the later-gestation fetal sheep. Journey of Endocrinology 174: 27–36.

Kerr, J.B., Loveland, K.L., O'Bryan, M.K. and De Kretser, D.M. 2006. Cytology of the testis and intrinsic control mechanisms. In: J.D. Neil, Knobil, T.M. Plant (eds), Knobil and Neill's Physiology of Reproduction. Vol. 1, Third Edition. Chapt. 18: 827–947. St Louis: Elsevier Academic Press.

Kim, J., Ghosh, S., Weil, A. and Zirkin, B. 2001. Caspase-3 and caspase-activated deoxyribonuclease are associated with testicular germ cell apoptosis resulting from reduced intratesticular testosterone. Endocrinology 142(9): 3809–3816.

Kimura, M., Itoh N., Takagi, S., Takumi, S., Takahashi, A., Masumori, N. and Tsukamoto, T. 2003. Balance of Apoptosis and Proliferación of Germ Cells Ralated to Spermatogenesis in Aged Men. Journal of Andrology 24(2): 185–191.

Lalau, J.D., Aubert, M.L., Carmignac, D.F., Gregoire, I. and Dupouy, J.P. 1990. Reduction in testicular function in rats: II. Reduction by dexamethasone in fetal and neonatal rats. Neuroendocrinology 51: 289–293.

Liggins, G.C. and Howie, R.N. 1972. A controlled trial of antepartum glucocorticoid treatment for prevention of the respiratory distress syndrome in premature infants. Pediatrics 50: 515–25.

Nyirenda, M.J., Lindsay, R.M., Kenyon, C.J., Burchell, A. and Seckl, J.R. 1998. Glucocorticoid exposure in late gestation permanently programs rat hepatic phosphoenolpyruvate carboxykinase and glucocorticoid receptor expression and causes glucose intolerance in adult offspring. Journal of Clinical Investigation 101: 2174–2181.

Ortega, O.O., Salvetti, N.R., Amable, P., Dallard, B.E., Baravalle, C., Barbeito, C.G. and Gimeno, E.G. 2007. Intraovarian Localization of Growth Factors in Induced Cystic Ovaries in Rats. Anat. Histol. Embryol. 36: 94–102.

Page, K., Sottas, C.H. and Hardy, M. 2001. Prenatal Exposure to Dexamethasone Alters Leydig Cell Steroidogenic Capacity in Immature and Adult Rats. Journal of Andrology 22(6): 973–980.

Pedrana, G., Sloboda, D., Pérez, W., Newnham, J. Bielli, A. and Martin, G. 2008a. Effects of pre-natal glucocorticoids on testicular development in sheep. Anatomia, Histologia, Embryologia 37(5): 352–358.

Pedrana, G., Mernies, B., Pérez, W., Vitarella, F., Baravalle, C., Velásquez, M., Bielli, A., Martin, G.B. and Ortega, H. 2008b. Estudio inmunohistoquímico de la actividad apoptótica en testículos fetales de ovinos tratados in utero con betametasona. Veterinaria. Montevideo 43 (171), 36.

Pentikäinen, V., Erkkila, K. and Dunkel, L. 1999. Fas regulates germ cell apoptosis in the human testis in vitro. American Journal of Physiology-Endocrinology and Metabolism 276: 310–316.

Rhind, S. 2004. Effects of maternal nutrition on fetal and neonatal reproductive development and function. Animal Reproduction Science 82–83: 169–181.

Rodriguez, I., Ody, C., Araki, K., Garcia, I., and Vassalli, P. 1997. An early and massive wave of germinal cell apoptosis is required for the development of functional spermatogenesis. EMBO Journal 16: 2262–2270.

Russell, L.D. & Peterson, R.N. 1984. Determination of the elongate spermatid-Sertoli cell ratio in various mammals. Journal of Reproduction and Fertility 70: 635–641.

Said, T., Gaglani, A. and Agarwal, A. 2010. Implication of apoptosis in sperm cryoinjury. Reproductive BioMedicine Online 21(4): 456–462.

Sapolsky, R., Meaney, M. and Mc Ewen, B. 1985. The development of the glucocorticoid receptor system in the rat limbic brain. III. Negative-feed-back regulation. Developmental Brain Research 18: 169–173.

Seckl, J. 2004. Prenatal glucocorticoids and long-term programming. European Journal of Endocrinology 151: 49–62.

Sloboda, D., Newnham, J. and Challis, J. 2000. Effects of repeated maternal betamethasone administration on growth and hypothalamic–pituitary–adrenal function of the ovine fetus at term. Journal of Endocrinology 165: 79–91.

Sloboda, D.M., Newnham, J.P. and Challis, J.R.G. 2002. Repeated maternal glucocorticoid administration and the developing liver in fetal sheep. Journal of Endocrinology 175: 535–543.

Squires, E. 2006. Endocrinología animal aplicada. Zaragoza: Acribia.

Tangalakis, K., Lumbers, E.R. and Moritz, K.M. 1992. Effect of cortisol on blood pressure and vascular reactivity in the ovine fetus. Experimental Physiology 77: 709–717.

Ward, I. and Weisz, J. 1980. Maternal stress alters plasma testosterone in fetal males. Science 207: 328–329.

Yazawa, H., Sasagawa, I. and Nakada, T. 2000. Apoptosis of testicular germ cells induced by exogenous glucocorticoid in rats. Human Reproduction. 15: 1917–1920.

Computational Vision and Medical Image Processing – Tavares & Natal Jorge (eds)
© 2012 Taylor & Francis Group, London, ISBN 978-0-415-68395-1

Colourquantisation as a preprocessing step for image segmentation

H. Palus & M. Frąckiewicz
Silesian University of Technology, Gliwice, Poland

1 INTRODUCTION

Colour image quantisation is the process of transformation of a true colour image (typically eight bit onto each colour component) into an image consisting of a small number of specially selected colours (colour palette). New colours are selected by minimizing the colour difference between the original image and the quantised image. In other words, this is a special case of vector quantisation realized in three-dimensional colour space.

Colour quantisation is also very often used as an auxiliary operation in colour image processing. On example it can reduce the complexity of image segmentation process. In literature we can find examples such uses of colour quantisation as preprocessing in image segmentation.

The paper will be organized as follows. In Section 2, we will review former works that have been done to investigate a sense of colour quantisation in image segmentation. The idea of proposed experiment and final results will describe in Section 3 and Section 4 and finally we will conclude the paper in Section 5.

2 RELATED WORKS

Ten years ago the first important work about using colour quantisation in image segmentation process was published (Deng & Manjunath 2001). Deng and Manjunath proposed JSEG technique composed from two independent steps: colour quantisation by modified Generalized Lloyd Algorithm (GLA) and spatial segmentation based on quantised colours. This quantisation technique contained a special PGF denoising, quantising in perceptual CIELUV colour space and merging close clusters with the use of a threshold value (Deng et al., 1999). Authors emphasized the importance of good quality of quantisation technique and recommended the use of 10–20 colours in the images of natural scenes. Unfortunately, the colour quantisation technique is sensitive on selected value of parameter (a threshold of the quantisation). Improper threshold badly affects the result of quantisation and leads to incorrect segmentation.

In last years JSEG technique was many times modified. This also applies to colour quantisation technique. Good example is JSEG version with variance-based quantisation method (Celebi et al., 2005) that is faster than modified GLA. In other paper (Wang Y.-G. et al., 2006) special attention has been paid to the need of searching better colour quantisation algorithms for JSEG technique. Another modified version of JSEG uses an adaptive mean-shift clustering technique (AMS) for non-parametric colour quantisation (Wang Y. et al., 2006).

Sometimes attention is paid to decreasing the computational costs and reducing the sensitivity of segmentation to the noise data (Dong & Xie 2005; Ilea & Whelan 2008). The authors of both papers demonstrated that colour reduction by using a self-organizing map (SOM) simplifies further segmentation. Similarly some method of colour texture segmentation start with a simple uniform colour quantisation (Weng et al., 2005).

The colour quantisation is used for many years as preprocessing in segmentation of complex document images (Zhong et al., 1995). Additionally, recently developed techniques automatically estimate the final number of colours in segmentd image (Nikolaou & Papamarkos 2009).

The colour quantisation is also a simplification step in video segmentation (Smith M. & Khotanzad A. 2006). A large number of unique colours in several frames of a image sequence is reduced to few quantised colours.

3 IDEA OF EXPERIMENT AND USED TOOLS

In an experiment the results of segmentation preceded by a colour quantisation have been compared with segmentation without such preprocessing step. Below we present tools for colour quantisation, image segmentation and evaluation of segmentation results, that were selected for this experiment.

3.1 *Techniques for colour quantisation*

In this paper were considered two colour quantisation techniques based on clustering of pixels: the classic *k-means* technique (KM) (MacQuenn 1967) and new *k-harmonic means* technique (KHM) proposed by Zhang (Zhang 2000). The usefulness of both techniques for colour image quantisation has been show by authors of this paper in work (Frąckiewicz & Palus 2011).

$$KHM(X, C) = \sum_{i=1}^{n} \frac{k}{\sum_{j=1}^{k} \frac{1}{\|x_i - c_j\|^p}} \quad (1)$$

The KHM technique requires defining an internal parameter p, which usually fulfils following condition: $p \geq 2$. We used here the value $p = 2.7$. The fuzzy membership (2) of pixel to cluster $m(c_j|x_i)$ was here applied and similarly was applied the dynamic weight function $w(x_i)$ (3), what means different influence an individual pixel x_i on calculating the new values c_j in each next iteration.

$$m(c_j \mid x_i) = \frac{\|x_i - c_j\|^{-p-2}}{\sum_{j=1}^{k} \|x_i - c_j\|^{-p-2}} \quad (2)$$

$$w(x_i) = \frac{\sum_{j=1}^{k} \|x_i - c_j\|^{-p-2}}{\left(\sum_{j=1}^{k} \|x_i - c_j\|^{-p}\right)^2} \quad (3)$$

The KHM technique, basing on formulae (2) and (3), uses the following formula for calculating new cluster centres:

$$c_j = \frac{\sum_{i=1}^{n} m(c_j \mid x_i) w(x_i) x_i}{\sum_{i=1}^{n} m(c_j \mid x_i) w(x_i)} \quad (4)$$

Both quantisation techniques are used here with the same deterministic initialization method marked as *SD*. This method uses a size of pixel cloud of a colour image. First, the mean values and standard deviations (*SD*) for each *RGB* component of all image pixels are calculated. Then, around the point of mean colour is constructed a rectangular cuboid with side lengths equal to $2\sigma_R$, $2\sigma_G$ and $2\sigma_B$. We assume that it lies within the RGB cube.

Next, the main diagonal of cuboid is divided into k equal segments. The centres of these diagonal segments are used as initial cluster centres.

As a background for the quantisation techniques described above were applied two simpler splitting techniques. The splitting techniques divide the colour space into smaller subspaces and then a colour palette is built by choosing representative colours from subspaces. We used here a technique

implemented in IrfanView ver.4.0 and designated as IV and more complicated Wu's algorithm implemented in Ximagic plugins.

3.2 *Region-based image segmentation*

Of the many techniques developed for image segmentation, the unseeded region growing (USRG) technique, described by Palus (Palus 2006), has been selected. This is a typical bottom-up technique. It is based on the concept of region growing without seeds needed to start the segmentation process. At the beginning of the algorithm each pixel has its own label (one-pixel regions). Neighbouring pixels are merged into regions, if their attributes, for example colours, are sufficiently similar. This similarity is often represented by a homogeneity criterion. If a pixel satisfied the homogeneity criterion, then the pixel can be included to the region. After such inclusion, the region's area and mean colour are updated. For this updating recurrent formulae are used.

Two simple raster scans of the colour image are applied in this technique: one pass from the left to the right and from the top to the bottom can be followed by an additional reverse pass over the image. The pixel aggregation process results in a set of regions characterized by their mean colours, their sizes and lists of pixels that belong to proper regions.

The typical homogeneity criterion based on the Euclidean metric has following form:

$$\sqrt{\left(R - R^*\right)^2 + \left(G - G^*\right)^2 + \left(B - B^*\right)^2} \leq d \quad (5)$$

where: R, G, B are colour components of tested pixel, R^*, G^*, B^* are colour components of mean colour of creating region and d is the parameter, that is very important for segmentation results. If the value of parameter d increases, then the number of regions R in the segmented image simultaneously decreases. Too low value of parameter d is lead to oversegmentation and too high value is a reason of undersegmentation. The version of the algorithm described here, works in the RGB colour space.

The segmentation of good quality images result also in a large number of small regions on the edges of objects. The USRG technique removes these regions from the segmented image by post-processing. It is not difficult task, because after segmentation the technique has at its disposal a list of regions that can be sorted according to their area. A threshold value of the area of small region A depends on the image. After merging of small region, the mean colour of new region is computed and a label of small region pixels is changed. In result of such postprocessing, the number of regions in the segmented image significantly decreases.

3.3 *Tool for evaluation of image segmentation*

Among different methods we can find empirically defined function used for evaluation of segmentation results (Borsotti et al., 1998):

$$Q(I) = \frac{1}{10000\,(M \cdot N)} \sqrt{R} \sum_{i=1}^{R} \left[\frac{e_i^2}{1 + \log A_i} + \left(\frac{R(A_i)}{A_i} \right)^2 \right] \quad (6)$$

where I is the segmented image, $M \cdot N$ is the size of the image, R is the number of regions in the segmented image, A_i is the area of the region i, $R(A_i)$ is the number of regions having an area equal to A_i and e_i is the colour error of region i. The colour error in RGB space is calculated as the sum of the Euclidean distances between colour components of pixels of region and components of average colour, which is an attribute of this region in the segmented image. The colour errors in different colour spaces are not comparable and therefore are transformed back to the RGB space. First term of Eq. (6) is a normalization factor, the second term penalizes results with too many regions (oversegmentation), and the third term penalizes results with non-homogeneous regions. Last term is scaled by the area factor because the colour error is higher for large regions. The main idea of using this kind of function can be formulated as follows: the lower the value of $Q(I)$, the better is the segmentation result.

4 EXPERIMENTAL RESULTS

Preliminary tests were carried out on five images with relatively easy defined number of output colours. For test image Chart (Fig. 1a) we assumed the number of clusters $k = 25$, $k = 20$ for test image DNA (Fig. 1d) and $k = 10$ for other test images (Fig. 1b, 1c, 1e). In all cases, the quantisation process used 15 iterations. The following parameter values were applied in the USRG segmentation technique: for image Chart—$d = 25$, $A = 1000$, for image Objects—$d = 25$, $A = 1000$, for image Book—$d = 25$, $A = 10$, for image DNA—$d = 10$, $A = 500$ and for image Eye—$d = 20$, $A = 100$.

The data in Table 1 shows that not every method of colour quantisation, carried out as preprocessing step in the process of segmentation, leads to improved segmentation result. Good example is a case of IV technique: all $Q(I)$ values are higher than $Q(I)$ for segmentation without quantisation. A much better impact on the segmentation have

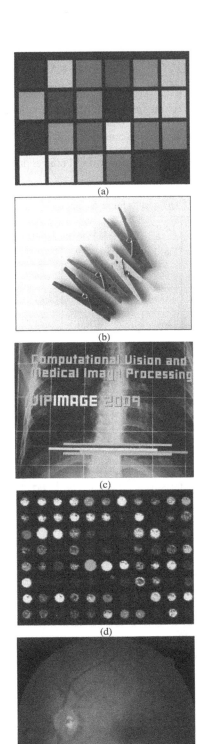

Figure 1. Test images used in the experiment: (a) Chart, (b) Objects, (c) Book, (d) DNA, (e) Eye.

133

the Wu's algorithm. The KHM technique reduces the values of $Q(I)$ index but the KM technique, on the contrary, can in some cases increase it significantly. All this means that poorly quantised images badly affect the final result of segmentation.

It is easy to see that the usefulness of colour quantisation in segmentation process depends on the value of parameter k (number of clusters). Tables 2 and 3 show for two test images how, in the case of KHM, the number of clusters k affects the value of $Q(I)$. From these tables, one can see that for each of the tested images, there is a range of values of k which improves the image segmentation by initial colour quantisation.

5 CONCLUSIONS

We proposed and preliminary tested an idea to use initial colour quantisation as preprocessing step for colour image segmentation. The performance of segmentation can be limited by the quality of colour quantisation. Therefore, our approach needs a good quantisation technique e.g., researched segmentation technique works better for KHM quantisation technique than KM technique. It is also important to properly select the size of the palette to the image.

It has long been known that the significant reduction of the number of image colours before segmentation simplifies and accelerates the execution of this difficult operation. In this paper we searched for the conditions of additional improvement in image segmentation preceded by a colour quantisation. The further research will be focused on establishing the conditions and parameters of the tested approach.

Our study uses different images acquired from relatively simple scenes without significant highlights and shadows. For more complex images results will not be so good. Therefore, an interesting question is what kind of colour images need to be quantised before the segmentation. Perhaps the estimation of image segmentation difficulty will help answer this question (Liu et al., 2011).

Table 1. Q(I) results for tested images.

Image	USRG	IV+ USRG	Wu+ USRG	KM+ USRG	KHM+ USRG
Chart	617	823	759	959	**478**
Objects	998	8139	1204	650	**409**
Book	387	477	415	463	**348**
DNA	4647	8592	**881**	944	2628
Eye	613	1325	397	386	**287**

Table 2. Dependence of Q(I) on assumed number of clusters.

Chart, k=	10	15	20	25
USRG	617			
KHM+USRG	2312	839	**467**	**478**
Chart, k=	30	35	40	45
USRG	617			
KHM+USRG	**445**	682	756	725

Table 3. Dependence of Q(I) on assumed number of clusters.

Objects, k=	5	8	10	15
USRG	998			
KHM+USRG	2142	**637**	**409**	1506
Objects, k=	20	25	30	35
USRG	998			
KHM+USRG	1608	1504	721	1183

ACKNOWLEDGEMENTS

This work was supported by Polish Ministry for Science and Higher Education under internal grant BK-208/RAu1/2011 for Institute of Automatic Control, Silesian University of Technology.

REFERENCES

Borsotti, M., Campadelli, P. & Schettini, R. 1998. Quantitative evaluation of color image segmentation results, *Pattern Recognitions Letters* vol. 19, no. 8, 741–747.

Celebi, M.E., Aslandogan, Y.A. & Bergstresser, P.R. 2005. Unsupervised border detection of skin lesion images, Proceedings of the International Conference on Information Technology: Coding and Computing (ITCC'05), vol. II, 123–128, Las Vegas, NV, USA.

Deng, Y.N. & Manjunath, B.S. 2001. Unsupervised segmentation of color-texture regions in images and video, *IEEE Transactions on Pattern Analysis and Machine Intelligence*, vol. 23, no. 8, 800–810.

Dong, G. & Xie, M. 2005. Color clustering and learning for image segmentation based on neural networks, *IEEE Transactions on Neural Networks*, vol. 16, no. 4, 925–936.

Deng, Y.N., Kenney, C., Moore, M.S. & Manjunath, B.S. 1999. Peer group filtering and color image quantization. Proc. of IEEE Intl. Symposium on Circuits and Systems VLSI, vol. 4, 21–24, Orlando, FL, USA.

Frąckiewicz, M. & Palus, H. 2011. KM and KHM clustering techniques for colour image quantisation. In Joao Manuel R.S. Tavares & R.M. Natal Jorge (eds), *Computational Vision and Medical Image Processing: Recent Trends*, Springer, Dordrecht, 161–174.

Ilea, D.E. & Whelan, P.F. 2008. CTex—an adaptive unsupervised segmentation algorithm based on colour-texture coherence, *IEEE Transactions on Image Processing*, vol. 17, no. 10, 1926–1939.

Liu, D., Xiong, Y., Pulli, K. & Shapiro, L. 2011. Estimating image segmentation difficulty, Proceedings of 7th International Conference on Machine Learning and Data Mining (MLDM 2011), New York, USA.

Mac Queen, J. 1967. Some methods for classification and analysis of multivariate observations. In L.M. Le Cam & J. Neyman (eds.), Proceedings of the Fifth Berkeley Symposium on Mathematics, Statistics, and Probabilities: vol. 1, 281–297, Berkeley and Los Angeles, CA, USA.

Nikolaou, N. & Papamarkos, N. 2009. Color reduction in complex document images, *International Journal of Imaging Systems and Technology*, vol. 19, iss.1, 14–26.

Palus, H. 2006. Color image segmentation: selected techniques. In Lukac R. & Plataniotis K.N., (eds.), *Color image processing: methods and applications*, CRC Press, Boca Raton, 103–128.

Smith, M. & Khotanzad, A. 2006. Unsupervised object-based video segmentation using color and texture features, Proc. of IEEE Southwest Symposium on Image Analysis and Interpretation, 124–128, Denver, CO, USA.

Wang, Y.-G., Yang, J. & Chang, Y.-C. 2006. Color-texture image segmentation by integrating directional operators into JSEG method, *Pattern Recognition Letters*, vol. 27, no. 16, 1983–1990.

Wang, Y., Yang, J. & Peng N. 2006. Unsupervised color-texture segmentation based on soft criterion with adaptive mean-shift clustering, *Pattern Recognition Letters*, vol. 27, no. 5, 386–392.

Weng, S.-K., Kuo, C.-M. & Kang, W.-C. 2005. Unsupervised texture segmentation using color quantization and color feature distributions, Proc. of Intl. Conference on Image Processing, vol. 3, 1136–1139, Genoa, Italy.

Zhang, B. 2000. Generalized k-harmonic means—boosting in unsupervised learning. *Technical Report HPL-2000–137*. Hewlett-Packard Labs, Palo Alto, CA, USA.

Zhong, Y., Karu, K. & Jain, A.K. 1995. Locating text in complex color images, *Pattern Recognition*, vol. 28, no. 10, 1523–1535.

Computational Vision and Medical Image Processing – Tavares & Natal Jorge (eds)
© 2012 Taylor & Francis Group, London, ISBN 978-0-415-68395-1

Reconstruction of a stratified flow inside a duct using X-ray transform for constant by parts functions

Alberto R. Teixeira & Nilson C. Roberty
Nuclear Engineering Program—COPPE—UFRJ—Brazil

ABSTRACT: This work presents a methodology for reconstruction of constants by parts functions. The paper focus in one application of this methodology for identify the phases of the stratified multiphase flow (oil-water-gas) in a duct. The principle physics is based in attenuation of X ray. Each element of the composed have a specific cross section contributing with the loss of the intensity of X ray. In this study, an parallel beam for the cases of two dimension is used to enforce the ideas. Then, in three dimensions, each ray generates one algebraic equation. The experiment shows that with a single view it is possible to obtain information of a stratified flow and reconstruct it only if there is enough number of rays transversing the medium.

1 INTRODUCTION

Many industrial and medical applications involves the reconstruction of functions from a small number of views given by many function projections related with its Radon, fan beam and cone beam associated with the X ray propagation. These functions in the reconstruction process that represents the radiation attenuation coefficients estimation are frequently associated with characteristic sub-domains inside the whole function domain. These homogeneous parts may results from the manufacture process, or from some natural stratification or segregation of components inside the body. By collecting a-priori information about the support and the value of these characteristics parts, the number of constant parameters needed to resolves the uniqueness problem of reconstruction may be reduced. In the case of parallel two dimensional X ray beam, where the projection may gives us this additional information, the procedure consists in inspect its discontinuities and back projection it accordingly. The support of the possibles parts are located inside the convex polygonal domains that results from these lines intersection. The same method may be applied for divergent beam in two or three dimensions. In this case we need to know the source position in order to back project the rays accordingly in a divergent way. Note that in three dimensions, the projections discontinuity determination problem is substituted by the projections images contour determination. The kind of software appropriated to implement shape from shadow X ray based support determination are based on decomposed solid geometry. The second part of this constant by part reconstruction method is based on ray tracing. By determining the length of the intersection of a ray starting at the source and ending in the detector, we may weight the contribution of each characteristic part of the function to the detector intensity measurement. Each ray generates one algebraic equation that will compose the system with the unknown source intensity. The system may be solved with algorithms based on least square method and related regularizations procedures to infer the appropriated intensities in the support of each part of the function. The technique of X ray attenuation is often used in the petroleum industry because of its robustness and noninvasive nature, and can perform these measurements without changing the operational conditions. The two views are arranged at an of 90 degrees to each other, the intention is to measure the attenuation of the beam that is influenced by changes in the composition of the flow. The information flows in the oil-water-gas system are usually obtained by subject interpretation from visual observations which may lead to misinterpretations. Therefore, a noninvasive system that identifies the flow regime without subjective evaluation is very important.

2 MODEL PHYSICAL CONCEPT

Since we are supposing to know only a small amount of projections, such as only one or two views, we must give more information about the support of the function. The first possibility is derive it from the analysis of the projections.

Projections are X ray shadows of the cross section and characteristic parts of the constant by parts function representing the extinction coefficient of the material may be identified by analyzing the contours inside these radiographies. Contours in the two dimension projection of the three dimensional object and derivatives in one dimensional projection of the two dimensional object section. Figure 1 exemplifies the two dimensional situation. The source of the parallel beam rays used to form the projection must be consider at the ∞. We may note that the back projection of the derivative location will determines variables sized strips in which the values of the function are changing. Two or more views will make possible the determination of the convex envelop of the constants parts elements of the functions. If in addition we has some a-priori information that is independent of the projections, such as that the function represents an stratified medium as in the main application of this work, it will be easier the function support characterization.

2.1 The X ray attenuation model

Along an ray, the radiation can be absorbed by various known processes, depending on its nature and energy and also on the characteristics of the medium through which it propagates. There are situations in which the scattering process gives an important contribution to detectors measurements. In this case the appropriated modeling of the radiation propagation is done through the radiative transport equation. Since we are supposing ray collimation, we will neglected the scattering process and consider only the extinction process. In this special case, the problem simplifies considerably, and the attenuation of the ray along its trajectory is exponential, and we may identify the X ray transform with the logarithm of the ray attenuation

$$\int_{\mathbb{R}^1} \sigma\,(\xi + t\theta)\,dt = -\log\left(\frac{I(E, \xi, \theta)}{I_0(E, \xi, \theta)}\right) = b\,(\xi, \theta) \quad (1)$$

where $(\xi, \theta) \in \pi_\theta \times \mathbb{R}^{d-1}$ are, respectively, the trace of the X ray in an plane containing the $\mathbb{R}^d$ origin with normal along its direction. $I_0(E, \xi, \theta)$ is the initial source beam intensity for an specific photon energy E that decreases along the ray trajectory to $I(E, \xi, \theta)$ in the detector position. Data with energy variation of the extinction cross section of important materials utilized in the oil-gas industry can be found in [2]. When $d = 2$, the X ray transform is equivalent to the Radon transform used in the tomography. In general, we may have the parallel ray or divergence ray geometry. In our model,

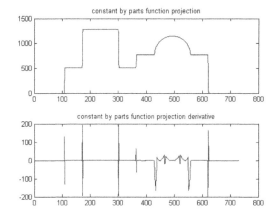

Figure 1. Projection and its derivative.

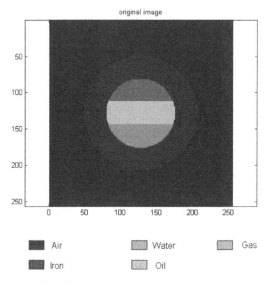

Figure 2. Water oil gas inside the duct.

we are consider only a small number of views, and collecting each ray as an algebraic equation to form a system to be solved in order to reconstruction the constant by parts function representing the unknown material.

3 MODEL GEOMETRY

We consider as an application two beams of X ray to the identification of a multiphase flow with gas, oil and water inside a metallic duct.

Due to the difference in the densities of the mixtures components, the three fluid mixture flow stratifies induced by gravity, which gives an important a-priori information about the constant by part cross section that will be reconstructed. We have used this information to model an linear system used with the reconstruction algorithm whose weight matrix parameters are determined with an computational algorithm.

3.1 Synthetic data generation

Numerical data has been produced with the simulated direct problem in two situations. In the first we consider only one view and collect the data in a direction parallel to the level of the flow stratification. Based on the experimental three dimensional divergent beam whose geometry is showed in Figure 3, we computed the set of data with photon energy $180 \, KeV$. These data are used to test our methodology for identification of the interface between the three phases of fluid inside the duct. We proceed the synthesization of the data by calculating the integral in equation X ray transform [7] with a prescribed three phase constant by parts distribution of extinction cross section. The position of source detector pair are respectively, $\{(x_s^{(j)}, x_d^{(j)}); \ j = 1, 2\} = \{((0, 0, 64),$ $(-16*8: 8: 16*8, -16*8: 8: 16*8, -64)); ((64, 0, 0),$ $(-64, -16*8: 8: 16*8, -16*8: 8: 16*8))\}$ for the case of 2×429 rays crossing the duct, and $\{(x_s^{(j)}, x_d^{(j)});$ $j = 1, 2\} = \{((0, 0, 64), (-8*8: 4: 8*8, -8*8: 4: 8*8,$ $-64)); ((64, 0, 0), (-64, -8*8: 4: 8*8, -8*8: 4: 8*8))\}$ for the case of 2×825 rays crossing the duct, which corresponds to two sets with two groups of divergent beams data with source rotated by $\pi/2$. The duct axis in the direction x_2, as shown schematically in figure 3. The external and internal pipe radius are respectively, 36 and 24 and the x_3 level of water and air are −10 and 10, respectively. The oil layer is situated between these two level. For each source the set of detector positions distributed in a plane tangent the cylinder with radius 64 and axis equal x_2 collects the values of X ray integral along these pairs of directions. These kind of data are known in the literature as the optical thickness between the source and the detector. The related experiments investigated will be named, the lateral and top experiments for the 429 and 825 rays per view cases.

4 ALGEBRAIC PROBLEM FORMULATION

For a radiation energy E fixed, let us consider the following problem: Giving some set of data

$$\{b(\xi, \theta), \xi \text{ and } \theta \text{ associated with a set of rays}\}$$

to find the constant by part function σ solution to the system formed with the respective associated X ray optical thickness Equation (1).

By using the a-priori information about the support of the function that represents the cross section to be reconstructed, our problem becomes the following linear algebraic system problem:

Problem 4.1 (Algebraic Linear System) *For a set of rays associated with* (ξ, θ),

- *given:*

$$\{b(\xi, \theta)\}, \ \delta_{n, i(\xi, \theta)} \text{ and } \gamma_{i(\xi, \theta)}, i = 1, ..., I(\xi, \theta)\}$$

- *to find* σ_n *such that*

$$\sum_{n=1}^{N} \sum_{i=1}^{I(\xi, \theta)} \sigma_n \delta_{n, i(\xi, \theta)} (\gamma_{i(\xi, \theta)} - \gamma_{i(\xi, \theta)-1}) = b(\xi, \theta) \quad (2)$$

5 LINEAR SYSTEM INVERSION

Let us give a matrix representation to the problem by defining:

$$A_{(\xi, \theta)}^n = \sum_{i=1}^{I(\xi, \theta)} \delta_{n, i(\xi, \theta)} (\gamma_{i(\xi, \theta)} - \gamma_{i(\xi, \theta)-1}) \quad (3)$$

and write the problem as:

Problem 5.1 (Algebraic Linear System) *Fixed the photon energy E. For a set of rays associated with* (ξ, θ),

- *given:*

$$b(\xi, \theta) = -\log\left(\frac{I(E, \xi, \theta)}{I_0(E, \xi, \theta)}\right)$$

- *to find* σ_n *such that*

$$\sum_{n=1}^{N} A_{(\xi, \theta)}^n \sigma_n = b(\xi, \theta) \quad (4)$$

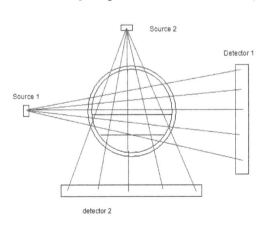

Figure 3. Divergent beam experimental set.

The physical system modeled by equations (1) when a discrete number of X rays attenuations are measured constitutes an inverse problem with discrete data [4] whose theory has been extensively studied and constitutes an main chapter in the inverse problem subject. The system given by equations (4), in which the consequences of the stratification in the model has been introduced, can have repeated lines and can be singular if not enough lines cross the domain of the function to be reconstructed or if they cross in an inappropriate angle of incidence. The remotion of repeated lines of this system can be easily done but has been noted to have no influence the solution. Figure 4 shows the singular values of the weight matrix to be used in the reconstruction for the problem with 2×429 rays with top and lateral views. Note that this problem presents singular behavior and has an illdetermined rank that does not change if we removes the repeated lines. It is Figure 5 shows the singular values of the weight matrix for problems with 825 rays in one lateral view. Note that the non singular behavior of the lateral weight matrix in contrast with the hight singular behavior of the top view matrix. For another hand, the singular values of the weight matrix for lateral view has been observed when the number of rays crossing the duct are not enough for reconstruction with only one view, even if it is a lateral one. The singularity presents in the problem is associated with the compacticity of the X ray operator has been removed by the adoption of the constant by parts representation to cross sections, and the singular behavior that remains is due to data incompleteness. Techniques based on singular values truncation may be adopted when the system is not so big, which is the case of the present work.

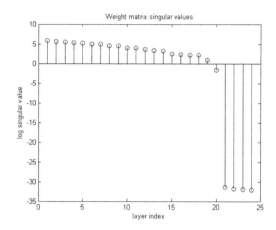

Figure 4. Weight matrix singular values decomposition.

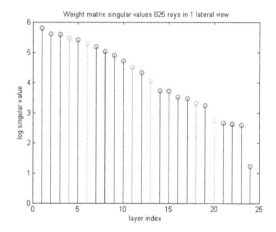

Figure 5. Weight matrix singular values decomposition for 1 lateral view with 825 rays.

5.1 The regularization problem

Through the inverse of a linear system can be constructed by using the Moore-Penrose pseudo inverse, for which non existence and non uniqueness are removed by least squares projection of the data in the operator range and factorization of indeterminate solutions due to non trivial operator null, respectively, when the operator presents compactness, such as the observed in the present $3D$ X ray transform based system, the operator range is not closed and the problem presents instability in the presence of numerical or experimental noise. The most common techniques that are adopted to solve these kind of problem are the singular value decomposition method, also known as spectral cut-off, the Tikhonov regularization method, which is a kind of optimization penalized by the noise level and the Landwebwer iterative method associated with some discrepancy based stopping rule. All these methodology are fundamentally based on the idea that the unstably problem must be substituted by an problem that will give an stable but approximated solution to the original problem. The error is committed with noise level that the original problem presents and the higher the noise level the worst the approximation will expected to be. The relation between the original and the approximated problem is controlled by a small parameter ε, which acquires different meaning, depending on the regularization method that we are using, but that is always related with the noise to signal ratio associated with the data been used.

5.2 The singular value decomposition method

The singular value decomposition method is a standard linear algebra procedure to find the decomposition of matrix $A = VDU^T$ in system (4). The matrices V and U are orthonormal and forms a basis for, respectively, the domain and the range of the matrix (operator) A, that is, they are square matrices with size equal the number of lines (m) and columns (n) of A, respectively. On other hand, the matrix D is an diagonal $n \times m$ matrix whose entries are the singular values of matrix A. The main idea in the svd regularization method for solution of problem (5.1) is constructed the regularized pseudo inverse:

$$x_\varepsilon^\dagger = A_\varepsilon^\dagger b \tag{5}$$

where

$$A_\varepsilon^\dagger = U D_\varepsilon^\dagger V^T \tag{6}$$

and $D_\varepsilon^\dagger$ is an diagonal $n \times m$ matrix with inverse entries of the diagonal $m \times n$ matrix D truncated by the rule $\mu^2 \le \epsilon(\delta)$. When the squared singular value μ^2 becomes less than the parameter ε which is of the same order of the noise level δ, this value is not invert and is ruled as zero in the inverse. Figures 6 and 7 shows multiphase flow interface and cross sections values for the case with one lateral view and 825 X rays for noise levels 1% and 5%, respectively. In this case in which the angle and the number of rays are adequetely, no cut off is necessary and the reconstruction is straight forward.

Note that is a common sense in the singular value decomposition regularization method that by truncation we means the removal of the higher frequencies components of the representation of the solution by neglecting the small singular values and doing the pseudo inversion without them.

5.3 The Thikhonov regularization method

We again consider the top and laterals views in the 2×429 rays problem in order to investigate the application of the Tikhonov regularization method, which is based on the following optimization problem:

Problem 5.2 (Tikhonov regularization Problem) *Fixed the photon energy E. For a set of rays associated with (ξ, θ), to find the extinction coefficient x which is solution of the following minimization problem*

$$\min\{\| Ax - b \|^2 + \epsilon \| x \|^2\} \tag{7}$$

The parameter ε is the Tikhonov regularization parameter (noise to signal ratio) and is choose in a such way that the error due to modification of the original problem doesn't compromises the stabilities benefits introduced by the improvement of the numerical condition number of the algebraic matrices problem.

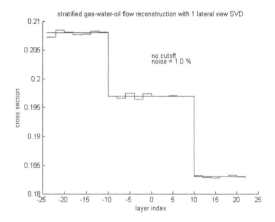

Figure 6. Svd cross section reconstruction for 1 lateral view with 1% noise.

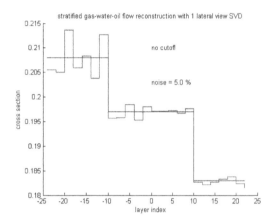

Figure 7. Svd cross section reconstruction for 1 lateral view with 5% noise.

For small size systems such that given by the X ray transform Equation (2), the solution can also be written formally with Equations (5) and (6), but the diagonalized Tikhonov regularized pseudo inverse $D_\epsilon^\dagger$ is an diagonal $n \times m$ matrix with entries $\lambda_\varepsilon = \frac{\mu}{\mu^2 + \varepsilon}$.

5.4 The L curve method to the noise to signal parameter ϵ best determination

The L curve method for determination of the best regularization parameter ϵ for the Tikhonov solution $x_{\epsilon,\delta}^\dagger$ when noised data b^δ are not known exactly but with within the noise level $\|b - b^\delta\| \le \delta$ is based on the monotonicity of the curvature of the the following curve

$$\varepsilon > 0 \mapsto (f(\varepsilon), g(\varepsilon)) := (\|Ax_{\varepsilon,\delta}^\dagger - b^\delta\|^2, \|x_{\varepsilon,\delta}^\dagger\|^2) \tag{8}$$

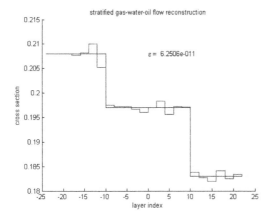

Figure 8. Cross section reconstruction by Tikhonov method under at L curve knee.

relating the norm of residual in the data space and the norm of the pseudo inverse in the signal space. Following [5], in the case of small size systems we can use svd to express these quantities in terms of the singular values:

$$\|Ax_{\varepsilon,\delta}^{\dagger} - b^{\delta}\|^2 = \sum_{i=1}^{N} \frac{\varepsilon^2}{(\mu_i^2 + \varepsilon)^2} |v_i^T b^{\delta}|^2 \qquad (9)$$

$$\|x_{\varepsilon,\delta}^{\dagger}\|^2 = \sum_{i=1}^{N} \frac{\mu_i^2}{(\mu_i^2 + \varepsilon)^2} |v_i^T b^{\delta}|^2 \qquad (10)$$

The complete range of regularizations parameter $1 \geq \varepsilon \geq 6,2506e - 011$ practically do not influence the reconstructions for the no noise data case. The stably reconstruction at the ε parameter lower bound $6,2506e - 011$ is slight better than the other reconstruction. For a lower $\varepsilon = 3,7276e - 011$ the reconstruction became instable.

6 CONCLUSIONS

The interface and cross sections values associated with the three phase stratified flow (oil-water-gas) can be reconstructed with only one lateral view if a sufficiently number of X rays is provide. The experiments presents has shown that the hypotheses of constant by parts cross section adopted in the model is enough to resolved the compactness issue that frequently generates ill-posed rank

discrete problems. So, the problem becomes rank deficient only when insufficient data are provides. If this is not the case, the reconstruction for noised data can be conducted with conventional linear algebra solvers.

REFERENCES

[1] Roberty N.C. 'Introdução à Regularização de Problemas Inversos', Lecture in the 'Curso Intensivo de Matemática Aplicada e Computação na Engenharia', Coppe/Ufrj, 2010.
[2] Hubbell, J.H. and Seltzer, S.M. 'Tables of X-Ray Mass Attenuation Coefficients and Mass Energy-Absorption Coefficients from 1 keV to 20 MeV for Elements Z = 1 to 92 and 48 Additional Substances of Dosimetric Interest', http://www.nist.gov/physlab/data/xraycoef, 1996.
[3] Hu, B. et al. 2005, "Development of an X-ray computed tomography (CT) system with sparse sources: application to three-pahase pipe flow visualization", Experiments in fluids, Vol. 39, pp. 667–678.
[4] Bertero, M., De Mol, C. and Pikes, E.R. 'Linear inverse problems with discrete data: II. Stability and regularisation', Inverse Problems, 4 (1988) 573–594.
[5] Engl, H.W. and Grever, W. "Using the L curve for determining optimal regularization parameters", Numer Math, 69; 25–31 (1994).
[6] Salgado, C.M., Schirru, R., Brandão, L.E.B. and Pereira, M.N.A. 2009. "Flow regime identification with MCNP-X Code and artificial neural network", Proceedings of the 2009 International Nuclear Atlantic Conference-INAC 2009, ABEN,Rio de Janeiro, Brazil, ISBN: 978-85-99141-03-8.
[7] Kak, A.C. and Slaney, M. "Principles of Computerized Tomographic Imaging", IEEE Press, New York, 1987, Editorial Board.
[8] Hussein, E.M.A. and Han, P. 1995. "Phase volume-fraction measurement in oikl-water-gas flow using fast neutrons", Nuclear Geophysis, Vol. 9, pp. 229–234149–167.
[9] Froystein, T. Kvandal, H. and Aakre, H. 2005. "Dual energy gamma tomography system for high pressure multiphase flow", Vol. 16, pp. 99–112.
[10] Hansen, P.C. 1998. "Rank-Deficient and Discrete I11-Posed Problem", ISBN 0-89871-403-6.
[11] Kaper, G.H., Leaf, G.K. and Linderman, A.J. 1975. "Formulation of a Ritz-Garlekin type procedure for the approximate solution of the neutron transport equation", Vol. 50, pp. 42–65.
[12] Salgado, C.M., Brandão, L.E.B., Pereira, c. M.N., Ramos, R., Silva, A.X. and Schirru, R. "Prediction of volume fractions in three-phase flows using nuclear technique anaad artificial neural network", Applied Radiation and Isotopes, doi:10.1016/j.apradiso.2009.02.093-Reference ARI4470(2009).

Computational Vision and Medical Image Processing – Tavares & Natal Jorge (eds)
© 2012 Taylor & Francis Group, London, ISBN 978-0-415-68395-1

Parallelization environment of digital images processing for medical applications

C.A. Bravo Pariente & P.E. Ambrósio
Universidade Estadual de Santa Cruz, Bahia, Brasil

ABSTRACT: This work describes the work in progress on the development of a project focused on the implementation of a parallel environment for digital image processing aimed to support medical applications. The project's overall objective is to develop and make publicly available to the scientific community a platform of high performance computing aimed on the massive processing of images with emphasis on applications in areas of medicine, such as computed mammography, computed tomography and radiography in general.

1 INTRODUCTION

Digital Image Processing (DIP) allows the automation of the processing of large amounts of information which is usually associated with the representation of images in digital format. For example it is possible to specify objective criteria for the image processing avoiding possible bias caused by human subjectivity. Another advantage of the digital image processing is the velocity of the data manipulation. Last, but no least important, there are techniques which allows the comparison of a new image with an older one, pointed out the differences between both, allowing to describe and analyze the evolution of the phenomena represented on those images.

From the standpoint of medical applications the interest in the techniques of image processing is focused in the following requirements:

– Identification of the general contours and mapping of two-dimensional images of organs.
– Fusion of images to improve the accuracy of a diagnosis.
– Three-dimensional visualization and animation of organs functioning.
– Visualization of flat sections of organs under study.
– Monitoring of functional aspects such as motion, contraction, etc.

There are well established image processing algorithms to handle these problems but, in general, all of them are computationally demanding tasks and require, therefore, specialized equipment and software. Of course, there are proprietary solutions for these applications which usually include a set of software and dedicated hardware for medical applications, but such solutions are not always available to researchers in medical fields that could make use of resources of this type.

Moreover, the classical image processing algorithms have an ideal structure for parallelization because it is possible to apply pattern recognition strategies and local operators in restricted areas of a digital image, this way distributing the processing of a digital object between the various available processors in a parallel computing environment.

This work describes a project which proposes to meet the characteristics mentioned above by providing an environment for processing digital images to be offered as a free service over the web to the general research community, and particularly of medical areas.

Internally the processing will take advantage of parallelization techniques that can be applied in image processing algorithms using a cluster of computers to maximize the performance of the image processing algorithms allowing also define several experiments with the same data set via parameters specified by the user.

The project described in this work is under development in the Departamento de Ciencias Exatas e Tecnológicas da Universidade Estadual de Santa Cruz, Ilhéus, Bahia, BRASIL with funding from FAPESB under contract n° BOL0584/2010.

The rest of this document is organized in the following manner: section 2 offers an overview of the project; section 3 describes software and hardware resources allocated for the project; section 4 is a brief summary of the development already done; section 5 summarize conclusions and future work of the project; the text finalizes with the references used in this work.

2 OVERVIEW OF THE PROJECT

This section is devoted to describe the different parts of the project. All parts are projected in such a way to offer well defined APIs to interoperation. This way it is easy to add new functionalities in the form o a new module for implement a new feature (for example, a new codec to add a new image file format) or replace an older version of a module. The project is divided in three main parts: a) parallel image processing (PIP) algorithms; b) job scheduler; and c) remote user interface. These three parts are depicted in the Figure 1 and described below.

2.1 *The parallel image processing algorithms*

The algorithms chosen to be parallelized are of two classic areas of image processing: histogram manipulation and edge-detection. In each case were selected seven different algorithms widely used to process digital images.

For the histogram manipulation these algorithms are: negative, bright enhancement, bright attenuation, threshold, histogram splitting and histogram equalization. For edge detection were selected the algorithms: first derivative, Roberts, Sobel, Prewitt, Gaussian noise (with two different convolution masks) and Laplacian of Gaussian, Velho (2009).

In order to keep independence between the data and the transformations operated by the above algorithms in sequential and parallel versions, the codification and decodification of the matrix of pixels of a image was planned as a separate module. This makes easy to add new image file formats and allow to concentrate the develop on the characteristics of each transformations and the nuances of the parallel project. Also, such a separation makes easy the inclusion of new parallel image processing algorithms in the system.

The project includes the development of a module to acts as an interface to compose the parallelized algorithms in such a way to make possible

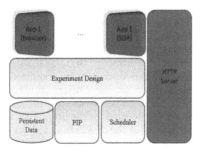

Figure 1. The general architecture of the proposed system.

specify the successive application of two of more algorithms to an image, allowing the user define several parameters as threshold level or bright enhancement and, after that, apply an edge-detection masks.

2.2 *The job scheduler*

Since the project aims to run parallel algorithms on large data sets, ideally with several different parameters for each experiment on the same data set, the project include the development of a subsystem to orderly schedule the execution of each experiment and identify the data results with the original running parameters and submitting user.

Since the system is develop to offer service for multiple users, it is also necessary to provide a module to implement a mechanism to attach each experiment request with a specific user and keep track of the requested experiments, the running jobs and the results data sets; also, a policy of limited time storage will be implemented by this module. The intend is prepare a FIFO spool of requested experiments. Experiments results will be published as soon as the experiment ends.

The above description corresponds to the operation of the scheduler from a local user point of view; for the remote users will be implemented a wrapper offering scheduler primitives.

2.3 *Experiments design layer for remote users*

Since the project aims to offers to the users with an environment to execute a large number of experiments, the project includes the development of a *experiment design layer*, allowing a remote user to provide all the necessary information to the experiments to be requested.

This layer will be programmed as a web-based application running on the top of a local http server. In particular the web interface will make transparent to the user the activation of the scheduler to run the requested experiments. On the other side, this web-interface must supply mechanism of upload to the server massive data, including resume options to avoid loss of data by network problems. In the same way, the user will be able to download from the server the data resulting of the requested experiments, when these experiments complete and the resulting data become available.

The data results will be stored for a fixed space of time and after that will be deleted; in the mean time the user will receive notice of the non-downloaded data becoming obsolete. There is no plan to create users accounts, but the experiments will be attached to a valid email and the request of a set of experiment will be protected with standard captcha mechanism.

As usual with two-tier applications, the web-based interface, avoids the necessity of distribute—and keep updated- a proprietary client for use the system, since the remote users will access the system only through web-browser applications. Also, the architecture chosen allows planning an extension of the system (but this is not included in the original project) to offer web service-based request of experiments and recollection of results.

3 MATERIALS AND METHODS

This section is devoted to describe the software and hardware infrastructure allocated to the project.

3.1 The basic codec

Throughout this paper we consider the RGB color space with 256 levels per channel and the image are encoded in the JPEG format. In order to test the develop were considered only images of 256×256 pixels.

To extract the values of the RGB channels of the images, a decoder was developed based on the JPEGLIB library of the Independent JPEG group (2010); when supplied with a JPEG image as a parameter, this decoder creates four files $R.txt$, $G.txt$, $B.txt$ and $RGB.txt$; Each of the first three files contain an array of 256 rows and 256 columns in which the value at coordinates (x, y) represents the channel value at these coordinates. In the $RGB.txt$ file, each line represents one pixel stating its coordinates x, y and the respective values of the three RGB channels in these coordinates, so that this file has 65,536 rows. In the four files, the values are separated by TAB.

3.2 Parallelization developing and running environment

The development platform for parallelization and compilation is a Beowulf-type development cluster, codename COCOA. This cluster is configured with a server node, five client nodes and a node for system administration training; for physical access, the cluster has a KVM switch, for switching of video, keyboard and mouse between the server and client nodes. Remote access is gained through an SSH server (Secure Socket Layer) OpenBSD (2009). The communication between client nodes and the server is accomplished through a Gigabit Ethernet board; equipments are protected by four UPSs. The OS installed is Linux Debian Sarge 3.1 rev 2. We used the C programming language offered by the gcc 4.2.1 The FSF Foundation, (2010). For the parallelization of the algorithms we used MPI (Message Passing Interface) Open MPI org. (2009).

For production, the project counts with another Beowulf-type BULL cluster, codename CACAU, with 20 nodes each one with a 64 bit processor of 8 cores, amount to 160 cores; all processors are Intel ® Xeon ® cpu e5430 of 2.66 ghz. This cluster has also 320 Giga RAM and storage with a total capacity of 8.5 Tb. Fast inter nodes communication is provided by an Infiniband board and external communications through a gigabit Ethernet board. The operational system is Red Hat Enterprise Linux 5; for parallelization this cluster has installed the Intel C compiler 11.1, Intel-MPI library 4.0, and PBS 10.0 for schedule jobs to the cluster.

3.3 Visible human data for experiments

In order to test the parallel algorithms massive quantities of data need to be available. In the context of our project the ideal set of data must be publicly available, come from medical areas, have been taken at high resolution and be of high number of bits per pixel.

All these requirements are met by the data from the Visible Human Project, Banvard (2002). The Visible Human Male data sets, released between November 1994 and November, 1995, consists of MRI, CT, and anatomical images of a male and a female human beings. These data were obtained under a standard agreement signed between the researcher, the project coordinator and the National Library of Medicine U.S.

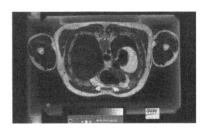

Figure 2. A typical image from the visible human data.

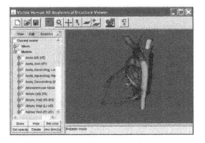

Figure 3. Virtual human server viewer.

In the context of the project these data sets are intended to be used in a twofold way: in performance tests and in the construction of voxel phantoms for physiological system.

From its publication the data sets of the visible human project have been used as a base for 3D reconstruction and visualization of the original data through web applications such as Visible Human Server by Hersch et al. (2000), and Visible Human Viewer by Chang (1998). The main difference between such systems and the one proposed in this project is that we plan allowing the user to retarget the voxel phantom obtained from the visible human dataset, using geometric deformations, to accommodate data from a patient's CT, MRI or radiography.

4 SOFTWARE DEVELOPMENT ALREADY DONE

This section is devoted to describe the software development already done in the scope of the project.

4.1 Parallelization of histogram manipulation algorithms

For the histogram manipulation the algorithms selected for parallelization are: negative, bright enhancement, bright attenuation, threshold, histogram splitting and histogram equalization.

Only the seventh of these algorithms requires, in the parallel version, two rounds of communication: one for distribute the pixels matrix of a channel in order to compute the original histogram frequencies and another to use those histogram frequencies to compute the equalized histogram. The division of the processing between the master and the client nodes is depicted in the Figure 4. The other algorithms can be modeled using only one round of communication.

In the case of the first six algorithms this amounts to a distribution of the rows of the pixels matrix from the master to compute and posterior recollection of the computed new frequencies and new matrix of pixels.

4.2 Parallelization of edge detection algorithms

For edge detection were selected the algorithms: first derivative, Roberts, Sobel, Prewitt, Gaussian noise (with two different convolution masks) and Laplacian of Gaussian.

As in the case of the first six histogram manipulation algorithms, the parallel version of these algorithms can be modeled with a simple round of communication between the master node and the compute nodes.

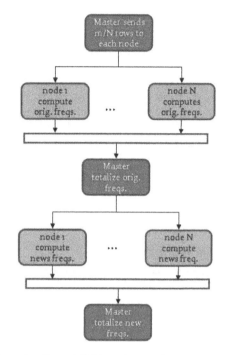

Figure 4. General division of processing and communication for parallel histogram equalization.

But, because of the nature of the convolution masks, some additional processing must be done by the master to match the boundary rows between parcels computed by different compute nodes.

Specifically, the local mask application on the rows received by the compute nodes leave alone the four boundaries (first row and column and last row and column), without defined values and the choose was that the master provide the necessary post-processing.

In the case of rows which do not include the first and last row of the original pixels matrix, the master can simply compute the missing values using the adequate entries of the pixels matrix around the entries of the boundary rows.

On the other cases, for 3x3 convolution masks, when the missing values are on the first or last row of the original matrix of pixels, the master computes the entry (i, j) as the mean value between the values at entries $(i + 1, j - 1)$ and $(i + 1, j)$, for the first row and the mean value between the values at entries $(i - 1, j - 1)$ and $(i - 1, j)$, for the last row. Mask of side greater than 3 are filled up in analogous manner beginning the interpolation of rows missing entries with the missing row closest to know values received from some compute node. Of course this strategy guarantee smooth changes between successive entries in the firsts or last rows of the matrix of pixels, but inevitably induces noise in the operators with mask greater than 3. The rightmost and leftmost columns are treated in a similar manner to the upper and bottom rows.

The overhead of the post-processing of the boundary rows between groups of rows processed by different computes nodes must be taken into account in order to decide how many rows each compute node must receive. In fact the post-processing in charge of the master can take as much computations as those made by a compute node, so it is natural to look for a balance between the time complexity of an individual compute node and the time complexity associated to the post-processing in charge of the master. This objective can be achieved by requiring that the rows of the matrix of pixels must be shared between, at most, half of the available compute nodes. This way the total amount of post-processing computing operations is dominated by the complexity of the general case of a compute node.

4.3 *Composition of the parallelization version of the algorithms*

In order to make easy the use of the system, an interface module between the algorithms was developed which made the user able to use the results of an algorithm as input to another. In this section we present some results of the interface module between the following algorithms: i) Histogram equalization followed by the operator of Roberts; ii) Gaussian operator followed by the operator of Roberts; iii) Laplacian of Gaussian operator followed by Roberts operator.

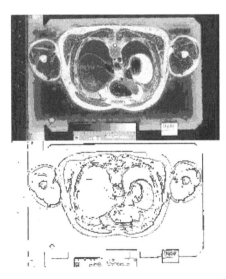

Figure 5. Histogram equalization followed by Roberts operator.

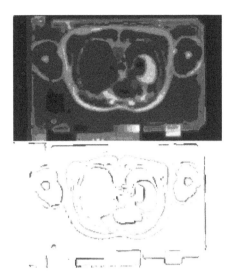

Figure 6. Gaussian operator followed by Roberts operator.

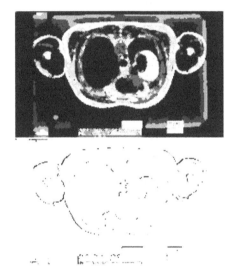

Figure 7. Application of Laplacian of Gaussian followed by Roberts operator.

The above algorithms were combined using the interface module by passing manually the arguments; for the remote users, the web interface will provide a facility to specify such combinations, allowing to supply several parameters values, in order to schedule tandem execution of different algorithms in large data sets.

For testing the algorithms, was chosen the image a_vm1484.png, which corresponds to a horizontal section of the chest of an adult male which is part of the Visible Human data set.

To obtain the voxel phantom the general plan is make a batch processing of a representative sample using different combinations of the algorithms to identify the contours of the skeletal system or the cardiac muscle, for example; the resulting data will be statistically profiled in order to identify parameters which make us able to reject false positive in the processing of the whole data set.

4.4 *Use of the visible human data set*

The visible human data sets are freely available through an agreement which must be signed between the United States Library of Medicine and the interested research institution. The documents required to establish such agreement were sent by postal mail on December 2010 and the application was approved on February 2011. Since then the download of both datasets are on the way in low priority velocity and must be completed in the next weeks. In the meantime, some specific images from the male thorax are selected to tests. The already mentioned web-based systems, Visual Human Server and Visible Human Viewer, available to explore the visible human data set, function only as 2D/3D viewers or 3D organs navigators, but the medical user has no option to resize the data to match the body size of a specific patient.

While this approach is well fitted to didactical activities in undergraduate level, it would be better that a voxels phantom can be resized up to the discretion of the medical user, in such a way that a medical doctor can superimpose CT data of a specific patient and those from the visible human project so that he can count with a realistic 3D reconstruction of the internal organs of interest. In order to meet this objective it is planned the segmentation of the images of the visible human in such a way that principal human body systems, such as skeletal and circulatory, can be reconstructed in a voxel phantom. Geometric deformations adequate to resize this voxel phantom such as described by Dong et al. (2002) will be implement to allow a remote user to use this voxel phantom as a template and resize it according to his necessities.

5 CONCLUSION AND FUTURE WORK

The implemented modules provide a basic framework for the project but must be extended in order to offer more versatility to the users; in particular new codecs for TIFF and DICOM file formats must be included into the system in order to attend the most common data in the field of medical images; these extensions must provide support for 12 bits and 16 bits grayscale images which are common on medical databases.

The integration between the parallel version of the histogram manipulation algorithms and the parallel versions of the edge-detect algorithms is in progress; this module will be completed on the next month; once integrated, the whole set will be installed on the production cluster and the development will be concentrated on the job scheduler in its local and remote version; this work must be completed by the end of 2011. The first semester of 2012 will be dedicated to the user interface which will allow remote users to submit jobs and review the work in progress of jobs already submitted. The whole system must be on the air for public access on the second semester of 2012.

REFERENCES

Banvard Richard, A. The Visible Human Project® Image Data Set From Inception to Completion and Beyond, Proceedings CODATA 2002: Frontiers of Scientific and Technical Data, Track I-D-2: Medical and Health Data, Montréal, Canada, October, 2002.

Delp, S.L., Anderson, F.C., Arnold, A.S., Loan, P., Habib, A., John, C.T., Guendelman, E. & Thelen, D.G. OpenSim: Open-source Software to Create and Analyze Dynamic Simulations of Movement. IEEE Transactions on Biomedical Engineering. (2007).

Dong, F. Clapworthy, G.J. Krokos, M.A. Yao, J. "An Anatomy-Based Approach to Human Muscle Modeling and Deformation," IEEE Transactions on Visualization and Computer Graphics, vol. 8, no. 2, pp. 154–170, Apr.–June 2002, doi:10.1109/2945.998668.

Hersch, R.D., Gennart, B., Figueiredo, O., Mazzariol, M., Tarraga, J., Vetsch, S., Messerli, V., Welz, R. & Bidaut, L. *The Visible Human Slice Web Server: A first Assessment.* Proceedings IS&T/SPIE Conference on Internet Imaging, San Jose, Ca, Jan. 2000, SPIE Vol. 3964, 253–258. Available at: http://visiblehuman.epfl.ch/index.php

Independent JPEG Group. *Free library for JPEG image compression. Version: release 8b of 16-May-2010.* Access on Mai 5th, 2010. URL: http://www.ijg.org/

NBCGIB DCET UESC. *Plataforma de Alto Desempenho para Solução de Problemas em Bioinformática.* URL: http://labbi.uesc.br/nbcgib/pt/administracluster/cadcluster

OpenBSD. *OpenSSH.* Access on May 2009. URL: http://www.openssh.com/

Open MPI org. Open MPI. URL: http://www.open-mpi.org/

The FSF Foundation. *GCC, the GNU Compiler Collection.* Access on April 2010. URL: http://gcc.gnu.org/

Velho, L., Frery, A. & Gomes, J. 2009. *Image Processing for Computer Graphics and Vision.* London: Springer.

Yuh-Jye Chang, Paul Coddington and Karlie Hutchens. Viewing the Visible Human using Java and the Web, Proc. of Asia Pacific Web (APWeb) '98, Beijing, Sept 1998, eds. Y. Yang et al., (International Academic Publishers, 1998).

Computational Vision and Medical Image Processing – Tavares & Natal Jorge (eds)
© *2012 Taylor & Francis Group, London, ISBN 978-0-415-68395-1*

Fovea and optic disc detection in retinal images

José Pinão
University of Coimbra, Coimbra, Portugal

Carlos M. Oliveira
Critical Health, S.A., Coimbra, Portugal

ABSTRACT: This work presents a new method to detect fovea and optic disk in retinal images. The proposed method consists of five steps: selection of an area in the image where the optic disk is located using Sobel operator, extraction of optic disk boundaries applying the Hough transform to detect center and diameter of optic disk, detection of the ROI (region of interest) where the fovea is located based on the optic disk center and its diameter, detection of the fovea within the ROI. The developed algorithm has been tested in a proprietary dataset with 1464 images (with ground truth generated by experts) and with some public datasets.

Keywords: Biomedical image processing, digital images, filtering, image segmentation, anatomical structure

1 INTRODUCTION

Image analysis of retinal photographs is a common procedure in diagnosis and treatment of some eye diseases such as glaucoma and diabetic retinopathy (Lalonde et al., 2001) (Singh and Sivaswamy 2008) (Chutatape). Moreover, optic disk detection is required to enable detection of other structures present in the retinal image (Lalonde et al., 2001). Furthermore some processing algorithms can have their performance improved by masking the optic disk since it is one of the brightest regions. The Foveal region is responsible for high acuity color vision. The ability to assess the location of lesions relative to the fovea is an important factor to diagnosis (Singh and Sivaswamy 2008). The proposed method uses some anatomic features to do the detection in field 1 (centered in optic disk) and field 2 (centered in fovea) namely: vertical orientation of vessels near the optic disc, the brightness region with a circular or slightly elliptical shape of the optic disk, vessels and fovea darkness and the fact that the fovea is located in an approximate distance of two and a half optic disk diameters from its center (Sinthanayothin et al., 1999).

2 CONCEPTUAL MODEL

The first step of this method is to smooth the image in order to homogenize the image of the fundus of the eye and to resize the image to a processing size, by setting the height to 576 pixel, while keeping the aspect ratio. Applying then the Sobel operator (Equation 1) to the red channel enables one to get the horizontal derivative of the image for the purpose of defining a ROI where the optic disk is located:

$$G_y = \begin{bmatrix} 1 & 2 & 1 \\ 0 & 0 & 0 \\ -1 & -2 & -1 \end{bmatrix} * A \qquad (1)$$

The major response from this operator will occur where there are more vessels with vertical orientation. In the vicinity of the optic disc, since there are vessels crossing which which branch upwards and downwards, the Sobel operator will produce a higheramplitude response.

In Figure 1 it is observed the Sobel operator response which commonly exhibits a peak in the optic disk region. This is due to vertical dark blood vessels crossing the bright optic disk and where there is a major response due to the presenceof blood vessels. The ROI is defined where the response is higher as a square image centred on the peak, with an area of 31,25% of the whole image. If the source image is field 2, the optic disk is located near of the margins. In these cases, the ROI does not intercept the center of the image and will have an area of 25% of the image size. Otherwise the ROI keeps a size of 31,25%.

Within the ROI a new binarization process is then applied. Frequently the optic disk shape is slightly elliptic. Hence, in order to obtain the best

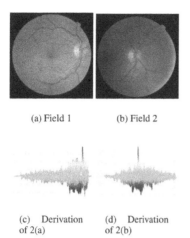

(a) Field 1   (b) Field 2

(c) Derivation   (d) Derivation
of 2(a)   of 2(b)

Figure 1. Sobel operator derivation in retinography images.

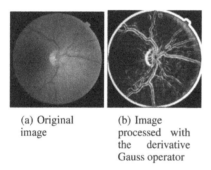

(a) Original   (b) Image
image   processed with
    the derivative
    Gauss operator

Figure 2. Derivative Gaussian operator effect.

results with Hough transform (detailed below), ROI binarization is performed after applying a derivative Gaussian filter. By choosing an appropriate standard deviation for the derivative Gaussian filtering kernel, one can control the thickness of gradient change. The derivative Gaussian filter is applied to each color channel individually, and the final filterresponse is chosen as the maximum individual color response for each position. This increased thickness enables the Hough (circle) transform to better detect the optic disk (a thinner transition would weaken the Hough transform result). Initial testing showed that when using a standard deviation of 2 for the derivative Gaussian filter kernel, a peak of performance on the results of the Hough circle transform is achieved.

After the normalisation of the Gaussian image with a sigmoid function the image is binarized with the function implemented in matlab im2bw. The normalization method was initially proposed by *Sinthanayothin et al*.

With the aim of isolating the optic disk in ROI, in a first step, the vessels are to be erased. This is achieved using the following procedure. The optic disk is the portion of the image where there is a higher contrast between vessels (dark structures) and bright area in the vicinity. A median filter with a kernel size larger than the blood vessels thickness masks vessels and renders the optic disk more clearly isolated in the ROI. In images with a height of 576 pixels, a kernel with size of 31×31 proved to be of efficacy. A subtraction is then performed between the existing Optic disk ROI and the resulting image from processing with median filter. After a normalization operation, a mask for the vessels is obtained. Finally a subtraction between the obtained ROI from the derivative Gaussian filter operation with the vessels mask is performed (Figure 3). A threshold based in the median of the output image is than applied to binarize it.

The last step will perform a quantitization of the ROI. Prior to this operation, the ROI image is normalized following the principle detailed in (Sinthanayothin et al., 1999). The optic disk ROI is then quantized in 32 levels. Distinct intensity levels, which in some images are present within the optic disk, can causes artificial boundaries to be detected by the Sobel operator. From studying test images it was found that the optic disk boundary typically has an intensity between 87,5% and 71% of the full scale value. Hence all the areas with a intensity the higher then 87,5% are set to zero. To keep the ROI as clean as possible additionally the pixels with an intensity lower then 71% are also set to zero to remove some undesired noise. This step improves significantly the performance of the algorithm.

The Hough transform allows the detection of shapes in images. In this case it is used to detect circular shapes within the ROI. With this transform relevant information such as the optic disk center and diameter is obtained (Figure 4).

With the information obtained about the optic disk center and diameter, it is possible to define a ROI for the fovea. Anatomically, the fovea is located approximately at 2.5 diameters from the optic disk center. Based on this information the image is masked and the darkest area in that ROI is searched for (Figure 5).

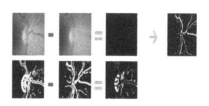

Figure 3. Vessels erased with median filter.

150

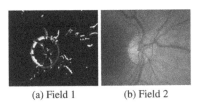

(a) Field 1   (b) Field 2

Figure 4. Optic disk detection with the Hough transform.

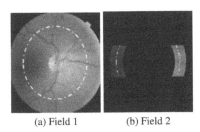

(a) Field 1   (b) Field 2

Figure 5. Sobel operator derivation in retinography images.

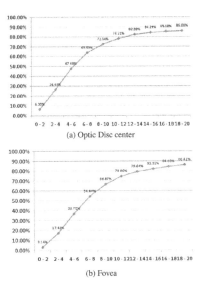

(a) Optic Disc center

(b) Fovea

Figure 6. Cumulative chart of percent images for the local dataset by difference (Euclidean distance) from ground truth in pixels.

3 ANALYSIS

The technique described above was tested on a proprietary dataset and on four public datasets: Messidor, ROC, Utrech and Stare. The proprietary dataset has 1464 non-mydriatic anonymous images from a Diabetic Retinopathy Screening Programme in Portugal. For the proprietary dataset tests, a detection was considered correct when optic disk center and fovea had at most an Euclidean distance of 20 pixels from the ground truth in images with size of 768×576. Regarding radius, a coefficient between ground truth and radius detected with an interval between 0.9 and 1.1 was admitted as correct. The method herein described obtained the following results: Optic disk center was correctly detected in 1259 images (86%), 912 (62.30%) for optic disk radius and 1265 (86.41%) regarding fovea location. Figure 6 shows two cumulative charts indicating the detection performance for optic disk center and fovea location as a function of the acceptable error margin (in pixels) in relation to a ground truth that has been marked by experienced ophthalmologists.

Another important feature about the developed code is the low average time processing per image. Average processing time took 10.9452 seconds in a computer with 2 Quad CPU 2.85 GHz, 1.98 Gb of RAM.

For the public datasets, the analysis performed on the results had some changes due the absence of ground truth. Fovea detection was not assessed, and detection of optic disk was admitted as correct if the center was detected within the optic disk boundary. Messidor (http://messidor.crihan.fr/index-en.php) is a dataset constituted by 1200 eye fundus color images acquired by 3 ophthalmologic departments using non-mydriatic retinographs with a 45 degree field of view. Each one was captured using 8 bits per color plane. ROC dataset (http://roc.healthcare.uiowa.edu/) has 100 images all taken from patients with diabetes without known diabetic retinopathy. The images are a random sample of all patients that were noted to have 'red lesions'. For the Utrech dataset (http://www.isi.uu.nl/Research/), the photographs were obtained from a diabetic retinopathy screening program in The Netherlands. Forty photographs have been randomly selected to creat the dataset, 33 do not show any sign of diabetic retinopathy and 7 show signs of mild early diabetic retinopathy. Stare dataset (www.perl.clemson.edu/stare/nerve) is constituted by 81 images: 31 healthy retinas and 50 containing pathological lesions of various types and severity. Stare dataset hasa significant number of images with a deformed optic disk due to some diseases, so it is not the best dataset to test these algorithms. Not with standing it is a widely tested dataset in this field. The results for all this public datasets are represented in Table 1.

Except for the stare dataset, the method herein proposed generated excellent results on detection. In a significant number of images in the STARE dataset, the detection failed due a bad detection of the ROI. To improve the performance for this last dataset, the vessel mask was also made use of when selecting the ROI. Since the optic disk is always crossed by vessels, the Sobel operator output is set to zero in regions where no vessels are present in the vicinity. With this change, there occur less wrong detections of the ROI. This new approach improved significantly the results for the stare dataset. (Table 2).

4 EXAMPLES

In this section a sample of each dataset is presented. Each sample is representative of the quality of the images for each dataset and the respective detection achieved by the developed method. For the

Table 1. Results for the public datasets.

Dataset	Optic disk detected	
	Images	%
Messidor	1156	96,33
ROC	98	98,00
Utrech	39	97,50
Stare	47	58,02

Table 2. Optic disk detection results for the proposed and literature methods with the Stare dataset.

Optic disk detection methods	Stare dataset
Highest average variation (Sinthanayothin et al., 1999)	42.0%
Largest brightest connected objects (Walter 2001)	58,0%
Average OD-images model—based (Osareh et al.)	58,00%
Developed method with normal calculation of the ROI	**58,0%**
Resolution pyramid using a simple Haar-based discrete wavelet transform (ter Haar 2005)	70,4%
Hausdorff—based template matching, piramidal decomposition & confident assignment (Lalonde et al., 2001)	71,6%
Hough transform applied only to pixels close to the retinal vasculature (ter Haar 2005)	71,6%
Developed method with mask of vessel to calculate the ROI	**74,1%**
Fuzzy convergence (Hoover and Goldbaum 2003)	89,0%
Fitting the vasculature orientation on a directional model (ter Haar 2005)	93,8%
A geometrical model of the vessel structure structure using 2 parabolas (Foracchia et al., 2004)	97,5%
Vessels direction matched filter (Youssif et al., 2008)	98,8%

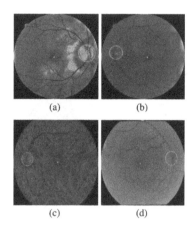

Figure 7. Images of the proprietary dataset.

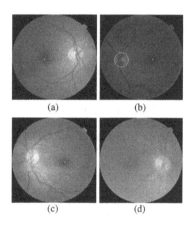

Figure 8. Images of the Messidor dataset.

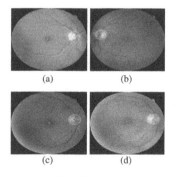

Figure 9. Images of the Utrech dataset.

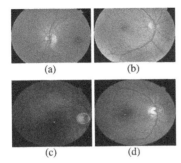

(a)   (b)

(c)   (d)

Figure 10.   Images of the ROC dataset.

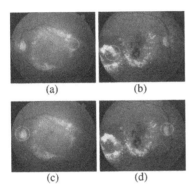

(a)   (b)

(c)   (d)

Figure 11.   Images of the Stare dataset.

case of the Stare dataset (Figure 11), Figure 11(a) and 11(b) are processed with the method which ROI is calculated without the vessels mask and Figure 11(c) and 11(d) with it.

5   CONCLUSIONS

A new fully automatic method is proposed in this work to detect the fovea and optic disk center and radius in retinal images. Comparing with the literature, this method is one of the few that detects both the center and the radius of the optic disk. This algorithm was developed with a particular concern to be both a fast method and to keep interesting levels of detection performance. For all the datasets tested, this proposed methodology revealed to be a powerful tool to detect the structures mentioned.

The optic disc was particularly reliably detected and may be examined in the future for patterns of disease such as glaucoma. Beyond the reach a excellent accuracy, this model revealed extremely fast comparing with the literature models that had better results with the Stare dataset (Youssif et al., 2008) (Foracchia et al., 2004) (Hoover and Goldbaum 2003) (ter Haar 2005). These ones are

based in detecting the main arcades position which do a gross estimate of optic disk center and can not detect theoptic disk radius or the fovea. The proposed method successfully detects fovea and optic disk in over 86% and 86.41% respectively, of 1464 images in the Proprietary Diabetic Retinopathy Screening Programme dataset. However if there are a significant number of exudates in retinal images, there is a significant probability to do an erroneous ROI detection of the optic disk. Making use of the vessel mask as mentioned in the calculation of the ROI, this error is reduced.

Future work will test the approach with the vessel mask in the calculation of the ROI with more datasets to understand the real effect of this modification.

REFERENCES

Chutatape, O. Automatic location of optic disk in retinal images. *Proceedings 2001 International Conference on Image Processing (Cat. No. 01CH37205)*, 837–840.

Foracchia, M., Grisan, E., Ruggeri, A. and Member, S. (2004). Detection of Optic Disc in Retinal Images by Means of a Geometrical Model of Vessel Structure. *IEEE Trans Med Imaging 2004 23*, 1189–1195.

Hoover, A. and Goldbaum, M. (2003, August). Locating the optic nerve in a retinal image using the fuzzy convergence of the blood vessels. *Medical Imaging, IEEE Transactions on 22*(8), 951–958.

Lalonde, M., Beaulieu, M. and Gagnon, L. (2001, November). Fast and robust optic disc detection using pyramidal decomposition and Hausdorff-based template matching. *IEEE transactions on medical imaging 20*(11), 1193–200.

Osareh, a., Mirmehdi, M., Thomas, B. and Markham, R. Comparison of colour spaces for optic disc localisation in retinal images. *Object recognition supported by user interaction for service robots*, 743–746.

Singh, J. and Sivaswamy, J. (2008). Fundus Foveal Localization Based on Image Relative Subtraction-IReS Approach. *cvit.iiit.ac.in*.

Sinthanayothin, C., Boyce, J.F., Cook, H.L. and Williamson, T.H. (1999, August). Automated localisation of the optic disc, fovea, and retinal blood vessels from digital colour fundus images. *The British journal of ophthalmology 83*(8), 902–10.

ter Haar, F. (2005). Automatic localization of the optic disc in digital colour images of the human retina. *Utrecht University*.

Walter, T. (2001). Segmentation of color fundus images of the human retina: Detection of the optic disc and the vascular tree using morphological techniques. *Medical Data Analysis*, 282–287.

Youssif, a.R., Ghalwash, a.Z. and Ghoneim, a.R. (2008, January). Optic disc detection from normalized digital fundus images by means of a vessels' direction matched filter. *IEEE transactions on medical imaging 27*(1), 11–8.

Computational Vision and Medical Image Processing – Tavares & Natal Jorge (eds)
© *2012 Taylor & Francis Group, London, ISBN 978-0-415-68395-1*

Displacement measurements with block motion algorithms

G. Almeida & J. Fonseca
Universidade Nova de Lisboa, FCT, Monte da Caparica, Portugal

F. Melício
ISEL, Lisboa, Portugal

ABSTRACT: The traditional methodology used for displacement measurements in civil engineering requires a large volume of equipment and a very complex procedure. The goal of using digital image processing techniques is to calculate the displacement or the strain field without contact using a simple low cost camera. Digital Image Correlation is a method that examines consecutive images taken during the deformation period and detects the movements based on a mathematical correlation algorithm. Using image-processing techniques it is possible to measure the whole area of interest and not only a few points of the test materials as when using the conventional methodology. In this paper, block-matching algorithms are used in order to compare the results from DIC with data obtained using linear voltage displacement transducer sensors during the load test. Several laboratory tests were done in order to validate the adopted approach and measure the effectiveness of the solution.

1 INTRODUCTION

The accurate measurement of deformations, displacements, strain fields and surface defects is a challenge in many material tests in Civil Engineering. Traditionally, these measurements require complex and expensive equipment and time consuming calibration.

When conventional methodology is used the number of measured points takes on a huge importance because they increase the need for hardware, the time to get the setup ready and the costs. Using image analysis techniques the density of the measured points can be very high without changing the equipment. As an example, a trivial image of 1024 by 1024 pixels can be used to obtain a continuous information field with more than 4000 analysis points.

Since the 80's, when Digital Image Correlation (DIC) was first conceived (Peters & Ranson 1982; Sutton et al., 1983; Chu et al., 1985; Sutton et al., 1991), several works have been developed in order to obtain an optimized and accurate algorithm. DIC is also very flexible because it is possible to apply this technique to several types of digital images such as photography, optical and microscopy.

The analysis of the deflection using image processing depends on the texture of the material. Since concrete is typically homogenous (or at least too homogenous for detailed image analysis) it is necessary to paint the beam under analysis with a pattern that allows detailed movement detection. In our experiments white non-plastic matt ink was used as a bottom layer and a black pattern was sprayed on top of it.

In order to obtain an efficient measuring system it is essential to study the influence of the speckle pattern applied, the image contrast, the size of the analysis block and the resolution of the images on the final measurement precision (Reu et al., 2009).

A deep study of the efficiency of a random speckle pattern and its influence on the measured in-plane displacements with respect to the subset size was presented in (Lecompte et al., 2006).

Our goal is to compare the traditional observations using LVDT (Linear Variable Differential Transformer) displacement sensors with a measuring system using digital image techniques. The results of the image processing approach are compared with the results obtained with standard sensors normally used in civil engineering laboratory tests.

The block matching Simple and Efficient Search algorithm (SES) was first applied (Almeida et al., 2010). In this paper SES is compared with the Adaptive Rood Pattern Search (ARPS) that has been used in order to study the influence of the speckle pattern. Both algorithms were applied to images from real tests with concrete beams and Plexiglass bars. The Plexiglass bars were used in order to create a more controllable environment where the *ground truth* was easier to find and different speckle patterns were easily changed.

2 BLOCK MOTION ALGORITHM

In this paragraph the two block motion algorithms, SES and ARPS, used in this work are presented. With both these algorithms the Cross Correlation (CC) function was used, as reported in (Barranger et al., 2010).

2.1 Three—step search

The general idea of Three-Step Search algorithm (TSS) is to start the search at the middle of the search window with a step size, S. The least cost makes it the new search origin and the step size will be $S = S/2$. This procedure is repeated until $S = 1$.

The Simple and Efficient Search algorithm (SES) presented by (Jianhua & Liou 1997) is a variation of the classical TSS algorithm.

The SES algorithm has two phases in order to reduce computation time taking advantage of the uniformity of the pattern.

In each phase the number of steps of the algorithm is dependent on the search window. Phase 1 consists on selecting the search direction quadrant (Figure 1).

To choose the search quadrant it is necessary to compute the cross correlation function (CC) for the three locations A, B and C. With the following four rules the most promising quadrant is selected:

If $CC(A) \geq CC(B)$ and $CC(A) < CC(C)$
    quadrant I is selected;
If $CC(A) < CC(B)$ and $CC(A) < CC(C)$
    quadrant II is selected;
If $CC(A) < CC(B)$ and $CC(A) \geq CC(C)$
    quadrant III is selected;
If $CC(A) \geq CC(B)$ and $CC(A) \geq CC(C)$
    quadrant IV is selected.

After selecting the most promising quadrant it is necessary to calculate the other points that will help deciding the best block match. This is the second phase.

In Figure 2 the initial search patterns of phase 1 (black dots) and phase 2 (white squares) are indicated. The goal of this phase is to find the location

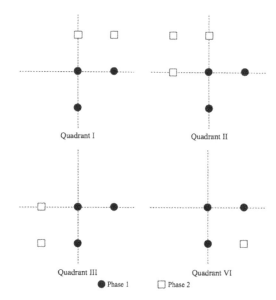

Figure 2. Search patterns for each select quadrant in phase 1 and 2.

with the smallest error considering the previously selected quadrant. This process is iterated with the points A, B and C inside the new search window until a null displacement is found.

2.2 Adaptive rood pattern search

The adaptive rood pattern search algorithm implemented on this work was based on the proposal by (Nie & Kai-Kuang 2002).

In most cases the adjacent blocks have similar motions. The blocks on the immediate left, above, above-left and above right of the current block are the most important to calculate the predicted the motion vector (MV). Four types of region of support can be used. In this paper the motion vector predicted is based on the immediate left of the current block.

For the initial search, the ARPS algorithm evaluates the four endpoints in a symmetrical rood pattern plus the predicted motion vector (MV) (see Figure 3).

The four arms of the rood pattern are of equal length and its initial size is equal to the length of the predicted motion vector.

It is therefore necessary to compute the cost function in each search point. As for the SES algorithm the cross correlation was also used has cost function.

The minimal matching error (MME) point found in the current step will be the starting search center for the next iteration. The algorithm repeats

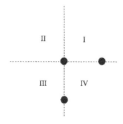

Figure 1. Phase 1 search quadrants.

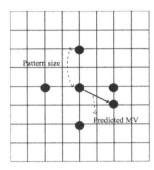

Figure 3. The adaptive rood pattern.

itself until the MME coincides with the center of the rood pattern.

3 RESULTS

For the evaluation of the developed system three different structures were tested:

- a concrete T-beam 3 m wide by 0.3 m high was tested until rupture in a 4-point bending test system;
- a concrete beam 0.6 m wide by 0.15 m high was tested until rupture;
- a Plexiglass bar 0.43 m wide by 0.032 m high.

Both concrete beams followed a monotonic loading history. The deflection measurement was supported by standard 100 mm LVDT sensors displayed along the longitudinal direction of the beam. The data from the LVDT sensor at the mid-span was used for the comparison with the data obtained from the image analysis system.

Image acquisition was done with a digital Cannon EOS 400D camera with a resolution of 3888 × 2592 and two spotlights of 500 W.

The T-beam was prepared with an underlying cover of white matt ink on top of which a super-imposed random speckle pattern was manually applied using a large brush with black matt ink. On the Plexiglass bars, due to its reduced size, painting was done with an ink spray.

Table 1 shows the data acquisition parameters.

All the digital measurements were done at a distance without any particular calibration, with a low cost support and easy setup.

The experiments with concrete beams were done until rupture on a destructive test while the Plex-iglass bar rested undamaged allowing its reuse.

In Figure 4 it is possible to see the initial and final stage of the load tests with the concrete beams and the Plexiglass.

Figures 5 and 6 show the results obtained from the concrete beams with the ARPS algorithm.

Table 1. Data acquisition parameters.

Test name	Number of photos	Interval between photos [s]	Resolution [Pixel/cm]
TSC1	50	30	35
NS10000_04	65	5	95
Plexiglass	33	5	205

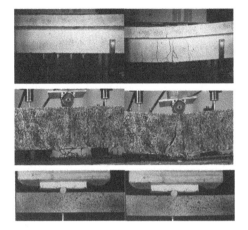

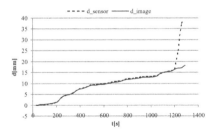

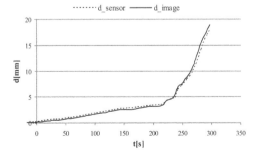

Figure 4. Images of the tests: initial shape (left) and the final shape (right). Concrete beams: TSC1 (top) and NS10000_04 (middle). Plexiglass bar (bottom).

Figure 5. Displacement vs. time for TSC1 T-beam.

Figure 6. Displacement vs. time for NS10000_04 beam.

157

These graphs represent the displacement versus time at the middle of the beam.

On Figure 5 (TSC1 beam) it is possible to see that, for larger displacement, the intervals of 30 s between photos was insufficient to follow the major cracks that appear around second 1200.

On Figure 6 (NS10000_04 beam) the intervals between the photos was 5 s and it is possible to see that the system is able to follow the major displacements.

Some other patterns, which were applied identically, didn't show so good results.

In order to study a variation of random speckle pattern, several tests were done with a Plexiglass bar. With this small bar it was much easier to repeat the tests because it takes less time to setup up and the bar was undamaged. This way it was possible to test different resolutions, intervals of photos and speckle patterns.

One of the important issues is the size of the block used in the algorithm and also the search window, p. For the results presented in this paper the p used was half of the block size. Both algorithms were used with different block sizes. The data obtained with a block of 32×32 pixels was identified by b_32 at the graph. The same terminology was used for blocks with the size of 50, 64 and 100 pixels.

In Figures 7 and 8 is shown the displacement versus time with different sizes of blocks and also

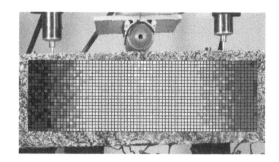

the data obtained from the LVDT sensor. The region of interest was at the middle of the beam, i.e., the same place as the sensor.

As we can see, the pattern applied and the block size are related and are both important for achieving accurate results. With a large pattern and a small block size it is not possible to follow the pattern because the pattern is often not recognisable. Also, if we choose a small pattern and a small block size (small enough to follow the pattern) the computation time can be too high.

For the same pattern and for each block motion algorithm there is an ideal size of block. If the block size is too small it is not possible to identify the pattern that we want to follow and if the block size is too large it is more time consuming.

The results show that the ARPS algorithm was faster and more accurate than SES. For the ARPS the best result was achieved with a block size of 64. With the TSS algorithm the result wasn't acceptable for any block size. However, even in this case the block size of 64 is the most suitable.

With the information obtained with image processing it is possible to calculate the displacement map for the entire area, Figure 9.

A grid of blocks was marked on the entire region of interest. The ARPS algorithm was processed and the values of displacements for each block calculated. In order to visualize where the largest displacements were one color was associated for each displacement. The dark regions indicated the regions where the displacements were lower and the light regions where the displacements were higher.

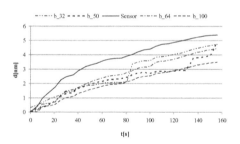

Figure 7. Displacement vs. time with the SES algorithm for different block sizes.

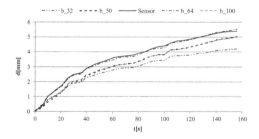

Figure 8. Displacement vs. time with ARPS algorithm for different block sizes.

4 CONCLUSIONS

The comparison between the measurements from LVDT sensors and the measurements obtained from image processing techniques are very similar with a lower investment and much faster and easier setup when compared with the traditional methodologies used in Civil Engineering.

We currently have errors between 0.4 and 1.4 mm depending on the speckle pattern applied and the photos resolution.

The results obtained in this study show that it is possible to use Digital Image Correlation with confidence on the whole area of a T-beam. Additionally, the tests with the Plexiglass increase the confidence in the best application of the random speckle pattern, the best block size and also the best resolution.

The cost function used was the cross correlation for both algorithms.

The ARPS is approximately twice as fast as TSS and its results more accurate. The decreasing of interval between photos showed an improvement in results.

The results obtained with ARPS were more accurate than with SES. For both algorithms the block size is very important. For the ARPS algorithm the best block was with 64×64 pixels. The ARPS algorithm will be used in future tests with concrete beams.

With the data obtained with this algorithm it is possible to calculate the map of displacements and the strain map for the entire beam.

The achieved results were accurate and indicated that it is possible to calculate other Civil Engineering measurements such as the map of displacements, the strain map.

ACKNOWLEDGMENTS

Professor Carlos Chastre from the Civil Engineering Department of the Universidade Nova de Lisboa conducted all the tests. We must acknowledge him for his suggestions and for provision of the data evaluated in this study. The data from the sensors was obtained from the tests done in conjunction with the Phd student Hugo Biscaia.

REFERENCES

Almeida, G., Biscaia, H., Melicio, F., Chastre, C. & Fonseca, J. (2010). Displacement Estimation of a RC Beam Test based on TSS algorithm. *Information Systems and Technologies (CISTI), 2010 5th Iberian Conference on* Santiago de Compostela.

Barranger, Y., Doumalin, P., Dupré, J.C. & Germaneau, A. (2010). Digital Image Correlation accuracy: influence of kind of speckle and recording setup. *ICEM 14 – 14th International Conference on Experimental Mechanics*, EPJ Web of Conferences. **Volume 6, 2010:** 7.

Chu, T.C., Ranson, W.F., Sutton, M.A. & Peters, W.H. (1985). "Applications of Digital. Image-Correlation Techniques to Experimental Mechanics." *Experimental Mechanics* **25**(3): 232–244.

Jianhua, L. & Liou, M.L. (1997). "A simple and efficient search algorithm for block-matching motion estimation." *Circuits and Systems for Video Technology, IEEE Transactions on* **7**(2): 429–433.

Lecompte, D., Sol, H., Vantomme, J. & Habraken, A. (2006). Analysis of speckle patterns for deformation measurements by digital image correlation. *SPIE*. Nimes,France, Proceedings of SPIE. **Vol. 6341:** E1–E6.

Nie, Y. & Kai-Kuang, M. (2002). "Adaptive Rood Pattern Search for Fast Block-Matching Motion Estimation." *IEEE TRANSACTIONS ON IMAGE PROCESSING* **11**(12): 8.

Peters, W.H. & Ranson, W.F. (1982). *DIGITAL IMAGING TECHNIQUES IN EXPERIMENTAL STRESS ANALYSIS*. Optical Engineering.

Reu, P.L., Sutton, M., Wang, Y. & Miller, T.J. (2009). Uncertainty quantification for digital image correlation. *Proceedings of the SEM Annual Conference*. S. f. E.M. Inc. 2009. Albuquerque New Mexico USA.

Sutton, M., Turner, J., Bruck, H. & Chae, T. (1991). "Full-field representation of discretely sampled surface deformation for displacement and strain analysis." *Experimental Mechanics* **31**(2): 168–177.

Sutton, M.A., Wolters, W.J., Peters, W.H., Ranson, W.F. & McNeill, S.R. (1983). Determination of displacements using an improved digital correlation method. *Image and Vision Computing*. **1**: 133–139.

Computational Vision and Medical Image Processing – Tavares & Natal Jorge (eds)
© *2012 Taylor & Francis Group, London, ISBN 978-0-415-68395-1*

Automatic segmentation of the secondary austenite-phase island precipitates in a superduplex stainless steel weld metal

Victor H.C. Albuquerque
Universidade de Fortaleza, Centro de Ciências Tecnológicas, Fortaleza, Brazil

Rodrigo Y.M. Nakamura & João P. Papa
Departamento de Computação, UNESP—Universidade Estadual Paulista, Bauru, Brazil

Cleiton C. Silva
Departamento de Engenharia Metalúrgica e Materiais, Universidade Federal do Ceará, Fortaleza, Brazil

João Manuel R.S. Tavares
Universidade do Porto, Faculdade de Engenharia, Porto, Portugal

ABSTRACT: Duplex and superduplex stainless steels are class of materials of a high importance for engineering purposes, since they have good mechanical properties combination and also are very resistant to corrosion. It is known as well that the chemical composition of such steels is very important to maintain some desired properties. In the past years, some works have reported that γ_2 precipitation improves the toughness of such steels, and its quantification may reveals some important information about steel quality. Thus, we propose in this work the automatic segmentation of γ_2 precipitation using two pattern recognition techniques: Optimum-Path Forest (OPF) and a Bayesian classifier. To the best of our knowledge, this if the first time that machine learning techniques are applied into this area. The experimental results showed that both techniques achieved similar and good recognition rates.

1 INTRODUCTION

Duplex and superduplex stainless steels are a important class of materials for engineering, which have an exceptional corrosion resistance and good mechanical properties combination (Nilsson 1992). The success of these alloys is associated to the microstructural balance of phases, in which ferrite and austenite have approximately the same proportions. All these characteristics have motivated the use of duplex and super-duplex stainless steels in a wide variety of industrial sectors, such as chemical ones, petrochemical and oil & gas (Tavares et al., 2010; Bastos et al., 2007).

The balance of phases is influenced by the chemical composition of the alloys, and also by the cooling rate experimented during its production (Hemmer and Grong 1999; Hemmer et al., 2000). However, depending on the manufacturing process, this proportion can be changed and then the properties degraded. One of the most important processes used in the manufacturing and repairing of pipes and equipments for industrial applications is the welding, in which the steel is subjected to a high cooling rate. The high temperature reached during the welding cycle causes the austenite dissolution, and consequently one may observe an increasing in the ferrite content, harming the toughness and ductility (Kotecki and Hilkes 1994; Hertzman et al., 1997). In multipass welding, the reheated zone by deposition of subsequent weld beads causes, as main microstructural changes, the dissolution of chromium nitrides and also the precipitation of secondary austenite (γ_2) (Ramirez et al., 2004; Ramirez et al., 2003).

Some works have reported that γ_2 precipitation improves the toughness of the duplex and super-duplex stainless steels (Lippold and Al-Rumaih 1997; Lee et al., 1999). On the other hand, the low chromium, molybdenium and nitrogen contents of the γ_2 are harmful to corrosion resistance (Nilsson and Wilson 1993; Nilsson et al., 1995). Based on these aspects, it is very important to quantify the amount of γ_2 in welded joints, especially in fusion zone, in order to improve the weld quality. However, this quantification is not straightforward, mainly because the secondary austenite formed is more evident when the precipitates are located inside the ferrite grain, with needles shape and also with the presence of γ_2 islands. Thus, the quantification of such islands is usually carried out by manual operations using all purpose image analysis softwares, demanding a long time and user experience.

In this paper, we propose the automatic segmentation of γ_2 islands using machine learning techniques, focusing on the Optimum-Path Forest (OPF) (Papa, Falcão, and Suzuki 2009) and a Bayesian classifier (Duda, Hart, and Stork 2000). As far as we know, this is the first time that OPF is applied into this domain, as well as any other computational technique, once that these precipitates have never been automatically segmented up to date.

The remainder of the paper is organized as follows. Section 2 revisits the classifiers, and Section 4 discuss the experimental results. Finally, Section 5 states the conclusions.

2 MACHINE LEARNING BACKGROUND

This section addresses a review about the pattern recognition techniques applied.

2.1 *Optimum-path forest classifier*

The OPF classifier works by modeling the problem of pattern recognition as a graph partition in a given feature space. The nodes are represented by the feature vectors and the edges connect all pairs of them, defining a full connectedness graph. This kind of representation is straightforward, given that the graph does not need to be explicitly represented, allowing us to save memory. The partition of the graph is carried out by a competition process between some key samples (*prototypes*), which offer optimum paths to the remaining nodes of the graph. Each prototype sample defines its optimum-path tree (OPT), and the collection of all OPTs defines de optimum-path forest, which gives the name to the classifier (Papa, Falcão, and Suzuki 2009).

The OPF can be seen as a generalization of the well known Dijkstra's algorithm to compute optimum paths from a source node to the remaining ones (Dijkstra 1959). The main difference relies on the fact that OPF uses a set of source nodes (prototypes) with any path-cost function. In case of Dijkstra's algorithm, a function that summed the arc-weights along a path was applied. For OPF, we used a function that gives the maximum arc-weight along a path, as explained before.

Let $Z = Z_1 \cup Z_2$ be a dataset labeled with a function λ, in which Z_1 and Z_2 are, respectively, a training and test sets such that Z_1 is used to train a given classifier and Z_2 is used to assess its accuracy. Let $S \subseteq Z_1$ a set of prototype samples. Essentially, the OPF classifier creates a discrete

optimal partition of the feature space such that any sample $s \in Z_2$ can be classified according to this partition. This partition is an optimum path forest (OPF) computed in $\Re^n$ by the image foresting transform (IFT) algorithm (Falcão, Stolfi, and Lotufo 2004).

The OPF algorithm may be used with any *smooth* path-cost function which can group samples with similar properties (Falcão, Stolfi, and Lotufo 2004). Particularly, we used the path-cost function f_{max}, which is computed as follows:

$$f_{max}(\langle s \rangle) = \begin{cases} 0 & \text{if } s \in S, \\ +\infty & \text{otherwise} \end{cases}$$
$$f_{max}(\pi \cdot \langle s,t \rangle) = \max\{f_{max}(\pi), d(s,t)\}, \quad (1)$$

in which $d(s, t)$ means the distance between samples s and t, and a path π is defined as a sequence of adjacent samples. As such, we have that $f_{max}(\pi)$ computes the maximum distance between adjacent samples in π, when π is not a trivial path.

The OPF algorithm assigns one optimum path $P^*(s)$ from S to every sample $s \in Z_1$, forming an optimum path forest P (a function with no cycles which assigns to each $s \in Z_1 \backslash S$ its predecessor $P(s)$ in $P^*(s)$ or a marker *nil* when $s \in S$. Let $R(s) \in S$ be the root of $P^*(s)$ which can be reached from $P(s)$. The OPF algorithm computes for each $s \in Z_1$, the cost $C(s)$ of $P^*(s)$, the label $L(s) = \lambda(R(s))$, and the predecessor $P(s)$.

The OPF classifier is composed of two distinct phases: (i) training and (ii) classification. The former step consists, essentially, into finding the prototypes and computing the optimum-path forest, which is the union of all OPTs rooted at each prototype. After that, we pick a sample from the test sample, connect it to all samples of the optimum-path forest generated in the training phase and we evaluate which node offered the optimum path to it. Notice that this test sample is not permanently added to the training set, i.e., it is used only once. The next sections describe in more detail this procedure.

2.1.1 *Training*

We say that S^* is an optimum set of prototypes when OPF algorithm minimizes the classification errors for every $s \in Z_1$. S^* can be found by exploiting the theoretical relation between minimum-spanning tree (MST) and optimum-path tree for f_{max} (Allène, Audibert, Couprie, Cousty, and Keriven 2007). The training essentially consists in finding S^* and an OPF classifier rooted at S^*.

By computing an MST in the complete graph (Z_1, A), we obtain a connected acyclic graph whose nodes are all samples of Z_1 and the arcs are undirected and weighted by the distances d between adjacent samples. The spanning tree is optimum in the sense that the sum of its arc weights is minimum as compared to any other spanning tree in the complete graph. In the MST, every pair of samples is connected by a single path which is optimum according to f_{max}. That is, the minimum-spanning tree contains one optimum-path tree for any selected root node.

The optimum prototypes are the closest elements of the MST with different labels in Z_1 (i.e., elements that fall in the frontier of the classes). By removing the arcs between different classes, their adjacent samples become prototypes in S^* and OPF can compute an optimum-path forest with minimum classification errors in Z_1. Note that, a given class may be represented by multiple prototypes (i.e., optimum-path trees) and there must exist at least one prototype per class.

2.1.2. Classification

For any sample $t \in Z_2$, we consider all arcs connecting t with samples $s \in Z_1$, as though t were part of the training graph. Considering all possible paths from S^* to t, we find the optimum path $P^*(t)$ from S^* and label t with the class $\lambda(R(t))$ of its most strongly connected prototype $R(t) \in S^*$. This path can be identified incrementally by evaluating the optimum cost $C(t)$ as:

$$C(t) = \min\{\max\{C(s), d(s,t)\}\}, \forall s \in Z_1. \quad (2)$$

Let the node $s^* \in Z_1$ be the one that satisfies Equation 3 (i.e., the predecessor $P(t)$ in the optimum path $P^*(s)$). Given that $L(s^*) = \lambda(R(t))$, the classification simply assigns $L(s^*)$ as the class of t. An error occurs when $L(s^*) \neq \lambda(t)$.

2.2 Bayesian Classifier

Let $p(\omega_i|x)$ be the probability of a given pattern $x \in \Re^n$ to belong to class ω_i, $i = 1, 2, ..., c$, which can be defined by the Bayes Theorem (Jaynes 2003):

$$p(\omega_i \mid x) = \frac{p(x \mid \omega_i)P(\omega_i)}{p(x)}, \quad (3)$$

where $p(x|\omega_i)$ is the probability density function of the patterns that compose the class ω_i, and $p(\omega_i)$ corresponds to the probability of class the ω_i itself.

A Bayesian classifier decides whether a pattern x belongs to the class ω_i when:

$$p(\omega_i \mid x) > p(\omega_j \mid x), i, j = 1, 2, ..., c, i \neq j, \quad (4)$$

which can be rewriten as follows by using Equation 3:

$$p(x \mid \omega_i)P(\omega i) > p(x \mid \omega_j)P(\omega_j), i, j = 1, 2, ..., x, i \neq j \quad (5)$$

As one can see, the Bayes classifier's decision function $d_i(x) = p(x|\omega_i)P(\omega_j)$ of a given class ω_i strongly depends on the previous knowledge of $P(x|\omega_i)$ and $P(\omega_i)$, $\forall i = 1, 2, ..., c$. The probability values of $P(\omega_i)$ are straightforward and can be obtained by calculating the histogram of the classes, for instance.

However, the main problem is to find the probability density function $p(x|\omega_i)$, given that the only information we have is a set of patterns and its corresponding labels. A common practice is to assume that the probability density functions are Gaussian ones, and thus one can estimate their parameters using the dataset samples (Duda, Hart, and Stork 2000). In the n-dimensional case, a Gaussian density of the patterns from class ω_j can be calculated by:

$$p(x \mid \omega_i) = \gamma exp\left[-\frac{1}{2}(x - \mu_j)^T C_i^{-1}(x - \mu_j)\right], \quad (6)$$

in which

$$\gamma = \frac{1}{(2\pi)^{n/2}|C_i|^{1/2}}, \quad (7)$$

and μ_i and C_i stand for, respectively, to the mean and the covariance matrix of class ω_i. These parameters can be obtained by considering each pattern x that belongs to class ω_i using:

$$\mu_i = \frac{1}{N_i} \sum_{x \in \omega_i} x \quad (8)$$

and

$$C_i = \frac{1}{N_i} \sum_{x \in \omega_i} (xx^T - \mu_i\mu_i^T), \quad (9)$$

in which N_i means the number of samples from class ω_i.

3 MATERIALS AND METHODS

In order to evaluate the performance of the machine learning algorithms for automatic identification of the secondary austenite islands in microstructure of superduplex stainless steels, multipass welds were performed using gas metal arc welding process (G*MAW). A testing bench with an industrial robot and an electronic welding power supply was used to produce the sample. The alloy used was the UNS S32750 (SAF 2507) superduplex stainless steel pipes with 19 mm thickness as base metal and as filler metal was AWS ER 2594.

Samples for metallographic evaluation were extracted from welded joints and conventionally prepared through mechanical grinding and polishing using silicon carbide sand paper and diamond past, respectively. An electrochemical etching to reveal the microstructure was carried out using an aqueous solution with 40% vol. of nitric acid (HNO_3) and applying a potential of 2.0 V during 40 seconds.

We used optical microscopy images with 200× and 1000× of magnifications. These images were previously labeled by a technician into positive (γ_2 islands) and negative (background) samples. Figure 1 displays these images.

Now, imagine an interactive classification tool in which the user can select same positive and negative samples in order to classify the remaining image. After that, the use may want to refine the classification process by marking another set of samples, and then to execute the process again. In most applications, one know that the effectiveness of classification is strongly related with the training set size, since we have more information to train the classifier. In this work, we would like to simulate this user behavior by randomly selecting some samples for training, and then to classify the remaining image. The percentages used for training were: 30% and 50%.

In this work, each pixel to be classified was described by a texture kernel around its neighborhood and also by its gray value. In order to extract texture information, we applied the Gabor filter

(Feichtinger and Strohmer 1997), which can be mathematically formulated as follows:

$$G(x,y,\theta,\gamma,\sigma,\lambda,\psi) = e^{\frac{x'^2+y'^2\sigma^2}{2\sigma^2}} \cos\left(2\pi\frac{x'}{\lambda}+\psi\right), \quad (10)$$

where $x'=x\cos(\theta)+y\sin(\theta)$ and $y'=x\sin(\theta)+y\cos(\theta)$. In the above equation, λ means the sinusoidal factor, θ represents the orientation angle, ψ is the phase offset, σ is the Gaussian standard deviation and γ is the aspect spatial ratio.

The main idea of Gabor filter is to perform a convolution between the original image I and $G_{\theta,\gamma,\sigma,\lambda,\psi}$ in order to obtain a Gabor-filtered representation as:

$$\hat{I}_{\theta,\gamma,\sigma,\lambda,\psi} = I * G_{\theta,\gamma,\sigma,\lambda,\psi}, \quad (11)$$

in which $\hat{I}_{\theta,\gamma,\sigma,\lambda,\psi}$ denotes the filtered image. Thus, one can obtain a filter bank of Gabor filtered images by varying its parameters. We used a convolution filter of size 3 × 3 with the following Gabor parameters that were empirically chosen and based on our previous experience:

- 6 different orientations: θ = 0°, 45°, 90°, 135°, 225° and 315°;
- 3 spatial resolutions: λ = 2.5, 3 and 3.5. Notice that, for each one of λ values, we applied different values for σ, say that σ = 1.96, 1.40 and 1.68;
- ψ = 0 and
- γ = 1.

Once we get the Gabor-filtered images (one can see that we have 6 × 3 = 18 images), we then compute the texture features at pixel p as the set of corresponding gray values among these images. Thus, each pixel is described by 19 features, being 18 of them related with texture and the remaining one is the original gray value. After classification process, we applied a 3 × 3 mode filter in order to postprocessing the image.

In regard to the pattern recognition techniques, for OPF we used the LibOPF (Papa, Suzuki, and Falcão 2009), which is a free tool to the design of classifiers based on of optimum-path forest. For Bayesian classifier (BC) we used our own implementation.

4 EXPERIMENTAL RESULTS

We describe in this section the results obtained. Figures 2 and 3 display, respectively, the images classified with BC and OPF.

In order to emphasize the importance of mode filter, Figure 4 displays the image of Figure 1a

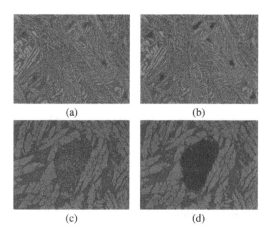

(a)   (b)

(c)   (d)

Figure 1. Microscopic images used in the experiments: original images with magnifications of (a) 200× and (c) 1000×, and the respectively manual segmentations in (b) and (d).

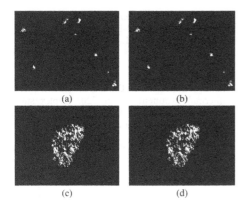

(a)   (b)

(c)   (d)

Figure 2. Classified images with BC using: (a) 30% and (b) 50% for training and (c) 30% and (d) 50% for training. The images (a)-(b) and (c)-(d) refer, respectively, to the original images in Figure 1a and Figure 1c.

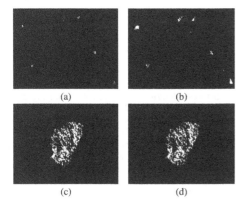

(a)   (b)

(c)   (d)

Figure 3. Classified images with OPF using: (a) 30% and (b) 50% for training and (c) 30% and (d) 50% for training. The images (a)-(b) and (c)-(d) refer, respectively, to the original images in Figure 1a and Figure 1c.

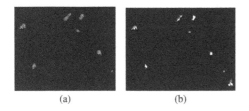

(a)   (b)

Figure 4. Figure 1a classified: (a) without and (b) with the mode filter.

classified by BC with and without mode filter. Notice that the image in Figure 4b is equal to the image of Figure 2a.

One can see that the results obtained using 30% of the whole image for training are better when we used the BC classifier in case of Figure 1a.

Table 1. Recognition rates for the image in Figure 1a. The most accurate classifiers are bolded.

Classifier	Training %	Accuracy
OPF	30	68.51%
BC	30	69.14%
OPF	50	77.31%
BC	50	75.96%

Table 2. Recognition rates for the image in Figure 1c. The most accurate classifiers are bolded.

Classifier	Training %	Accuracy
OPF	30	70.62%
BC	30	69.85%
OPF	50	79.13%
BC	50	82.41%

Using 50% the results appear to be similar. In regard to Figure 1c, both classifiers achieved close results using 30% and 50% for training. It is important to shed light over that, for both techniques, the mode filter played an important role to filter the images after classification. Table 1 displays the recognitionrates for Figure 1a.

One can see that BC outperformed OPF using 30% of the whole image for training, while OPF outperformed BC the second case, i.e., using 50% of the samples to train the classifiers. Table 2 displays the recognition rates for Figure 1c.

The OPF classifier achieved better results than BC using 30% for training, while the latter outperformed in case of 50%. However, one can see that the results are very similar for both classifiers using 30% and 50% for training in the employed images.

5 CONCLUSIONS

This paper was concerned on the problem of γ_2 island segmentation, which can provide important information about steel's quality and mechanical properties. In order to do that, we applied two supervised pattern recognition techniques, Optimum-Path Forest (OPF) and a Bayesian classifier (BC), on two labeled images with 200× and 1000× of magnifications, respectively.

Aiming to simulate an user behavior to select positive and negative samples, we conducted experiments with 30% and 50% of the whole images for training, to further classify the remaining pixels. The training samples were randomly chosen, and described by their gray values and texture features. In regard to recognition rates, both classifiers achieved similar results. A mode filter was applied to enhance the quality of images after classification.

Thus, we may conclude that the results were very promising, since this was the first work that addressed the problem of automatic segmentation of γ_2 islands in secondary austenite-phase precipitates.

ACKNOWLEDGMENTS

The authors are grateful to FAPESP grant #2009/16206-1. The first author thanks National Council for Research and Development (CNPq) and Cearense Foundation for the Support of Scientific and Technological Development (FUNCAP) for providing financial support through a DCR grant to UNIFOR.

REFERENCES

Allène, C., Audibert, J.Y., Couprie, M., Cousty, J. and Keriven, R. (2007). Some links between min-cuts, optimal spanning forests and watersheds. In *Mathematical Morphology and its Applications to Image and Signal Processing (ISMM'07)*, pp. 253–264. MCT/INPE.

Bastos, I.N., Tavares, S.S.M., Dallard, F. and Nogueira, R.P. (2007). Effect of microstructure on corrosion behavior of superduplex stainless steel enviroment conditions. *Scripta Materialia (Oxford)* 57, 913–916.

Dijkstra, E.W. (1959). A note on two problems in connexion with graphs. *Numerische Mathe-matik 1*, 269271.

Duda, R.O., Hart, P.E. and Stork, D.G. (2000). *Pattern Classification*. Wiley-Interscience Publication.

Falcão, A.X., Stolfi, J. and Lotufo, R.A. (2004). The image foresting transform theory, algorithms, and applications. *IEEE Transactions on Pattern Analysis and Machine Intelligence 26*(1), 19–29.

Feichtinger, H.G. and Strohmer, T. (1997). *Gabor Analysis and Algorithms: Theory and Applications* (1st ed.). Birkhauser Boston.

Hemmer, H. and Grong, O. (1999). A process model for the heat-affected zone microstructure evolution in duplex stainless steel weld-ments: Part i. the model. *Metallurgical and Materials Transactions A 30*(11), 2915–2929.

Hemmer, H., Grong, O. and Klokkehaug, S. (2000). A process model for the heat-affected zone microstructure evolution in duplex stainless steel weldments: Part ii. application to electron beam welding. *Metallurgical and Materials Transactions A 31*(13), 1035–1048.

Hertzman, S., Brolund, B. and Ferreira, P. (1997). An experimental and theoretical study of heat-affected zone austenite reformation in three duplex stainless steels. *Metallurgical and Materials Transactions A 28*(2), 277–285.

Jaynes, E.T. (2003). *Probability Theory: The Logic of Science*. Cambridge University Press.

Kotecki, D.J. and Hilkes, J.L.P. (1994). Welding processes for duplex stainless steels. In *Proceedings of the Fourth International Conference on Duplex Stainless Steels*, Volume 2, Glasgow, Scotland.

Lee, K.M., Cho, H.S. and Choi, D.C. (1999). Effect of isothermal treatment of saf 2205 duplex stainless steel on migration of δ/γ interface boundary and growth of austenite. *Journal of Alloys and Compounds 285*(1–2), 156–161.

Lippold, J.C. and Al-Rumaih, A.M. (1997). Toughness and pitting corrosion of duplex stainless steel weld heat affected zone microstructures containing secondary austenite. In *Proceedings of the Conference of Duplex Stainless Steels*, Maastrisht, The Netherlands, pp. 1005–1010.

Nilsson, J.O. (1992). Overview: Super duplex stainless steels. *Materials Science and Technology 8*, 685–695.

Nilsson, J.O. and Wilson, A. (1993). A. influence of isothermal phase transformation on toughness and pitting corrosion of superduplex stainless steel saf 2507. *Materials Science and Technology 9*(6), 545–554.

Nilsson, J.O., Karlsson, L. and Andersson, J.O. (1995). Secondary austenite formation and its relation to pitting corrosion in duplex stainless steel weld metal. *Materials Science and Technology 11*(3), 276–283.

Papa, J.P., Falcão, A.X. and Suzuki, C.T.N. (2009). Supervised pattern classification based on optimum-path forest. *International Journal of Imaging System and Technology 19*(2), 120–131.

Papa, J.P., Suzuki, C.T.N. and Falcão, A.X. (2009). *LibOPF: A library for the design of optimum-path forest classifiers*. Software version 2.0 available at: http://www.ic. unicamp.br/~afalcao/LibOPF

Ramirez, A.J., Brandi, S.D. and Lippold, J.C. (2004). Secondary austenite and chromium nitride precipitation in simulated heat affected zones of duplex stainless steels. *Science and Technology of Welding and Joining 9*(4), 301–313.

Ramirez, A.J., Lippold, J.C. and Brandi, S.D. (2003). The relationship between chromium nitride and secondary austenite precipitation in duplex stainless steels. *Metallurgical and Materials Transactions A 34A*(8), 1575–1597.

Tavares, S.S.M., Scandian, C., Pardal, J.M., Luz, T.S. and da Silva, F.J. (2010). Failure analysis of duplex stainless steel weld used in flexible pipes in off shore oil production. *Engineering Failure Analysis 17*, pp. 1500–1506.

Computational Vision and Medical Image Processing – Tavares & Natal Jorge (eds)
© 2012 Taylor & Francis Group, London, ISBN 978-0-415-68395-1

Discrete t-norms in noisy image edge detection

M. González-Hidalgo, S. Massanet & A. Mir
Department of Mathematics and Computer Science, University of the Balearic Islands
Palma de Mallorca, Spain

ABSTRACT: Image edge detection is one of the most important pre-processing steps in many image processing techniques. In this paper, an edge detection algorithm for noisy images using a fuzzy morphology based on discrete t-norms is proposed. It is shown that this algorithm is robust when it is applied to different types of noisy images. It improves the results of other well-known fuzzy morphological algorithms such as the ones based on the Łukasiewicz t-norm, uninorms and umbra approach. This comparison is made using some different objective measures for edge detection and noise removal. The filtered results and the edge images obtained with our approach improve the values obtained by the other approaches.

1 INTRODUCTION

Edge detection is a fundamental low-level image processing operation, which is essential to carry out several higher level operations such as image segmentation, computer vision, motion and feature analysis and recognition. Its performance is crucial for the final results of the image processing techniques. A lot of edge detection algorithms have been developed over the last decades. These different approaches vary from the classical ones (Pratt 2007) based on a set of convolution masks, to the new techniques based on fuzzy sets (Bustince, Barrenechea, Pagola, and Fernandez 2009).

The fuzzy mathematical morphology is a generalization of binary morphology (Serra 1988) using techniques of fuzzy sets (see (Bloch and Maître 1995), (Nachtegael and Kerre 2000)). Mathematical morphology, either crisp or fuzzy, provides an alternative approach to image processing based on the shape concept represented by the so-called structuring element (see (Serra 1988)). The fuzzy operators used to build a fuzzy morphology are conjunctors (usually t-norms, or recently conjunctive uninorms in (González-Hidalgo, Mir-Torres, Ruiz-Aguilera, and Torrens 2009b)) and implicators. As gray-scale images are not represented in practice as functions of $\mathbb{R}^n$ into [0,1] but as discrete functions, discrete fuzzy operators can also be used. In (González-Hidalgo, Massanet, and J. Torrens 2010) and (González-Hildago, and Massanet 2011a), the algebraic properties usually required to a morphology in order to become a "good" one were proved using discrete t-norms as conjunctors and their residual implicators.

Among the techniques used for edge detection, several have been designed based on residuals and morphological gradients obtained from the crisp or fuzzy mathematical morphology. See for example, (González-Hidalgo, Mir-Torres, Ruiz-Aguilera and Torrens 2009a) and (Jiang, Chuang, Lu, and C.-S-Fahn 2007) and references therein. All these works show that the morphological gradients remain relevant and useful in the analysis and image processing. In this work the feasibility of alternate filters will be studied, from opening and closing of the fuzzy morphology based on discrete t-norms (studied in detail in González-Hidalgo and Massanet 2011a)). There, the authors used the alternate filters to reduce the noise and here we will use them in the design of an edge detection algorithm for noisy images reaching a compromise between elimination and smoothing of noise and the detection of the features of the images. In this work, we study the performance of this algorithm in presence of salt and pepper noise. Moreover, the behaviour of this algorithm is investigated depending on the amount of noise in the images. Some different objective measures are used to evaluate the filtered results, the recently defined Structural Similarity Index Measurement (SSIM) (see (Wang, Bovik, Sheikh, and Simoncelli 2004)) and the fuzzy *DI*-subsethood measure $EQ_{\sigma DI}$ (see Bustince, Pagola, and Barrenechea 2007). In addition, Pratt's figure of merit (Pratt 2007) and the ρ-coefficient (Grigorescu, Petkov, and Westenberg 2003) are used as performance measures to evaluate the edge images obtained. It can be noticed that the discrete approach outperforms the other considered fuzzy morphological approaches.

2 PRELIMINARIES

We will suppose the reader to be familiar with the basic definitions and properties of the fuzzy discrete logical operators that will be used in this work, specially those related to discrete t-norms and discrete residual implicators (see (Mayor and Torrens 2005)). From now on, the following notation will be used: $L = \{0, ..., n\}$ a finite chain, I will denote a discrete implicator, C a discrete conjunctor, N the only strong negation on L which is given by $N(x) = n - x$ for all $x \in L$, T a discrete t-norm, I_T its residual implicator, A a gray-scale image and B a gray-level structuring element that takes values on L.

Definition 1. *The* fuzzy discrete dilation $D_C(A, B)$ *and the* fuzzy discrete erosion $E_I(A, B)$ *of A by B are the gray-scale images defined as*

$$D_C(A, B)(y) = \max_x C(B(x - y), A(x)),$$
$$E_I(A, B)(y) = \min_x I(B(x - y), A(x)).$$

Definition 2. *The* fuzzy discrete closing $C_{C,I}(A, B)$ *and the* fuzzy discrete opening $O_{C,I}(A, B)$ *of A by B are the gray-scale images defined as*

$$C_{C,I}(A, B)(y) = E_I(D_C(A, B), -B)(y),$$
$$O_{C,I}(A, B)(y) = D_C(E_I(A, B), -B)(y).$$

Note that the reflection $-B$ of a N-dimensional fuzzy set B is defined by $-B(x) = B(-x)$, for all $x \in \mathbb{Z}^N$.

Obviously a discrete t-norm is a conjunctor. Thus, these operators and their residual implicators can be used to define fuzzy discrete morphological operators using the previous definitions. In (González-Hidalgo, Massanet, and J. Torrens 2010) and (González-Hidalgo and Massanet 2011a), the discrete t-norms that have to be used in order to preserve the morphological and algebraic properties that are satisfied by the classical morphological operators were fully determined. Among these properties, we highlight the following ones:

- The fuzzy dilation D_T is increasing in both arguments, the fuzzy erosion E_{I_T} is increasing in their first argument and decreasing in their second one, the fuzzy closing C_{T,I_T} and the fuzzy opening O_{T,I_T} are both increasing in their first argument.
- If $B(0) = n$ the fuzzy dilation is extensive and the fuzzy erosion is anti-extensive $E_{I_T}(A, B) \subseteq A \subseteq D_T(A, B)$. The fuzzy closing is extensive and the fuzzy opening is anti-extensive: $O_{T,I_T}(A, B) \subseteq A \subseteq C_{T,I_T}(A, B)$.

Moreover, the fuzzy closing and the fuzzy opening are idempotent, i.e.:

$$C_{T,I_T}(C_{T,I_T}(A, B), B) = C_{T,I_T}(A, B),$$

and $O_{T,I_T}(O_{T,I_T}(A, B), B) = O_{T,I_T}(A, B).$

- Among other discrete t-norms, the nilpotent minimum that is given by

$$T_{nM}(x, y) = \begin{cases} 0 & \text{if } x + y \le n, \\ \min\{x, y\} & \text{otherwise,} \end{cases}$$

guarantees also the duality between fuzzy morphological operators.

3 THE PROPOSED EDGE DETECTOR ALGORITHM

The main goal of this work is to develop an algorithm which can detect and preserve, in presence of noise, edges in images. We will use a residual operator from fuzzy opening and closing operations in order to detect edge images and, at the same time, denoise the image. Recall that a residual operator of two morphological operations or transformations is their difference. In previous works, (González-Hidalgo, Massanet, and J. Torrens 2010) and (González-Hidalgo and Massanet 2011a), the performance of fuzzy gradients and top-hat transformations based on discrete t-norms in order to detect edges in natural images was presented.

From the operation properties of the fuzzy morphology based on discrete t-norms, it is satisfied that

$$O_{T,I_T}(C_{T,I_T}(A, B), B) \subseteq C_{T,I_T}(A, B).$$

Let B be such that $B(0) = n$ and consider $F = O_{T,I_T}(C_{T,I_T}(A, B), B)$. So we have (see (González-Hidalgo, Massanet 2011a))

$$E_{I_T}(C_{T,I_T}(F, B), B) \subseteq C_{T,I_T}(F, B)$$
$$\subseteq D_T(C_{T,I_T}(F, B), B).$$

Then we can compute the next residual operator

$$\delta_{T,I_T}^{1+}(A, B) = D_T(C_{T,I_T}(F, B), B) \setminus E_{I_T}(C_{T,I_T}(F, B), B). \tag{1}$$

In Equation (1), the so called *alternate filters*, alternate composition of opening and closing, are involved. These alternate filters are used to remove and to smooth noise in (González-Hidalgo, Massanet 2011a). So, the proposed algorithm is the following one: first, we pre-process the image by an alternate filter in order to filter the noise and smooth the image, and then we apply a fuzzy gradient operator. Once the residual image (1) is obtained, the edge image is binarized applying the well-known Otsu's thresholding method (Otsu 1979) and then, we obtain edges of one pixel wide using Zhang and Suen's thinning algorithm (Zhang and Suen 1984). This method to transform the fuzzy edge image to a binary thin edge image gives the best results according to some performance measures (see (González-Hidalgo, Massanet 2011b)).

4 EXPERIMENTAL RESULTS AND ANALYSIS

In the following experiments, the nilpotent minimum discrete t-norm T_{nM} has been used. During these experimental results, the structuring elements B used for the fuzzy discrete morphological operators are represented by the matrices

$$B_1 = \begin{pmatrix} 0 & 255 & 0 \\ 255 & 255 & 255 \\ 0 & 255 & 0 \end{pmatrix} B_2 = \begin{pmatrix} 219 & 219 & 219 \\ 219 & 255 & 219 \\ 219 & 219 & 219 \end{pmatrix}.$$

The structuring element B_1 is a widely used 3×3 disk-shaped structuring element while B_2 has been already used in (Nachtegael and Kerre 2000). We compare the edge images with those obtained using the classical gray-scale morphology based on the umbra approach, and those obtained by the fuzzy approach based on the Łukasiewicz continuous t-norm, $T_L(x, y) = \max\{0, x + y - 1\}$ for all $x, y \in [0,1]$. The results are also compared to the ones obtained using an idempotent or a representable uninorm. The used idempotent uninorm is generated by the classical negation $N_C(x) = 1 - x$ and the representable one U_h by the additive generator $h(x) = \ln(x/1 - x)$. Note that we use the continuous counterpart of the structuring elements B for the morphology based on nilpotent t-norms scaled by e for the case of uninorms, where e is the neutral element of the uninorm.

For the comparison of the obtained edge images, some performance measures on edge detection have been considered. These measures need, in addition to the binary thin edge image (DE) obtained, a ground truth edge image (GT) that is a binary thin edge imagecontaining the true edges of the original image, i.e., the reference edge image. In this work, we will use the following measures to quantify the similarity between (DE) and (GT):

1. Pratt's figure of merit (Pratt 2007) defined as

$$FoM = \frac{1}{\max\{card\{DE\}, card\{GT\}\}} \cdot \sum_{x \in DE} \frac{1}{1 + ad^2},$$

where $card$ is the number of edge points of the image, a is a scaling constant and d is the separation distance of an actual edge point to the ideal edge points. In our case, we considered $a = 1$ and the Euclidean distance d.

2. The ρ-coefficient (Grigorescu, Petkov and Westenberg 2003), defined as

$$\rho = \frac{card(E)}{card(E) + card(E_{FN}) + card(E_{FP})},$$

where E is the set of well-detected edge pixels, E_{FN} is the set of ground truth edges missed by the edge detector and E_{FP} is the set of edge pixels detected but with no counterpart on the ground truth image. Since edges cannot always be detected at exact integer image coordinates, we consider that an edge pixel is correctly detected if a corresponding ground truth edge pixel is present in a 5×5 square neighborhood centered at the respective pixel coordinates, as it was considered in (Grigorescu, Petkov, and Westenberg 2003).

Larger values of FoM and ρ ($0 \leq FoM, \rho \leq 1$) are indicators of better capabilities for edge detection.

As we have already observed, the performance measures need a dataset of images with their ground truth edge images (edges specifications) in order to compare the outputs obtained by the different algorithms. So, the images and their edge specifications from the public dataset of the University of South Florida (Bowyer, Kranenburg, and Dougherty 1999), displayed in Figure 1, have been used. The salt and pepper noise in the images has been added using the standard functions of Matlab R2008a.

As in the case of edge detection, different objective measures can be used to evaluate the performance of a filter. Among them, we will use the SSIM (see (Wang, Bovik, Sheikh, and Simoncelli 2004)) and the fuzzy DI-subsethood measure $EQ_{\sigma DI}$ (see (Bustince, Pagola, and Barrenechea 2007)). Recently, SSIM was introduced under the assumption that human visual perception is highly adapted for extracting structural information from a scene. The SSIM is an alternative complementary framework for quality assessment based on the degradation of structural information. Let O_1 and F_2 be two images of dimensions $M \times N$. We suppose that O_1 is the original noise-free image

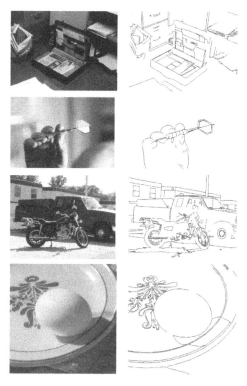

Figure 1. Original image (left) and its ground truth edge image (right).

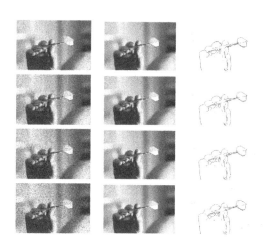

Figure 2. From top to down, corrupted image with salt and pepper noise with 0.02, 0.04, 0.06 and 0.08 (left), filtered image (center) and edge image (right) using T_{nM} and B_1.

and F_2 is the restored image for which some filter has been applied. The two measures are defined as follows:

$$SSIM(F_2, O_1) = \frac{(2\mu_1\mu_2 + C_1)}{(\mu_1^2 + \mu_2^2 + C_1)} \cdot \frac{(2\sigma_{12} + C_2)}{(\sigma_1^2 + \sigma_2^2 + C_2)},$$

where μ_k, $k = 1, 2$ is the mean of the image O_1 and F_2 respectively, σ_k^2 is the variance of each image, σ_{12} is the covariance between the two images, $C_1 = (0.01 \cdot 255)^2$ and $C_2 = (0.03 \cdot 255)^2$ (see (Wang, Bovik, Sheikh, and Simoncelli 2004) for details),

$$EQ_{\sigma DI}(F_2, O_1) = \frac{1}{MN} \sum_{i=1}^{M} \sum_{j=1}^{N} (255 - |O_1(i,j) - F_2(i,j)|).$$

Larger values of SSIM and $EQ_{\sigma DI}$ ($0 \leq SSIM, EQ_{\sigma DI} \leq 1$) are indicators of better capabilities for noise reduction and image recovery.

In Figure 2 we display the results obtained by the proposed fuzzy edge detection algorithm when four different salt and pepper noise functions, of parameter 0.02, 0.04, 0.06 and 0.08 respectively, were added to the image shown in Figure 1.

Note that there are also the filtered images by the alternate filter proposed. Our goal is to study the performance of the proposed algorithm when we increase the amount of noise present in the image. We can see as the edge images are little affected with the increase of noise and many features remain detected. In Table 1, we can observe that the performance measures on edge detection and noise removal remain high.

Finally, in order to compare our approach with the other fuzzy morphological ones, in Figures 3–5 we display the results obtained by the different methods. The original image was corrupted with a salt and pepper function of parameter 0.04, 0.05 and 0.06 respectively in each figure. The visual observation of the results clearly suggests that the discrete approach using T_{nM} performs better than the other used methods. The edge images obtained with T_{nM} contain the main edges of the original images without being distorted by the presence of the noise in the initial images. Although the other methods remove the noise quite well, they do not obtain some main edges of the original images. Note that the edge images obtained by the continuous Łukasiewicz t-norm are almost white, i.e., few edges are detected, specially in Figure 5 where no part of the egg is detected.

However, a visual comparison is not enough in order to compare these several methods. Therefore, some objective performance measures such as FoM and ρ have been computed for each of the obtained edge images in Figures 3–5 and they are displayed in Tables 2–4. The obtained values are in accordance with the visual results. The two computed measures give better values to the edge images obtained by the discrete approach using

Table 1. Measures from the results of Figure 2.

Noise	Filtered image		Edge image	
	SSIM	$EQ_{\sigma DI}$	FoM	ρ
0.02	0.997392	0.9936	0.5474	0.6787
0.04	0.997088	0.9933	0.5415	0.6779
0.06	0.996757	0.9930	0.5302	0.6707
0.08	0.995656	0.9925	0.5146	0.6701

Table 2. Measures from the results of Figure 3.

Measures	T_{nM}	T_L	Umbra	Idem. uninorm	Rep. uninorm
FoM	0.4635	0.1019	0.2353	0.4251	0.2528
ρ	0.6488	0.1633	0.394	0.6203	0.3884

Table 3. Measures from the results of Figure 4.

Measures	T_{nM}	T_L	Umbra	Idem. uninorm	Rep. uninorm
FoM	0.4371	0.1081	0.2905	0.3829	0.2821
ρ	0.5689	0.1665	0.4527	0.5149	0.4001

Table 4. Measures from the results of Figure 5.

Measures	T_{nM}	T_L	Umbra	Idem. uninorm	Rep. uninorm
FoM	0.5597	0.0051	0.1846	0.4824	0.1955
ρ	0.8102	0.0091	0.3438	0.6785	0.3303

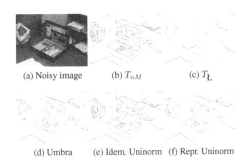

(a) Noisy image   (b) T_{nM} (c) T_L

(d) Umbra   (e) Idem. Uninorm   (f) Repr. Uninorm

Figure 3. Original corrupted image "briefcase" and edge images obtained by the different approaches.

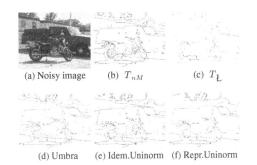

(a) Noisy image   (b) T_{nM} (c) T_L

(d) Umbra   (e) Idem.Uninorm   (f) Repr.Uninorm

Figure 4. Original corrupted image "vehicles" and edge images obtained by the different approaches.

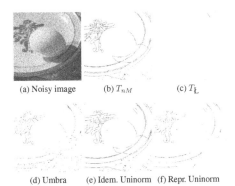

(a) Noisy image   (b) T_{nM} (c) T_L

(d) Umbra   (e) Idem. Uninorm (f) Repr. Uninorm

Figure 5. Original corrupted image "egg" and edge images obtained by the different approaches.

T_{nM} and they give the lowest values to the ones obtained by the Łukasiewicz t-norm. With respect to the rest of the compared methods, both visual and numerical comparisons indicate that the idempotent uninorm is not so far away of T_{nM} providing also notable edge images. Finally, not sogood results can be obtained with the umbra approach and the representable uninorm. So, summarizing both visual and numerical observations ensure that the discrete approach outperforms the other methods.

5 CONCLUSIONS AND FUTURE WORK

In this work, an edge detection algorithm based on the fuzzy morphology using discrete t-norms, derived as a residual operator from the basic morphological operations, has been proposed. Such algorithm is able to detect edges and contours, and preserve them. To evaluate the performance of the algorithm, comparison experiments with other well known approaches were carried out according to some performance measures. The results indicate that the proposed algorithm is robust against noisy images. Experimental results show that it outperforms other fuzzy morphological edge detection methods in detecting detailed edge features. Moreover, these edges can be preserved even though the image is corrupted by noise. Future work consists on one hand, in the study of the behaviour of the algorithm for other types of noise and, on the other hand in the selection of the size, shape, direction of the structuring element adapted to the edge features of the image and how we can improve performance.

ACKNOWLEDGEMENTS

This paper has been partially supported by the Spanish Grant MTM2009-10320 with FEDER support. The authors would like to thank H. Bustince and his group of the Public University of Navarra for his kindly support.

REFERENCES

Bloch, I. and Maître, H. (1995). Fuzzy mathematical morphologies: a comparative study. *Pattern Recognition 28*, 1341–1387.

Bowyer, K., Kranenburg, C. and Dougherty, S. (1999). Edge detector evaluation using empirical ROC curves. *Computer Vision and Pattern Recognition 1*, 354–359.

Bustince, H., Barrenechea, E. Pagola, M. and Fernandez, J. (2009). Interval-valued fuzzy sets constructed from matrices: Application to edge detection. *Fuzzy Sets and Systems 160*(13), 1819–1840.

Bustince, H., Pagola, M. and Barrenechea, E. (2007). Construction of fuzzy indices from fuzzy DI-subsethood measures: application to the global comparison of images. *Information Sciences 177*, 906–929.

Gonzàlez-Hidalgo, M. and Massanet, S. (2011a). Closing and opening based on discrete t-norms. applications to natural image analysis. Accepted in EUSFLAT-LFA 2011.

González-Hidalgo, M. and Massanet, S. (2011b). Towards an objective edge detection algorithm based on discrete t-norms. Accepted in EUSFLAT-LFA 2011.

González-Hidalgo, M., Massanet, S. and Torrens, J. (2010). Discrete t-norms in a fuzzy mathematical morphology: Algebraic properties and experimental results. In *Proceedings of WCCI-FUZZ-IEEE*, Barcelona, Spain, pp. 1194–1201.

González-Hidalgo, M., Mir-Torres, A., Ruiz-Aguilera, D. and Torrens, J. (2009a). Edge-images using a uninorm-based fuzzy mathematical morphology: Opening and closing. In J. Tavares and N. Jorge (Eds.), *Advances in Computational Vision and Medical Image Processing*, Number 13 in Computational Methods in Applied Sciences, Chapter 8, pp. 137–157. Netherlands: Springer.

González-Hidalgo, M., Mir-Torres, A. Ruiz-Aguilera, D. and Torrens, J. (2009b). Image analysis applications of morphological operators based on uninorms. In *Proceedings of the IFSA-EUSFLAT 2009 Conference*, Lisbon, Portugal, pp. 630–635.

Grigorescu, C., Petkov, N. and Westenberg, M.A. (2003). Contour detection based on nonclassical receptive field inhibition. *IEEE Transactions on Image Processing* 12(7), 729–739.

Jiang, J.-A., Chuang, C.-L., Lu, Y.-L. and Fahn, C.-S. (2007). Mathematical-morphology-based edge detectors for detection of thin edges in low-contrast regions. *IET Image Processing 1*(3), 269–277.

Mayor, G. and Torrens, J. (2005). Triangular norms in discrete settings. In E. Klement and R. Mesiar (Eds.), *Logical, Algebraic, Analytic, and Probabilistic Aspects of Triangular Norms*, Chapter 7, pp. 189–230. Amsterdam: Elsevier.

Nachtegael, M. and Kerre, E. (2000). Classical and fuzzy approaches towards mathematical morphology. In E.E. Kerre and M. Nachtegael (Eds.), *Fuzzy techniques in image processing*, Number 52 in Studies in Fuzziness and Soft Computing, Chapter 1, pp. 3–57. New York: Physica-Verlag.

Otsu, N. (1979). A threshold selection method from gray-level histograms. *IEEE Transactions on Systems, Man and Cybernetics 9*, 62–66.

Pratt, W.K. (2007). *Digital Image Processing* (4 ed.). Wiley-Interscience.

Serra, J. (1982,1988). *Image analysis and mathematical morphology, vols. 1, 2*. London: Academic Press.

Wang, Z., Bovik, A.C. Sheikh, H.R. and Simoncelli, E.P. (2004). Image quality assessment: From error visibility to structural similarity. *IEEE Transactions on Image Processing 13*(4), 600–612.

Zhang, T.Y. and Suen, C.Y. (1984). A fast parallel algorithm for thinning digital patterns. *Commun. ACM 27*, 236–239.

Computational Vision and Medical Image Processing – Tavares & Natal Jorge (eds)
© 2012 Taylor & Francis Group, London, ISBN 978-0-415-68395-1

An object-based image analysis approach to spine detection in CT images

Michael Schwier, Teodora Chitiboi, Lars Bornemann & Horst K. Hahn
Fraunhofer MEVIS, Institute for Medical Image Computing, Bremen, Germany

ABSTRACT: While computer assistance became common in medical practice, some of the most challenging tasks that remain unsolved are in the area of automatic detection and recognition. The human visual perception is in general far superior to computer vision algorithms. Object-based image analysis is a relatively new approach that aims to lift image analysis from a pixel-based processing to a semantic region-based processing of images. It allows to effectively integrate reasoning processes and contextual concepts into the recognition method. In this paper we present an approach that applies object-based image analysis to the task of detecting the spine in CT images. We show that with this method region-based features, contextual information and domain knowledge, especially concerning the typical shape and structure of the spine and its components, can be used effectively in the analysis process.

1 INTRODUCTION

Nowadays computer assistance is common in medical practice. From the acquisition of images such as computed tomography (CT) or magnetic resonance imaging (MRI) to the diagnosis and planning of interventions, image processing and analysis methods play an important role. One of the most challenging tasks in medical image analysis is the development of automatic detection and recognition algorithms.

It is striking how hard it is to teach a computer to recognize structures which for the human vision do not pose any particular difficulties. The advantage of the human vision can—at least partly—be explained considering that it is based on a different perception concept: We perceive an image neither as a whole nor as an array of pixels, but instead we identify individual objects (even only abstract shapes/regions) and evaluate them in their context. Furthermore another important aspect of our human vision is that we employ domain knowledge: We have an idea about what image content to expect in a certain context.

The idea of the object-based image analysis approach is to lift image analysis from the limitations of pixel-based processing to a level of semantic processing, which is closer to the way humans comprehend an image.

We applied this approach to the task of detecting the spine in CT images to evaluate its applicability to medical images. The recognition of the spine is a typical problem that is easily solved by a human, but has not yet been conclusively solved by a computer algorithm. Some of the tasks that

would benefit from a spine detection are: detection of bone metastases and spine fractures, assessment of spinal deformities, or support of radiological reporting by vertebrae labeling. Many of the published methods addressing this problem are based on MR images like the recent work of Tang and Pauli (Tang and Pauli 2011) who use an active-shape model approach combined with an atlas based registration to detect the spine curve. Other approaches use curve-fitting, statistical models or atlas based matching.

In this paper we want to show the applicability of object-based image analysis to the task of detecting the spine in CT images. In our approach we aim to detect the spine in the sagittal slices which lie along the centerline of the vertebral bodies from the 2nd cervical vertebra to the 5th lumbar vertebra.

2 THE CONCEPT OF OBJECT-BASED IMAGE ANALYSIS

The basic idea of object-based image analysis is to partition the image into regions to gain a structuring that corresponds to the way humans comprehend an image. Then on each of these regions features that exhibit meaningful information are calculated. An object in the sense of object-based image analysis is an abstract representation of an image region and its features. But not only do the objects in themselves bear semantic information, also the spatial context of the objects is considered and mapped. In this way a high level formalized representation of the image is created. On this object-based image representation it is now possible to formulate reasoning processes which are based on domain knowledge and can easily consider contextual information. This means to create rules and decision concepts to iteratively explore the data space, merge objects into semantically more significant entities and finally recognize structures in the image.

Object-based image analysis is a relatively new approach and is rarely used in medical image analysis, while it is more common in the field of geographic information science (Shackelford and Davis 2003). Hay and Castilla (Hay and Castilla 2006) tried a first formal definition of object-based image analysis and discussed its strengths and weaknesses.

Further approaches that follow a similar concept are described in (Maillot et al., 2004) and (Renouf et al., 2007). However, their concept is different from ours, since they follow a top-down approach: A domain expert provides an abstract concept definition and the required segmentation and feature calculations are automatically derived from that. We believe though, that in general it is not feasible to match a concept based on real word experience directly to features derived from an image. The object-based image analysis concept follows a bottom-up approach, which requires to consider the artificial nature of the features we are actually able to calculate on images and to build reasoning concepts based on that.

It is important to mention that object-based image analysis is not intended to replace pixel-based image processing, but to enhance it. Object-based image analysis should represent a follow-up stage when pixel-based methods reach their limits and when it becomes important to incorporate semantic concepts and domain knowledge into the analysis process.

For a long time no general concept existed on how to put object-based image analysis into practice in an actual implementation. Therefore we proposed a generic implementation concept that is founded on the relational data model to manage objects and to formulate reasoning processes (Homeyer et al., 2010). The object-based spine detection algorithm described later in this paper (section 3.2) is based on our implementation of this concept.

As mentioned before, the prerequisite for object-based image analysis is an appropriate over-segmentation of the image. Typically an adaptation of the watershed transformation (Vincent and Soille 1991) or a region merging method like the one described by Redding et al. (Redding et al., 1999) are feasible, preceded by an appropriate filtering of the image. However, depending on the task and the image, customized segmentation methods might also be considered.

Of course object-based image analysis is not applicable to every problem. However, if the task is to detect and/or segment a structure that can be visually perceived by a human, it should be considered as a valuable addition to commonly employed pixel based methods.

3 SPINE DETECTION ALGORITHM

In the following we will describe the required pre-segmentation of the image in section 3.1 and subsequently in section 3.2 the object-based reasoning process that leads to the final detection of the spine.

The required image input for the described method is a full upper body CT scan in a sagittal reformation.

3.1 Pre-segmentation

As a first step an anisotropic enhancement filtering is applied to the image to gain a smoothing of the image and an enhancement of edges. The employed filtering is a combination of steerable low pass and high pass filters as described in (Granlund and Knutsson 1995. For optimal performance in the spatial domain, the filter kernels were pre-computed and optimized following the procedure described in (Knutsson et al., 1999).

On the resulting image we apply the Sobel operator followed by a morphological closing operation. This results in an image that delineates the edges of bone structures well enough for subsequently performing a watershed transformation, that creates an appropriate over segmentation of the image. Our watershed implementation is based on the method described in (Hahn and Peitgen 2003).

The watershed transformation of the 3D CT images is performed on a per-slice basis on the sagittal reconstruction. Thus the resulting regions only span in x and y direction but they exist in the 3D space.

During the pre-segmentation step we can already disregard all regions that do not lie close to bone structures. Not considering those regions in the further processing saves computation time and simplifies the object-based detection algorithm.

To get a mask that covers only bone structures and their vicinity first a simple thresholding selects all voxels with a value above 180 Hounsfield Units (HU). On the resulting mask image a strong dilation is performed, followed by a connected components analysis to keep only the biggest structure. Now again a strong dilation is performed, which results in a coarse mask of the main bone structures and their vicinity. Some gaps might still occur in the mask, thus a connected components analysis is performed on the background voxels and all small enclosed components are included in the mask.

The resulting mask is now used to limit the regions created by the watershed transformation. See Fig. 1b for an example of a pre-segmentation.

3.2 Detection algorithm

The object-based detection algorithm is composed as a set of rules and concepts that formulate an iterative reasoning process. The result is a set of objects classified as part of the spine. We consider O the initial set of 2D segments of the pre-segmentation as a set of objects in the sense of object-based image analysis. Thus, each object $o \in O$ holds features to be used in the reasoning process. We will use the following notation for features of an object: $o.feature$.

The first step in the detection is to find some objects $S \subset O$ that are clearly part of the spine, which then will serve as seeds for the further detection. Thus the features of the objects must identify them unambiguously. For this we are aiming to find segments of the lumbar vertebral bodies and the lower thoracic vertebral bodies on the slides crossing the center of the spine. Because of their size, shape and usually good delineation they are easily distinguishable. This is done by the following rule:

$$S = \{o \in O \,|\, o.size > 950 \text{ mm}^2$$
$$\wedge o.size < 2050 \text{ mm}^2$$
$$\wedge o.stddev < 200 \text{ HU}$$
$$\wedge o.mean > 80 \text{ HU}$$
$$\wedge o.lower\_quartile > -20 \text{ HU}$$
$$\wedge o.eccentricity < 0.1$$
$$\wedge o.compactness > 0.5\}$$

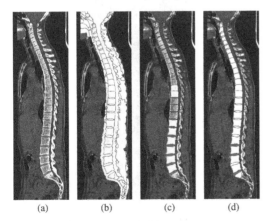

| (a) | (b) | (c) | (d) |

Figure 1. Steps of the algorithm. (a) Initial image. (b) Pre-segmentation. (c) Seed objects. (d) Final result.

The calculation of the eccentricity of an object o follows the definition given in (Burger and Burge 2009):

$$o.eccentricity = \frac{[\mu_{20}(o) - \mu_{02}(o)]^2 + 4 \cdot [\mu_{11}(o)]^2}{[\mu_{20}(o) + \mu_{02}(o)]^2}$$

with μ_{pq} being the central moments of the binary image region that is defined by o (for details on central moments see e.g. (Burger and Burge 2009)).

The compactness feature computation is based on the isoperimetric inequality, which connects an object's area to its perimeter, stating that for any planar object $4\pi Area \leq Perimeter^2$, equality being achieved in case of a circle. Thus $o.compactness$ is defined as:

$$o.compactness = \frac{4\pi \cdot o.size}{o.border\_size^2}$$

Naturally, vertebral bodies are considered to have a rather regular, compact shape.

The features $o.mean$, $o.lower\_quartile$ and $o.stddev$ refer to the intensity statistics of the objects. While $o.mean$ simply states that the average pixel intensity should correspond to a spine structure, a low value of $o.stddev$ and the $o.lower\_quartile$ reinforce this statement by excluding objects with a higher proportion of dark pixels than expected in a vertebral segment. The thresholds for these rules were determined by investigating the feature space of ground truth objects with usual data mining techniques. See Fig. 1c for an example of a seed selection.

As mentioned before, our goal is to detect the spine in CT slices along the centerline of the spine, in which all vertebral bodies are visible. The automatic selection of these slices from a full size CT can be achieved by analyzing the distribution of seed objects over all sagittal slices of the image. We are aiming to determine a continuous sequence of 4 to 13 slices that offer a complete view of the spine, are located around the centerline of the spine, and are suited for applying the further steps in the detection process.

In order to find those central slices we consider the histogram of the number of detected seed objects per slice. In the optimal case the histogram would resemble a Gaussian distribution, with a maximum number of seed objects present on the slices around the center of the spine. In practical cases though, the distribution may be noisy due to poor contrast and noise in the image as well as structural changes to the spine which cause the pre-segmentation to create regions that do not meet the strict seed objects criteria. Therefore a linear average filter is applied to the histogram. In this filtered histogram the position of the maximum number of seeds is determined. If the maximum is present more than once in the histogram, then the mid-position between the first and last occurrence of the maximum is considered. Then we span an interval around this position until the first histogram position with a number of seeds lower than half of the real maximum (see Fig. 2 for examples on the histogram analysis). For the further processing only the slices that correspond to that interval will be considered.

Next we iterate through all objects in the set S, trying to reconstruct the spine step by step in vertical direction, starting from the seeds. For each object $s_i \in S$ we consider N_i the set of direct and secondary neighbors as candidates for extension. We call an object $e \in O$ a secondary neighbor of s_i if there is another object $d \in O$, such that e is a direct neighbor of d and d is a direct neighbor to s_i. At this stage, an object's neighborhood extends only on the same slice.

All objects in N_i are classified according to their relative spatial position to s_i. During this step we are especially making use of domain knowledge: Since we assume that all $s \in S$ are parts of the spine and we know how the human spine is shaped, we can now limit the candidates in N_i to only those that lie in directions relative to s_i where the spine should continue. For that we have created a heuristic model expressing the relations between a spine object (which can be a vertebral body or spinal disc) and its neighboring spine segments. The model describes for each object s_i, according to its axial position on the spine, the distance and angular ranges where its upper and lower neighboring segments are likely to be found. The distance constraints are based on the observation that the size of vertebral bodies decrease with their vertical position from lumbar to cervical area, and thus the distance between bigger consecutive objects situated in the lower part of an image should be larger than between the smaller consecutive objects situated on the top part. The angular constraints are described as piecewise linear functions of the axial position along the spine, in clockwise and counter-clockwise directions. As illustrated in Fig. 3 the angular constraints are based on statistical observations to account for the spinal curves in the lumbar, thoracic and cervical areas.

As a result of this step, from the set N_i we can extract all objects that meet the local spacial and orientation criteria for being part of the spine, as set N_i^+. Next for all objects in N_i^+, their shape and intensity statistics are evaluated. For this our heuristic model also contains locally adaptive identification criteria for spine objects, according to their axial position along the spine. The model is based on the knowledge that their intensity is always

bright and the spine segments are larger along the inferior parts of the spine and become smaller towards the cervical part. While the larger vertebrae are more compact, the smaller ones are more elliptical and slightly elongated in the sagittal direction. Also, the vertebral bodies are distinguishable from the spinal discs, not only by their intensity, which can be misleading when the boundaries are not well defined, but also by their shape: vertebral bodies are more compact, while spinal discs are flat and have an almost horizontal principal axis. In oder to quantify these observations, we introduce a new feature $o.ellipticity$ which measures the ratio between the object's surface area and the area of an ellipse that has the same perimeter as the object and the same ratio between principal axis and secondary axis:

$$o.ellipticity = \frac{o.size}{ellipse\_area}$$

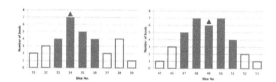

Figure 2. Examples for the histogram analysis to detect the central slices: The triangle marks the maximum position or the mid position between the first and last maximum occurrence. The solid bars indicate the interval of slices which will be considered for the further processing.

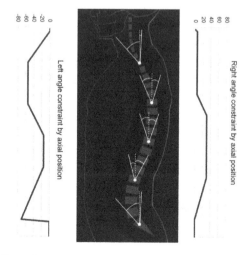

Figure 3. Exemplary illustration of the heuristic model for the angular constraints depending on the axial position.

176

In our model, the spine segments fall into three categories:

- Large vertebrae, regularly shaped and positioned on the lower part of the spine;
- Small vertebrae, or small fragments of vertebrae, positioned relatively high up the spine, and either very compact or very elliptical;
- Spinal discs, also relatively small, and regardless of their sagittal position, with the principal axis oriented close to horizontal.

Therefore, the features used to express these criteria are: *o.size* for the area of the object, *o.mean*, *o.lower_quartile* and *o.stddev* for its intensity, *o.eccentricity*, *o.compactness* and *o.ellipticity* for the shape and *o.principal_axis* for orientation.

Each object of N_i^+ classified as part of the spine is added to the set of seeds S, which is iterated until each $s_i \in S$ has been processed. The heuristic also takes into account that some vertebrae might be partitioned in more than one region by the pre-segmentation, or that some vertebra can be fused together. Also the algorithm can jump over a small vertical section of the spine where the spinal bodies are not well enough defined, for example due to image contrast, or not even existent, for example due to a fracture, and resume the detection and iterative reconstruction of the spine once the vertebrae are visible again.

At the end of this iterative reconstruction, some small segments belonging to the spine might have been overlooked because of feature values that fall out of range. However, some possible gaps in the resulting spinal mask can be filled by including in the segmentation all relatively small objects which share all (or most) of their border with neighboring already marked segments.

Up to this point the segmentation algorithm has considered each slice independently. However, additional domain knowledge can be employed, such as confidence gained by identifying spine objects in neighboring CT slices, as well as the knowledge that they need to form large continuous structures. In order to do this, we first choose three consecutive slices containing the most complete segmentation of the spine. Since the cervical part of the spine is the most narrow, being visible in the fewest number of slices, we choose for reference the slices where the reconstructed spine expands the highest in sagittal direction. A high confidence mask is then built by overlapping the three consecutive segmentation results and marking all spine segments that are present in at least two slices. This mask is then propagated starting from the reference slices in both directions, at each step finding pairs of overlapping spine segments. Through this process we can identify possible false positives and fill in missing vertebras that could not

be detected during the slice-wise approach. Finally, the segmentation results over the entire set of slices are united and merged by neighborhood criteria. This enables us to exclude small remote segments which are disconnected from the spine.

4 EVALUATION

For our evaluation we used 10 upper body CT scans without contrast agent. The images included pathologically changed spines as well as healthy spines. On 7 of the images the spine was included completely, while on 3 images the cervical vertebrae were not included due to the acquired field of view.

We evaluated our method on the sagittal slices along the centerline of the spine on which all vertebral bodies are visible. We compared for which of the visible vertebral bodies in the original image the corresponding segments covering them were correctly classified as "spine". For now our method is designed to detect only the free vertebral bodies, therefore we excluded the sacrum and the coccyx, though sometimes the upper part of the sacrum is detected already (see Fig. 1d). Since the "Atlas"(1st cervical vertebra) surrounds the "Axis" (2nd cervical vertebra) and only the latter is mainly visible along the centerline, we counted only the "Axis".

Table 1 shows that for all but two cases all vertebral bodies were correctly detected (see also Fig. 1d). The one missing in cases 3 and 4 was the "Axis". This was due to irregularities in their shape that were not covered by our model. Also the gap closing and z-overlap strategies could not find them, because the "Axis" lies at the topmost end of the spine. Furthermore in some cases vertebral discs were ignored during the analysis, due to the fact that during the pre-segmentation the

Table 1. Lists how many of the vertebrae actually visible in the test images were found by our method.

Vertebrae		
Case	total	found
1	23	23
2	23	23
3	23	22
4	23	22
5	23	23
6	23	23
7	23	23
8	18	18
9	18	18
10	17	17

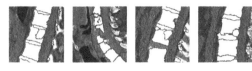

Figure 4. Difficult cases successfully detected.

respective segment leaked into surrounding tissue (see Fig. 1d for an example).

Our approach could also handle cases, where single vertebral bodies were over segmented or degenerated (e.g., fractures). See Fig. 4 for some examples. Furthermore in none of the images any objects out of the spine structure were included (no false positives).

5 CONCLUSIONS

The application of object-based image analysis to the task of detecting the spine in CT images shows promising results (see also Fig. 5 for some examples). This approach allowed us to formulate a reasoning process that utilizes domain knowledge and contextual concepts, which leads to a robust recognition of the spine along its vertebral bodies.

During our evaluation we only found a few issues, namely missing the "Axis" in two cases and missing some vertebral discs. The latter case can probably be solved easily by splitting the objects that lie in the gaps of the detected spine into smaller objects and re-evaluating them.

Currently our method is designed as a pure detection algorithm. Therefore it is sufficient to detect the spine only on the sagittal slices along its centerline, because thus we already gain the spatial position of the whole spine and even a good approximation of the position of the single vertebrae. For many applications it would be desirable though, to get a full 3D reconstruction of the spine and each individual vertebra. Therefore our main goal now is to use the current algorithm and extend it to perform an automatic detection and 3D segmentation of the spine and vertebrae, founded on an object-based image analysis approach.

Another current limitation we intend to overcome is that the input images are required to only contain roughly the area between the neck and pelvis. For example, on full body scans our method would fail, because the assumptions about the axial positions used in the heuristic model would not be valid.

Nevertheless the current algorithm could already be used, for example, to provide an automatic vertebra labeling to support radiological reporting.

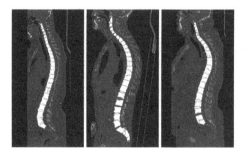

Figure 5. Some examples of the detection results.

REFERENCES

Burger, W. and Burge, M.J. (2009). *Principles of Digital Image Processing: Core Algorithms*. Springer.

Granlund, G. and H. Knutsson (1995). *Signal Processing for Computer Vision*. Kluwer Academic Publishers.

Hahn, H. and Peitgen, H.-O. (2003). IWT—Interactive Watershed Transform: A hierarchical method for efficient interactive and automated segmentation of multidimensional gray-scale images. In *Proc. SPIE Medical Imaging*, Volume 5032, pp. 643–653.

Hay, G.J. and Castilla, G. (2006). Object-based image analysis: strengths, weaknesses, opportunities and threats (SWOT). In *Proc. 1st International Conference on Object-based Image Analysis (OBIA 2006)*.

Homeyer, A., Schwier, M. and Hahn, H.K. (2010). A generic concept for object-based image analysis. In *Proc. International Conference on Computer Vision Theory and Applications*, Volume 2, pp. 530–533.

Knutsson, H., Andersson, M. and Wiklund, J. (1999). Advanced filter design. In *11th Scandinavian Conference on Image Analysis*.

Maillot, N., Thonnat, M. and Boucher, A. (2004). Towards ontology-based cognitive vision. *Machine Vision and Applications 16*(1), 33–40.

Redding, N., Crisp, D., Tang, D. and Newsam, G. (1999). An efficient algorithm for Mumford-Shah segmentation and its application to SAR imagery. *Proc. Conference on Digital Image Computing: Techniques and Applications*, 35–41.

Renouf, A., Clouard, R. and Revenu, M. (2007). How to formulate image processing applications. In *Proc. International Conference on Computer Vision Systems*.

Shackelford, A. and Davis, C. (2003). A combined fuzzy pixel-based and object-based approach for classification of high-resolution multispec-tral data over urban areas. *IEEE Transactions on GeoScience and Remote sensing 41*(10), 2354–2363.

Tang, Z. and Pauli, J. (2011). Fully automatic extraction of human spine curve from MR images using methods of efficient intervertebral disk extraction and vertebra registration. *International Journal of Computer Assisted Radiology and Surgery 6*, 21–33.

Vincent, L. and Soille, P. (1991). Watersheds in digital spaces: An efficient algorithm based on immersion simulations. *IEEE Transactions on Pattern Analysis and Machine Intelligence 13*(6), 583–598.

Computational Vision and Medical Image Processing – Tavares & Natal Jorge (eds)
© 2012 Taylor & Francis Group, London, ISBN 978-0-415-68395-1

Comparing different filtering and enhancement methods to evaluate the impact on the geometry reconstruction for medical images

A.J. João, A.M. Gambaruto & A. Sequeira

CEMAT, Departamento de Matemtica, IST, Lisbon, Portugal

ABSTRACT: Among various diseases related to the cardiovascular system the most studied are aneurysms, atherosclerosis and embolisms. These diseases include a variety of disorders and conditions that affect the heart and blood vessels. According to Ministério da Saúde of Portugal (Portal da Sade), cardiovascular diseases represent 40% of all the deaths in Portugal, and stroke being the main killer among women and men.

The nature of cardiovascular diseases involves a number of factors that include the biochemistry and haemodynamics, as well as genetic predisposition amongst others. These factors are specific to each individual and in order to perform meaningful numerical simulations to aid in the diagnosis, prognosis and therapy choice, accurate patient specific data acquisition is necessary. Here we focus on effects of errors stemming from uncertainty in *in vivo* medical imaging will alter the reconstructed conduit geometry and as a consequence the computed haemodynamics.

In this study the effects of filtering, enhancement and segmentation of medical images are examined with relation to the geometry. Different image processing methods were chosen and tested and the most suitable combination of approaches is discussed. The impact of the vessel geometry has to be considered taking into account clinically relevant information that may change the perception of the clinician; these are commonly fluid dynamic parameters on and near the vessel wall that have been widely correlated to disease.

1 INTRODUCTION

There are several studies over the past decades that which indicate that cardiovascular diseases such as aneurysms and atherosclerosis are directly related with the heamodynamic properties of the lumen wall (Caro et al., 1971) (Ku et al., 1985) (Lei et al., 2001) (Caro et al., 1992). These are typically the wall shear stress (Caro et al., 1971), the gradient oscillatory number (Shimogonya et al., 2008), oscillatory shear index (Ku et al., 1985), aneurysm formation indicator (Mantha et al., 2006) and near-wall residence time (Himburg et al., 2004). The reasons why fluid parameters on the vessel wall are related with disease sites are mainly the evidence that endothelial cells respond to signalling forces from fluids as well as considerations of transport and diffusion, hence interaction with the vessel and surroundings. Despite of the significance of heamodynamics parameters on the vessel lumen wall in the analysis of the disease, there has been relatively little study on the pre-processing of the medical images used to reconstruct the geometry for computational models, that subject to uncertainty due to limited imaging resolution and random noise, can result in noticeable differences in the reconstructed vessel surface definition and hence the computed flow field.

It is the aim of this work to illustrate the need for care in medical image filtering and enhancement in the reconstruction procedure prior to the numerical simulations of the haemodynamics.

2 METHODS

2.1 Filtering methods

2.1.1 Anisotropic diffusion

The anisotropic diffusion method, proposed by Perona-Malik (Perona & Malik, 1990), simulates the process of creating a scale-space, where an image generates a parameterised family of successively blurred images based on a diffusion process. Each of the resulting images are used as a convolution between the image and a 2D isotropic Gaussian filter. The conductance coefficients are chosen to be a decreasing function of the signal gradient. This process is a linear and space-invariant transformation of the initial image.

$$\frac{\partial}{\partial_t} I(x, y, t) = \nabla[c(x, y, t)\nabla I(x, y, t)] \tag{1}$$

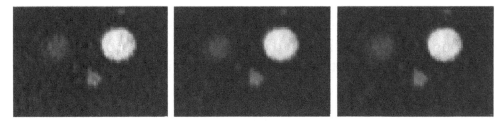

Figure 1. (Left) original image—sample slice of peripheral bypass graft; (Middle) image filtered using anisotropic diffusion; (Right) image filtered using forward and backward anisotropic diffusion.

where $I(x, y, t)$ denotes the image pixel at position (x, y), t refers to the interaction step and $c(x, y)$ is the monotonically decreasing conductivity function, that depends on the image gradient magnitude as:

$$c_1(x, y, t) = e^{-\left(\frac{|\nabla I(x,y,t)|}{\beta}\right)^2} \tag{2}$$

or

$$c_2(x, y, t) = \frac{1}{1 + \left(\frac{\|\nabla I(x,y,t)\|}{\beta}\right)^2} \tag{3}$$

2.1.2 Forward and backward anisotropic diffusion

The goal of forward and backward diffusion is to emphasise the extrema, if they indeed represent singularities and are not result of noise. It can be understood as moving back in time along the scale space or more generally, reversing the diffusion process.

Even though, mathematically we could simply use a inverse linear diffusion, by changing the sign of the conductance coefficient to negative, this process has proven to be unstable. In order to avoid this instability a higher gradient value for the inverse diffusion coefficient is used. (Smolka et al., 2002)

$$c_1(x, y, t) = 2e^{-\left(\frac{|\nabla I(x,y,t)|}{\beta_1}\right)^2} - e^{-\left(\frac{|\nabla I(x,y,t)|}{\beta_2}\right)^2} \tag{4}$$

or

$$c_2(x, y, t) = \frac{2}{1 + \left(\frac{\|\nabla I(x,y,t)\|}{\beta_1}\right)^2} - \frac{1}{1 + \left(\frac{\|\nabla I(x,y,t)\|}{\beta_2}\right)^2} \tag{5}$$

where $\beta_1 < \beta_2$.

In this way, when the singularity exceeds a given threshold it stops affecting the process.

2.2 Contrast enhancement methods

2.2.1 Histogram equalisation

The histogram equalisation algorithm enhances the contrast of an input image by transforming its intensity values, so that the histogram of the output image approximately matches a specified histogram.

Initially it takes the cumulative histogram of the image to be equalised and normalises it to 255. Finally it used the normalised cumulative histogram as the mapping function of the input image.

2.2.2 Local histogram equalisation

On the other hand, local histogram equalisation enhances the contrast on small regions of the images, called tiles, rather than the whole image, as in histogram equalization.

Each tiles contrast is enhanced in order to match the output histogram with the one specified a priori. Then, the neighbouring tiles are combined using interpolation to eliminate induced boundaries.

The resultant contrast can be limited to avoid amplifying noise that can be present in the original image, mainly in homogeneous areas.

2.2.3 Unsharp masking

In the Unsharp masking method, the enhanced image $H(x, y)$ is obtained from the input image $I(x, y)$ as

$$H(x, y) = I(x, y) + \lambda F(x, y) \tag{6}$$

where $F(x, y)$ is the correction signal computed as the output of linear high-pass filter and λ the positive scaling factor which controls the contrast enhancement level acquired as the output image.

2.2.4 Multiscale retinex

The centre-surround multiscale retinex method is considered the trade-off between dynamic range compression and rendition. The main challenge

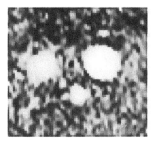 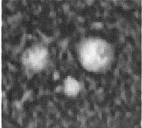 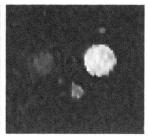

Figure 2. (Left) image enhanced using histogram equalisation; (Middle) image enhanced using local histogram equalisation; (Right) image enhanced using unsharp masking.

is to choose the suitable scale in the Gaussian formula G.

Multiscale retinex is an extension of the Singlescale retinex method and the enhanced image is considered as linear combination of the weighted enhanced image under different scales.

$$H_i(x,y) = \sum \omega_n \{\log I_i(x,y) - \log[G_n(x,y) * I_i(x,y)]\}$$
(7)

where N is the number of scales, ω_n represents the weighting factor of each scale.

3 CONCLUSIONS

Results indicate that image processing and especially preprocessing can substantially alter the quality of the image to improve desired object extraction. This removes a certain level of uncertainty in the segmentation process. Nevertheless, care must be taken to choose appropriate and robust schemes.

In this work, a survey of different methods is undertaken and both geometry and CFD variations are analysed.

ACKNOWLEDGEMENTS

The authors kindly acknowledge the Biomedical Flow Group, Aeronautics Department, Imperial College London, for providing the medical data. This work has been partially supported by the research centre CEMAT/IST through FCTs funding program, and by the FCT project UTAustin/CA/0047/2008 and UTAustin/CA/0047/2008.

REFERENCES

Caro, C.G., Fitz-Gerald, J.M. & Schoreter, R.C. 1971. Atheroma and arterial wall shear: observations, correlation and proposal of a shear dependent mass transfer mechanism for atherogenesis. Proc. R. Soc. London B177, pp. 109–159.

Caro, C.G., Doorly, D.J., Tarnawski, M., Scott, K.T., Long, Q. & Dumoulin, C.L. 1996, Non-planar curvature and branching of arteries and non-planar-type flow Proc. R. Soc. Lond. 452:85–197.

Cheng, H.D. & Shi, X.J. 2004. A simple and effective histogram equalization approach to image enhancement. Digital Signal Processing, 14(2):158–170.

Gerig, G., Kubler, O., Kininis, R. & Jolesz, F.A. 1992. Nonlinear Anisotropic Filtering of MRI Data. IEEE Transactions on Medical Imaging, 11(2):221–232.

Himburg, H.A., Grzybowski, D.M., Hazel. A.L., LaMack, J.A., Li, Z. & Friedman, M.H. 2004. Spatial comparison between wall shear stress measures and porcine arterial endothelial permeability. AJP Heart and Circulatory Physiology 286:1916–1922.

Ku, D.N., Giddens, D.P., Zarins, C.K. & Glagov, S. 1985. Interactive multi-resolution modeling on arbitrary meshes. Arteriosclerosis. 5(3):293–302.

Lei, M., Giddens, D.P., Jones, S.A., Loth, F. & Bassinouny, H. 2001. Pulsatile flow in an end-to-side vascular graft model: comparison of computations with experimental data. ASME Journal of Biomechanical Engineering. 123:80–87.

Mantha, A., Karmonik, C., Benndorf, G., Strother, C. & Metcalfe, R. 2006. Hemodynamics in a cerebral artery before and after the formation of an aneurysm. American Journal of Neuroradiology, 27(5):1113–1118.

Perona, P. & Malik, J. 1990. Scale-space, edge detection using anisotropic diffusion. IEEE Transactions on Pattern Analysis and Machine Intelligence. 12(7):629–639.

Pietro, P. & Jitendra, M. 1990. Scale-Space and edge detection using anisotropic diffusion. IEEE Transactions on Pattern Analysis and Machine Intelligence, 12(7):629–63.

Polesel, A., Ramponi, G. & Mathews, J.V. 2000. Image Enhancement via Adaptive Unsharp Masking. IEEE Transactions on Image Processing, 9(3):505–510.

Russ, J. 2007. Image Processing Handbook (Fifth Edition) . New York: CRC Press.

Smolka, B. & Szczepanski, M. 2002. Forward and backward anisotropic diffusion filtering for color image enhancement. IEEE Digital Signal Processing. 2:927–930.

Zuiderveld, K. 1994. Contrast Limited Adaptive Histogram Equalization. Graphic Gems IV. San Diego: Academic Press Professional. 474–485.

181

Computational Vision and Medical Image Processing – Tavares & Natal Jorge (eds)
© 2012 Taylor & Francis Group, London, ISBN 978-0-415-68395-1

Fast identification of individuals based on iris characteristics for biometric systems

J.G. Rogeri, M.A. Pontes, A.S. Pereira & N. Marranghello
Department of Computer Science and Statistic, IBILCE, Sao Paulo State University (UNESP), São Jose do Rio Preto—SP, Brazil

A.F. Araujo & João Manuel R.S. Tavares
Faculdade de Engenharia, Universidade do Porto (FEUP)/Instituto de Engenharia Mecânica e Gestão Industrial (INEGI), Porto, Portugal

ABSTRACT: Nowadays, systems based on biometric techniques have a wide acceptance in many different areas, due to their levels of safety and accuracy. A biometric technique that is gaining prominence is the identification of individuals through iris recognition. However, to be proficiently used these systems must process their recognition task as fast as possible. The goal of this work has been the development of an iris recognition method to produce results rapidly, yet without losing the recognition accuracy. The experimental results show that the method is quite promising.

1 INTRODUCTION

Due to the increasing rate of violence in almost all the world, the biometric techniques are gaining attention both in academic and commercial areas, because in this type of technique the access keys are physical or behavioral characteristics of individuals.

One of the biometric techniques that has attained considerable attention in recent years is the identification of individuals through iris recognition, due to some characteristics of this region of the human body, such as: suffers light change over time, is fairly well protected, and presents many particular details.

There are several iris-based recognition methods, some of which are very accurate. However, when it comes to restricted area access systems, a high processing speed is also required, as long as delayed outcomes potentially generate service delays.

A fundamental step for the recognition of individuals through the iris is the exact localization of the iris to be analyzed in the input image. Failures in this process can lead to recognition errors, jeopardizing overall system reliability. However, the precise segmentation of this region is usually unfeasible as it often demands high computational costs.

This paper aims at developing a method to locate the iris with minimal computational cost. To achieve this goal, we do not use well-known techniques, such as Daugman integro-differential operator and Hough transform, which despite being proven effective, have high computational costs. Instead, our method is based on histogram variations, morphological operators, and distance calculations.

In section 2 we present the two main methods used in the segmentation of the input iris images.

Afterwards, in section 3 we discuss in details the implementation achieved as well as the tools used for iris localization.

In section 4 we present the experimental tests performed, then we discuss the results obtained, and compare our results to the ones reported in the literature.

Finally, in section 5, we draw the conclusions.

2 RELATED WORK

For the location of the iris in eye images, two methods are widely used: the Hough Transform and Daugman Integro-Differential Operator.

2.1 *Hough transform*

Patterns free from noise and discontinuities are hardly found in images. Hough Transform has been an efficient technique for the detection of approximately circular shapes in digital images [5].

To achieve this goal it uses a process of accumulation of votes, in which the votes are allocated to the crossing points of the possible circles in the

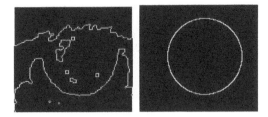

Figure 1. Example of the application of the Hough Transform: (a) segmented image of a human eye, (b) circle detected by the Hough Transform.

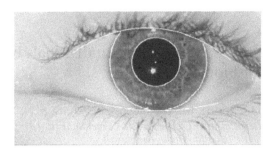

Figure 2. Image of an iris located by the method of Daugman [1].

input image. For this, it defines a mapping between the image space and the parameter space. The votes are accumulated in an array, and a possible circle is detected when a high amount of votes is attained.

Most studies using the Hough Transform start from images already preprocessed, for example, from image with the edges previously detected, in order to make the process simpler and quicker, since, despite high rates of identification of circles in images, the Hough Transform has a high computational cost, making it barely indicated for cases requiring a very fast processing.

Equation 1 shows how x and y coordinates on the plane, points a and b as the center of the circle that is being sought and r as radius. The parameter space is discretized and represented as an array of integers or cells, where each position in the array corresponds to a range of parameters in the real space. Wanted all circles (a, b, r) passing through each point (x, y).

$$r^2 = (x - a)^2 + (y - b)^2 \qquad (1)$$

Figure 1 shows an example of using the Hough Transform, where Figure 1(a) is the original image, obtained from segmenting one image of a human eye, and Figure 1(b) is the image obtained after using the Hough Transform, i.e., the circle detected.

As can be seen in Figure 1, the Hough transform, when associated with an efficient segmentation method can produce good results in the identification of the iris in images.

2.2 Integro-differential operator

Another method widely referenced for the localization of the iris in images is the Integro-Differential operator, proposed by Daugman [1]. This operator is given by the equation 2.

$$\max \left| G_\sigma(r) * \frac{\partial}{\partial r} \oint_{(r,x_o,y_o)} r, x_0, y_0 \frac{I(x,y)}{2\pi r} ds \right| \qquad (2)$$

where, $I(x, y)$ is the image containing the eye to be analyzed, r is the radius and $x0$, $y0$ are the coordinates of the iris center. In this equation, the symbol* denotes the image convolution and is a function of smoothing with a Gaussian filter of scale σ. Looking over the image domain by the maximum value of the partial derivative with respect to the radius r, the normalized integral of the contour of the image along a circular arc ds [1].

According to Daugman [1], with this technique it is possible to estimate separately the parameters of the iris and pupil, delimiting the inner contour of the iris with the pupil and the outer with the sclera. In Figure 2 the iris has been limited by the Daugman operator.

3   FAST IRIS LOCATION

The identification process consists in the image segmentation to separate the region of interest of the iris.

This work proposes to use only the inner region of the iris, discarding the outer region. Two reasons led to this decision:

1. The internal region of the iris, closest to the pupil, is one that concentrates most of the specific features of every human being, while the external region, nearer the sclera, has a smaller number of specific features [8].
2. The process of segmentation of the iris is usually one of the most computational expensive steps of the common recognition process. The use only the inner region of the iris reduces the processing time for separating the region of interest without losing the most important features for the iris recognition.

In this work, due to using only the inner region of the iris, is not necessary the location of the boundary between the iris and sclera. Targeting the boundary between the pupil and the iris is possible to separate the region of interest for the achievement of the following processes.

As the pupil has lower intensity than the rest of the image, we can use the histogram equalization followed by thresholding and a sequence of morphological operations to perform the segmentation of the boundary between the pupil and iris. The use of morphological operations instead of edge detection operators makes the segmentation process faster, which is highly relevant when one intends to use the iris recognition system in real time.

The sequence of talks used in the segmentation process of the pupil are: 1) histogram equalization, which aims to achieve a better distribution of the gray levels over the input image, causing a higher differentiation of the intensities presented; 2) thresholding the equalized image, aiming to separate the image regions with gray levels below a certain value, by using as threshold the average value obtained from the pixels in the central region of the image; 3) dilation, used to remove potential sources of low intensity that are not part of the pupil; 4) opening, which aims to repair possible faults in the region of the pupil caused by applying the dilation operator; and 5) extraction of borders, used to let the edges of the image. Figure 3 presents an example of applying these tasks to an original image: Figure 3(a) corresponds to the original image; Figure 3(b) shows the image after histogram equalization; Figure 3(c) presents the thresholded image; Figure 3(d) has the image after dilation; Figure 3(e) shows the image after applying the open operator; Figure 3(f) presents the image after the extraction operation of the borders; and Figure 3(g) shows the original image overlapped with the pupil identified. It should be noted that the circle visible on Figure 3(g) resulted from the last morphological operation that extracted the border presented in Figure 3(f).

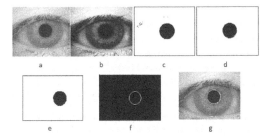

Figure 3. Process of pupil identification: (a) original image, (b) image after histogram equalization, (c) thresholded image (d) image after the dilation, (e) image after opening operation, (f) image after the borders operation, (g) original image overlapped with the detected circle of the iris.

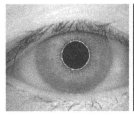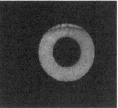

Figure 4. Identification of the iris region of interest: (a) image with the pupil identified, (b) identified region of interest of the iris.

After locating the pupil, we must find the region of interest of the iris for further recognition. Having the outline of the pupil, the process of separating the region of interest of the iris becomes simpler.

Three different approaches were taken for testing the definition of the iris region of interest, as follows:

1. Region of interest defined by a distance corresponding to the length of the radius of the pupil. Such a distance has been circularly applied all over the iris from its border with the pupil so defining the iris region of interest.
2. Region of interest defined by a distance corresponding to a fixed amount of pixels. Such a distance has been circularly applied all over the iris from its border with the pupil. In this case the distance has been empirically determined from the analysis of the image database to be 50 pixels, as this distance must be proportional to the spatial resolution of the used images. Tests were conducted using fixed distances between 20 pixels and 80 pixels, being 50 the number of pixels for this distance that led to the best results during the recognition process.
3. Region of interest defined through a percentage inversely proportional to the distance from the border of the iris with the pupil to the border of the iris with the sclera. The number of pixels was kept approximately constant during comparisons, disregarding eventual dilation or contraction of the pupil.

After applying some tests on the database, we decided to use the fixed distance approach to locate the region of interest, as this one presented the best results. Such results are presented in section 4. Figure 4 shows an example of the region of interest located in the iris.

4 TESTS AND RESULTS

For the experimental tests, we used the images of the iris database of the Chinese Academy of

Sciences—Institute of Automation (CASIA). The choice of this image database is due to the fact that it has been used for testing in the works used in this work for comparison purpose. We also used two different computational platforms during the tests:

- Machine I: Personal computer with Intel Pentium 4 processor, at 2.4 GHz, and 256 Mb RAM, using Microsoft Windows XP and Matlab version 6.1.
- Machine II: Notebook with Intel I3 processor, at 2.4 GHz, and 4 GB of RAM, using Microsoft Windows 7 and Matlab version 7.8.

To locate the region of interest of the iris three different models were tested, as described in section 3. Table 1 displays the results obtained from the three models with respect to the localization of the region of interest accuracy ratio. It can be seen that the model based on a fixed region around the pupil presented the best results, thus being used as the method of choice for the present work.

The worst results presented by the model based on the length of the radius of the pupil are related to cases were the pupil is too dilated, in which case the radius of the pupil is larger than the radius of the iris. In such occurrences, the method takes regions of the sclera as regions of interest of the iris.

The worst results obtained from the method that takes a percentage of the whole iris are due to the difficulty in finding the border between the iris and the sclera. In this case the border is incorrectly guessed for several of the images.

The location of the region of interest of the iris represented in an eye image is one of the most complex processes in recognition of people through the iris and, without doubt, the process that requires the highest computational cost. The reduction of the recognition area of the iris, as reported in section 3, gives to the proposed algorithm a high gain with respect to the time necessary to carry out the recognition process. Moreover, the need for detecting only the border between the iris and pupil makes the localization relatively simple and provides a high accuracy.

Table 2 shows a comparison between the accuracy rates in localizing the iris in the image of the database used between the proposed method and other methods used as reference. It can be

Table 1. Accuracy in iris localization.

Method	Accuracy (%)
1. Length of the radius of the pupil	99.60
2. Fixed amount of pixels	100.00
3. Percentage inversely proportional	82.75

Table 2. Comparison between the accuracy rates in localizing the iris.

Method	Accuracy (%)
Proposed	100.00
Wildes[4]	99.50
Daugman[1]	98.60
Masek[3]	82.53

Table 3. Segmentation processing time.

Method	Time (s)
Proposed	0.82
Wildes[4]	1.98
Daugman[1]	6.56
Masek[3]	23.37

observed that the proposed method is the only that had localized successfully the region of interest in all testing images.

Table 3 presents the comparison in terms of the average computational time required to locate the region of interest in the testing images. We can verify that the proposed method requires a time lower than the other methods for locating the region of interest of the iris, which is due to a decrease in the region to be analyzed. It should be noted the high computational time required by the Masek method. This method uses as a basis for the exact location of the iris the Hough Transform, which despite being proven effective for locating circles in images, is very computationally expensive.

The times shown in Table 3 were obtained using Machine I. Performing the test of the proposed method using the Machine II, the average computational was 0.27 seconds.

5 CONCLUSION

The recognition of individuals based on biometric techniques has gained great prominence in recent years. Among these techniques the one that presents the most interesting results is the recognition of individuals through iris features.

However, most existing methods have the drawback of high computational costs, mainly because segmentation of the iris from the rest of the input image is needed.

In this paper we presented a method in which the segmentation process can be performed with minimal computational cost, and that could identify successfully all the irises in the testing image database used. We could verify that the proposed method is very promising, primarily for its excellent performance with respect to the required computational effort and especially for not failing to identify the region of interest in all of the testing images used.

In spite of the main goal of the described work having been the speed up of the iris segmentation process, it should be noted an important outcome that was also obtained, which may lead to a promising future research: using only the region of the iris nearest to the pupil, a 99.42% level of accuracy over the entire image database as achieved.

ACKNOWLEDGMENTS

The authors are thankful to FUNDUNESP—Fundação para o Desenvolvimento da UNESP—Brazil and FAPESP—Fundação de Amparo à Pesquisa do Estado de São Paulo—Brazil for the financial support.

REFERENCES

[1] Daugman, J. How Iris Recognition Works. IEEE Trans. on Circuits and Systems for Video Technology, 14(1) 21–30, 2004.

[2] Gonzales e, A.C. & Woods, R.E. Digital Image Processing—3ª Edition. Pearson Prentice Hall, São Paulo, Brazil, 2010.

[3] Masek, L. Recognition of Human Iris Patterns for Biometric Identification. Master's Degree Dissertation. School of Computer Science and Software Engineering, The University of Western, Australia, 2003.

[4] Wildes, R. Iris recognition: an emerging biometric technology. Proceedings of the IEEE, 85(9) 1348–1363, 1997.

[5] Duarte, G.D. Use of the Hough Transform to detect circles in digital images. Available www2.pelotas.ifsul.edu.br/glaucius/tese/artigo10.pdf accessed in september of 2010.

[6] Ma, L., Tan, T., Wang e, Y. & Zhang, D. Personal identification based on iris texture analysis. IEEE Transactions on Pattern Analysis and Machine Intelligence, 25(12) 1519–1533, 2003.

[7] Daugman, J. Wavelet Demodulation Codes, Statistical Independence, and Pattern Recognition. Available at: citeseerx.ist.psu.edu/viewdoc/download?doi = 10.1.1.46.2202.pdf, acessed in september 2010.

[8] Pereira, M. A Proposal to the Reliability Increase of Iris Recognition System and its Implementation via Genetic Algorithms. Master's Degree Dissertation. Department of Eletrical Engineering, University of Uberlândia. 2005.

[9] Cui, Y., Wang, T., Tan, L. Ma & Sun, Z. A Fast and Robust Iris Localization Method Based on Texture Segmentation. Center for Biometric Authentication and Testing, National Laboratory of Pattern Recognition, Chinese Academy of Sciences, Beijing, P.R. China, 2004.

[10] Ma, L. Tan, T., Wang, Y. & Zhang, D. Efficient Iris Recognition by Characterizing Key Local Variations. IEEE Transactions on Image Processing, 13(13) 739–750, 2004.

Computational Vision and Medical Image Processing – Tavares & Natal Jorge (eds)
© 2012 Taylor & Francis Group, London, ISBN 978-0-415-68395-1

Monitoring feet temperature using thermography

D. Bento & F.C. Monteiro
Polytechnic Institute of Bragança, ESTiG/IPB, C. Sta. Apolonia, Bragança, Portugal

A.I. Pereira
Polytechnic Institute of Bragança, ESTiG/IPB, C. Sta. Apolonia, Bragança, Portugal
ALGORITMI, Minho University, Campus de Azurém, Guimarães, Portugal

ABSTRACT: Studies show that regular monitoring of feet temperature may limit the incidence of disabling conditions such as foot ulcers and lower-limb amputations. Infrared thermometry and liquid crystal thermography were identified as the leading technologies in use today. In this study, we analysed the maximum temperature and tested some mathematical models for the foot temperature distribution.

1 INTRODUCTION

Diabetic foot (DF) ulcers are one of the major complications in diabetics, seriously affecting the quality of their lives. The possibility to measure the different aspects of DF and its ulcerative pathology gives to clinicians the chance to both evaluate and weigh up the different components contributing to the genesis and evolution of the cases and to monitor their clinical course as a consequence of the therapeutic interventions. Therefore, it is necessary to establish methods of prevention or early diagnosis for diabetic foot complications (Nishide et al., 2009).

The DF lesions are a combination of several risk factors acting simultaneously and can be triggered by peripheral diabetic neuropathy, peripheral vascular diseases and biomechanical changes. The decrease in sensory function in the foot and limitation of joint mobility are some early signs for the appearance of foot ulcers, meaning high risk of developing inflammations or other complications. These changes can be assessed using various techniques, thus preventing the appearance of ulcers and reducing the risk of foot amputation.

The use of thermal techniques to evaluate diabetic foot has largely remained a research topic (Lavery et al., 2004, Sun et al., 2006, Armstrong et al., 2007, Nagase et al., 2011). The authors believe that thermal techniques can be significantly useful in diabetic foot assessment, with the intent of determining risk of foot ulceration.

Recent advances of physiological imaging techniques have prompted us to use thermography for screening skin temperature, deep tissue edema or fluid collection due to inflammation (Nishide et al., 2009). Infrared thermography is one of the leading technologies in use today. This technology is feasible for temperature monitoring of the foot and can be used as a complement to current practices for foot examinations in diabetes.

In this study, we used thermal plantar images in patients without diabetes to support a mathematical model for foot normal temperature distribution.

2 MATERIALS AND METHODS

2.1 Subjects

This study includes healthy volunteers, recruited from Polytechnic Institute of Bragança, representing a feet healthy population who were between 21 to 43 years old. This preliminary study includes a set of fifteen thermographic images.

2.2 Protocol

The subjects were guided to keep resting supine position without shoes or socks for 10 minutes, before measurement, to stabilize the feet temperature.

The images were collected by a thermal camera (FLIR 365) positioned at a fixed distance of 1 metre of subject's feet. A plate of rigid foam was placed over the ankles to isolate the temperature of feet from the rest of the body. The total duration of data acquisition process did not exceed 15 minutes.

2.3 Image processing

Infrared thermography is a real-time temperature measurement technique used to produce a coloured visualization of thermal energy emitted by skin.

However, temperature discrimination threshold, on the foot, could be a difficult process due to the large temperature variation between the feet and the background.

As we can see from Figure 1, the large temperature variation in the image produces small colour variations of skin temperature.

Through the application of image processing techniques it is possible to obtain images with a better contrast of the structures in question. In order to isolate the feet from the background, we apply image segmentation, based on region growing, followed by a histogram expansion using only the temperature values of the feet, obtaining discriminative images, as showed in Figure 2.

2.4 Characterize foot regions

Interpretation of the colour patterns according to the anatomic temperature distribution is thought to aid in evaluating and diagnosing foot complications.

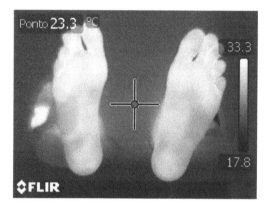

Figure 1.   Thermal infrared image.

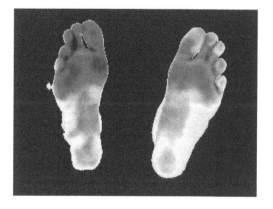

Figure 2.   Improving the temperature discrimination.

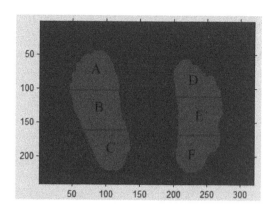

Figure 3.   Foot regions.

With the numerical data, obtained through image processing, we defined main areas by measuring each foot (length and width) and divided it in three regions. Considering the left foot, Region A is the upper region; Region B is the central region and the lower region was defined as Region C.

In a similar way, Regions D, E and F were defined for the right foot, as represented in Figure 3.

3   NUMERICAL RESULTS AND DISCUSSION

In this study, we used fifteen feet images. Nine of them follow the same pattern for the maximum temperature while the other six do not have a defined pattern.

Figure 4 shows the maximum temperature value, for each region, from the set of nine images which follow a pattern.

We can observe that the maximum temperature value was obtained at Region A and D (the upper regions of the feet) which agrees with other results presented in the literature.

In this preliminary study, we tested three nonlinear mathematical models for the temperature distribution. The parameters i, j represent the pixels positions.

$$f_1(x,i,j) = x_1 ij + x_2 i^2 + x_3 j^2 + x_4 i + x_5 j + x_6 \quad (1)$$

$$f_2(x,i,j) = x_1 \sin(x_2 i + x_3) + x_4 \sin(x_5 j + x_6) + x_7 \quad (2)$$

$$f_3(x,i,j) = x_1 \sin^2(x_2 i + x_3) + x_4 \sin^2(x_5 j + x_6) + x_7 \quad (3)$$

It was observed that the best mathematical function that approximates the temperature distribution was the function f_2. The evaluation was done using the nonlinear least method combined with l_1 penalty method.

190

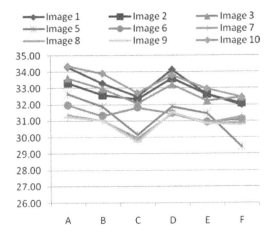

Image 1   Image 2   Image 3
Image 5   Image 6   Image 7
Image 8   Image 9   Image 10

Figure 4. Absolute temperature maximum values.

4 CONCLUSIONS AND FUTURE WORK

High temperature gradients between foot regions may predict the onset of neuropathic ulceration, which makes temperature monitoring a way to reduce the risk of ulceration.

In this study, we observed that the temperature maximum value, in general, is obtained in the upper regions of the foot.

A preliminary study indicates that the best mathematical model to approximate the temperature distribution is a sine sum function. Future prospective observation is needed to confirm our mathematical model or some variation of it.

REFERENCES

Armstrong, D., Holtz-Neiderer, K., Wendel, C. et al., 2007. Skin temperature monitoring reduces the risk for diabetic foot ulceration in high-risk patients, *The American Journal of Medicine* 120: 1042–1046.

Lavery, L., Higgins, K., Lactot, D., Constantinitides, G., Zamorano, R., Armstrong, D., et al., 2004. Home monitoring of foot skin temperatures to prevent ulceration, *Diabetes Care* 27(11): 2642–2647.

Nagase, T., Sanada, H., Takehara, K., Oe, M., Iizaka, S., Ohashi, Y., Oba, M., Kadowaki, T. & Nakagami, G. 2011. Variations of plantar thermographic patterns in normal controls and non-ulcer diabetic patients: novel classification using angiosome concept, *Journal of Plastic, Reconstructive & Aesthetic Surgery* 64(7): 860–866.

Nishide, K., Nagase, T., Oba, M., Oe, M., Ohashi, Y., Iizaka, S., Nakagami, G., Kadowaki, T. & Sanada, H. 2009. Ultrasonographic and thermographic screening for latent imflammation in diabetic foot callus. *Diabetes Research and Clinical Practice* 85(3): 304–309.

Sun, P.C., Lin, H.D., Jao, SH., Ku, Y.C., Chan, R.C. & Cheng, C.K. 2006. Relationship of skin temperature to sympathetic dysfunction in diabetic at-risk feet. *Diabetes Research and Clinical Practice* 73(1): 41–46.

Computational Vision and Medical Image Processing – Tavares & Natal Jorge (eds)
© *2012 Taylor & Francis Group, London, ISBN 978-0-415-68395-1*

Identification of foliar diseases in cotton crop

A.A. Bernardes, J.G. Rogeri, N. Marranghello & A.S. Pereira
Department of Computer Science and Statistics, IBILCE, Sao Paulo State University (UNESP),
Sao Jose do Rio Preto—SP, Brazil

A.F. Araujo & João Manuel R.S. Tavares
Department of Mechanical Engineering (DeMec), Faculty of Engineering, University of Porto(FEUP)
Institute of Mechanical Engineering and Industrial Management(INEGI), Porto, Portugal

ABSTRACT: The pathogens manifestation in plantations are the largest cause of damage in several cultivars, which may cause increase of prices and loss of crop quality. This paper presents a method for automatic classification of cotton diseases through feature extraction of leaf symptoms from digital images. Wavelet transform energy has been used for feature extraction while Support Vector Machine has been used for classification. Five situations have been diagnosed, namely: Healthy crop, Ramularia disease, Bacterial Blight, Ascochyta Blight, and unspecified disease.

1 INTRODUCTION

This work aims at identifying foliar diseases in cotton plantations. This cultivar is of great economic importance to Brazil, being one of the pillars of the textile industry, which consumes around one million tons of cotton fiber per year [1, 2].

The primary goal of the developed system has been to identify the existence of pathogens in cotton foliars. Once a disease is identified it has to be automatically classified through further processing of the corresponding image. The pathogens used in our tests are among those most frequently occurring in Brazil, which are very aggressive, rapidly spreading throughout the plantations, and that can be fought against only by the use of chemicals [1, 2, 3, 4]. Three diseases were used during the classification stage, as follows: Ramularia (RA), Bacterial Blight (MA), and Ascochyta Blight (AS). Alternatively we allowed the system to classify an image as not belonging to any of these classes (NONE).

In this work we used both RGB and HSV standards, as well as I3a and I3b channels, and grey level (GL) images. The color channels I3a and I3b are obtained from a transformation of the I1I2I3 color standard [5]. The energy of the wavelet transform was computed for each sub-band to build feature vectors that were utilized during the training phase of the support vector machine (SVM) used for image classification.

1.1 *Generation of I3a and I3b channels*

Channels and I3a and I3b were created from changes carried out by Campbell [5] on the color channel of I1I2I3 model defined by Ohta et al. [6].

1.2 *Wavelets and image processing*

Currently, the application of wavelet transform has proven very efficient to perform complex analysis of non-stationary signals, with respect to time-frequency signal. There is a considerable increase in its application in a variety of biosignals, such as in neurophysiological signal analysis, medical signals and image diagnosis, pulmonary microvascular pressure estimation, mammograms, signal compression, brain signals analysis, and classification of voice disorders [7].

1.3 *Support Vector Machine*

Support Vector Machine (SVM) is a classification technique that is becoming increasingly used in science, when high performance computation is required for practical applications. The outcome of such a technique is often superior to results obtained by other machine learning algorithms such as Artificial Neural Networks [8, 9, 10]. SVMs have been used for pattern recognition, image processing, machine learning, bioinformatics, among others [11].

2 MATERIAL

A total of 420 images were used in this research. One ser of images was provided by phytopathologist Dr. Nelson Dias Suassuna, researcher at Embrapa

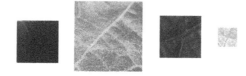

Figure 1. Images of healthy leaf area of cotton [12, 13].

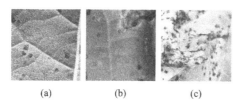

(a)   (b)   (c)

Figure 2. Severity degree of MA cotton disease: (a) initial; (b) intermediate; and (c), advanced stages of infection [12].

Cotton, in Campina Grande, Paraiba, Brazil [12]. This database was complemented by another set of images from the Forestry Images website [13].

Size, brightness, contrast and resolution of the images are quite different, resulting in a very heterogeneous database. To illustrate the database items some images of healthy regions of cotton leaves are shown in Figure 1. Opposite to this some images of infected leaves with varying degrees of disease severity are shown in Figure 2. Figure 2(a) displays the leaf area at an early stage of MA disease; Figure 2(b) presents the infected leaf, at an intermediate stage; and Figure 2(c) shows the advanced stage.

3 PROPOSED METHOD

The classification process was divided into two phases:

- **Phase 1:** Finding the best feature vector for each class;
- **Phase 2:** Create the final classification system from the best results obtained in the previous phase.

3.1 *Phase 1: Finding the best feature vector*

This phase is aimed at finding the best feature vector to represent each of the classes to be considered during classification. To achieve this goal the following steps were accomplished:

- Decomposition of images into multiple channels (R, G, B, H, S, V, I3a, I3b, and GL);
- Application of the discrete wavelet transform (DWT) up to the third level;
- Computation of the energy for each sub-band and compose the feature vector;

- Creation of the SVM classification environment;
- Listing of the images used for training and testing;
- Evaluation of the best feature vectors.

3.1.1 *Decomposition of the image*
The decomposition of the images is the first process the system executes. In this stage an image is decomposed into nine channels, namely: R, G, B, H, S, V, I3a, I3b and GL.

3.1.2 *Application of the discrete wavelet transform*
Discrete Wavelet Transform (TWD) decomposition is applied up to the third level. When an image is decomposed as such it will have ten sub-bands, as illustrated in Figure 3. Note that each sub-band is identified by a number between 1 and 10. Region A1 and sub-bands 8, 9 and 10, are generated by the first level of decomposition of the DWT. Region A2 and sub-bands 5, 6 and 7 refer to the second level of decomposition, and the third level is formed by the sub-bands 1, 2, 3 and 4.

3.1.3 *Computation of the energy for each sub-band*
After applying the DWT to the three levels, the energy for each wavelet sub-band is computed. Each value obtained is inserted into a feature vector as the one illustrated in Figure 4. The vector in this figure consists of ten elements, each of them is identified by a number corresponding to the number of the sub-band in Figure 3. The energy value computed for each sub-band is stored in the corresponding vector element.

3.1.4 *Creation of an SVM classification environment*
The network architecture used is shown in Figure 5. Note that 10 input elements are used. To each input element is assigned the value of the element of the corresponding characteristic

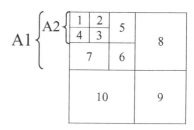

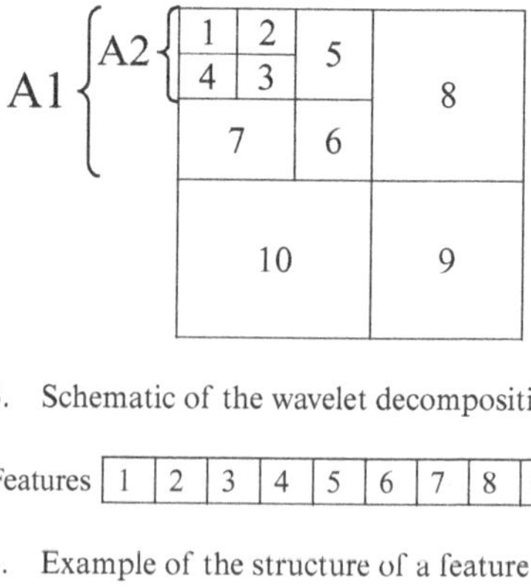

Figure 3. Schematic of the wavelet decomposition.

Vector Features	1	2	3	4	5	6	7	8	9	10

Figure 4. Example of the structure of a feature vector.

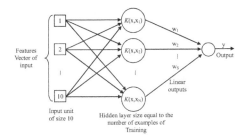

Figure 5.   Architecture of SVM used.

Table 1.   Coefficients and support numbers used.

Coefficient name	Number of support	Abbreviation used
Beylkin	18	Bey18
Coiflets	12 e 30	Coi12 e Coi30
Daubechies	4, 14, 34, 64 e 74	Dau4, Dau14, Dau34, Dau64 e Dau74
Haar	1	*Haar*
Symmlets	8 e 16	Sym8 e Sym16
Vaidyanathan	24	Vai24

vector. In the hidden layer there are a number of neurons (N) equal to the number of training examples, making the net convergence easier [8, 9]. The Gaussian function has been used as the network mapping function (kernel).

3.1.5 *Listing of the images used for training and testing*

The classification process was divided into two different steps:

- **Step 1:** Label the leaf images as healthy (SA) or injured (LE).
- **Step 2:** Find the best descriptor (feature vector) representing each class. It is performed only among the three types of pathogens (**RA, MA and AS**), which an image can be classified.

To find the best descriptor for each class, 12 wavelets were used. Table 1 displays the name of the wavelet coefficients, followed by the number of its support, and the abbreviations used in this work, which associates the name of a coefficient to a support number. The 12 wavelets were identified as: Bey18, Coi12, Coi30, Dau4, Dau14, Dau34, Dau64, Dau76, Haar, Sym8 and Vai24.

3.1.6 *Evaluation of the best feature vectors*

First, 108 feature vectors are obtained. Then they are classified either as LE or as SA. After that the percentage of correct answers of the 108 feature vectors for the classes RA, MA and AS is computed. The best feature vectors for each class are listed in

Table 2.   Best results achieved between the classes.

Class name	Channel	Coefficient	Percentage of correct
SA	H	Vai24	96,2%
LE	H	Vai24	100%
MA	I3b	Coi12 e Sym16	97,1%
RA	H	Dau4	88,6%
AS	H	Bey18	88,6%

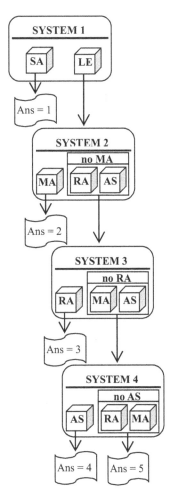

Figure 6.   Final classification system.

Table 2. Among classes SA and LE the best feature vector that separated the two classes was in the channel H, by using the wavelet Vai24, which for SA achieved 96.2% correct guesses, and for LE it reached 100% accuracy. For class MA the best result was in I3b channel coefficients, on Coi12, Sym16, which reached 97.1% accuracy. Class RA achieved 88.6% accuracy using the feature vector of channel H and wavelet Dau4. It can also be seen in Table 2 that the AS class presents the best result, achieving 88.6% accuracy in channel H, using coefficient wavelet Bey18.

3.2 Creating the final classification system

In the previous section the best descriptors (feature vectors) for each class were identified. This section describes the methodology to compose the final classification system.

Figure 6 illustrates the general classification structure. Observe that four different classification systems were created. Each system was trained and tested with the best feature vectors, as discussed in the previous section.

4 RESULTS AND DISCUSSION

Among 210 images used for the tests, 188 images were correctly classified (101 SA images, 34 MA images, 28 RA images, and 25 AS images) corresponding to slightly over 89.5% correct guesses.

For the healthy class (SA), which comprises 105 images, 101 were correctly classified, corresponding to about 96.2% of correct guesses. Table 3 displays the percentage of healthy image classification for each diagnosis. Note that 3.8% are false positives, half of which were classified as belonging to class Bacterial Blight, and another half as Ramularia Disease.

For Bacterial Blight class, 34 of the 35 images were correctly classified. Table 4 displays some details for this classification, where it can be seen that 97.1% of images were correctly classified, and only 2.9% were false positives.

For Ramularia class 28 of the 35 images were correctly classified. Table 5 shows details of "Ramularia" classification for each diagnosis. Note that 80% of the images were correctly classified, and 20% were false positives, being 8.6% classified as MA, 11.4% classified as AS, and no

Table 3. Test results for 105 "Healthy" images.

SA	False positive			
	MA	RA	AS	NONE
96,2%	1,9%	1,9%	0,0%	0,0%

Table 4. Test results for 35 "Bacterial Blight" images.

MA	False positive			
	SA	RA	AS	NONE
97,1%	0,0%	0,0%	0,0%	2,9%

Table 5. Test results for 35 "Ramularia" images.

RA	False positive			
	SA	MA	AS	NONE
80,0%	0,0%	8,6%	11,4%	0,0%

Table 6. Test results for 35 "Ascochyta Blight" images.

AS	False positive			
	SA	MA	RA	NONE
71,4%	0,0%	11,4%	14,3%	2,9%

images were classified as healthy or as presenting no known disease.

For the Ascochyta Blight class 25 of the 35 images were correctly classified. Table 6 displays the details of image classification for the "Ascochyta Blight" set. Note that 71.4% of images were correctly classified, and 29.6% were false positives, being 11.4% classified as MA, 14.3% classified as RA, and 2.9% classified as not belonging to any known class.

Note from the healthy (SA) class of tables 3 through 6 that no images of injured leaves was classified as healthy. Thus, it follows that all 105 infected images, namely with pathogens Bacterial Blight, Ascochyta Blight and Ramularia, were classified as injured, achieving 100% accuracy of image separation, and consequently resulting in no false positive.

5 COMPARISON TO RELATED WORKS

The present work has taken cotton culture as its subject. As far as we could determine no other research took such a cultivar as subject in the same sense we took.

Huang [14] presented a study on rubber trees with four different diagnosis (healthy, and three diseases) achieving a score of 97.2% correct guesses for injured leaves. A problem with Huang's work is the fact that only injured leaves were used.

Abduhlah et al. [15] classified three pathogens for rubber trees achieving 80% of correct guesses. However, Abdulah and co-workers' tests considered only one kind of pathogens.

Meunkaewjinda et al. [16] examined three diagnoses (healthy, and two diseases) for grape cultivars. In their study they achieved 86.3% correct guesses.

Phadicar and Sil [17] studied rice crops achieving 92% of correct diseases classification. However, only two classes were used for this study.

6 CONCLUSIONS

216 feature vectors were generated for our study, half of which used to identify the best feature vectors within SA and LE classes, and the other half used to find the best among MA, RA, and AS classes.

The best feature vectors were used during the final system classification. After sorting the healthy (SA) images out, the image set of supposedly infected leaves was classified within one of the four other sub-classes, namely: MA, RA, AS, and NONE. The final results achieved were: 96.2% accuracy for the SA class, 97.1% accuracy for the MA class, 80% accuracy for the RA class, and 71.4% accuracy for the AS class.

Moreover, the present work achieved better results with respect to other cultivars. Considering it used a small amount of samples to train the SVM, it produced descriptors adequately representing each class, even using a heterogeneous database, and it produced appropriate classification of a fairly large number of classes with almost 90% accuracy.

ACKNOWLEDGMENTS

The authors are thankful to FUNDUNESP—Fundação para o Desenvolvimento da UNESP—Brazil and FAPESP—Fundação de Amparo à Pesquisa do Estado de São Paulo—Brazil for the financial support.

REFERENCES

[1] Oliveira, M.C. Agricultural Protection Agency of Goias (Agrodefesa). Program of Prevention and Control of Pests in Cotton. Available at: http://www.agrodefesa.go.gov.br/index.php?option=com_content&view=article&id=74. Accessed on January, 2010.

[2] Galbieri, R. Behavior of Cotton Genotypes in the Presence of Pathogens and Nematodes. Master Dissertation (Tropical and Subtropical Agriculture), Campinas, SP—Brazil, 2007. (in Portuguese).

[3] Kimati, H.; Amorim, L.; Bergamin Filho, A., Camargo L.E.A. and REZENDE, J.A.M. Handbook of Phytopathology. Vol. 2: Diseases of Cultivated Plants. Sao Paulo: Agronomic Ceres Ltda, 1997.

[4] Curvelo, C.R.S., Rodrigues, F.A., Berger, P.G. and Rezende, D.C. Scanning electron microscopy of the infectious process of Ramularia aureola on cotton leaves. Trop. Plant Pathol. [online]. v. 35, n. 2, pp. 108–113, 2010. ISSN: 1982–5676.

[5] Camargo, A., Smith, J.S. An image-processing based algorithm to automatically identify plant disease visual symptoms. Biosystems Engineering, v. 102, n. 1, pp. 9–21, 2009.

[6] Ohta, Y., Kanade, T. and Sakai, T. Color information for region segmentation. Computer Graphics and Image Processing. Department of Information Science, Kyoto, Japan, v. 13, n. 3, pp. 222–241, July, 1980.

[7] Addison, P.S., Walker, J. and Guido, R.C. Time-frequency analysis of biosignals, Engineering in Medicine and Biology Magazine, IEEE, v. 28, n. 5, pp.14–29, September—October, 2009.

[8] Souza, L.M. Intelligent Detection in Laryngeal Pathologies Based on Support Vector Machines and Wavelet Transform. Master Dissertation (Applied Computational Physics)—University of Sao Paulo at Sao Carlos, SP, Brazil, 2011. (in Portuguese).

[9] Bisognin, G. Using Support Machine to Prediction of Protein Tertiary Structure. Master Dissertation (Applied Computing)—University of Vale do Rio dos Sinos, Sao Leopoldo, RS - Brazil, 2007. (in Portuguese).

[10] Fonseca, E., Guido, R.C., Scalassara, P.R., Maciel, C.D. and Pereira, J.C. Wavelet Time-frequency Analysis and Least-Squares Support Vector Machine for the Identification of Voice Disorders. Computers in Biology and Medicine, Elsevier, v. 37, n. 4, pp. 571–578, 2007.

[11] Yu, Z., Wong, H. and Wen, G.A. Modified Support Vector Machine and its Application to Image Segmentation. Image and Vision Computing, v.29, pp. 29–40, 2011.

[12] Suassuna, N.D. Private Communication. Brazilian Company of Agricultural Research, Campina Grande, PB—Brazil.

[13] FI. Forestry Images. A joint project of the Center for Invasive Species and Ecosystem Health, USDA Forest Service and International Society of Arboriculture. The University of Georgia—Warnell School of Forestry and Natural Resources and College of Agricultural and Environmental Sciences. Available at: http://www.forestryimages.org. Accessed on August, 2010.

[14] Huang, K. Application of artificial neural network for detecting Phalaenopsis seedling diseases using color and texture features. Comput. Electron. Agric. v. 57, n. 1, pp. 3–11, May, 2007.

[15] Abdullah, N.E.; Rahim, A.A.; Hashim, H.; and Kamal, M.M. Classification of Rubber Tree Leaf Diseases Using Multilayer Perceptron Neural Network, Research and Development. SCOReD 5th Student Conference. pp. 1–6, 11–12 December, 2007.

[16] Meunkaewjinda, A., Kumsawat, P., Attakitmongcol, K. and Srikaew, A. Grape leaf disease detection from color imagery using hybrid intelligent system. Electrical Engineering/Electronics, Computer, Telecommunications and Information Technology, 2008. ECTI-CON 2008. 5th International Conference on v. 1, pp. 513–516, 14–17 May, 2008.

[17] Phadikar, S. and Sil, J. Rice Disease Identification using Pattern Recognition Techniques; Proceedings of the 11th International Conference on Computer and Information Technology (ICCIT 2008), Khulna, Bangladesh. pp. 420–423, 25–27 December, 2008.

Computational Vision and Medical Image Processing – Tavares & Natal Jorge (eds)
© *2012 Taylor & Francis Group, London, ISBN 978-0-415-68395-1*

A local invariant features approach for classifying acrosome integrity in boar spermatozoa

L. Fernández Robles, V. González-Castro, O. García-Olalla, M.T. García-Ordás & E. Alegre
University of León, Spain

ABSTRACT: In this work we have used a number of texture descriptors to characterize the acrosome state of boar sperm cells, which is a key factor in semen quality control applications. Laws masks, Legendre and Zernike moments, Haralick features extracted from the original image and from the coefficients of the Discrete Wavelet Transform, and descriptors based on interest points using the Speeded-Up Robust Features (SURF) method have been evaluated. Classification using kNN show that the best results were obtained by SURF, with an overall hit rate of 94.88% and, what is more important, a higher hit rate in the damaged (96.86%) than in the intact class (92.89%). These results make this descriptor very attractive for the veterinary community.

1 INTRODUCTION

Proper semen quality assessment is an important problem for medical and veterinarian research. The porcine industry is one of the most important fields where it is applied with the purpose of obtaining better individuals for human consumption in each generation.

For several years the Computer-Assisted Semen Analysis (CASA) systems have been used for assessing the seminal quality [3]. Currently these systems analyse the motility, concentration and provide some simple geometric measures of the spermatozoa's head to characterize abnormal head shapes, obtaining an assessment of the studied sample based on these values. However, there are three valuable criteria, used by veterinary experts, that these systems do not measure automatically. Those are the number and presence of proximal and distal droplets, the vitality of the sample based on the presence of dead or alive spermatozoa and the integrity of the acrosome membrane.

Nowadays, the evaluation of the acrosome integrity of the spermatozoon heads is carried out manually, using stains and there are not any computerassisted tools for that analysis. This manual assessment has several drawbacks such as its high cost in terms of time, its lack of objectivity, or the requirement of specialized veterinarian staff and equipments. Hence, it would be very interesting to get an automatic classification of the acrosomes as intact or damaged.

Texture analysis and classification have been used in the literature applied to a wide range of fields with high performance [11] but there are few computer vision works which deal with boar sperm analysis. Moreover, computer-based systems designed for semen analysis tasks should reliably segment the heads of the spermatozoa [5], extract the patterns which characterize them and finally classify those patterns in order to estimate how many damaged acrosomes are present in the sample.

In this way, Alegre et al. [1] used Learning Vector Quantization (LVQ) to classify the acrosome integrity achieving a minimum error rate of 6.8%. In [14], Suárez et al. used statistic texture descriptors to classify boar sperm images applying discriminant analysis. The best results, with an error rate of 13.81%, were obtained using the QDA classifier. In [4], González et al. used a discrete wavelet Transform (DWT) and several texture descriptors to classify the acrosome integrity obtaining an error rate of 7.91%.

Using local features, we can avoid segmentation which represents by itself an unsolved problem. The development of image matching by using a set of local interest points can be traced back to the work of Moravec [10] on stereo matching using a corner detector. The Moravec detector was improved by Harris and Stephens [6] to make it more repeatable under small image variations and near edges. However, it was Lowe [9], with SIFT, who satisfactorily introduced invariance to the local features approach. This detector based on DoG (Difference of Gaussians), performs extremely well in matching and image retrieval probably due to a good balance between spatial localization and scale estimation accuracy.

The rest of the paper is organized as follows: In section 2 the methods used for determine the acrosome quality are presented. The results are introduced in section 3 and finally the conclusions of this work are presented in section 4.

2 METHODS

2.1 *Image preprocessing*

A digital camera connected to a phase-contrast microscope with a 100× magnification was used to capture boar semen images with a resolution of 780 × 580 pixels. Therefore, most of the spermatozoa come from different takings, which means that illumination is not completely constant, leading to a robust method to illumination changes. Information about the sample preparation can be found in [12].

Two snapshots of the same spermatozoa, one in real color under fluorescent illumination and other in grey scale under positive phase contrast illumination, are taken without moving the position of the sample. The heads of the grey scale images are then cropped and labeled as damaged or intact based on the real color fluorescent image. Overlapped heads cannot be analysed, so they are discarded from the set of images. Luckily, due to the conditions under which the sample is obtained, overlapped heads do not appear frequently.

After they are labeled, each head is registered automatically in order to assure scale and rotation invariance. First of all, the heads are rotated to its vertical position. This is performed by relating an sperm head with an ellipse and correcting the orientation of the major axis to achieve verticality. Then, the image is right and left cropped leaving head's pixels untouched. Afterwards, the coordinates of the tail are detected. Evaluating if the tail is placed in the bottom half or in the top half of the image will let us know if the spermatozoa has its head up or down respectively. In the second case, the image is flipped, leading to equal orientations. Then, the image is up and down cropped leaving head's pixels intact.

Once all images have the same orientation, our goal is to modify them to achieve the same dimensions. Dimensions of the present set of images are stored and the median of these measures is calculated. Other statistics were implemented— maximum and minimum values, mean, mode and standard deviation—but worst results were obtained. Finally, bad registered images are manually discarded.

After all this process we have a set of 856 intact and 861 damaged heads. Figure 1 shows 3 intact and damaged registered sperm heads.

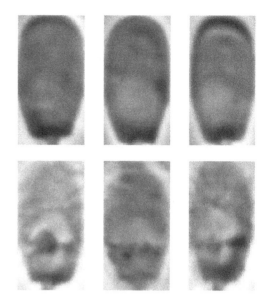

Figure 1. Intact (upper row) and damaged (lower row) registered acrosomes.

2.2 *Description methods*

The first descriptor is made up of 13 out of the 14 features proposed by Haralick, all except the Maximal Correlation Coefficient, and it is called Haralick henceforth.

We have also computed the same features from the GLCMs (Grey Level Co-occurrence Matrix) of the original image together with the coefficients of the first level decomposition of the wavelet transform yielding a 65 features vector. When the transform is applied on an image, four matrices of coefficients are obtained: approximations and horizontal, vertical and diagonal details (LL1, LH1, HL1, HH1). The first one holds almost all the energy of the image, while the other three hold the high frequency details. We will call it WCF13.

The third one was Laws [7] method that consists on applying convolutions with several filters to images, yielding such many images as convolutions are carried out. Let be I the initial image and g_1, g_2, ..., g_n a set of filters.

A generic image resulted after the convolution is defined by $J_n = I * g_n$. Kernels used are defined for neighbourhoods of 5 × 5, so a 16 feature vector is obtained for each image pixel. Subsequently, vectors are reduced from 16 to 9 features. Let be $F_k[i,j]$ the result of applying the k-th mask on the pixel (i, j), then the map E_k of the texture energy for the filter k is define as:

$$E_k(r,c) = \sum_{j=c-7}^{c+7} \sum_{i=r-7}^{r+7} |F_k(i,j)|$$

As fourth descriptor, Legendre moments were used. These moments allow new applications as the reconstruction of an image from the mathematical features provided by these moments. Shu and Yu [13] present an efficient method for computation of Legendre moments. Legendre moments are defined by:

$$\lambda_{p,q} = \frac{(2p+1)(2q+1)}{4} \int_{-1}^{1} \int_{-1}^{1} P_p(x)P_q(y)f(x,y)dxdy$$

where P_p y P_q are the Legendre polynomials.

The fifth method, Zernike moments [8] were used because they yield rotation, scale and translation invariance. As Zernike moments are orthogonal, the reconstruction of the original function from the obtained one is simplified. The low order moments represent the global shape of a pattern and the higher order the detail. When the Zernike moments of the image are suitable for a large number of terms, then the reconstruction of the input image function can be achieved with high accuracy.

Finally, the SURF (Speeded-Up Robust Features) [2] method, based on local features, was employed. A Hessian matrix-based measure $(H(x,\sigma))$ for the interest point detection, defined in Equation 1, has been used.

$$H(x,\sigma) = \begin{bmatrix} L_{xx}(x,\sigma) & L_{xy}(x,\sigma) \\ L_{xy}(x,\sigma) & L_{yy}(x,\sigma) \end{bmatrix} \quad (1)$$

To describe each interest point a Haar wavelet-based descriptor is used. An oriented quadratic grid with 4×4 square sub-regions is laid over the interest point. For each square, the wavelet responses are computed. The 2×2 sub-divisions of each square correspond to the actual fields of the descriptor. These are the sums d_x, $|d_x|$, d_y and $|d_y|$, computed relatively to the orientation of the grid. Hence, each sub-region has a four-dimensional descriptor vector V for its underlying intensity structure:

$$V = \left(\sum d_x, \sum d_y, \sum |d_x|, \sum |d_y| \right) \quad (2)$$

Concatenating the descriptor vectors for all 4×4 sub-regions, this results in a features vector of length 64.

3 RESULTS

K-Nearest Neighbors method with leave-one-out was used to classify the images. It consists of taking one element of the test set and finding the k nearest

elements to it. The class assigned to that element is the most repeated one in those k elements.

Figures 2, 3 and 4 show the interest points matched by SURF between the same image, two intact acrosomes in Figure 3 and two damaged acrosomes in Figure 4. It is remarkable that in intact acrosomes interest points are mostly found in the top half of the head whereas in damaged acrosomes they are found in the whole image. This is perhaps due to the irregular texture present at the half bottom of damaged acrosomes.

We randomly take a set of 70% of images of each class for training and the rest for testing, computing errors with odd k numbers between 1 and 15. This process is repeated 10 times in order to achieve robustness to random choices. The final error rate is the average of the error rates during those 10 runs.

The proximity between the patterns is computed using the Euclidean distance through all evaluated methods.

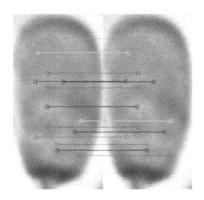

Figure 2. Interest points matched between the same image. Image best viewed in color.

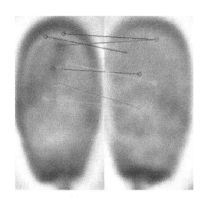

Figure 3. Interest points matched between two intact acrosomes. Image best viewed in color.

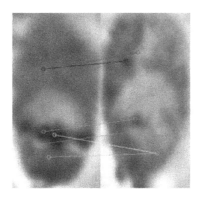

Figure 4. Interest points matched between two damaged acrosomes. Image best viewed in color.

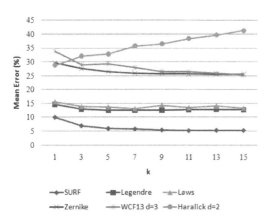

Figure 5. Mean errors (%) against k for each descriptor.

$$d(P_1, P_2) = \sqrt{(x_2 - x_1)^2 + (y_2 - y_1)^2} \qquad (3)$$

The lowest error rate is yielded by SURF with k = 11 (5.12%), outperforming the rest of traditional texture descriptors for every k considered as it is shown in Figure 5.

As shown in Figure 6, SURF always produces a lower hit rate of intact heads (92.89%) in relation to the hit rate of damaged heads (96.86%). The high variability presented by damaged acrosomes leading to more significant interest points where as the intact ones present a similar distribution could be the reason. And even more important, the rest of global methods out perform the recognition of intact heads over the damaged ones except for Haralick in which both rates are quite similar (Figure 7).

In Table 1, the best classification hit rates of the mentioned descriptors are shown, with the number k of neighbors considered in each case and with the better distance obtained for Haralick and WCF13.

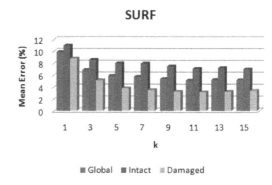

Figure 6. Global, intact and damaged mean errors (%) against k with SURF and Euclidean distance.

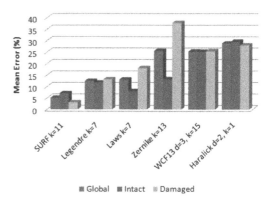

Figure 7. Best global, intact and damaged mean errors (%) for each descriptor.

Table 1. Best hit rates of each assessed descriptor and number of neighbors (k) used.

Descriptors	K	Global (%)	Intact (%)	Damag. (%)
SURF	11	94,88	92,89	96,86
Legendre	7	87,55	88,24	86,86
Laws	7	86,95	91,98	81,94
Zernike	11	74,46	86,80	62,21
WCF13 d = 3	15	74,76	74,90	74,61
Haralick d = 2	1	71,22	70,39	72,05

It can be observed again that SURF achieved better results than the evaluated texture descriptors, obtaining a hit rate of 94.88%.

4 CONCLUSIONS

This work demonstrate the success of applying a computer vision approach to classify images of boar sperm heads as intact or damaged acrosome.

We assessed SURF, an interest point based algorithm which relies on local invariant feature description against global texture methods: Haralick, WCF13 and Zernike, Laws and Legendre moments; classifying with k-Nearest Neighbors and Euclidean distance. Our experiments have obtained error rates when classifying our data set as intact or damaged. Results show global, intact and damaged error rates for each of the above methods. It was observed that hit rates of SURF with k = 11 (94.88%, 92.89% and 96.86% respectively) outperform the rest of methods. Haralick achieved the worst results with an error rate of 28,78%.

Furthermore, using SURF, misclassifications of sperm heads with intact acrosome are lower than in the case of heads with damaged acrosome. On the contrary, texture descriptors achieved the opposite situation (a higher recognition with damaged acrosomes). Future works can adopt a combination of both global and local invariant descriptors in order to improve their individual results.

In conclusion, the best results were obtained using SURF with a hit rate of 94.88%, which proves the interest of this approach for semen quality control according to veterinarian community.

ACKNOWLEDGEMENTS

This work has been supported by grants DPI2009-08424 and PR2009-0280 from the Spanish Government.

The authors would like to thank CENTROTEC for providing the semen samples and for their collaboration in the images acquisition.

REFERENCES

[1] Alegre, E., Biehl, M., Petkov, N. and Sánchez, L. (2008). "Automatic classification of the acrosome status of boar spermatozoa using digital image processing and LVQ", Comput. Biol. Med., vol. 38, no. 4, Elmsford, NY, USA, Pergamon Press, Inc., pp. 461–468.

[2] Bay, H., Ess, A., Tuytelaars, T. and Van Gool, L. (2008). "Speeded-Up Robust Features (SURF) ", Comput. Vis. Image Underst., 110 (3), pp. 346–359.

[3] Didion, B. (2008). "Computer-assisted semen analysis and its utility for profiling boar semen samples". Theriogenology, in Proceedings of the VIth International Conference on Boar Semen Preservation, 70(8), 1374–1376.

[4] González, M., Alegre, E., Aláiz-Rodráguez, R. and Sánchez, L. (2008). "Acrosome integrity classification of boar spermatozoon images using DWT and texture descriptors", Computational Vision and Medical Imaging Processing, pp. 165–168.

[5] González-Castro, V., Alegre, E., Morala-Argáello, P. and Suarez, S.A., (2009) "A combined and intelligent new segmentation method for boar semen based on thresholding and watershed transform", International Journal of Imaging 2 (S09), pp. 70–80.

[6] Harris, C. and Stephens, M. (1988). "A combined corner and edge detector", Fourth Alvey Vision Conference, Manchester, UK, pp. 147–151.

[7] Laws, K. (1979). "Texture energy measures" In Image Understanding Workshop, DARPA.

[8] Liao, S. and Pawlak, M. (1997). "Image analysis with Zernike moment descriptors". Electrical and Computer Engineering. IEEE 1997 Canadian Conference on., 2, pp. 700–703.

[9] Lowe, D. (2004). "Distinctive image features from scale-invariant keypoints", International Journal of Computer Vision, 2(60), pp. 91–110.

[10] Moravec, H. (1981). "Rover visual obstacle avoidance", International Joint Conference on Artificial Intelligence, Vancouver, Canada, pp. 785–790.

[11] Perner, P., Perner, H. and Muller, B. (2002). "Texture classification based on the boolean model and its application to hep-2 cells", Proc. 16th International Conference on Pattern Recognition, 2, pp. 406–409.

[12] Sanchez, L., Petkov, N. and Alegre, E. (2006). "Statistical approach to boar semen evaluation using intracellular intensity distribution of head images", Cellular and Molecular Biology, 52 (6), pp. 38–43.

[13] Shu, H., Luo, L., Bao, X. and Yu, X. (2000). "An efficient method for computation of legendre moments". Graphical Models, 62, pp. 237–262.

[14] Suárez, S.A., Alegre, E. Casteján-Limas, M. and Sánchez, L. (2008). "Use of statistic texture descriptors to classify boar sperm images applying discriminant analysis", Computational Vision and Medical Imaging Processing, pp. 197–201.

Computational Vision and Medical Image Processing – Tavares & Natal Jorge (eds)
© *2012 Taylor & Francis Group, London, ISBN 978-0-415-68395-1*

Analysis of mixing of a clothoid based passive micromixer: A numerical study

F. Pennella, S. Ripandelli, L. Ridolfi, F. Mastrangelo, M.A. Deriu, F.M. Montevecchi & U. Morbiducci
Politecnico di Torino, Turin, Italy

M. Rasponi
Politecnico di Milano, Milan, Italy

M. Rossi & C.J. Kähler
Institut für Strömungsmechanik und Aerodynamik LRT-7, Universität der Bundeswehr München, Deutschland

ABSTRACT: A computational study of a novel passive micromixer is presented. In this work, we analysed a Clo-plus micromixer designed to achieve efficient mixing and characterized by a process of construction that can use a single planar soft lithography step. Mixing studies were carried out at different Reynolds numbers ranging from 1 to 100. The preliminary results suggest that at Re> 50, the Clo-plus micromixer is characterized by a good mixing because of stronger Dean secondary flow and recirculation effect.

1 INTRODUCTION

Mixing in micromixers is crucial in optimizing biochemical reactions but, even though most mixing techniques have been built up, mixing in microfluidic system continues to be an important challenge. Microfluidic systems are characterized mostly by laminar flow and cannot take advantage of turbulence. In the absence of turbulence mixing support, the design of microchannels becomes important. In literature, micromixers are classified as either active or passive. Active micromixers make use of external power sources to enhance mixing, such as external variable-frequency pumping (Niu et al., 2003) or ultra-sound agitation (Yang et al., 2001).

On the contrary, passive micromixers take advantage of geometric characteristic of the microchannel, in fact several geometries have been proposed to induce mixing, e.g., microchannel with grooves (Stroock et al., 2002). In planar micromixers, other examples are curved microchannels. In the curved microchannel, Dean vortices enhance fluid convective mixing due to the centrifugal forces. In literature, there are zigzag microchannels (Mengeaud et al., 2002), spiral (Sudarsan et al., 2006) and rhombic microchannels (Chung et al., 2007) which take advantage of Dean vortices. In this work, the Clo-plus microchannel mixer was analysed and its mixing efficiency was evaluated.

In particular, 3D numerical simulations were used to understand vortice phenomena and fluid mixing mechanism.

2 MATERIALS AND METHODS

2.1 *Micromixer design*

Figure 1 shows the proposed Clo-plus micromixer.

The micromixer is characterized by three inlets, four units and the channel outlet. Widths of the

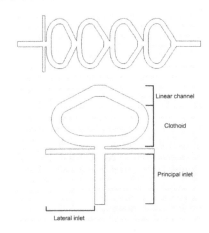

Figure 1. Clo-plus geometry used in this study.

principal-inlet and lateral-inlet are fixed at 200 and 100 μm, respectively. The width of the unit channel is 200 μm. The length of the unit cell is fixed at 1 mm. Channel depth in this design is fixed at 75 μm. Each unit is characterized by two clothoid channels and two straight channels. In the clothoid channel, the curvature increases linearly with the curvilinear coordinate, then, when a costant Reynolds number is applied, the Dean number increases with the curvature. In fact, the dimensionless Dean number Dn is proportional to curvature k

$$Dn = \frac{uD}{\upsilon}\sqrt{\frac{D}{R}} = \text{Re } \sqrt{kD}$$

where Re is diameter based Reynolds number, D is the hydraulic diameter, u the average velocity, υ the fluid kinematic viscosity, k the duct curvature. Dean (Dean 1928) demonstrated that the flow in a curved channel undergoes secondary flow formation when Dn number exceeds a threshold of about 36: in particular, the flow undergoes a progressive centrifugal displacement of the maximal axial velocity, leading to the onset of vortices because of the unbalance of the centrifugal force and radial gradient of static pressure.

2.2 Numerical simulation

In this work, the incompressible Navier–Stokes equation and a convection–diffusion equation for a concentration field using the commercial solver Fluent 6.2 (ANSYS Inc) are solved. Two kinds of species flow into the microchannels through the main inlet and side-inlets. The main inlet is for water and the other two side inlets are for water with dye rhodamine-b. In this research, the values of the ρ and υ are 998 kg m^{-3} and 0.001003 kg m^{-1} s^{-1}. Diffusion coefficient of the rhodamine-b is 4E-10 m^2 s^{-1}. Fluid was assumed steady-state and incompressible. No-slip boundary condition was imposed at the wall. Body force is negligible and is not accounted in the simulation. Boundary conditions of constant flow velocities and fixed pressure were assigned at the inlets and outlet of the micromixer. The molar concentration of two fluid species was set as 0 and 1, respectively. Uniform mixing was achieved as the molar intensity of two species reached the value of 0.5. Simulations were performed to calculate the velocity field at 13 different Re (range 1–100). 3D micromixer model is constructed by GAMBIT. Total number of grid cells is around 2722794 cells.

2.3 Metrics

In order to quantify the degree of mixing, the mixing efficiency (ME) can be calculated by the expression

$$ME = 1 - \sqrt{\frac{1}{N}\sum_{i=1}^{N}\left(\frac{c_i - c}{c}\right)^2}$$

where N is the number of points where the flow field has been numerically solved, c_i is the mole fraction of solute in the ith point, and c is the average mole fraction of solute (Chung et al., 2007).

3 RESULTS AND DISCUSSION

Flow field and mixing process of the micromixer are investigated by 3D numerical simulations at different Reynolds numbers (Re).

Figure 2 shows mixing efficiency of the Clo-plus micromixer at different Reynolds numbers in correspondence of three section-planes.

It can be noticed that level of mixing does not increase regularly with Reynolds number, even though it grows in function of distance that flows cover along the microchannel.

In accord with our expectation, ME grows significantly from the first section to the exit one. It is important to observe the role played by mixing cell in function of the Reynolds number. When the flow does not cross the first mixing-cell the value of ME remain stable and does not modify itself even though Reynolds number become greater. On the other hand when the flow crosses the first two mixing-cells, the value of mixing efficiency increases. At Re > 20, the effect of Dean vortices influences the fluid mixing.

Mixing efficiency is approximately 40% at Re = 20, whereas, at Re = 100, becomes over 80%. It can be noticed that both for the Plane B and Plane C there is a peak at Re = 75. This is an

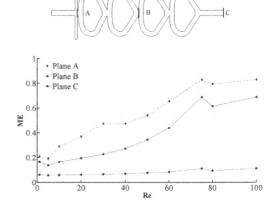

Figure 2. Mixing efficiency plot at different Re numbers.

important feature for our micromixer. In fact, this characteristic can offer the possibility to work with gradient of velocity and pressure lower than those obtained working with Re = 100 obtaining the same value of ME. Finally, it is possible to observe at Re = 5 that ME has the lower value in Plane B and Plane C. This result is interesting but not new, in fact in others work other researchers observed the same results employing geometry more different from clothoidic one. In fact, whereas at Re = 1 mixing is dominated by molecular diffusion and at Re > 10 there is the influence of convective phenomena, at Re = 5 there exists a sort of equilibrium between convective phenomena and diffusion ones.

Figure 3(a-b) shows the cross-sectional concentration distributions of the first Clo-plus microchannels cell at Re = 10 and Re = 100, respectively. At Re = 10, the level of mixing is very low and the interfaces between two species are slightly distorted: this result can be observed seeing sections plotted along the channel that show the level of concentration. At Re = 100, the results obtained are very different (Figure 3-b): it is possible to observe the sections plotted that show the

level of mixing reached and it can be noticed that interface between two species are much distorted by the stronger centrifugal forces. As fluid flow passes through the clothoid channels, one pair of the counter-rotating Dean vortices will be created to disturb the fluid. The centrifugal force pushes the outer fluid toward the inside of the micromixer and the inner fluid toward the upper and lower walls of microchannel. This continuous bending channel can enhance mixing.

Figure 4 shows concentration distribution of the exit section for different Reynolds numbers from 1 to 100. It can be noticed that up to Re = 60 the interface distortion increases due to the clothoid-based structure of the cell that induces stretching. After Re = 60, it is impossible to distinguish the interface because there is homogeneous concentration distribution with a value of the mole concentration equal to 0.5.

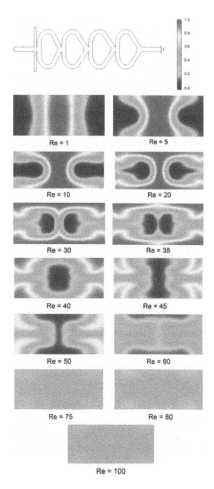

Figure 4. Concentration distribution of the exit at different Re.

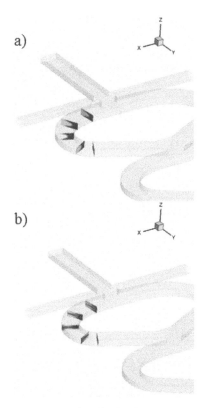

Figure 3. Concentration distribution at Re = 10 (a) and Re = 100 (b).

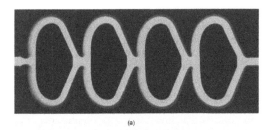

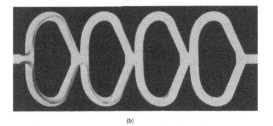

Figure 5. Mixing evaluated in laboratory for Re = 10 (a) and Re = 100 (b) the clearer blue represents the dye rhodamine-b.

Figure 5 (a-b) shows two images of clotho-plus micromixer working at Re = 10 (a) and Re = 100 (b). The clearer fluid is normal water with a chemical dye sensible to the light, while pure water is represented with a dark blue. When the channel is completely coloured by clearer fluid mean that an higher level of mixing is reached. The analysis proposed in figure 5 proves that results obtained from numerical simulation are useful for a preliminary study: for higher value of Reynolds number, higher ME is reached, while for lower ones the two fluids remain separated.

According to the results of the numerical simulations, this Clo-plus microchannel shows a good mixing efficiency computationally and experimentally. Because of enhancement by vortices, over 80% mixing efficiency can be achieved at Re > 75.

REFERENCES

Chung, C.K. & Shih, T.R. 2007. A rhombic micro-mixer with asymmetrical flow for enhancing mixing. In Journal of Micromechanics and Microengineering 17: 2495–2504.

Dean, W.R. 1928. The stream-line motion of fluid in a curved duct. In Philos. Mag. 5: 673–695.

Mengeaud, V. et al. 2002. Mixing processes in a zigzag microchannel: finite element simulations and optical study. Analytical Chemistry; 74: 4279–4286.

Niu, X. & Lee, Y. 2003. Efficient Spatial-Temporal Chaotic Mixing in Microchannels. In J. Micromech. Microeng., 13, 454.

Stroock, A.D. et al. 2002. Chaotic mixer for microchannels. In Science 295: 647–650.

Sudarsan, A.P. & Ugaz, V.M. 2006. Fluid mixing in planar spiral microchannels. In Lab on chip 6: 74–82.

Yang, Z., Matsumoto, S., Goto, H., Matsumoto, M. & Maeda, R. 2001. Ultrasonic Micromixer for Microfluidic Systems. Sensors and Actuators, A93, 266.

Computational Vision and Medical Image Processing – Tavares & Natal Jorge (eds)
© 2012 Taylor & Francis Group, London, ISBN 978-0-415-68395-1

Flow visualization of trace particles and Red Blood Cells in a microchannel with a diverging and converging bifurcation

V. Leble & C. Fernandes
ESTiG, IPB, C. Sta. Apolonia, Braganca, Portugal

R. Dias & R. Lima
ESTiG, IPB, C. Sta. Apolonia, Braganca, Portugal
CEFT, FEUP, R. Dr. Roberto Frias, Porto, Portugal

T. Ishikawa & Y. Imai
Department of Bioengineering & Robotics, Grad. School Engineering, Tohoku University, Aoba, Sendai, Japan

T. Yamaguchi
Department of Biomedical Engineering, Grad. School Engineering, Tohoku University, Aoba, Sendai, Japan

ABSTRACT: This paper aims to investigate the effect of both diverging and converging bifurcations on the flow behaviour of Pure Water (PW) and Red Blood Cells (RBCs). A confocal micro-PTV system is used to visualize and measure the flow characteristics of the working fluids. The results show no formation of a Cell-Free Layer (CFL) around the apex of the bifurcation. In contrast, there is a clear formation of a triangular CFL just downstream of the confluence apex. As a result, this triangular CFL seems to play an important role on the in vitro blood flow characteristics at this region.

1 INTRODUCTION

Blood flow behaviour in both *in vivo* and *in vitro* environments has been investigated for several years [1–4]. However, studies performed by Suzuki et al. [3] and Pries, et al. [4] have found conflicting results between *in vivo* and *in vitro* experiments with respect to the blood rheological properties. Potential causes for the observed *in vivo/in vitro* discrepancies are the effect of the endothelial surface layer, the presence of white blood cells and the complex microvascular networks composed by diverging and converging bifurcations [2]. In order to better understand the observed discrepancies we need to investigate in more detail the effect of both diverging and converging bifurcations on the rheological properties of blood. Therefore, the aims of the present paper is to visualize and measure the flow characteristics of both trace particles suspended in pure water and *in vitro* blood in a diverging and converging bifurcation. The experimental flow visualizations and measurements will be performed by means of a confocal system combined by image analysis techniques from ImageJ.

2 MATERIALS AND METHODS

2.1 Working fluids and microchannel geometry

Two working fluids were used in this study: pure water (PW) with fluorescent trace particles of 1 μm and Dextran 40 (Dx-40) containing about 14% (14Hct) of human RBCs. The washed RBCs were fluorescently labelled with a lipophilic carbocyanine derivative dye, chloromethylbenzamido (CM-Dil, Molecular Probes), using a previously described procedure [5].

The polydimethylsiloxane (PDMS) microchannels used in this study were fabricated using a soft lithography technique [6] and consist of a diverging bifurcation and converging bifurcation (also known as confluence). Fig. 1 shows the dimensions of both diverging and converging bifurcations used in the present study.

2.2 Experimental set-up

The confocal micro-PTV system used consists of an inverted microscope combined with a confocal scanning and a diode-pumped solid state (DPSS)

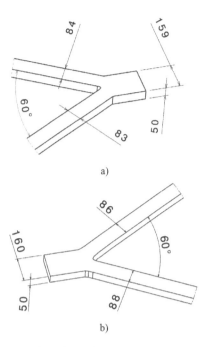

Figure 1. Dimensions of the a) diverging and b) converging bifurcation used in this study. The channel dimensions are in μm.

laser with an excitation wavelength of 532 nm and a high-speed camera. The PDMS microchannel was placed on the microscope stage with a surrounding temperature of about 37°C. By using a syringe pump the flow rate of the working fluids could be controlled by adjusting the injection speed. The flow rates were kept constant and approximately the same for both fluids. Hence, the Reynolds number (Re) used for PW and *in vitro* blood was Re ≈ 0.04 and Re ≈ 0.008, respectively. For the Re used in this study, the flow of PW inside the microchannel can be assumed as a steady, laminar flow of a Newtonian, incompressible fluid (Stokes flow). Therefore, change in the flow rate of PW to achieve the Re of *in vitro* blood will not influence the trajectories of trace particles. Thus, the comparison of trajectories of both fluids is applicable. More detailed information about the experimental set-up, microchannel fabrication and RBC labelling used in this study can be found elsewhere [1, 5, 6].

2.3 *Image analysis*

All the confocal images were recorded around the middle of the PDMS microchannel with a resolution of 640 × 480 pixels, at a rate of 100 frames/s. The recorded images were transferred to the computer and then evaluated in the image processing program ImageJ (NIH) [7] by using the manual tracking MtrackJ plugin [8] and automatic ParticleTracker 2D plugin [9] to track the trace particles in PW and RBCs in D × 40, respectively.

3 RESULTS AND DISCUSSION

In this section we present the flow visualizations results and investigate the effect of both diverging and converging bifurcation on the trace particles in PW (see Figs. 2a and 3a) and on labelled RBCs (see Figs. 2b and 3b).

For the case of trace particles in PW (Figs. 2a and 3a) we observed that the trajectories were almost symmetric and do not present so many fluctuations for both geometries. These results are consistent with the Stokes flow regime. In contrast, for the case of labelled RBCs the trajectories are more asymmetric when compared with PW trajectories. Additionally, we can also observe several fluctuations on their trajectories.

From Fig. 3a we also observed that the trace particles tend to flow very close to the inner walls

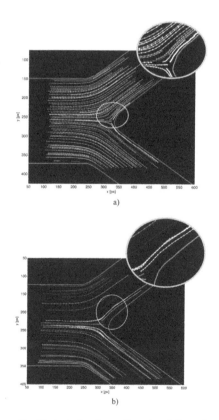

Figure 2. Trajectories in a diverging bifurcation of a) fluorescent particles in PW and b) labelled RBCs in D × 40.

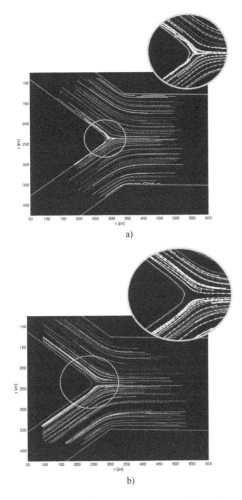

a)

b)

Figure 3. Trajectories in a converging bifurcation of a) fluorescent particles in PW and b) labelled RBCs in D × 40.

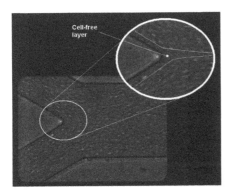

Figure 4. a) Original image of *in vitro* blood showing the triangular CFL formed in the region just downstream of the confluence apex.

and as a result they tend to flow in the centre of the microchannel, just downstream of the confluence apex. However, for the case of labelled RBCs we could not measure any trajectory passing in this centre region (see Fig. 3b). This is due to the existence of a cell-free layer (CFL) in both inner walls and a consequent formation of a triangular CFL in the region of the confluence apex (see Fig. 4). As this triangular CFL seems to play an important role on the *in vitro* blood flow characteristics, a detailed quantitative study, to clarify the CFL effect in the velocity profiles, is currently under way.

ACKOWLEDGEMENTS

The authors acknowledge the financial support provided by: PTDC/SAU-BEB/108728/2008, PTDC/SAU-BEB/105650/2008 and PTDC/EME-MFE/099109/2008 from the FCT (Science and Technology Foundation) and COMPETE, Portugal.

REFERENCES

[1] Lima, R., Ishikawa, T., Imai, Y., Takeda, M., Wada, S. & Yamaguchi, T. Radial dispersion of red blood cells in blood flowing through glass capillaries: role of haematocrit and geometry. *Journal of Biomechanics* **41**, 2188–2196, 2008.

[2] Maeda, N. Erythrocyte rheology in microcirculation. *Japanese Journal of Physiology* **46**, 1–14, 1996.

[3] Suzuki, Y., Tateishi, N., Soutani, M. and Maeda, N. Deformation of erythrocytes in microvessels and glass capillaries: effects of erythrocyte deformability. *Microcirculation* **3**, 49–57, 1996.

[4] Pries, A., Secomb, T., et al, Resistance to blood flow in microvessels in vivo. *Circulation Research* **75**, 904–915, 1994.

[5] Lima, R., Ishikawa, T., Imai, Y., Takeda, M., Wada, S. and Yamaguchi, T. Measurement of individual red blood cell motions under high hematocrit conditions using a confocal micro-PTV system. *Annals of Biomedical Engineering*, **37**, 1546–59, 2009.

[6] Lima, R., Fernandes, C.S. et al., "Microscale flow dynamics of red blood cells in microchannels: an experimental and numerical analysis", In: Tavares and Jorge (Eds), Computational Vision and Medical Image Processing: Recent Trends, Springer, **19**, 297–309, 2011.

[7] Abramoff, M., Magelhaes, P. and Ram, S. Image Processing with ImageJ. *Biophotonics International* **7**, 11, 36–42, 2004.

[8] Meijering, E., Smal, I. and Danuser, G. "Tracking in Molecular Bioimaging". *IEEE Signal Processing Magazine*. **3**, 23, 46–53, 2006.

[9] Sbalzarini, I.F. and Koumoutsakos, P. Feature Point Tracking and Trajectory Analysis for Video Imaging in Cell Biology, Journal of Structural Biology 151(2): 182–195, 2005.

Computational Vision and Medical Image Processing – Tavares & Natal Jorge (eds)
© 2012 Taylor & Francis Group, London, ISBN 978-0-415-68395-1

Does fluid shear stress represent the degree of a Red Blood Cell deformation?

M. Nakamura
Department of Mechanical Engineering, Saitama University, Japan

S. Wada
Department of Mechanical Engineering and Bioengineering, Osaka University, Japan

ABSTRACT: Deformation of a Red Blood Cell (RBC) in a high-shear flow was numerically investigated. The simulation of RBC in a parallel shear flow showed that the maximum strain of the RBC membrane increased monotonically with an increase in fluid shear. In contrast, in a complex flow, no consistency was found between the maximum of the area strain and a hemolysis index. Those results addressed the importance of considering an RBC deformation for accurately predicting hemolysis.

1 INTRODUCTION

A Red Blood Cell (RBC) is elastic and deforms into various shapes by undergoing fluid forces while flowing. Upon excessive deformation, an RBC is damaged and hemolysis, the breaking open of RBC, can occur. Plasma free hemoglobin released by the destruction of RBC represents severe pathological conditions in vital organ systems including esophageal spasm, abdominal pain, erectile dysfunction and even thrombosis (Rother et al. 2005).

Extensive efforts have been made to establish the way of estimating hemolysis from a flow field of interest (Bludszuweit, 1995). Although a good correlation was reported between the proposed hemolysis index and the amount of hemoglobin in a simple flow condition, the index is practically useless as flow becomes more complex (Wurzinger et al. 1986)

In this study, we investigated the deformation of an RBC in simple and complex flows to demonstrate that a conventional hemolysis index does not reflect RBC deformation in a complex flow.

2 METHODS

2.1 *Modeling of RBC membrane*

The RBC has no nucleus and thus its mechanical nature is mostly concerned with that of the membrane. The RBC membrane consists of a lipid bilayer and its underlying structure of cytoskeleton, called spectrin. The spectrin is anchored firmly to the membrane via various trans-membrane proteins, which results in a high resistance against shear (in-plane) deformation. In contrast, the lipid bilayer is highly fluidic and thus relatively less contributive to the shear deformation. In addition, as both lipid bilayer and spectrin networks have thickness, they exhibit resistance to bending.

A spring network model was adopted to express those mechanical natures of the RBC membrane (Wada and Kobayashi, 2003). As shown in Figure 1 (a), the RBC is firstly expressed as a sphere with the diameter of 6.5 μm. Figure 1 (b) magnifies the RBC membrane, showing that neighboring meshes are connected with bending springs while nodal points at the vertex of a mesh are linked by a stretching spring.

Deformation of the membrane results in an increase of elastic energies. We modeled the stretching energy W_s as

$$W_s = \frac{1}{2}k_s\sum_{l=1}^{N_s}\left(L_l - L_{l0}\right)^2 \tag{1}$$

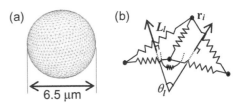

Figure 1. (a) RBC model and (b) a mechanical model of RBC membrane.

where k_s is a spring constant for stretching, N_s is the number of stretching springs, L_{l0}, L_l are length of spring at the natural state and after deformation. Similarly, the bending energy W_b is modeled as

$$W_b = \frac{1}{2} k_b \sum_{l=1}^{N_b} L_l \tan^2\left(\frac{\theta_l}{2}\right) \quad (2)$$

where k_b is a spring constant for bending, N_b is the number of bending springs and θ_l is the contact angle between neighboring elements.

The RBC membrane resists its area change because the total number of lipid molecules in the RBC membrane is constant. Here, we considered area changes of both the whole membrane and each element of the membrane. The former represent the situation where lipid molecules can move freely over the cytoskeletal membrane, while the latter does the situation where movement of lipid molecules is confined to a local element. We express the elastic energy due to an area change as

$$W_A = \frac{1}{2} k_A \left(\frac{A - A_0}{A_0}\right)^2 A_0 + \frac{1}{2} k_a \sum_{e=1}^{N_e} \left(\frac{A_e - A_{e0}}{A_{e0}}\right)^2 A_{e0} \quad (3)$$

where A is the total area of RBC membrane, A_e is the area of each element, subscript 0 denotes the natural state, N_e is the number of elements consisting of RBC membrane and k_A and k_a are coefficients for global and local area constraint.

To assure incompressibility of the RBC, we need to introduce an energy-like function for the volume V

$$W_V = \frac{1}{2} k_V \left(\frac{V - V_0}{V_0}\right)^2 V_0 \quad (4)$$

where V_0 is a desired volume. By vector analyses, energies (1)–(4) can be written as a function of the positional vector of nodes $\mathbf{r}_i$. Therefore, the problem of determining the RBC shape is equivalent to calculating positional vectors of nodes which minimizes the total elastic energy $W = W_s + W_b + W_A + W_V$ with respect to $\mathbf{r}_i$.

2.2 Modeling of fluid forces

Fluid forces $\mathbf{F}^F$ act on a RBC externally from plasma and internally from hemoglobin due to a difference in the velocity between a RBC and fluid flow. For simplicity, we here assume that a RBC does not affect flow and implement one-way coupling for flow-RBC where flow is pre-defined.

From Newton's viscosity law and conservation of the fluid momentum, tangential $\mathbf{f}_{e,t}^{out}$ and normal

$\mathbf{f}_{e,n}^{out}$ components of the external forces working on element e are modeled as

$$\mathbf{f}_{e,n}^{out} = \rho Q \Delta \mathbf{u}_n^e, \quad (5)$$

$$\mathbf{f}_{e,t}^{out} = \mu_{out} A_e \Delta \mathbf{u}_t^e / \delta \quad (6)$$

where $\Delta \mathbf{u}^e$ is the velocity difference between external fluid and element e, ρ is the density of external fluid, Q is flow rate passing through element e, μ_{out} is the viscosity of external fluid. δ is equivalent boundary layer thickness which is estimated as $\delta = 4a/9$ based on Stoke's theory. The internal force $\mathbf{f}^{in}$ was modeled in a similar way to $\mathbf{f}^{out}$.

2.3 Modeling of the interaction with the wall

As a RBC comes closer to the wall, a fluid pressure between the RBC and the wall elevates. We here use a potential function to represent this pressure elevation, given by

$$\Psi_i = k_n \left(\pi y_i / 2 - \tan\left(\pi y_i / 2\right)\right) \quad (0 < d_i < \delta) \quad (7)$$

where $y_i = (d_i - \delta)/\delta$ and d_i is the distance between node i on the RBC and the wall. This potential function works only when the RBC falls below distance δ from the wall.

2.4 Solving method

The behavior of a RBC was calculated by solving the motion equation of each node. For node i, it is given by

$$m\ddot{\mathbf{r}}_i = \mathbf{F}_i^E + \mathbf{F}_i^F + \mathbf{F}_i^R \quad (8)$$

where m is a mass, a dot means a time derivative, $\mathbf{F}^E$ is an elastic force of the membrane, $\mathbf{F}^F$ is a fluid force and $\mathbf{F}^R$ is a repulsive force from the wall. According to the virtual work principle, $\mathbf{F}^E$ and $\mathbf{F}^R$ working on node i are gained by

$$\mathbf{F}_i^E = -\frac{\partial W}{\partial \mathbf{r}_i} \quad (9)$$

and

$$\mathbf{F}_i^R = -\frac{\partial \Psi_i}{\partial \mathbf{r}_i} \quad (10)$$

2.5 Parameters

Constants are basically determined from experimental data (see Wada and Kobayashi, 2003). Used values are: $k_A = 4500 \ \mu N/m$, $k_a = 500 \ \mu N/m$,

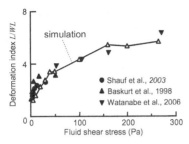

Figure 2. Relationship between shear stress and L/W in steady Couette flow.

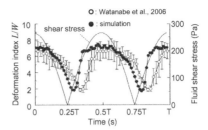

Figure 3. Relationship between shear stress and L/W in unsteady Couette flow.

$k_V = 5 \cdot 10^7$ μN/m², $k_b = 1 \cdot 10^{-4}$ μN, $a = 3.3$ μm, $\mu_{out} = 0.003$ Pa·s, $\mu_{in} = 0.005$ Pa·s. To express an increase in stretching resistance with elongation of spectrin, a spring constant k_s is defined as a function of stretching ratio λ;

$$k_s = k_{s0} \exp\{\alpha(\lambda - \beta)\} \qquad (11)$$

where α and β are constants. In this study, they were set by trial and error to achieve satisfactory match between the simulation and the experiments (Baskurt et al. 1998, Shauf et al. 2003, Watanabe et al. 2006). As presented in Figure 2, the simulation results were well congruent with the experimental data when constants in eq. (11) were set as $\alpha = 2.5$, $\beta = 1$.

3 RESULTS

3.1 Basic behaviour of the RBC model

The RBC model was put in the steady Couette flow which gives a constant shear γ in the space between two parallel plates. The motion of the RBC varied depending on the magnitude of shear; it tank-treaded, tumbled or did both. The tumbling occurred at low shear roughly smaller than 20 s⁻¹. As the shear rate γ elevated, the RBC started to show tank-treading of the membrane. A transition from tank-treading to tumbling occurs at the shear rate of 20–40 s⁻¹.

The RBC in a cyclically reversing unsteady Couette flow at 5 Hz was also investigated. Figure 3 plots temporal variations of fluid shear stress and L/W. As seen, the simulation results of deformation index L/W was consistent with experimental results (Watanabe et al. 2006).

3.2 Deformation of the RBC in Couette flows

The maximum of the first principal strain over the RBC membrane for various fluid shears was plotted against the fluid shear stress of Couette flow in Figure 4. As seen, the maximum of area strain of the RBC membrane increased monotonically with an increase in fluid shear stress.

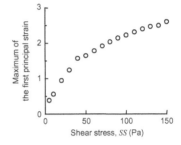

Figure 4. Relationship between shear stress and L/W in unsteady Couette flow.

3.3 Deformation of the RBC in bifurcation flows

The RBC behavior in bifurcation flow was simulated. A distance from the inlet to the apex of bifurcation is 230 μm. The flow channel bifurcates symmetrically at the angle of 45 degrees. The bifurcation apex is described by an arc with a radius of 23 μm. Velocity in the flow channel was obtained by numerically solving Navier-Stokes and continuity equations with STAR-CD (CD-Adapco, Japan). A fully-developed flow with a mean velocity of 1 m/s was applied at the inlet.

Given the flow, we calculated the behavior of a RBC which was initially placed near the center of the inlet. Figure 5 presents the snapshots of RBC (a) at the inlet, (b) in the entrance (c) in the bifurcation and (d) on the wall. Color represents the area strain of the membrane. As seen, in the entrance, the RBC exhibited a spindle shape. As it came closer to the wall, the head portion of RBC started to collapse. Upon striking on the wall, the RBC deformed significantly with demonstrating a locally high area strain (1.81 at maximum). The shape of RBC when impinging on the wall was similar to the one observed in experiments (Yagi et al. 2009).

The maximum of the area strain over the membrane at each time instant was plotted against SS in Figure 6. SS is an index that scalarizes a fluid shear stress tensor at the point of interest, and

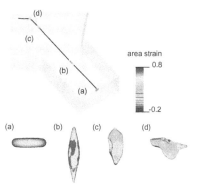

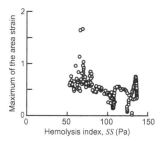

Figure 5. Snapshots of RBCs with the contour plot of the area strain in bifurcation flow.

Figure 6. Plot of the maximum area strain against hemolysis index SS in the bifurcation flow.

fluid-mechanically equivalent to the fluid shear stress plotted as the value of x-axis of Fig. 1. This index has been conventionally used for evaluating hemolysis (Bludszuweit, 1995). As seen in Fig. 3, there was no consistent tendency between the maximum of area strain and SS.

4 DISCUSSION

Quantitative evaluation of hemolysis is essential in de-signing artificial organs. Although the maximum principal strain is well correlated with the fluid shear stress in the simple flow as presented in Fig. 4, their relation becomes chaotic in the complex flow as in Fig. 6. This is attributable to a fact that the RBC appeared to behave as a visco-elastic material in which the shape was determined not only fluid force acting on it at that moment but also its deformation history. In other words, it is basically impossible to estimate the mechanical state of RBC membrane solely from fluid mechanical data of the macroscopic flow field. This would be the reason why conventional hemolysis indices have limitations in their accuracy. For amelioration of the predictive accuracy, it is requisite to take into account deformation of individual RBCs in a flow field.

The simulation conditions of bifurcation flow were almost the same as Yagi et al. (2009). who observed that the RBC leaked protoplasm upon the impingement on the wall in *in vitro* experiments. According to molecular dynamics simulations (Koshiyama et al. 2011), when the lipid bilayer is stretched at strain of 1.4~1.6, spatial distributions of the lipid molecules are unbalanced and thereby a pore which penetrates the lipid bilayer is formed. This suggests that hemolysis can occur at the strain larger than 1.5. As described, our simulation showed that the area strain reached 1.8 upon the impingement on the wall. This implies that the leakage of protoplasm observed by Yagi et al. (2009) would be attributable to a local stretch of the RBC membrane. These results suggest that hemolysis could be estimated by evaluating the area strain of RBC membrane.

5 CONCLUSION

In conclusion, the results address the necessity to consider RBCs deformations for better evaluation of hemolysis. The present model would be useful to establish the hemolysis simulator based on the analysis of RBC deformations.

REFERENCES

Baskurt, O., Gelmont, D., Meiselman, H. 1998 Red blood cell deformability in sepsis. *Am. J. Respir. Crit. Care Med.*, 157: 421–427.
Bludszuweit, C. 1995 Three-dimensional numerical prediction of stress loading of blood particles in a centrifugal pump. *Artif. Organs*, 19: 590–596.
Koshiyama, K. & Wada, S. 2011. Molecular dynamics simulations of pore formation dynamics during the rupture process of a phospholipid bilayer caused by high-speed equibiaxial stretching. *J. Biomech.* (in press)
Rother, R.P., Bell, L., Hillmen, P. et al. 2005 The clinical sequelae of intravascular hemolysis and extracellular plasma hemoglobin: a novel mechanism of human disease. *JAMA*, 293: 1653–1662.
Schauf, B., Aydeniz, B., Bayer, R. et al. 2003 The laser diffractoscope – a new and fast system to analyse red blood cell flexibility with high accuracy. *Lasers Med. Sci.*, 18: 45–50.
Wada, S., Kobayashi, R. 2003. Numerical simulation of various shape changes of a swollen red blood cell by decrease of its volume. *J. Soc. Mech. Eng. Trans. A*, 69: 14–21 (in Japanese).
Watanabe, N., Kataoka, H., Yasuda, T. et al. 2006 Dynamic deformation and recovery response of a red blood cell to cyclically reversing shear flow: effects of frequency of cyclically reversing shear flow and shear stress level. *Biophys. J.* 91: 1984–1998.
Wurzinger, L., Opitz, R., Eckstein, H. 1986 Mechanical blood trauma – an overview. *Angeiologie*, 19: 81–87.
Yagi, T., Wakasa, S., Tokunaga, N. et al. 2009 Single-cell real-time imaging of flow-induced hemolysis using high-speed microfluidic technology. *Proc. 11th international congress of the IUPESM*, in CD.

Computational Vision and Medical Image Processing – Tavares & Natal Jorge (eds)
© *2012 Taylor & Francis Group, London, ISBN 978-0-415-68395-1*

Flow of Red Blood Cells through a microfluidic extensional device: An image analysis assessment

T. Yaginuma, A.I. Pereira & P.J. Rodrigues
ESTiG, IPB, C. Sta. Apolonia, Bragança, Portugal

R. Lima
ESTiG, IPB, C. Sta. Apolonia, Bragança, Portugal
CEFT, FEUP, R. Dr. Roberto Frias, Porto, Portugal

M.S.N. Oliveira
CEFT, FEUP, R. Dr. Roberto Frias, Porto, Portugal

T. Ishikawa
Department of Bioengineering and Robotics, Graduate School of Engineering, Tohoku University, Aoba, Sendai, Japan

T. Yamaguchi
Department of Biomedical Engineering, Graduate School of Engineering, Tohoku University, Aoba, Sendai, Japan

ABSTRACT: The present study aims to assess the deformability of Red Blood Cells (RBCs) under extensionally dominated microfluidic flows using an image based technique. For this purpose, a microchannel having a hyperbolic shaped-contraction was used and the images were captured by a standard high-speed microscopy system. The images acquired display RBCs with various light intensity levels and image analysis was used to quantify the Deformation Index (DI) of the RBCs considering these light intensity differences. Additionally, the velocities of different intensity-level RBCs flowing along the centerline of the channel were measured using particle tracking velocimetry. The preliminary results at two different flow rates reveal a highly deformable nature of RBCs when submitted to strong extensional flows. It was also observed that the low intensity cells exhibit a slightly higher velocity than intermediate intensity cells, which we attribute to the cells being located in different planes.

1 INTRODUCTION

Red Blood Cells (RBCs) are known as a highly deformable blood component that plays an important role in delivering oxygen to the tissues in microcirculation. According to Mokken et al. (1992) the capacity of RBCs to deform is related to three main characteristics: the viscoelastic properties of its membrane; the high surface area-to-volume ratio associated with its biconcave discoid shape; and the viscosity of its intracellular solution. A variation of any of these factors can have a significant impact on RBC deformability leading to serious health consequences. In particular a decrease in RBC deformability can result in impaired perfusion of the peripheral tissues. Furthermore, it has been reported that the elastic characteristics as well as the shape of RBCs are important factors to explain the etiology

of certain pathologies (Mokken et al. 1992). As a consequence, there has been a number of studies on RBC deformability, which use, among others, techniques such as RBC filtration (Gueguen et al. 1984), laser diffraction ellipsometry (Shin et al. 2004) and rheoscopy (Dobbe et al. 2002). Most of these studies focus on the effect of shear flow. However, extensionally-dominated flows are often found in the human circulatory system, namely when there is a change in the cross-sectional area, e.g. in stenoses and in the transition from vessels to catheters (Selby et al. 2003, Fujiwara et al. 2009). In this study, we use an image analysis to characterize the velocity and deformation index of RBCs flowing through microchannels having a hyperbolic shape (Fig. 1). The shape of the channels was chosen so that the fluid at the centerline is submitted to a strong extensional flow and experiences a nearly constant strain rate (Oliveira et al. 2007).

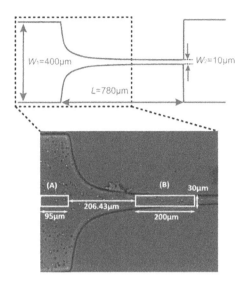

Figure 1. Geometry and dimensions of the PDMS hyperbolic microchannel.

Typically, the images captured by standard microscopy systems using a high speed camera display RBCs with various light intensity levels, but to the best of our knowledge, few studies have considered this difference in the analysis. Therefore, our investigation on RBC behavior is based on an image analysis performed considering the different RBC intensity levels. The results obtained for different flow rates indicate the highly deformable nature of RBCs under strong extensional flows.

2 MATERIALS AND METHODS

2.1 Working fluids and microchannel geometry

The working fluid examined was composed of Dextran 40 (Dx40) containing ~1% of human RBCs (i.e., hematocrit, Hct~1%). The blood used was collected from a healthy adult volunteer, and EDTA (ethylenediaminetetraacetic acid) was added to the collected samples to prevent coagulation. The blood samples were then submitted to washing and centrifuging processes and were then stored hermetically at 4°C until the experiments were performed at a temperature of ~37°C. All procedures were carried out in compliance with the guidelines of the Ethics Committee on Clinical Investigation of Tohoku University.

The microchannels containing the hyperbolic contraction were produced in polydimethylsiloxane (PDMS) using standard soft-lithography techniques from a SU-8 photoresist mold. The molds were prepared in a clean room facility by photo-lithography using a high-resolution chrome mask. The geometry and dimensions of the micro-fabricated channels are shown in Fig. 1. The channel depth, h, was constant throughout the PDMS chip and the width of the upstream and downstream channels was the same, $W_1 = 400$ μm. The minimum width in the contraction region is $W_2 = 10$ μm, defining a total Hencky strain of $\varepsilon_H = \ln(W_1/W_2) = \ln(40)$.

For the microfluidic experiments, the channels were placed on the stage of an inverted microscope (IX71, Olympus, Japan) and the temperature of the stage was adjusted by means of a thermo plate controller (Tokai Hit, Japan) to 37°C. The flow rate of the working fluids was controlled using a syringe pump (KD Scientific Inc., USA), and two different flow rates were examined: 9.45 μL/min and 66.15 μL/min. The images of the flowing RBCs were captured using a high speed camera (Phantom v7.1, Vision Research, USA) and transferred to the computer to be analyzed. An illustration of the experimental set-up is shown in Fig. 2.

2.2 Image analysis

The original data obtained from the experiments are the digital video sequences captured at the frame rate of 4800 frames/s with the exposure time of 2 μs. This corresponds to the frame intervals of 208 μs. For the image analysis, firstly, the captured videos were converted to a sequence of static images (stack), with a resolution of 800 × 600 pixels each.

Then, in order to reduce the dust and static artifacts in the images, an averaged background image was created from the original images and subtracted from the stack. This process eliminates all the static objects from the images including the microchannel walls, which resulted in images having only the flowing RBCs visible. To enhance the image quality, image

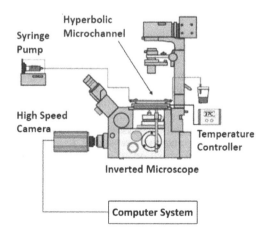

Figure 2. Experimental set-up.

filtering such as *Median* operation with the mask size of 3×3 pixels and *Brightness/Contrast* adjustment was applied using ImageJ (NIH). Finally, the grey scale images were converted to binary images adjusting the threshold level. ImageJ default threshold method based on IsoData method was applied first and then the level was adjusted manually for the optimal binarization. For instance, the ImageJ default threshold set the min. value as 0 and the max. value as 68 automatically for the images of flow rate 9.45 µL/min, but the max. value was slightly raised to 70 manually in order to obtain better binary images to analyze. This means the pixels with intensity levels in the range of 0–70 were set to be 0 (black) and the pixels with intensity levels greater than 70 were set to be 255 (white). This segmentation process yields regions of interest with RBCs as black circular objects (with or without holes inside) against a white background. More details about the intensity levels of the RBCs are described in Section 3.2.

To analyze the deformation index, the cells were measured in two pre-defined regions, (A) and (B) as shown in Fig. 1. Region (A) is located upstream of the hyperbolic contraction and region (B) comprises a narrow part of the contraction region. Both regions are located axially along the centerline of the channel.

The flowing cells selected for measurement in region (A) were tracked and identified in region (B). In other words, the same cells were measured twice, once in region (A) and another in region (B) in order to examine the DI transition of identical cells.

The *Analyze Particles* function in ImageJ (NIH) was used for measuring the cells dimensions. This command counts and measures objects in binary images according to the pre-defined measurement settings (e.g. centroid, width, length, etc.). Some parameters such as *Area* and *Circularity* are useful to ignore out-of-interest objects. In the current work, the area of the objects was limited to 17–50 µm² and the circularity to 0.5–1.0. These settings reasonably ignore the apparent deviant objects such as out-of-focus cells, aggregated cells, and so on.

Finally, the RBC deformation was characterized by the deformation index (DI) as $(A_{Major} - A_{Minor})/(A_{Major} + A_{Minor})$, where A_{Major} and A_{Minor} refer to the major (primary) and minor (secondary) axis lengths of the ellipse best fitted to the cell. These values were obtained by the measurements obtained with *Analyze Particles* operation.

3 RESULTS AND DISCUSSION

3.1 *Deformation index*

Fig. 3 shows RBCs flowing through the PDMS hyperbolic microchannel in original images at

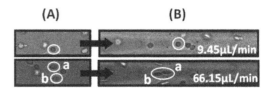

Figure 3. RBC deformation at different flow rates in region A and B.

different flow rates (9.45 µl/min and 66.15 µl/min) and in two pre-defined regions, (A) and (B). In Fig. 4 the average deformation index calculated based on the results of image analysis are shown for each case.

As can be seen in Fig. 4, for both flow rates, DI is higher in the hyperbolic contraction region (B) where the RBCs are submitted to a strong extensional flow. In the contraction region (B), DI increases substantially with the flow rate as a consequence of the higher strain rate to which the RBCs are submitted. These results evidence the highly deformable nature of RBCs under strong extensional flows.

3.2 *Intensity levels*

The images captured by a microscope with a high speed camera display RBCs with various light intensity levels (Fig. 5 (a)). When these are converted to binary images, they appear with rather different shape/size (Fig. 5 (b)). In this study, we distinguished RBCs by three levels of light intensity, corresponding to low (black), intermediate (grey) and high intensity (white), and the average deformation index was calculated for each class of RBCs. However, the results in Fig. 4 show only the low and intermediate intensity levels RBCs, as high intensity level cells were deemed to be out of focus for DI to be accurately determined—the different shape of the white cells can be clearly seen in Fig. 5 (b).

In Fig. 4 it is clear, that despite the shape of the grey cells being slightly more elongated than black cells, the differences are not very significant.

Additionally, we have quantified the flow velocities of the cells considering their intensity level. Fig. 6 presents our preliminary results of the cell flow velocities for the two intensity level groups considered for DI measurements: low intensity cells (black cells) and intermediate intensity cells (grey cells). As expected, the velocity increases as the cells travel through the hyperbolic microchannel at its centerline. Additionally, the velocities of intermediate intensity cells are higher than those of the low intensity cells. This result may be related to the fact that we are using

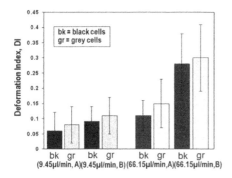

Figure 4. Comparison of deformation index at different flow rates in different regions.

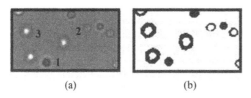

(a)   (b)

Figure 5. (a) Original image containing RBCs with various intensities: 1. low (black), 2. intermediate (grey) and 3. high (white), and (b) Corresponding binary image.

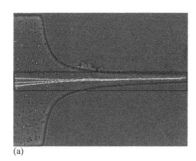

(a)

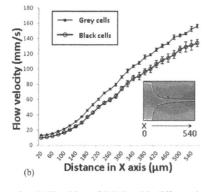

(b)

Figure 6. (a) Tracking of RBCs with different intensity levels for velocity measurements. (b) Axial velocity profiles of the low and intermediate intensity RBCs along the centerline at $Q = 9.45$ μl/min.

volume illumination, in which the depth-of-focus is determined by the characteristics of objective used. As a consequence, despite being centered at the mid-plane of the channel where the cell velocity is the highest, cells at different z-planes are also captured. In this case, we believe that the black cells are not truly located at the mid-plane and therefore its velocity is slightly lower than that of the grey cells. Following these preliminary results, further investigation on the cell velocities and deformation index in various regions of the microchannels under different flow conditions will be performed.

ACKNOWLEDGEMENTS

We thank Dr. Matsuki for help with blood sample collection. Additionally, we acknowledge the financial support provided by 2007 GlobalCOE Program "Global Nano-BME Education and Research Network", Japan. We are also thankful to FCT (Portugal) and COMPETE for financial support through projects PTDC/SAU-BEB/108728/2008, PTDC/SAU-BEB/105650/2008 and PTDC/EME-MFE/099109/2012.

REFERENCES

Abramoff, M., Magelhaes, P., Ram, S., 2004. Image processing with image. J. Biophotonics Int. 11, 36–42.
Dobbe, J.G.G., Hardeman, M.R., Streekstra, G.J., Strackee, J., Ince, C., Grimbergen, C.A., 2002. Analyzing red blood cell-deformability distributions. Blood Cells, Mol. Dis. 28, 373–384.
Fujiwara, H., Ishikawa, T. Lima, R., Matsuki, N., Imai, Y., Kaji, H., Nishizawa, M., Yamaguchi, T., 2009. Red blood cell motions in a high hematocrit blood flowing through a stenosed micro-channel. J. Biomech. 42, 838–843.
Gueguen, M., Bidet, J.M., Durand, F., Driss, F., Joffre, A., Genetet, B., 1984. Filtration pressure and red blood cell deformability: evaluation of a new device: erythrometre. Biorheology Suppl. 1, 261–265.
Mokken, F.Ch., Kedaria, M., Henny, Ch.P., Hardeman. M.R., Gelb, A.W., 1992. The clinical importance of erythrocyte deformability, a hemorrheological parameter, Ann. Hematol. 64, 113–122.
Oliveira, M.S.N., Alves, M.A., Pinho, F.T., McKinley, G.H., 2007. Viscous flow through microfabricated hyperbolic contractions. Exp. Fluids. 43, 437–451.
Shelby, J.P., White, J., Ganesan, K., Rathod, P.K., Chiu, D.T., 2003. A microfluidic model for single-cell capillary obstruction by Plasmodium falciparum-infected erythrocytes. PNAS. 100, 14618–14622.
Shin, S., Ku, Y., Park, M.S., Suh, J.S., 2004. Measurement of red cell deformability and whole blood viscosity using laser-diffraction slit rheometer. Korea-Australia Rheol. J. 16, 85–90.

Computational Vision and Medical Image Processing – Tavares & Natal Jorge (eds)
© 2012 Taylor & Francis Group, London, ISBN 978-0-415-68395-1

An automatic method to track Red Blood Cells in microchannels

D. Pinho
Polytechnic Institute of Bragança, ESTiG/IPB, C. Sta. Apolonia, Bragança, Portugal

F. Gayubo
Fundación CARTIF, División de Robótica y Visión Artificial, Parque Tecnológico de Boecillo, Valladolid, Spain

A. Isabel
Polytechnic Institute of Bragança, ESTiG/IPB, C. Sta. Apolonia, Bragança, Portugal
ALGORITMI, Minho University, Campus de Azurém, Guimarães, Portugal

R. Lima
Polytechnic Institute of Bragança, ESTiG/IPB, C. Sta. Apolonia, Bragança, Portugal
CEFT, FEUP, R. Dr. Roberto Frias, Porto, Portugal

ABSTRACT: Image analysis is extremely important to obtain crucial information about the blood phenomena in microcirculation. The current study proposes an automatic method for segmentation and tracking Red Blood Cells (RBCs) flowing through a 100 μm Glass capillary. The original images were obtained by means of a confocal system and then processed in Matlab using the Image Processing Toolbox. The automatic measurements obtained with the proposed automatic method are compared with a manual tracking method using a plugin from ImageJ.

1 INTRODUCTION

The study of the red blood cells (RBCs) flowing in microvessels and microchannels is very important to provide a better understanding on the blood rheological properties and disorders in microvessels [1–5]. In this kind of study, the image analysis is an essential part to obtain crucial information about the blood rheology. However, most of the data analysis procedures have been executed manually [1–3] which is an extremely time consuming task especially with a large amount of data. Additionally, manual tracking methods can also introduce user errors into the data. Hence, it is important to develop image analysis methods able to get the data automatically. The main purpose of this work is to develop an approach able to track the RBCs with x and y coordinates automatically. To accomplish it we tested filtering, segmentation and feature extraction functions available in MatLab.

2 MATERIALS AND METHODS

2.1 Experimental set-up

The confocal micro-PIV system used in this study consists of an inverted microscope (IX71;

Olympus) combined with a Confocal Scanning Unit (CSU22; Yokogawa), a Diode-Pumped Solid-State (DPSS) laser (Laser Quantum) with an excitation wavelength of 532 nm and a high-speed camera (Phantom v7.1; Vision Research) (Fig. 1). The glass capillary was placed on the stage of the inverted microscope and by using a syringe pump (KD Scientific) a pressure-driven flow was kept constant (Re ~ 0.008).

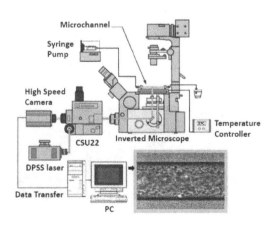

Figure 1. Experimental set-up.

More detailed information about this system can be found elsewhere [1].

2.2 *Image analysis*

The laser beam was illuminated from below the microscope stage through a dry 40× objective lens with a Numerical Aperture (NA) equal to 0.9. The confocal images were captured in middle of the capillary with a resolution of 640 × 480 pixel at a rate of 100 frames/s with an exposure time of 9.4 ms. Two image analyses methods were used in this study: method 1 (manual approach) and method 2 (automatic approach).

2.2.1 *Method 1*
A manual tracking plugin (MTrackJ) [6] of an image analysis software (ImageJ, NIH) [7] was used to track individual RBC. By using MTrackJ plugin, the bright centroid of the selected RBC was automatically computed through successive images for an interval of time of 10 ms. After obtaining x and y positions, the data were exported for the determination of each individual RBC trajectory.

2.2.2 *Method 2*
All frames were loaded and pre-processed using Matlab [8]. The region of interest was then cropped from the images with the function *imcrop*. The median function, *medfilt2*, with one mask 5 × 5 pixel,

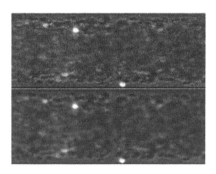

Figure 2. The region of interest (above) and the image filtered by using the median function *medfilt2*.

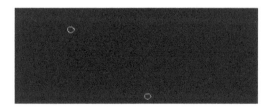

Figure 3. Result of the iterative *threshold* method and the filter *Sobel*.

was applied to eliminate most of the noise and to enhance the flowing object. In Fig. 2 we can see the result of these processing steps. In the next step, the images are subject to a segmentation filter, *Sobel*. With this segmentation it is possible to separate RBCs from the background, i.e. differentiate the area of interest (the RBCs) from the not-interest area (background image). This is possible using a *threshold* method, where a definition of one or more values of separation is enough to divide the image into one or more regions. The function *iterative threshold* was applied for the sequence of all the images.

The objects are defined with the *Sobel* filter (see Fig. 3), which shows only the edge of the objects. The *Sobel* computes an approximation of the gradient of the image intensity. At each pixel point in the image, the result of the *Sobel* operator is either the corresponding gradient vector or the norm of this vector.

3 RESULTS AND DISCUSSION

After the segmentation processing, the RBCs were tracked and sets of data (x and y positions) were obtained with the Matlab function (Fig. 4), stored in the image processing toolbox, *regionprops*. This function measures a set of properties (area, centroid, etc.) for each connected component (RBC) in the binary image.

In the Fig. 5 we can see the tracking of two RBCs, in a sequence of successive images, with an interval of 4 frames.

All of these image processes, presented in this work, are placed in an application, *RBC Data Tracking,* built in MatLab, in which all the steps can be done automatically.

Fig. 6 shows a qualitative comparison between method 1 (manual) and method 2 (automatic). The trajectories obtained from the proposed automatic method looks more smooth when compared with manual method.

Some deviations are observed between both methods. This may be due to the inaccuracy in manual tracking, especially for determination of the center of the RBCs, because the automatic method is more sensitive, even in the presence of small changes in the centroid.

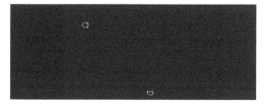

Figure 4. RBCs tracking and data extraction.

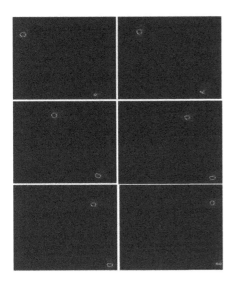

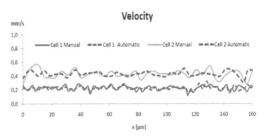

Velocity

Figure 7. Velocity of two cells by using both methods.

Fig. 7 shows the velocity of cell 1 and cell 2 calculated by data obtained from both methods. The results show good agreement between the two methods.

4 CONCLUSIONS

Although the automatic method presented in this study is a promising way to track the flowing RBCs, additional image analysis needs to be performed. Hence, detailed quantitative measurements of the RBC trajectories are currently under way and will be presented in due time.

In future work we are planning to explore more techniques to obtain quantitative measurements of the RBC trajectories, and more image analysis strategies need to be performed.

ACKNOWLEDGEMENTS

The authors acknowledge the financial support provided by: PTDC/SAU-BEB/108728/2008, PTDC/SAU-BEB/105650/2008 and PTDC/EME-MFE/099109/2008 from the FCT (Science and Technology Foundation) and COMPETE, Portugal.

Figure 5. RBCs tracking and data extraction in a sequence of 4 to 4 frames.

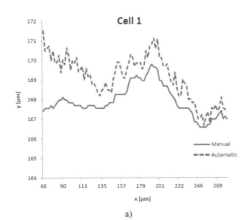

Cell 1

a)

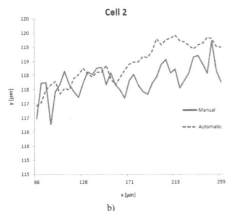

Cell 2

b)

Figure 6. Comparison of the manual (a) and automatic (b) methods.

REFERENCES

[1] Lima R, Ishikawa T, Imai Y, Takeda M, Wada S and Yamaguchi T. Measurement of individual red blood cell motions under high hematocrit conditions using a confocal micro-PTV system. *Annals of Biomedical Engineering* **37**, 1546–1559, 2009.
[2] Fujiwara H, Ishikawa T, Lima R, et al. Red blood cell motions in high-hematocrit blood flowing through a stenosed microchannel. *Journal of Biomechanics* **42**, 838–843, 2009.
[3] Suzuki Y, Tateishi N, Soutani M and Maeda N. Deformation of erythrocytes in microvessels and glasscapillaries:effectsoferythrocytedeformability. *Microcirculation* **3**, 49–57, 1996.

[4] Pries A, Secomb T, et al. Resistance to blood flow in microvessels in vivo. *Circulation Research* **75**, 904–915, 1994.

[5] Pinho D, et al. Red blood cells motion in a glass microchannel, Numerical Analysis and Applied Mathematics, Vol. 1281: 963–966, 2010.

[6] Meijering E, Smal I and Danuser G. Tracking in molecular bioimaging, *IEEE Signal Process. Mag.* **23**: 46–53, 2006.

[7] Abramoff M, Magelhaes P and Ram S. Image processing with imageJ, *Biophotonics Int.* **11:** 36–42, 2004.

[8] Steven L. Eddins. Rafael C. Gonzalez, Richard E. Woods, Digital Image Processing Using Matlab, 2002.

Computational Vision and Medical Image Processing – Tavares & Natal Jorge (eds)
© 2012 Taylor & Francis Group, London, ISBN 978-0-415-68395-1

Speech articulation assessment using dynamic Magnetic Resonance Imaging techniques

S.R. Ventura
School of Allied Health Science—Porto Polytechnic Institute, V.N. Gaia, Portugal

M.J.M. Vasconcelos & D.R. Freitas
Faculty of Engineering, University of Porto, Porto, Portugal

I.M. Ramos
Radiology Service, St. John Hospital and Faculty of Medicine, University of Porto, Porto, Portugal

João Manuel R.S. Tavares
Faculty of Engineering, University of Porto, Porto, Portugal

ABSTRACT: Magnetic Resonance Imaging (MRI) has been successfully applied on real-time analysis of the articulators during speech production along the whole vocal tract, with good signal-to-noise ratio and without ionizing effects. Because speech dynamic events need a minimal sampling rate, an improvement on the temporal resolution of MRI systems is demanded. Our aim is to describe a dynamic MRI technique to acquire and assess the main articulatory events during the production of some European Portuguese utterances. Hence, novel perceptions for dynamic MRI technique using a 3.0 Tesla System are presented in order to study the shape of the vocal tract during speech production.

Keywords: image analysis, medical imaging, speech production, dynamic techniques

1 INTRODUCTION

1.1 *Speech production analysis and challenges*

The speech production mechanism is a complex human motor activity that is able to achieve voice modulation and produce speech based mainly in the articulators' movements. The organs involved, mostly formed of soft tissues, such as the tongue, the lips, the velum and the pharynx, assume extremely important roles during speech production. In fact, these organs together with some bones, i.e. the palate and the jaw, modify the resonance cavities and the shape of the vocal tract in order to produce the sounds.

The human vocal tract's shape (Fig. 1) is different among subjects and presents a non-regular contour defined by the air-soft tissues' boundaries. This tube extends from the lips to the glottis, and is formed by four main structures: the oral cavity, the nasal cavity, the velum and the pharynx.

The tongue is the most important articulator, mainly because it is the largest one, and performs a wide range of slow and fast movements during speech production.

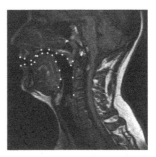

Figure 1. The shape of the vocal tract during the production of [ɛ] vowel in an image acquired by a 3.0 Tesla MR system.

Many approaches have been used to track and observe the movements of the articulators, in particular of the tongue, but most of them employ sensors (e.g. electromagnetic articulography) or the direct contact with the tongue and the palate (e.g. electropalatography).

Magnetic Resonance Imaging (MRI) has been successfully applied on real-time analysis of the articulators during speech production, along the whole vocal tract, with good signal-to-noise ratio and without ionizing effects. As such, several MRI techniques provided the calculation of cross-sectional areas and volumes directly from static postures during sustained articulations (Kim et al. 2009) or using multiple repetitions (Stone et al. 2001, Shadle et al. 1999).

Because speech dynamic events need a minimal sampling rate and considering the number of articulators involved, two challenges are demanded for the accurate examination, namely:

a. The development of a specific trigger for image acquisition to improve the temporal resolution of MRI systems;
b. Audio-recording in real-time during MRI acquisitions allowing sound acoustic analysis and imaging relationship.

Our aim is to describe a dynamic MRI technique to acquire and assess the main articulatory events during the production of some European Portuguese (EP) sounds.

The remaining of this paper is organized as follows. In the next section, the description of the MRI protocol, the speech corpus and the image analysis and assessment are described. Then, the articulatory measurements obtained for two subjects by using deformable models are presented and discussed. Finally, the conclusions and future outlooks are pointed out in the last section.

1.2 *Dynamic MRI techniques*

A few methods and applications of dynamic MRI have been presented concerning synchronized sampled method (Parthasarathy et al. 2007) or tagging technique (Stone et al. 2001), and achieving images at rates of 7 to 10 frames per second (Demolin et al. 2006, Stone et al. 2001, Mády et al. 2001, Engwall 2004) and even of 18 (Parthasarathy et al. 2007) and 24 frames per second (Narayanan et al. 2004). According to Shadle (1999), dynamic MRI is a potentially useful tool that allows the tracking of the vocal tract organs' movements. In addition, several morphological aspects can be studied as, for example, the motion of the tongue's surface or contour (Stone et al. 2001), the kinematic parameters of the tongue (i.e. velocity, principal strains) (Parthasarathy et al. 2007), the shape of the tongue (Avila-García et al. 2004) and characteristic distances (i.e. articulatory parameters) (Ventura et al. 2011, Echternach et al. 2010). In this area, dynamic MRI can also allow the assessment of articulatory impairments following surgery to structures of the oral cavity, such as for cancer treatment (Mády et al. 2001).

In a previous work, we presented a technique for the dynamic study of the vocal tract with MRI by using the heart's beat signal to synchronize and trigger the imaging acquisition process (Ventura et al. 2011). Our previous dynamic study revealed the existence of significant variability in sound productions among subjects. This variability is not only due to individual anatomic differences, but also to the peculiarities of each subject's movement and gesture control that was considered as being extremely individualized as was duly observed.

Due to the developments that have occurred in MRI, namely by the use of 3.0 Tesla magnetic fields, new applications and image refinements are expected, and consequently significant improvements on the quality of the data acquired with the articulatory events during speech production. Because speech dynamic events demand a minimal sampling rate around 20 Hz (Narayanan et al. 2004), an improvement on the temporal resolution of MRI systems is demanded, for example, by using k-space sampling strategies or more efficient triggering techniques.

1.3 *Vocal tract modeling*

The implementation of statistical methods to analyse data from speech production has proofed to be valuable in several studies. To name a few, (Harshman et al. 1977) used component analysis to identify a set of articulatory features of the tongue. Later, Maeda (1988) applied factor analysis in order to describe the lateral shapes of the vocal tract and (Stone et al. 1997) employed principal component analysis to examine the sagittal tongue's contours from ultrasound images.

The MRI of the vocal tract, associated with the use of statistical deformable models, has made possible the automatic extraction of the vocal tract's shape from the acquired images and the achievement of articulatory measurements that can be useful in the improving of computational speech models (Vasconcelos et al. 2010a, b).

2 METHODS

2.1 *Equipment, subjects and speech corpus*

The image data was acquired using a MAGNETOM Trio 3.0 Tesla MR system and two integrated coils (a 32-channel head coil and a 4-channel neck matrix coil), with the subjects in supine position.

According to the safety procedures for MRI, a questionnaire was performed for screening several contraindications. In addition, the subjects were previously informed and instructed about the study to be performed and the informed consent was obtained. Two young female volunteers, without articulatory disorders, were trained before the MRI exam to ensure the proper production of the intended sounds, and audio recordings were performed before image acquisition and in supine position.

The speech corpus consisted in two sequences of sounds of EP language, in two different articulatory contexts:

i. Vowel-Vowel articulation (VV);
ii. Set of Consonant-Vowel (CV) articulation during a word utterance.

The first articulatory context included the five oral vowels [a ɛ i ɔ u] and the second, the utterance word/pato/ (the English word "duck", IPA phonetic transcription [patu]). This choice was made considering the sounds familiarity, to any Portuguese subject, during the speech production, and because these sounds are easy to articulate. Furthermore, a coarticulation study was assessed, in the second utterance, stops on consonant-vowel context.

The two audio spectrograms in Figures 2 and 3 illustrate the two sequences of sounds of EP language recorded from the first subject. As can be

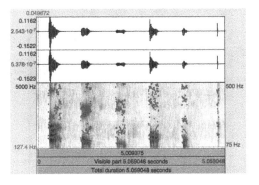

Figure 2. Spectrogram for the first articulatory context in PRAAT software.

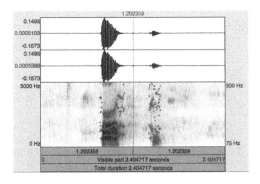

Figure 3. Spectrogram for the second articulatory context in PRAAT software.

verified, the vowels sequence utterance has a total duration of 5.05 seconds, and the word/pato/lasts 2.41 seconds.

2.2 Dynamic MRI technique

Concerning the data acquisition, two approaches were used: 1) firstly, rapid pulse sequences and, then, 2) a tagging technique. "Tagging" is a method that aids the tracking of objects' motion in MRI series. The inserted tags appear as dark regions in the images that move associated to the object under analysis. As such, this technique is particularly valuable in cardiac imaging, as the tissue of the heart's walls provides few natural features for motion tracking. For speech articulatory assessment, this technique is very difficult to use and more tests must be performed in order to improve temporal resolution and image quality intended for this purpose.

Hence, only rapid pulse sequences combined with parallel imaging were used and tested, through the compromise of the temporal resolution and signal-noise ratio of the MRI system.

Using a Flash Gradient-Echo Sequence, 100 midsagittal WT1 slices were acquired during 48 seconds for each repeated utterance. The MRI protocol parameters used are indicated in Table 1.

For the target utterance constituted by the five oral vowels, each sound occurred at least 13 to 37 times per sequence, according to the speed of speech and on the word length. The vowel [a] occurred 27 and 37 times per sequence for each subject. The vowels [ɔ u] were the sounds with lower occurrence rates.

For the second target word, each sound occurred at least 13 to 42 times per sequence, occurring for each subject the vowel [a] about 35 to 42 times and 13 to 16 times for the plosive consonant [t].

Table 1. MRI protocol parameters used in the dynamic study about speech production.

Parameters	2D dynamic imaging technique
TR (msecond)	6.4
TE (msecond)	2.44
Flip angle	10°
Number of averages	1
Slice thickness (mm)	6
Field of view (mm)	178×220
Matrix	156×192
Acceleration factor (parallel imaging)	4
Image resolution	0.873 *Pixel* per mm
Pixel spacing	1.146×1.146 mm

2.3 Deformable models

In order to perform a more robust analysis of the articulatory behavior during the speech production, statistical Point Distribution Models (PDMs) (Vasconcelos et al. 2008, 2010a) were used to automatically identify, i.e. segment, the vocal tract's key points in order to compute descriptive measures.

In the building of the PDMs (Cootes et al. 1992), the manual tracing of the key points was carried out by one of the authors with medical imaging knowledge and was realized on images sequentially displayed on the computer screen and later cross-checked by another author. The labeling method was performed according to the anatomic location of the vocal tract articulators (Fig. 2).

In the statistical modelling method used, all the training examples are aligned into a standard co-ordinate frame and a Principal Component Analysis is applied to the co-ordinates of the landmark points. This produces the mean position for each landmark, and a description of the main ways in which these points tend to move together (Vasconcelos et al. 2008, 2010a).

The local grey-level behavior of each landmark point can also be considered in the modeling of a shape (Cootes et al. 1993). Thus, statistical information is obtained about the mean and covariance of the grey values of the pixels around each landmark point. This information is used to construct the appearance models in Active Appearance Models that can be used to identify the modeled shape in new images.

Active Appearance Models were presented in (Cootes et al. 1998) and allow the building of texture and appearance models. These models are generated by combining a model of shape variation (a geometric model), with a model of the appearance variations in a shape-normalized frame. To identify the modelled shape in new images, the method uses the difference between the current estimate of appearance and the target image to drive an optimization process.

2.4 Image analysis and articulatory assessment

A total of 200 midsagittal MR images were acquired for each subject. Speech articulatory events were described considering seven distances measurements, as depicted in Figure 4. These measures represent the union of the major articulation points for consonants production (because vowels are produced without closure of the vocal tract) and pointed all articulatory (supraglottic) organs, as the lips, the tongue, the palate, the velum, the pharynx.

In order to automatically extract the landmarks of the images, active appearance models were built for each sequence of sounds for each subject (Cootes, 2004). The models were built from the first 20 images of each MRI sequence and later used to automatically label the others 80 images of the sequence.

For each subject, MRI data measurements were performed only when an articulatory posture occurred (based on visual assessment of the vocal tract's shape) and, to avoid errors in the analysis

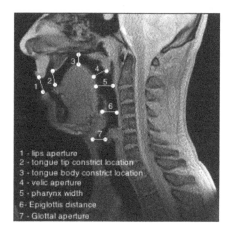

Figure 4. Articulatory measurements addressed on MR images during speech production.

Table 2. Articulatory measurements of the first articulatory context for the female subject 1.

	[a]		[ɛ]		[i]		[ɔ]		[u]	
	cm	SD	cm	SD	cm	SD	cm	SD	cm	SD
D1	1.051±	0.332	0.821±	0.145	1.055±	0.209	0.897±	0.176	0.872±	0.165
D2	1.363±	0.345	1.232±	0.132	1.048±	0.143	1.364±	0.236	1.130±	0.286
D3	1.274±	0.350	0.951±	0.201	0.635±	0.114	1.184±	0.323	0.927±	0.209
D4	1.288±	0.421	1.316±	0.244	1.488±	0.207	1.101±	0.238	0.949±	0.286
D5	1.154±	0.468	1.528±	0.252	2.137±	0.343	1.112±	0.347	1.226±	0.257
D6	0.984±	0.284	1.253±	0.190	1.606±	0.222	1.215±	0.251	1.126±	0.166
D7	0.901±	0.217	1.175±	0.288	1.108±	0.219	1.105±	0.243	1.044±	0.242

Measurements (cm); Standard Deviation (SD).

and automatic labeling process, rest positions (without speech activity) were excluded.

3 RESULTS

This study presents data concerning the vocal tract's shape during the utterance of sounds of two articulatory sequences and the quantification of seven articulatory parameters.

Considering the large set of images collected, the quantitative results are presented separately for each sound utterance and for each subject.

The analysis was based on the mean values and standard deviations of the seven distances extracted among the subjects, from each image sets that best represent each sound.

The results of the first articulatory context for each subject are presented in Tables 2 and 3.

Table 3. Articulatory measurements of the first articulatory context for the female subject 2.

	[a]		[ɛ]		[i]		[ɔ]		[u]	
	cm	SD	cm	SD	cm	SD	cm	SD	cm	SD
D1	0.940±	0.118	1.168±	0.087	1.218±	0.078	0.717±	0.184	0.585±	0.112
D2	1.084±	0.132	0.876±	0.073	0.837±	0.112	1.195±	0.083	1.165±	0.088
D3	1.399±	0.279	0.619±	0.181	0.479±	0.135	1.460±	0.111	0.910±	0.222
D4	1.016±	0.225	0.138±	0.161	1.310±	0.168	0.677±	0.127	0.662±	0.138
D5	1.146±	0.306	1.847±	0.141	2.187±	0.249	0.799±	0.108	1.104±	0.173
D6	1.058±	0.147	1.257±	0.175	1.318±	0.149	1.044±	0.126	1.176±	0.058
D7	0.823±	0.262	0.682±	0.107	0.576±	0.098	0.656±	0.084	0.787±	0.129

Measurements (cm); Standard Deviation (SD).

Table 4. Articulatory measurements of the second articulatory context for the female subject 1.

	[p]		[a]		[t]		[u]	
	cm	SD	cm	SD	cm	SD	cm	SD
D1	0.626±	0.186	1.002±	0.231	0.410±	0.070	0.650±	0.130
D2	1.046±	0.326	1.389±	0.185	0.599±	0.134	1.050±	0.205
D3	0.999±	0.225	1.232±	0.289	0.790±	0.100	0.887±	0.142
D4	0.901±	0.118	0.975±	0.153	1.063±	0.093	0.775±	0.148
D5	0.933±	0.264	0.789±	0.249	1.139±	0.073	1.069±	0.150
D6	1.043±	0.235	0.860±	0.245	1.260±	0.145	1.234±	0.164
D7	1.047±	0.288	0.832±	0.274	1.015±	0.166	0.943±	0.171

Measurements (cm); Standard Deviation (SD).

Table 5. Articulatory measurements of the second articulatory context for the female subject 2.

	[p]		[a]		[t]		[u]	
	cm	SD	cm	SD	cm	SD	cm	SD
D1	0.649±	0.168	0.887±	0.143	0.643±	0.262	0.620±	0.088
D2	0.851±	0.141	1.033±	0.247	0.460±	0.151	0.872±	0.128
D3	1.102±	0.216	1.250±	0.259	1.019±	0.173	0.963±	0.151
D4	0.838±	0.123	0.937±	0.091	0.933±	0.152	0.805±	0.147
D5	1.108±	0.142	0.976±	0.174	1.179±	0.083	1.223±	0.119
D6	1.172±	0.157	0.995±	0.229	1.138±	0.110	1.317±	0.158
D7	0.952±	0.318	0.793±	0.364	0.825±	0.093	1.126±	0.376

Measurements (cm); Standard Deviation (SD).

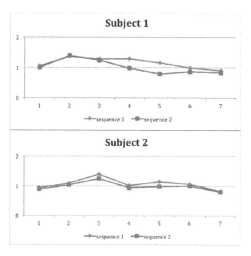

Figure 5. Comparative articulatory measurements performed for each female subject considering the target sound [a] in two different articulatory contexts: VV in sequence 1 and CV in sequence 2.

Comparing both subjects, higher distances are demonstrated concerning pharynx width (D5) during the utterance of the vowel [i] and in generally similar measurements can be observed. Except for the open-mid vowels [ɛ] and [ɔ], the global vocal tract's shape (based on the distance trajectory) and distances are fairly different among the subjects.

The results indicated in Tables 4 and 5 represent the measurements extracted from the images collected for the second articulatory context, the word [patu].

Comparing the several measurements obtained for each uttered sound, similar values can be observed for both subjects. Rather different measures are more frequent for each plosive consonant, namely the distances D1 to D3 to the consonant [t] and D2, D5 and D6 to the consonant [p].

Considering the higher occurrence of the target sound [a] (in times per sequence) in both articulatory contexts, a cross-parameter comparison was also performed in order to assess the effects of VV and CV articulation context, Figure 5.

As can be observed in Figure 5, in general, the values of the distances measured are fairly similar; however, a possible effect of the CV articulatory context in the distances measured, which are clearly lower for both subjects, can be seen.

4 CONCLUSIONS

We have compared the speech articulatory measurements attained in a large set of midsagittal images, acquired during speech production in a very reasonable acquisition time and with enough image resolution for analysis and subsequent quantitative assessment.

Each sound under analysis occurred at least 13 times per sequence during 48 seconds. The major drawback was revealed during the visual assessment of the images for the assemblage of images to each target sound.

By using deformable models in the image segmentation step, we improve the time spend in the process of measurements, as it passes from manual to automatic labelling and, instead of manually labelling 400 images, only 80 were manually annotated.

In line with the acoustic sounds duration, the sound [a] was imaged more times, and the associated measurements show a more linear distribution of all distances (from lips to glottis).

Higher discrepancies of values have been encountered in open-mid vowels, which means the tongue is positioned halfway between a closed vowel (e.g. the vowels [i] and [u]) and an open vowel (e.g. the vowel [a]). This could be related with some errors during the visual assessment of the vocal tract's shape for the assemblage of images to each target sound.

In the word [patu], major differences in the distances extracted were traced for both consonants between the subjects. This can be possible due to the characteristic short time duration of both plosive articulations and result of some measurement errors due to the difficulty of the automatic tracing of the landmark points concerning the lips and alveolar region.

Comparing with our previous works (Ventura et al. 2011 and Vasconcelos et al. 2010a) an improvement on the image acquisition protocol was achieved and more data concerning speech production using MRI was addressed. Hence, a large set of target sounds and articulatory parameters have been analyzed in two different articulatory contexts. Additionally, the statistical deformable models are now used to automatically extract the landmarks of the MR images and thus, to reduce the time employed to extract the trajectory distances of the vocal tract's shape under study.

Articulatory phonetics has long been a discipline with mainly qualitative analysis methods, but in the last decades the advances of MRI allowed the quantification of several articulatory parameters.

The knowledge obtained in this study represents a direct contribution to the improvement of speech synthesis algorithms considering the articulatory parameters measured, and can thereby allow novel perceptions about dynamic behavior of the articulators and co-articulation, namely on European Portuguese speech language.

In addition, these results could encourage researchers and give useful functional and non-invasive information concerning sounds articulation to be used in clinical practice.

In the future, an arrangement for simultaneous recording of speech and MRI of the vocal tract's shape will improve the accuracy of the results, namely for image-acoustic correlation of the target sounds.

ACKNOWLEDGMENTS

The images considered in this work were acquired at the Radiology Department of Hospital S. João EPE, in Portugal, and we would like to express our gratitude to the technical staff.

The first author would like to thank the support and contribution of the PhD grant from Escola Superior de Tecnologia da Saúde (ESTSP) and Instituto Politécnico do Porto (IPP), in Portugal.

The second author would like to thank the support of the PhD grant from *Fundação para a Ciência e Tecnologia* (FCT), with reference SFRH/BD/28817/2006.

This work was partially done in the scope of the project "Methodologies to Analyze Organs from Complex Medical Images—Applications to Female Pelvic Cavity", with reference PTDC/EEA-CRO/103320/2008, financially supported by FCT.

REFERENCES

Avila-García, M.S., Carter, J.N. & Damper, R.I. 2004. Extracting Tongue Shape Dynamics from Magnetic Resonance Image Sequences. *Transactions on Engineering, Computing and Technology* 2: 288–291.

Cootes, T.F., Taylor, C.J., Cooper, D.H. & Graham, J. 1992. Training models of shape from sets of examples in Proceedings of the British Machine Vision Conference, Leeds: 9–18.

Cootes, T.F. & Taylor, C.J. (1993). Active Shape Model Search using Local Grey-Level Models: A Quantitative Evaluation in *British Machine Vision Conference*, Guildford: BMVA Press.

Cootes, T.F. & Edwards, G. (1998). Active Appearance Models. *European Conference on Computer Vision*, Freiburg, Germany.

Cootes, T.F. *Build_aam.* 2004; Available at: http://www.wiau.man.ac.uk/~bim/software/am_tools_doc/download_win.html.

Demolin, D., Sampaio, A. & Metens, T. 2006. An MRI Study of Articulatory Compensation. *In 7th International Seminar on Speech Production*, Brazil: Ubatuba, São Paulo.

Echternach, M., Sundberg, J., Arndt, S., Markl, M., Schumacher, S. & Richter, B. 2010. Vocal Tract in Female Registers - A Dynamic Real-Time MRI Study. *Journal of Voice* 24(2): 133–139.

Engwall, O. 2004. From real-time MRI to 3D tongue movements. In 8th International Conference on Spoken Language Processing (INTERSPEECH 2004-ICSLP). Korea: Jeju Island.

Harshman, R.A., Ladefoged, P. & Golstein, L. 1977. Factor analysis of tongue shapes. *Journal of the Acoustical Society of America* (62): 693–707.

Kim, Y., Narayanan, S.S. & Nayak, K.S. 2009. Accelerated Three-Dimensional Upper Airway MRI Using Compressed Sensing. *Magnetic Resonance in Medicine* 61: 1434–1440.

Mády, K., Sader, R., Zimmermann, A., Hoole, P., Beer, A., Zei-lhofer, H. & Hannig, CH. 2001. Use of real-time MRI in assessment of consonant articulation before and after tongue surgery and tongue reconstruction. *In 4th Interna-tional Speech Motor Conference*. Netherlands: Nijmegen.

Maeda, S., 1988. Improved articulatory models. *Journal of the Acoustical Society of America* (84 S1): S146–S146.

Narayanan, S., Nayak, K., Lee, S., Sethy, A. & Byrd, D. 2004. An Approach to Real-time Magnetic Resonance Imaging for Speech Production. *Journal Acoustical Society of America* 115(4): 1771–1776.

Parthasarathy, V., Prince, Jl., Stone, M., Murano, Ez. & Nessaiver, M. 2007. Measuring tongue motion from tagged cine-MRI using harmonic phase (HARP) processing. *Journal Acoustical Society of America* 121 (1): 491–504.

Shadle, C.H., Mohammad, M., Carter, J.N. & Jackson, P.J.B. 1999. Multi-planar Dynamic Magnetic Resonance Imaging: New Tools for Speech Research. *In International Congress of Phonetics Sciences (ICPhS99)*. USA: San Francisco.

Stone, M., Cheng, Y. & Lundberg, A., 1997. Using principal component analysis of tongue surface shapes to distinguish among vowels and speakers. *Journal of the Acoustical Society of America* (101–5): 3176–3177.

Stone, M., Davis, E., Douglas, A.S., NessAiver, M., Gul-lapalli, R., Levine, W.S. & Lundberg, A. 2001. Modeling the motion of the internal tongue from tagged cine-MRI images. *Journal of the Acoustical Society of America* 109 (6): 2974–2982.

Stone, M., Davis, E., Douglas, A.S., & NessAiver, M. 2001. Modeling tongue surface contours from cine-MRI images. *Journal of Speech, Language, Hearing Research* 410: 1–40.

Vasconcelos, M.J.M. & Tavares, J.M.R.S. (2008). Methods to Automatically Built Point Distribution Models for Objects like Hand Palms and Faces Represented in Images. *Computer Modeling in Engineering and Sciences*, 36(3): 213–241.

Vasconcelos, M.J., Ventura, S.R., Freitas, D.R.S. & João Manuel R.S. Tavares. 2010a. Towards the Automatic Study of the Vocal Tract from Magnetic Resonance Images. *Journal of Voice:* in press.

Vasconcelos, M.J., Ventura, S.R., Freitas, D.R.S. & João Manuel R S Tavares. 2010b. Using Statistical Deformable Models to Reconstruct Vocal Tract Shape from Magnetic Resonance Images. *Proceedings of the Institution of Mechanical Engineers, Part H: Journal of Engineering in Medicine* 224(10): 1153–1163.

Ventura, S.R., Freitas, D.R. & João Manuel R.S. Tavares. 2011. Toward Dynamic Magnetic Resonance Imaging of the Vocal Tract During Speech Production. *Journal of Voice* 25(4): 511–518.

Computational Vision and Medical Image Processing – Tavares & Natal Jorge (eds)
© 2012 Taylor & Francis Group, London, ISBN 978-0-415-68395-1

The breast lesions characterization by b values variation in the DW-Magnetic Resonance Imaging

A. A. Fernandes
Centro Hospitalar Lisboa Central—Hospital de Santo António dos Capuchos/Escola Superior de Tecnologia da Saúde de Lisboa—Área Científica de Radiologia, Lisboa, Portugal

M.B. Ribeiro
Escola Superior de Tecnologia da Saúde de Lisboa—Área Científica de Radiologia/Departamento de Anatomia da Faculdade de Ciências Médicas da Universidade Nova de Lisboa, Lisboa, Portugal

J.C. Janardo
Escola Superior de Tecnologia da Saúde de Lisboa—Área Científica de Radiologia, Lisboa, Portugal

S.D. Jaguegivane
Radiology Department of Epsom and St. Helier University Hospitals NHS Trust, London, UK

M.E. Pereira
Departamento de Imagiologia do Centro Hospitalar Lisboa Central/Centro de Senologia Lisboa, Lisboa, Portugal

ABSTRACT: The DWI enables, by the b values variation, restriction of the water proton diffusion and provides a better characterization of the location, size and shape of lesions.

This study aimed to assess the impact of the DWI sequence, and their correlation between the ADC values and the histological results, on the characterization of malignant breast lesions.

The data collection includes 18 female aged between 38 and 71 years old, who presented with malignant breast lesions confirmed by histological reports. The DWI sequence was included to the MRI standard protocol to assess the ADC values.

The ADC values calculated in the centre of the malignant lesions, showed average values and Standard Deviation of $0.89 \pm 0.14 \times 10^{-3}$ mm²/s respectively. The combination of methods has a sensitivity of 100%.

The DWI technique proved to be a useful method that increases the diagnostic information in the characterization of malignant breast lesions.

1 INTRODUCTION

The breast is a modified gland of the skin, and is a part of the female reproductive system. It represents a purpose of feeding and sexuality, appearing in different shapes and sizes.[1,2]

The breast is a mass of glandular, fatty, and fibrous tissues distributed between the lobes and lobules, which end in the small ducts. (Fig. 1)

Breast cancer is the most common type of cancer in females, being responsible for 16% of death in this gender. Previous studies showed that 7,4 million of people have died with breast cancer in 2004 and if these tendencies be maintained it's estimated that in 2015 more than 83,2 million of people will suffer with breast cancer.[3]

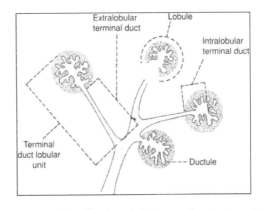

Figure 1. Classification of the breast microstructures.[3]

There are several types of breast carcinomas, whose diagnostics are made in an *in situ* or invasive state.[4,5]

At the moment, mammography is used as the first method to detect malignant breast lesions in early stage. However, the mammography technique presents a few disadvantages, such as the use of ionizing radiation and a low specificity in breasts with high density. This method allows the detection of the lesions but doesn't provide a good specificity about morphologic criteria.[2,6]

Ultrasound is performed as a complementary method to mammography, and the analysis of both methods demonstrates advantages, such as better sensitivity and specificity. It also allows the performance needed to the interventional procedures with the aim to obtain the best histological information. Even, with some advantages, ultrasound can't be used as a single method to diagnose breast lesions because it is operator dependent, presents a reduced image resolution and provides low contrast.[2,7]

To fight these limitations, in the most recent years, the great sensitivity and specificity of MRI for the diagnosis of malignant breast lesions (85% to 99%) made this technique an important benefit on the diagnosis of all pathological processes.

MRI has shown to be a method to complement other techniques, as it gives an excellent capacity in the demonstration of contrast between tissues through its different acquisition sequences, a detailed evaluation of size, dissemination and heterogeneity of the carcinoma, e.g. cancer staging.[6] (Table 1)

The breast MRI should be performed preferably between the 7th and 14th day of the menstrual cycle, to avoid false-positives. It is within this time frame that the best contrast among tissues is achieved, because the hormones have influence over them.[2,10,11]

Because of breath and cardiac motion artefacts breast MRI is a complex anatomy to study, so it is necessary to applies fast sequences like the BLADE weighting. The use of contrast (Gadolinium) is also necessary to show the angiogenesis of the tumour and the distribution of the contrast media across tissues to differentiate the malignant of the benign lesions.[10,11]

The diffusion weighted image was first applied in the early detection of cerebral ischemia. Nowadays the DWI sequence is used to complement almost all used sequences, showing important information for the detection of breast cancer, allowing the identification of biological features of the tissues, without using invasive or contrast methods. This leads the present research in the assessment of the capacity of the DWI to diagnose with high precision the malignant breast lesions and produce an empiric opinion about if this sequence should be, or not, included in the standard breast MRI protocol.[12–17]

The DWI is a phenomenon defined by the random movement of water protons, called Brownian movement, which is based in the dissipation of thermal energy. The DWI is based on SE (spin-echo) sequence weighted in T2 with application of diffusion gradients before and after the emission of the radiofrequency pulse. The power of the gradients is characterized by the amount and the variation of the b values. This value reflects the magnitude and sensibility of the DWI.[13,18–20]

There isn't a standard b value defined for the diagnoses of breast cancer.[19]

The suitable b value should be sufficient to suppress the fat tissue of the mammary gland allowing an adequate signal of the malignant lesion, usually using 3 b different values to obtain an Apparent Diffusion Coefficient (ADC) map (b values between 0 and 1000 s/mm^2).[14]

The water's degree of mobility in the biological tissues is characterized by the ADC, which is expressed in mm^2/s. This value refers that the quantitative measurement is proportional to the diffusion of water's molecules. The great cellular proliferation in malignant lesions increases the cellular density and this effect decreases the movement of water molecules between tissues and

Table 1. Types of the breast cancer.

I—Ductal carcinoma	II—Lobular carcinoma	III—Tubular carcinoma	IV—Medullar carcinoma	V—Colloid carcinoma
Represents 60 to 80% of the cases	Second more common type of breast carcinoma (15%)	2% of the breast carcinomas	6% of the breast carcinomas	Represents 2% of the carcinomas
Mass of high density	Multicentric and bilateral	Spiculated margins	Present in patient less than 50 years old	Present in older women
Spiculated margins	Spiculated mass with asymmetrical densities	Small dimensions	Maybe confused with fibroadenoma	Gelatinous type of mass

in the extra-cellular space, creating a low ADC value and a low intensity signal in the ADC map.[21]

The ADC value is achieved through the ADC map. It corresponds to the mean value of ROI (region of interest) multiplied by 10^{-3} mm^2/s. Therefore the ROI must be placed in the centre and margin of the lesion. The range of values of ADC between 1.21–2,58 × 10^{-3} mm^2/s will relates probably to a benign lesion as for the range of values between 0.34–1.19 × 10^{-3} mm^2/s the probability of the malignant lesions is higher. It is expected to establish a correlation between histological results and the ADC values to achieve a diagnosis with more accuracy.[9,18,22]

2 METHODS, MATERIALS AND PATIENTS

The experimental study included 75 female patients studied between November 2009 and June 2010. These patients have a range of ages between 38 and 71 years old, with a mean age of 54 years.[23]

The sample was a non probabilistic, with a rational choice. From the 75 patients, 18 were considered for this study, selected by the inclusion criteria "patients that presented malignant breast lesions confirmed by histological results, with a diameter equal or higher than 1 cm". All the patients underwent Breast MRI with the DWI sequence. The remaining patients were excluded from this study because they already had surgery, presented breast implants, already had undergone quimiotherapy/radiotherapy, had benign or no lesions.

The images were acquired with an MR system 1,5 T from Siemens® model Magnetom Avanto, using a bilateral breast coil. The patients were positioned in prone position, and the sequences used were: Axial T2 BLADE (TR/TE: 4200/90; FOV:350 mm; Slice Thickness: 3 mm) and Axial T1 dynamic, acquiring 1 series without contrast and 5 with contrast (TR/TE: 450/13; FOV:350 mm; Slice Thickness: 3 mm). (Table 2)

At last an EPI diffusion sequence was performed, in axial direction, on which the *b* values were: 50/400/800, with TR/TE of 1800/75, a FOV of 350 mm and a slice thickness of 3 mm. It is important to notice that the technical parameters were the usually used in the Hospital where this research was conducted.

The ADC values were automatically calculated by placing the ROI in the ADC map, on the centre and margin of the lesions, using the fibrous tissue value as a reference level. The software allowed the visualization of the mean value calculated by the ROI, corresponding to the ADC value (multiplied by 10-3). The ROI diameter was replicated in all the images, (0.2 cm^2) and placed in the image of the ADC map where the lesion was more evident.[12] (Figure 2)

Table 2. Acquisition sequences of the Breast MR protocol.

	Seq. 1	Seq.2	Seq. 3
Orientation	3 plains	TRA	TRA
Weighted	T1	T2	T1 Fat-sat
Sequence type	Scout view	BLADE	Dynamic

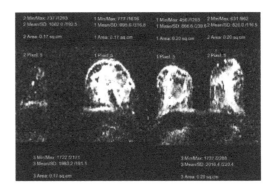

Figure 2. ROI's location in the ADC maps of 2 patients. (Image acquired by the authors after ethical procedures application).

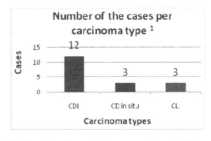

Graphic 1. Number of the cases founded by carcinoma type.
[1]CDI = Invasive ductal carcinoma; CLI = Invasive lobular carcinoma; CD in situ = Ductal carcinoma in situ.

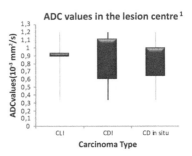

Graphic 2. ADC values achieved in the range of the malignant lesions values.
[1]CDI = Invasive ductal carcinoma; CLI = Invasive lobular carcinoma; CD in situ = Ductal carcinoma in situ.

Using the Excel program from Microsoft Office™ the results were reproduced in graphics and the average was also calculated. By the using the SPSS software package it was possible to calculate the standard deviation, sensibility and specificity.

3 RESULTS

By performing the analysis of the 18 cases, the ADC values obtained in the centre of the lesion were from 0,61 to $1,11 \times 10^{-3}$ mm²/s with a mean and standard deviation of $0,89 \pm 0,14 \times 10^{-3}$ mm²/s. The results obtained in the margin of the lesions presented values from 0,74 to $1,24 \times 10^{-3}$ mm²/s presenting a mean and standard deviation of $0,94 \pm 0,15 \times 10^{-3}$ mm²/s. For last the values acquired in the fibrous tissues showed results from 1,57 to 2.48×10^{-3} mm²/s with a mean and standard deviation of $1,91 \pm 0,29 \times 10^{-3}$ mm²/s. After analyzing the results of the ROI placed in the centre of the lesion it was possible to know that the sensibility of this sequence was of 100%.

4 DISCUSSION

The property of the DWI sequence in the characterization of the cellularity of the tissues has shown the utility of the MRI in the detection of malignant breast lesions.[20]

The differences in the cellular properties and the restriction of cellularity in malignant tissues produce a low diffusion and therefore low ADC values.[14,16,24]

There are few studies that performed measurements of the ADC values in breast lesions, however these presented a unconformity with the typical values obtained by the malignancy of the tissues.

Palle and Reddy showed, based on their studies, a range of values between $0.85–1.1 \times 10^{-3}$ mm²/s, however Wenkle et al demonstrated a range of $0.34–1.19 \times 10^{-3}$ mm²/s. This way, by performing this study, it was possible to see that the range established by Wenkle et al. is in agreement with the results achieved in this study. The ADC values were between 0,61 a $1,11 \times 10^{-3}$ mm²/s.[9,18]

It was also observed in this study that the invasive ductal carcinoma was the most common type of tumour, as 12 of the 18 cases presented this type of carcinoma. This result was also seen in other studies.

However the DWI sequence presents a few limitations, as it doesn't allow the characterization of lesions with a diameter inferior of 1 cm, as these lesions aren't visible in the ADC map and because the location of ROI's for the calculation of ADC values depends in the operator.[18]

The diffusion sequence presents another limitation, for the fact that it doesn't allow the differentiation of types of carcinomas. This study showed that the ADC values for the invasive ductal carcinoma were between 0,61 a $1,11 \times 10^{-3}$ mm²/s, and the values for the invasive lobular carcinoma were found between the range of 0,89 a $0,97 \times 10^{-3}$ mm²/s. So, it's not possible to correlate the ADC values among the different types of carcinomas.

It was observed that there is no agreement, for all the patients, between the results obtained in the centre and margin of the lesion. It was also possible to see that the age of the patients doesn't affect the ADC values.

5 CONCLUSIONS

To overcome the limitations of the Ultrasound and Mammography, the high sensitivity and specificity of MRI for the diagnosis of the malignant breast lesions, 85% to 99% respectively, led this method to a great role in the imaging departments.

Thus, MRI with Diffusion Weighted Image (DWI) appears as a complementary diagnostic method showing an excellent ability to extend the detailed assessment of the size, shape, distribution and heterogeneity of the carcinoma such as the local and the axilar loco regional staging trough the contrast between different tissues, given by MRI sequences protocol. The DWI enables, with its variety of b values, the assessment of the restriction of the water proton diffusion and more easily the lesions location.

The DWI is a series of Spin-Echo (SE) T2-weighted image with diffusion gradients applied before and after the pulse of the radiofrequency emission. The power of gradients is characterized by the b values. The magnitude of the water diffusion values and their sensibility reflects differences in image according to the lesion type.

This study aimed to assess the impact of the DWI sequence in the characterization of malignant breast lesions and evaluate if this sequence should be included in the breast MRI protocol. Also, after the application of the b values variation we propose the correlation of the ADC values and histological results.

After analyzing the results, it was possible to conclude that the DWI allows the characterization of breast malignant lesions, as it showed a sensivity of a 100%, recommending its introduction on the MRI standard breast protocol.

Even though this sequence shows a few limitations, it presents as a useful technique that should be studied and improved in the future. This way, posterior studies should be made to reduce the range of the ADC values for malignant and benign breast lesions, to allow a more specific characterization.

The reduced sample in this study and possibly the use of single equipment limited the results extrapolation. It will be possible to do a future research to try and overcome the weakness presented in this study.

REFERENCES

[1] Paredes E. Atlas of mammography. 3rd ed. Boston: Lippincott Williams & Wilkins. 2007. 704p.

[2] Koppans D. Breast imaging. 3rd ed. Boston: Lippincott Williams & Wilkins. 2007. 1136p.

[3] World Health Statistics. Part 1—Ten highlights in health statistics. In: OMS, 2008: disponivel em http://www.who.int/whosis/whostat/EN_WHS08_Part1.pdf.

[4] Winchester D, Winchester D. Atlas of clinical oncology: breast cancer. 1st ed. London: American cancer society, 2000. 607p.

[5] Hall J, Knaus J. The encyclopedia of visual medicine series: An Atlas of Breast Disease. 1st ed. New York: The Parthenon Publishing group, 2003. 88p.

[6] Charles-Edwards E, Souza N. Diffusion-weighted magnetic resonance imaging and its application to cancer. Cancer Imaging [Internet]. 2006 [cited 2010 Apr 12]; 6: 135–43. Available from: http://www.ncbi.nlm.nih.gov/entrez/query.fcgi?cmd=Retrieve&db=PubMed&dopt=Citation&list_uids=17015238.

[7] Saslow D, et al. American Cancer Society Guidelines for Breast Screening with MRI as an Adjunct to Mammography. CA Cancer J Clin [Internet]. 2007 Oct [cited 2010 Mar 25]; 57:75–89. Available from: http://caonline.amcancersoc.org/cgi/reprint/57/2/75.

[8] Harms S, Flamig D. Breast MRI. Journal of Clinical Imaging [Internet]. 2001 May 25 [cited 2009 Dec 22]; 25: 227–46. Available from: http://www.ncbi.nlm.nih.gov/pmc/articles/PMC1421307/pdf/20010500s00011p669.pdf.

[9] Wenkel E, et al. Diffusion Weighted Imaging in Breast MRI: Comparison of Two Different Pulse Sequences. Acad Radiol [Internet]. 2007 Jun 6 [cited 2009 Dec 28]; 14: 1077–83. Available from: http://www.academicradiology.org/article/S1076–6332%2807%2900329-7/pdf.

[10] Friedrich M. MRI of the breast: state of the art. Eur Radiol [Internet]. 1997 Nov 17 [cited 2009 Dec 28]; 8:707–25. Available from: http://www.springerlink.com/content/07 gwh3lk6t0aral5/fulltext.pdf.

[11] Morris E, Liberman L. Breast MRI: Diagnosis and Intervention. 1st ed. New York: Springer, 2005. 518p.

[12] Park M, et al. The Role of Diffusion-Weighted Imaging and the Apparent Diffusion Coefficient (ADC) Values for Breast Tumors. Korean J Radiol [Internet]. 2007 Nov 3 [cited 2010 Mar 25]; 8(5): 390–5. Available from: http://www.ncbi.nlm.nih.gov/pmc/articles/PMC2626812/pdf/kjr-8-390.pdf.

[13] Chavhan G. Mri Made Easy. 1st ed. Toronto: Anshan, 2007. 264p.

[14] Razek A, et al. Diffusion Weighted MR Imaging of the Breast. Acad Radiol. Forthcoming 2009.

[15] Stadlbauer A, et al. Diffusion-weighted MR imaging with background body signal suppression (DWIBS) for the diagnosis of malignant and benign breast lesions. Eur Radiol [Internet]. 2009 Oct [cited 2010 Feb 15]; 19(10): 2349–56. Available from: http://www.ncbi.nlm.nih.gov/entrez/query.fcgi?cmd=Retrieve&db=PubMed&dopt=Citation&list_uids=19415286.

[16] Pereira F, et al. The use of diffusion-weighted magnetic resonance imaging in the differentiation between benign and malignant breast lesions. Radiol Bras [Internet]. 2009 Set/Oct [cited 2010 Mar 30]; 42(5): 283–8. Available from: http://www.scielo.br/pdf/rb/v42n5/a05v42n5.pdf.

[17] Tozaki M, Maruyama K. Diffusion-Weighted Imaging for Characterizing Breast Lesions Prior to Biopsy. MAGNETOM Flash[Internet]. 2009 Feb [cited 2010 April 22]; 2: 66–71. Available from: http://www.medical.siemens.com/siemens/en_GLOBAL/gg_mr_FBAs/files/MAGNETOM_world/MAGNETOM_Flash/MAGNETOM_Flash_Issue41.pdf.

[18] Palle L, Reddy B. Role of diffusion MRI in characterizing benign and malignant breast lesions. Indian J Radiol Imaging [Internet]. 2009 Dec [cited 2010 Mar 25]; 19(4):287–90. Available from: http://www.ncbi.nlm.nih.gov/entrez/query.fcgi?cmd=Retrieve&db=PubMed&dopt=Citation&list_uids=19881104.

[19] Hendrick R. Breast MRI: Fundamentals and Technical Aspects. 1st ed. Chicago: Springer, 2008. 254p.

[20] Luypaert R, Boujraf S, Sourbron S, Osteaux M. Diffusion and perfusion MRI: basic physics. Eur J Radiol [Internet]. 2001 Apr [cited 2010 Mar 25]; 38(1):19–27. http://www.ncbi.nlm.nih.gov/entrez/query.fcgi?cmd=–Retrieve&db=PubMed&dopt=Citation&list_uids=11287161.

[21] Yili Z, et al. The value of diffusion-weighted imaging in assessing the ADC changes of tissues adjacent to breast carcinoma. BMC Cancer [Internet]. 2009 Jan 14 [cited 2009 Dec 28]; 1–10. Available from: http://www.ncbi.nlm.nih.gov/pmc/articles/PMC2633008/pdf/1471-2407-9–18.pdf.

[22] Wenkel E, et al. Diffusion Weighted Imaging in Breast MRI* —An Easy Way to Improve Specificity. MAGNETOM Flash[Internet]. 2007 [cited 2010 April 22]; 3: 28–32. Available from: http://www.medical.siemens.com/siemens/en_GB/rg_marcom_FBAs/files/brochures/MAGNETOM_Apr_2008/clinical_womens_health_breast_MRI_improve_specifity_wenkel_janka_university_hospiital_erlangen_nuernberg_Flash_Apr08.pdf.

[23] Fortin MF. O Processo de Investigação: Da concepção à realização. 5th ed. Salgueiro N, translator. Lisbon: Lusociência; 2009. 388p.

[24] Marini C, et al. Quantitative diffusion-weighted MR imaging in the differential diagnosis of breast lesion. Eur Radiol [Internet]. 2007 Mar 14 [cited 2010 Apr 14]; 17: 2646–55. Available from: http://www.springerlink.com/content/a43v1910380456r4/fulltext.pdf.

Computational Vision and Medical Image Processing – Tavares & Natal Jorge (eds)
© 2012 Taylor & Francis Group, London, ISBN 978-0-415-68395-1

Efficient lesion segmentation using Support Vector Machines

Jean-Baptiste Fiot
CEREMADE, UMR 7534 CNRS Université Paris Dauphine, France
CSIRO Preventative Health National Research Flagship ICTC, The Australian e-Health Research Centre—
BioMedIA, Royal Brisbane and Women's Hospital, Herston, QLD, Australia

Laurent D. Cohen
CEREMADE, UMR 7534 CNRS Université Paris Dauphine, France

Parnesh Raniga & Jurgen Fripp
CSIRO Preventative Health National Research Flagship ICTC, The Australian e-Health Research Centre—
BioMedIA, Royal Brisbane and Women's Hospital, Herston, QLD, Australia

ABSTRACT: Support Vector Machines (SVM) are a machine learning technique that has been used for segmentation and classification of medical images, including segmentation of White Matter Hyperintensities (WMH). Current approaches using SVM for WMH segmentation extract features from the brain and classify these followed by complex post-processing steps to remove false positives. The method presented in this paper combines the use of domain knowledge, advanced pre-processing (based on tissue segmentation and atlas propagation) and SVM classification to obtain efficient and accurate WMH segmentation. Features generated from up to four MR modalities (T1-w, T2-w, PD and FLAIR), differing neighbourhood sizes and the use of multi-scale features were compared. We found that although using all 4 modalities gave the best overall classification (average Dice scores of 0.54 ± 0.12, 0.72 ± 0.06 and 0.82 ± 0.06 respectively for small, moderate and severe lesion loads, using $3 \times 3 \times 3$ neighbourhood intensity features); this was not significantly different (p = 0.50) from using just T1-w and FLAIR sequences (Dice scores of 0.52 ± 0.13, 0.71 ± 0.08 and 0.81 ± 0.07 for the same lesion loads and feature type). Furthermore, there was a negligible difference between using $5 \times 5 \times 5$ and $3 \times 3 \times 3$ features (p = 0.93). Finally, we show that careful consideration of features and preprocessing techniques leads to more efficient classification which outperforms the one based on all features with post-processing, and also saves storage space and computation time.

Keywords: lesion, segmentation, classification, support vector machines, brain imaging

1 INTRODUCTION

WMH appear brightly on T2-weighted (T2-w) and Fluid Attenuated Inversion Recovery (FLAIR) MRI modalities. They are a possible risk factor for Alzheimer's Disease (AD), with progression associated with vascular factors and cognitive decline (Lao et al. 2008). To quantify these changes in large scale population studies, it is desirable to have fully automatic and accurate segmentation methods to avoid time-consuming, costly and non-reproducible manual segmentations. However, WMH segmentation using a single modality is challenging because their signal intensity range overlaps with that of normal tissue: in T1-weighted (T1-w) images, WMH have intensities similar to Grey Matter (GM), and in T2-w and PD images, WMH look similar to Cerebro-Spinal Fluid (CSF). The

FLAIR images have been shown to be most sensitive to WMH (Anbeek et al. 2004), but can also present hyper-intensity artifacts that can lead to false positives. To improve the WMH segmentation performance, additional discriminative information is extracted from multiple MR modalities.

The most successful lesion segmentation methods in the literature have been developed for the detection of multiple sclerosis lesions, with a recent grand challenge comparing the performance of various techniques (Styner et al. 2008). Lesion segmentation algorithms can be categorised into unsupervised clustering or (semi-)supervised voxel-wise classification. Unsupervised methods suffer from the issue of model selection. Supervised methods such as neural networks (Dyrby et al. 2008) and k-NN Anbeek (et al. 2004) have been proposed. Neural networks are efficient but setting their parameters is difficult. The k-NN method performs relatively well, but is computationally expensive.

We present an SVM based segmentation scheme inspired by the work in (Lao et al. 2008; Zacharaki et al. 2008). Lao et al. applied four steps: pre-processing (co-registration, skull-stripping, intensity normalisation and inhomogeneity correction), SVM training with Adaboost, segmentation and elimination of false positives. Our implementation utilises a similar but more advanced pre-processing pipeline and a simpler training procedure. As one of the primary causes of errors in other approaches is false positive cortical regions, we incorporate advanced pre-processing including patient specific tissue segmentation and atlas based population tissue priors to minimize the false positive regions that are usually found with naive classifier. As a result of this the advanced post processing required by other techniques (Lao et al. 2008) are not necessary. We also evaluated the relative value of each MRI acquisition protocol for segmentation. This scheme is quantitatively validated on a significantly larger dataset with healthy aging, mild cognitive impairment and AD subjects.

2 CLASSIFICATION AND SUPPORT VECTOR MACHINE THEORY

Lesion segmentation can be formulated as a binary classification problem. SVM (Schölkopf and Smola 2001) solves it in a supervised way: given l labelled features $(x_i, y_i) \in X \times \{-1,1\}$, it builds a function $f : X \to \mathbb{R}$ such that $y(\cdot) = sign(f(\cdot))$ is an optimal labeling function. The function f is computed via the optimization problem:

$$f^* = \underset{f \in H_K}{\arg\min} \frac{1}{l} \sum_{i=1}^{l} V(f(x_i), y_i) + \gamma \|f\|_K^2 \qquad (1)$$

where $K : X \times X \to \mathbb{R}$ is a Mercer Kernel, H_K its associated Reproducing Kernel Hilbert Space of functions $X \to \mathbb{R}$ and its corresponding norm $\|\|_K$, and V is the hinge loss defined as $V(f(x), y) = \max\{0, 1 - y \times f(x)\}$. The loss function V controls the labeling performance, and the second term controls the smoothness of the solution.

The optimization problem is convex because of the convexity of the hinge loss function. However as the objective function is not differentiable, the problem is reformulated with additional slack variables $\xi_1, ..., \xi_l \in \mathbb{R}$:

$$ff^* = \underset{\substack{f \in H_K \\ \xi_1,...,\xi_n \in \mathbb{R}}}{\arg\min} \frac{1}{l} \sum_{i=1}^{l} \xi_i + \gamma \| \ \|_K^2 \qquad (2)$$

subject to : $\xi_i \geq V(f(x_i), y_i) \forall i \in \{1, ..., l\}$

The Riesz representation theorem states that the solution of (1) exists in H_K, and can be written:

$$f^*(\cdot) = \sum_{i=1}^{l} \alpha_i K(., x_i) \text{ with } \alpha_i \in \mathbb{R} \qquad (3)$$

By plugging the expansion of f from (3) in (2), the optimisation problem becomes a finite dimension optimisation problem. Let the matrix K be defined as $K_{i,j} = K(x_i, y_j)$. The optimisation problem is now:

$$\underset{\substack{\alpha_1,...,\alpha_l \in \mathbb{R} \\ \xi_1,...,\xi_l \in \mathbb{R}}}{min} \frac{1}{l} \sum_{i=1}^{l} \xi_i + \gamma \alpha^T K \alpha \quad \text{subject to:}$$

$$\begin{cases} \xi_i - 1 + y_i \sum_{j=1}^{l} \alpha_j K(x_i, x_j) \geq 0 & \forall i \in \{1, ..., l\} \\ \xi_i \geq 0 & \forall i \in \{1, ..., l\} \end{cases} \qquad (4)$$

Let $\mu, \nu \in \mathbb{R}^l$ be the Lagrangian multipliers. The Lagrangian of this problem is:

$$L(\alpha, \xi, \nu, \mu) = \frac{1}{l} \sum_{i=1}^{l} \xi_i + \gamma \alpha^T K \alpha$$

$$- \sum_{i=1}^{l} \mu_i \left(\xi_i - 1 + y_i \sum_{j=1}^{l} \alpha_j K(x_i, x_j) \right) - \sum_{i=1}^{l} \nu_i \xi_i \qquad (5)$$

Solving $\nabla_\alpha L = 0$ leads to $\alpha_i^*(\mu, \nu) = \frac{y_i \mu_i}{2\gamma}$ $\forall i \in \{1, \&, l\}$. Solving $\nabla_\xi L = 0$ leads to $\mu_i + \nu_i = 1/l$. The Lagrance dual function is:

$$q(\mu, \nu) = \underset{\alpha, \xi \in \mathbb{R}^l}{\inf} L(\alpha, \xi, \nu, \mu)$$

$$= \begin{cases} \sum_{i=1}^{l} \mu_i - \frac{1}{4\gamma} \sum_{i,j=1}^{l} y_i y_j \mu_i \mu_j K(x_i, x_j) \text{ if} \\ \mu_i + \nu_i = \frac{1}{l} - \infty \text{ otherwise} \end{cases} \qquad (6)$$

The dual problem consists in maximising $q(\mu, \nu)$ subject to $\mu \geq 0, \nu \geq 0$, and is equivalent to:

$$\underset{0 \leq \mu \leq \frac{1}{l}}{max} \sum_{i=1}^{l} \mu_i - \frac{1}{4\gamma} \sum_{i,j=1}^{l} y_i y_j \mu_i \mu_j K(x_i, x_j) \qquad (7)$$

Therefore the problem that α must solve is:

$$\underset{\alpha_1,...,\alpha_l \in \mathbb{R}}{max} 2 \sum_{i=1}^{l} \alpha_i y_i - \sum_{i,j=1}^{l} \alpha_i \alpha_j K(x_i, x_j)$$

$$= \underset{\alpha_1,...,\alpha_l \in \mathbb{R}}{max} 2\alpha^T y - \alpha^T K \alpha \qquad (8)$$

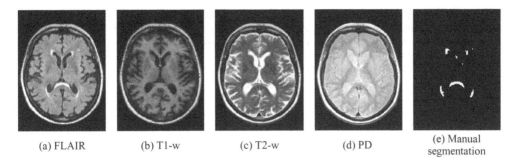

| (a) FLAIR | (b) T1-w | (c) T2-w | (d) PD | (e) Manual segmentation |

Figure 1. Axial slices from one subject illustrating the different MR modalities and manual segmentation. Lesions can be seen in the FLAIR and T2-w as a bright signal.

The training vectors with $\alpha_i \neq 0$ are called the support vectors. The optimization maximizes the margin, which is the distance between the decision boundary and the support vectors.

3 MATERIALS AND METHODS

3.1 Data

The dataset comes from the AIBL study (Ellis et al. 2009), where T1-w ($160 \times 240 \times 256$ image, spacing $1.2 \times 1 \times 1$ mm in the sagittal, coronal and axial direction, TR = 2300 ms, TE = 2.98 ms, flip angle = 9°), FLAIR ($176 \times 240 \times 256$, $0.90 \times 0.98 \times 0.98$ mm, TR = 6000 ms, TE = 421 ms, flip angle = 120°, TI = 2100 ms), T2-w ($228 \times 256 \times 48$, $0.94 \times 0.94 \times 3$, TR = 3000 ms, TE = 101 ms, flip angle = 150°) and PD ($228 \times 256 \times 48$ $0.94 \times 0.94 \times 3$, TR = 3000 ms, TE = 11 ms, flip angle = 150°) were acquired for 125 subjects. Lesions were manually segmented by PR, reviewed by a neuro-radiologist and used as ground truth in the classification.

3.2 Proposed algorithm

The proposed algorithm, summarised in Figure 2, consists of the following steps:

Pre-processing: images were rigidly co-registered (Ourselin et al. 2001), bias-field corrected (Salvado et al. 2006), smoothed using anisotropic diffusion and histogram equalised to a reference subject. T1-w images were segmented into WM, GM, CSF using an Expectation-Maximisation approach with priors (Acosta et al. 2009). For each modality, features were extracted within the mask defined below, and scaled to [0, 1]. Multi-modality features were created by concatenation of single modality features. Neighbourhood intensities features ($3 \times 3 \times 3$ and $5 \times 5 \times 5$ sizes) and pyramidal features (with 4 levels, taking one voxel per level, Gaussian kernel convolutions of $\sigma = \{0.5, 1, 1.5\}$) were tried.

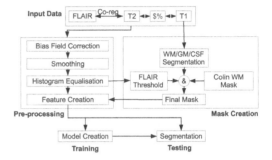

Figure 2. Summary of the WMH segmentation pipeline.

Mask creation: a global threshold on FLAIR images provides a high sensitivity, but poor specificity, which means it can be used to define areas of interest. To further reduce the areas of interest, we define the region W as the intersection of the dilated Colin WM mask (registered rigidly (Ourselin et al. 2001) then non-rigidly (Rueckert et al. 1999)) and the WM mask (defined from the segmentation of the previous step). Using the mean μ_W and standard deviation σ_W of the FLAIR intensities on W, an intensity threshold of $\mu_W + 2\sigma_W$ on W is used to define the mask M:

$$\begin{cases} \forall x \in W, M(x) = 1 \text{ if } FLAIR(x) > \mu_W \\ +2\sigma_W M = 0 \text{ everywhere else} \end{cases}$$

Training: a subset of 10 000 features, with half belonging to the lesion class, the other half belonging to the non-lesion class, randomly selected and equally distributed among the training samples was used to generate the classifiers. A Matlab implementation solving SVM in its primal formulation was used (Melacci 2009). The chosen kernel was the (gaussian) radial basis function. The width of the kernel and the regularisation weight were selected via a 10-fold cross validation.

Testing (Segmentation): the images in the test set were fully segmented within the mask created. Pixels outside this region were set to the non-lesion class. As post-processing, all the connected components of lesions with less than 10 voxels were removed.

3.3 Validation

The dataset was randomly split equally into training and test sets. A classifier was built using the training set, and then used to segment the test set. Then training set and test set were swapped, another classifier was built, and the rest of the segmentations were computed. Results were then merged. Model performances were compared using the Dice score (Dice 1945) DSC $= 2\lambda(S \cap GT)/\lambda(S) + \lambda(GT)$ (with S the computed segmentation, GT the ground truth and λ counting the number of voxels in a volume), the number of true/false positive/negative (TP, FP, TN, FN) voxels, the specificity ($TN/TN + FP$) and the sensitivity ($TP/TP + FN$) computed on the full image. Higher is better for DSC, TP, TN, sensitivity and specificity. Lower is better for FP and FN. Statistical significance was analysed via the p-values of paired t-tests (Ott and Longnecker 2008). We performed experiments to test the influence of the combination of modalities,

the influence of the feature type and the influence of using the mask in pre-processing instead of in the post-processing.

4 RESULTS

Figure 3 shows DSC, FP and TP for various combinations of modalities (using $3 \times 3 \times 3$ neighbourhood features). TN, FN, sensitivity and specificity are similar, so corresponding graphs are not displayed. As the overall lesion load impacts the segmentation performance, as previously report in (Anbeek et al. 2004), results are displayed for low (<3 mL), moderate (3–10 mL) and severe (>10 mL) lesion loads. When using one modality, FLAIR gives the best performance. Combining several modalities generates less FP and more TP. Table 1 indicates that the T1-w + FLAIR combination is statistically better than FLAIR on low and moderate lesion load, but T2-w + FLAIR is not. T1-w + T2-w + FLAIR combination is statistically better than FLAIR on the overall dataset. The model with the 4 modalities performs the best (Fig. 3), but not significantly better than T1-w + FLAIR (p = 0.50, see Table 1).

Figure 4 shows the performances of different feature types (using the 4 modalities). With neighbourhood intensity features, a $5 \times 5 \times 5$ size

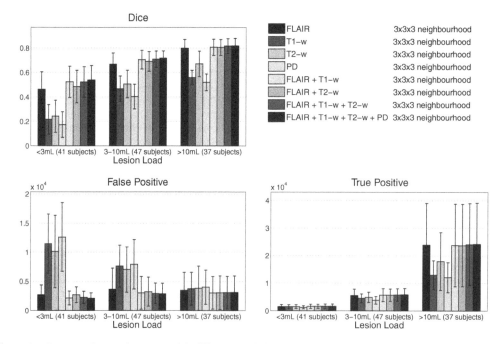

Figure 3. Segmentation performance with different modality combinations (using the $3 \times 3 \times 3$ neighbourhood intensity feature type).

Table 1. p-values of paired t-tests using $3 \times 3 \times 3$ features. Statistically significant differences ($p \ \alpha = 0:05$) in bold green.

Modalities		P-values of t-tests for lesion load in mL (number of subjects)			
Model 1	Model 2	<3 (35)	3–10 (47)	>10 (43)	Any (125)
FLAIR	FLAIR, T2-w	0.47	0.19	0.62	0.38
FLAIR	FLAIR, T1-w	0.047	0.032	0.57	0.070
FLAIR	FLAIR, T1-w, T2-w	0.048	0.014	0.26	0.047
FLAIR	FLAIR, T1-w, T2-w, PD	0.011	0.002	0.23	0.014
FLAIR, T1-w	FLAIR, T1-w, T2-w, PD	0.59	0.41	0.51	0.50

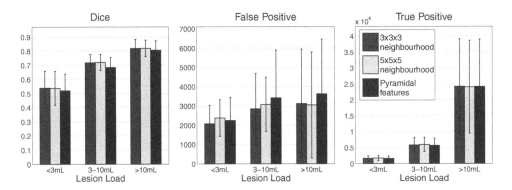

Figure 4. Segmentation performance with different feature types (using the 4 modalities).

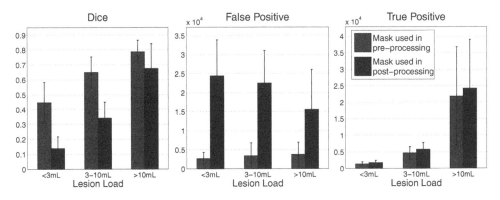

Figure 5. Using our mask M in the pre-processing gives better results than using it only as a post-processing step.

slightly increases the DSC compared to $3 \times 3 \times 3$, but the difference is not statistically significant (p = 0.93). Pyramidal features with 4 dimensions do not perform as well as neighbourhood intensity features, but the DSC difference is not statistically significant (p = 0.21 when compared with $3 \times 3 \times 3$ features, p = 0.18 with $5 \times 5 \times 5$).

As illustrated in Figure 5, using the mask in the pre-processing instead of post-processing

decreases FP dramatically and leads to a much better DSC. (Comparison using FLAIR and $3 \times 3 \times 3$ neighbourhood). The computation time in the prediction step being linear in the number of features to label, computing predictions for a significantly lower number of features (only within the mask) saves computation time. On average on the 125 patients, this represents a 41 times computation speed-up.

5 DISCUSSION

We have presented a machine learning scheme applied to the WMH segmentation problem. Our approach is inspired by the previous work on SVM but has a number of differences. It combines the use of tissue segmentation, atlas propagation techniques and SVM classification to get efficient and accurate segmentation results.

This work also quantifies the relative performance variations with regard to different modalities or feature types. Regarding the modalities, our results confirm that using all of the four modalities adds discriminative information and improves the segmentation results, as reported in (Lao et al. 2008). However, our quantitative results show that using only FLAIR and T1-w can give similar performance at a lower cost. One reason could be the lower axial resolution of our T2-w and PD images. Regarding the features types, there is a trade off between the complexity, storage place and computation time versus the performance.

As other important contribution of this work, the mask we define and use in the pre-processing has several positive impacts. First, it improves the classifier performance as the training features are selected in regions of interest, which leads to better classifiers. Second, computation time and storage space required are significantly lower (41 times lower on our dataset) as features and predictions are computed in a restricted area. Finally, using our mask in the pre-processing makes most of the complex post-processing steps required in current state-of-art methods redundant.

ACKNOWLEDGEMENTS

Data used in this article was obtained from the AIBL study funded by the CSIRO, www.aibl.csiro.au.

REFERENCES

Acosta, O., P. Bourgeat, M.A. Zuluaga, J. Fripp, O. Salvado, and S. Ourselin (2009). Automated voxel-based 3D cortical thickness measurement in a combined Lagrangian-Eulerian PDE approach using partial volume maps. *Medical Image Analysis* 13(5), 730–743.

Anbeek, P., K.L. Vincken, M.J.P. van Osch, R.H.C. Bisschops, and J. van der Grond (2004). Probabilistic segmentation of white matter lesions in MR imaging. *NeuroImage 21*(3), 1037–1044.

Dice, L.R. (1945, July). Measures of the amount of ecologic association between species. *Ecology* 26(3), 297–302.

Dyrby, T.B., E. Rostrup, W.F. Baar'e, E.C. van Straaten, F. Barkhof, H. Vrenken, S. Ropele, R. Schmidt, T. Erkinjuntti, L.-O. Wahlund, L. Pantoni, D. Inzitari, O.B. Paulson, L.K. Hansen, and G. Waldemar (2008). Segmentation of age-related white matter changes in a clinical multi-center study. *NeuroImage* 41(2), 335–345.

Ellis, K.A., A.I. Bush, D. Darby, D. De Fazio, J. Foster, P. Hudson, N.T. Lautenschlager, N. Lenzo, R.N. Martins, P. Maruff, C. Masters, A. Milner, K. Pike, C. Rowe, G. Savage, C. Szoeke, K. Taddei, V. Villemagne, M. Woodward, and D. Ames (2009). The Australian imaging, biomarkers and lifestyle (AIBL) study of aging: methodology and baseline characteristics of 1112 individuals recruited for a longitudinal study of Alzheimer's disease. *Int Psychogeriatrics* 21(4), 672–687.

Lao, Z., D. Shen, D. Liu, A.F. Jawad, E.R. Melhem, L.J. Launer, R.N. Bryan, and C. Davatzikos (2008). Computer-assisted segmentation of white matter lesions in 3D MR images using support vector machine. *Academic Radiology* 15(3), 300–313.

Melacci, S. (2009, September). Manifold regularization: Laplacian SVM. http://www.dii.unisi.it/~melacci/lapsvmp/index.html.

Ott, R.L. and M.T. Longnecker (2008, December). *An Introduction to Statistical Methods and Data Analysis* (6 ed.). Duxbury Press.

Ourselin, S., A. Roche, G. Subsol, X. Pennec, and N. Ayache (2001). Reconstructing a 3D structure from serial histological sections. *Image and Vision Computing* 19(1-2), 25–31.

Rueckert, D., L.I. Sonoda, C. Hayes, D.L. Hill, M.O. Leach, and D.J. Hawkes (1999, August). Nonrigid registration using free-form deformations: application to breast MR images. *IEEE transactions on medical imaging* 18(8), 712–721.

Salvado, O., C. Hillenbrand, S. Zhang, and D.Wilson (2006). Method to correct intensity inhomogeneity in MR images for atherosclerosis characterization. *Medical Imaging, IEEE Transactions on* 25, 539–552.

Schölkopf, B. and A.J. Smola (2001). *Learning with Kernels: Support Vector Machines, Regularization, Optimization, and Beyond (Adaptive Computation and Machine Learning)*. MIT Press.

Styner, M., J. Lee, B. Chin, M. Chin, O. Commowick, H. Tran, S. Markovic-Plese, V. Jewells, and S.Warfield (2008, sep). 3D segmentation in the clinic: A grand challenge II: MS lesion segmentation. In *MIDAS Journal, Special Issue on 2008 MICCAI Workshop - MS Lesion Segmentation*, pp. 1–5.

Zacharaki, E.I., S. Kanterakis, R.N. Bryan, and C. Davatzikos (2008). Measuring brain lesion progression with a supervised tissue classification system. In *Proceedings of MICCAI 2008*, pp. 620–627.

Computational Vision and Medical Image Processing – Tavares & Natal Jorge (eds)
© 2012 Taylor & Francis Group, London, ISBN 978-0-415-68395-1

Multimodality imaging population analysis using manifold learning

Jean-Baptiste Fiot
CEREMADE, UMR 7534 CNRS Université Paris Dauphine, France
CSIRO Preventative Health National Research Flagship ICTC, The Australian e-Health Research
Centre—BioMedIA, Royal Brisbane and Women's Hospital, Herston, QLD, Australia

Laurent D. Cohen
CEREMADE, UMR 7534 CNRS Université Paris Dauphine, France

Pierrick Bourgeat & Parnesh Raniga
CSIRO Preventative Health National Research Flagship ICTC, The Australian e-Health Research
Centre—BioMedIA, Royal Brisbane and Women's Hospital, Herston, QLD, Australia

Oscar Acosta
CSIRO Preventative Health National Research Flagship ICTC, The Australian e-Health Research
Centre—BioMedIA, Royal Brisbane and Women's Hospital, Herston, QLD, Australia
INSERM, U 642, Rennes, F-35000, France
Université de Rennes 1, LTSI, F-35000, France

Victor Villemagne
Department of Nuclear Medicine and Centre for PET, and Department of Medicine, University of Melbourne,
Austin Hospital, Melbourne, VIC, Australia
The Mental Health Research Institute, University of Melbourne, Parkville, VIC, Australia

Olivier Salvado & Jurgen Fripp
CSIRO Preventative Health National Research Flagship ICTC, The Australian e-Health Research
Centre—BioMedIA, Royal Brisbane and Women's Hospital, Herston, QLD, Australia

ABSTRACT: Characterizing the variations in anatomy and tissue properties in large populations is a challenging problem in medical imaging. Various statistical analysis, dimension reduction and clustering techniques have been developed to reach this goal. These techniques can provide insight into the effects of demographic and genetic factors on disease progression. They can also be used to improve the accuracy and remove biases in various image segmentation and registration algorithms. In this paper we explore the potential of some Non Linear Dimensionality Reduction (NLDR) techniques to establish simple imaging indicators of ageing and Alzheimers Disease (AD) on a large population of multimodality brain images (Magnetic Resonance Imaging (MRI) and PiB Positron Emission Tomography (PET)) composed of 218 patients including healthy control, mild cogniti ve impairment and AD. Using T1-weighted MR images, we found using laplacian eigenmaps that the main variation across this population was the size of the ventricles. For the grey matter signal in PiB PET images, we built manifolds that showed transition from low to high PiB retention. The combination of the two modalities generated a manifold with different areas that corresponded to different ventricle sizes and beta-amyloid loads.

Keywords: Population Analysis, Non Linear Dimensionality Reduction, Manifold Learning, Brain Imaging.

1 INTRODUCTION

Analysing trends and modes in a population, as well as computing meaningful regressions, are challenges in the field of medical imaging. A considerable amount of work has been done to simplify the use of medical images for clinicians, and summarising the information in just few imaging biomarkers, that would for example quantify and easily allow the interpretation of disease evolution. This is of great interest not only for clinical diagnosis, but also to study clinical studies and stratify cohorts during clinical trials.

Large medical databases challenge manual analysis of a population. Unbiased atlases can be used to describe a population (Lorenzen et al. 2005). (Blezek and Miller 2007) introduced the atlas stratification technique, discovering modes of variation in a population using a mean shift algorithm. (Sabuncu et al. 2009) introduced iCluster, a clustering algorithm computing multiple templates that represent different modes in the population. (Davis et al. 2007) demonstrated the use of manifold kernel regression to regress the images with regard to a known parameter, such as age. (Wolz et al. 2009) introduced the Learning Embeddings for Atlas Propagation technique, and showed that the use of manifold learning can improve the segmentation results compared to the simple use of image similarity in multi-atlas segmentation techniques. (Gerber et al. 2010) developed a generative model to describe the population of brain images, under the assumption that the whole population derive from a small number of brains. These techniques usually rely on computations of diffeomorphisms or transformations to compute distances between images. Alternatively it is also possible to use dimensionality reduction techniques directly on the image pixels intensities (Wolz et al. 2009), as we propose in this paper. Most dimensionality reduction techniques rely either on information theory or geometry. Information-based assumptions can be related to the maximum of variance (Principal Component Analysis (PCA), kernel Principal Component Analysis (kPCA)), entropy measure, etc. Geometric assumptions are either global (Multi Dimension Scaling (MDS), ISOmetric MAPping (ISOMAP)), or local (Local Linear Embeddings (LLE), Laplacian Eigenmaps (LEM), Hessian Eigenmaps (HEM), Diffusion Maps (DM), Local Tangent Space Alignment (LTSA). References to these algorithms can be found in (van der Maaten et al. 2007).

In this publication, we examine the use of NLDR techniques to analyse multi-modality brain images. AD is associated with the deposition in the brain of amyloid plaques, which can be imaged with PET using the Pittsburgh compound B markers (PiB), and with brain atrophy, which can be imaged with MRI T1 weighted (T1-w) images. We are investigating the use of manifold learning techniques for studying PET-PiB and T1-w.

2 MATERIAL AND METHODS

2.1 Data

The dataset is composed of 218 patients from the AIBL study (Ellis et al. 2009). T1-w (image matrix $60 \times 240 \times 256$, image spacing of $1.2 \times 1 \times 1$ mm in the sagittal, coronal and axial directions, TR = 2300 ms,

TR = 2.98 ms, TI = 900 ms, flip angle = 9°) and PiB (reconstructed image matrix $28 \times 128 \times 90$, $2 \times 2 \times 2$ mm spacing) scans were acquired.

2.2 Proposed algorithm

The proposed algorithm, summarised in Figure 1, consists of the following steps:

Pre-processing: PiB and MR images were affinely co-registered. All PiB Images were Standardised Uptake Value Ratio normalised to the mean uptake in the cerebellum crus region (Raniga et al. 2008). T1-w images were bias-field corrected in the mask creation process. T1-w images were then spatially normalised using an elderly brain atlas using affine and then non-rigid transformations. These transformations were then propagated to the PiB images. Noise was reduced in T1-w images using anisotropic diffusion, and in PiB images using a 2 mm Gaussian convolution.

Mask creation: using a subset of 98 MR images, an average elderly brain atlas and its associated probabilistic tissue priors (Grey Matter (GM), White Matter (WM) and Cerebro-Spinal Fluid (CSF)) were created from the segmentations obtained using citeAcosta2009 and a voting method. The segmentation of the atlas was used to create the mask used in the NLDR step (whole brain (union of WM, GM and CSF) or GM only).

NLDR: in this initial investigation, the NLDR was performed on the middle 2D slice using the mani Matlab implementation available at (Wittman 2005). Formally, NLDR performs the following operation: given n vectors $\{x_1, \ldots, x_n\} \in R^D$ and a target dimension $d < D$, n corresponding vectors $\{y_1, \ldots y_n\} \in R^d$ are computed, according to some

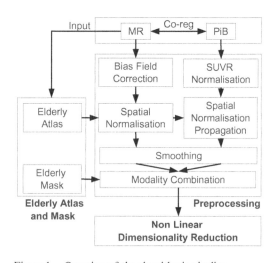

Figure 1. Overview of the algorithmic pipeline.

optimisation rules detailed below. In our study, the x_i are the brain images (the vector coordinates are the voxel intensities), the y_i are their low-dimension representations, n is the number of images, D is the input dimension (the number of non-zero voxels in the mask, common for all images), and d is the reduced dimension. Low dimension representation of population of T1-w, PiB and combined T1-w/PiB were then studied.

Initially LLE, LEM, HEM, and LTSA were investigated for multi modality brain imaging population analysis. LEM first builds a weighted adjacency graph and then solves an eigenvalue optimisation problem based on the Laplacian operator. The weighted adjacency graph is usually a graph of k Nearest Neighbours (kNN). In this graph, each image defines one vertex, and every image is connected with an edge to its kNN. Edges are bidirectional, and weighted based on distances between images, usually using the heat kernel. ISOMAP builds a weighted neighbourhood graph (usually kNN), then computes the weights between all pairs of points using shortest paths on graphs, and finally constructs the low-dimensional embedding via an eigenvalue problem. LLE builds a kNN graph, then computes the optimal weights minimising the sum of the errors of linear reconstructions in the high dimensional space, and finally solve an eigenvalue problem to map to embedded coordinates. HEM identifies the kNN, obtains tangent coordinates by singular value decomposition, and then computes the embedding coordinates using the Hessian operator and eigenanalysis. LTSA uses the tangent space in the neighbourhood of a data point (typically the kNN) to represent the local geometry, and then align those tangent spaces to construct the global coordinate system for the nonlinear manifold by minimizing the alignment error for the global coordinate learning.

Although we initially investigated several algorithms, we only report the LEM results as it was the only method we found to give stable manifold structures and that did not lead to numerical issues. In particular, HEM was found to have a prohibitive processing time. On our data, LLE had numerical stability problems that resulted from nearly-singular matrices (some eigenvalues being close to zero). LTSA did not reveal any meaningful manifold structures on our data. Moreover, several target dimensions were initially investigated, however we only report the results of 2D dimensional manifolds within, as they provided more stable and meaningful structures.

As the following results were computed using LEM (Belkin and Niyogi 2003), here are additional details about this algorithm. LEM aims is a distance-based dimensionality reduction algorithm. It aims at minimizing a weighted sum

of the distances in the final space (equation 1). The closer are the points in the original space, the higher are the weights.

$$\phi(Y) = \sum_{ij} w_{ij} \| y_i - y_j \|^2 \tag{1}$$

First a graph is built with edges connecting nearby points to each other. There are 2 variants: ε-graph (nodes i and j are connected if $\| x_i - x_j \|^2 \leq \varepsilon$) and K-NN graph (nodes i and j are connected if i is among the K nearest neighbors of j or j is the among K nearest neighbors of i). In this paper, the K-NN version is used. The default K parameter from (Wittman 2005) ($K = 8$) was used. The robustness of the manifold with regard to K was also analysed. Second the edge weights are computed. Two variants are available: heat kernel ($w_{ij} = e^{- \| x_i - x_j \|^2 / \sigma}$ if nodes i and j are connected, 0 otherwise) and simple-minded ($w_{ij} = 1$ if nodes i and j are connected, 0 otherwise). In this paper, we are using the simple-minded version (equivalent to a heat kernel version with $\sigma = \infty$). Third, the eigenmaps are computed. Let the the degree matrix D of W be the diagonal matrix with $d_{ii} = \sum_j w_{ij}$. The graph Laplacian L is computed by $L = D - W$. The optimization problem can be re-written:

$$\phi(Y) = 2Y^T L Y \tag{2}$$

The low dimensional representation can therefore be found by solving the generalized eigenvalue problem:

$$Lv = \lambda D v \tag{3}$$

for the d smallest nonzero eigenvalues. The d eigenvectors v_i corresponding to the smallest nonzero eigenvalues form the low-dimensional data representation Y.

3 RESULTS

The enlargement of the ventricles is one of the most obvious changes seen in MRIs of the brain as one ages. Figure 2 shows the LEM embeddings (i.e. the low dimension representation of the data) in dimension 2 with the MR images using a global tissue mask corresponding to the whole brain. A structure with two branches appears. The top branch corresponds to images with large ventricles, whereas the lower branch corresponds to smaller ventricles. Figure 3 shows that if only the central part of the brain image is used as input data (by eroding the mask), the structure of the manifold is conserved, with the same separation of ventricle sizes.

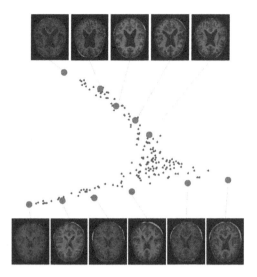

Figure 2. LEM embeddings using MR images registered with affine transformations and a global brain mask (218 images, input dimension: 23346, target dimension: 2). Several examples of corresponding images are also plotted showing increased ventricle size from bottom to top.

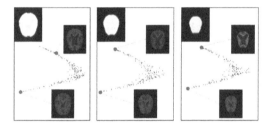

Figure 3. LEM Embeddings using MR images (registered using affine transformations) and global brain masks more and more eroded (218 images, target dimension: 2). The structure with two branches is conserved.

Amyloid load as observed using PET PiB is known to be related to AD. Figure 4 shows LEM embeddings in dimension 2 with PiB images. When using a global brain mask (input dimension: 23346) and images registered with affine transformations (Fig. 4a), the point cloud obtained has a similar structure as the one with MR images (Fig. 2) with two branches. The images in the bottom branch have increased PiB retention compared to the ones in the top branch. With a GM mask (input dimension: 12212) and images registered with affine transformations (Fig. 4b), the structure with two branches disappears. However, from top to bottom, the PiB retention increases. If the images are registered non-rigidly and a GM mask is used (Fig. 4c), there is a structure with 2 branches, the top branch with a low PiB retention, the other one with high PiB retention.

Figure 5a shows the LEM embeddings in dimension 2 of the data when combining the MR and PiB modalities, registered using affine transformations. Top left images have large ventricles, and bottom right images have a higher PiB retention. When images are registered non-rigidly, the structure with 2 branches appears again, and the PiB retention increases from top to bottom (Fig. 5b).

Table 1 illustrates the robustness with regard to the number of nearest neighbours K used in the neighbourhood graph. If K is too low or too high, the structure with two branches is destroyed. A value of K too high leads to jumps between different parts on the manifold.

4 DISCUSSION

In this paper, we investigated the use of LEM to model PET-PiB and MRI-T1-w to characterize the shape and appearance of images in a large clinical Alzheimer study. This can be particularly

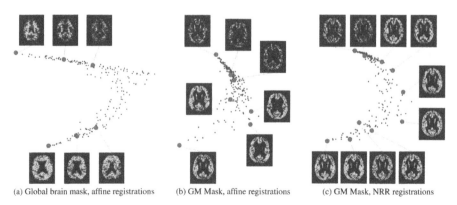

(a) Global brain mask, affine registrations   (b) GM Mask, affine registrations   (c) GM Mask, NRR registrations

Figure 4. LEM embeddings in dimension 2 using PiB images.

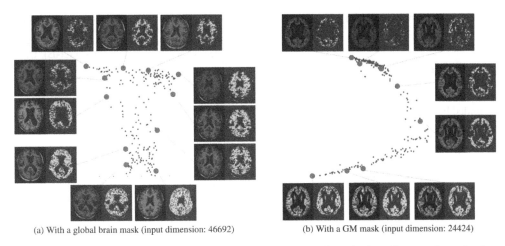

(a) With a global brain mask (input dimension: 46692)   (b) With a GM mask (input dimension: 24424)

Figure 5.   LEM embeddings in 2D using the combination MR + PiB (registered using affine transformations).

Table 1.   Test of robustness of LEM embeddings in dimension 2 with regard to K (number of Nearest Neighbours in the graph creation), using MR images and a global brain mask. If K is too low or too high, the structure with two branches gets destroyed.

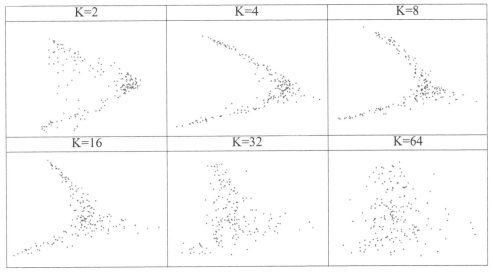

useful in atlas selection techniques, but can be applied in other areas. As far as shape analysis is concerned, NLDR techniques revealed that the ventricle size was the main variation in this population of brain images. The structure of the resulting 2D manifold with two branches was conserved when the cortical details were masked, leaving only the ventricles. This was expected as we used a L2 distance and many voxels were strongly affected with ventricle enlargement associated with the disease and ageing. To avoid biases from the ventricles (Fig. 4a), we examined

only the GM voxels when studying PiB intensity (Fig. 4b and Fig. 4c).

Many studies advice to use an image metric based on deformations to analyse population of images (Gerber et al. 2010). Nonetheless, we have shown that a simple Euclidean distance in LEM allowed identifying a low dimensional manifold structure corresponding to some anatomical and/or intensity variations. It is expected that using L2 distance would be less computationally expensive than deformation based approaches, such as diffeomorphic or elastic registrations.

This could offer faster processing especially for large databases.

ACKNOWLEDGEMENTS

Data used in this article was obtained from the AIBL study funded by the CSIRO, www.aibl.csiro.au.

REFERENCES

Acosta, O., P. Bourgeat, M.A. Zuluaga, J. Fripp, O. Salvado, and S. Ourselin (2009). Automated voxel-based 3D cortical thickness measurement in a combined Lagrangian-Eulerian PDE approach using partial volume maps. *Medical Image Analysis 13*(5), 730–743.

Belkin, M. and P. Niyogi (2003). Laplacian eigenmaps for dimensionality reduction and data representation. *Neural Comput. 15.*

Blezek, D.J. and J.V. Miller (2007). Atlas stratification. *Medical Image Analysis 11.*

Davis, B., P. Fletcher, E. Bullitt, and S. Joshi (2007, Oct.). Population shape regression from random design data. In *ICCV*, pp. 1–7.

Ellis, K.A., A.I. Bush, D. Darby, D. De Fazio, J. Foster, P. Hudson, N.T. Lautenschlager, N. Lenzo, R.N. Martins, P. Maruff, C. Masters, A. Milner, K. Pike, C. Rowe, G. Savage, C. Szoeke, K. Taddei, V. Villemagne, M. Woodward, and D. Ames (2009). The Australian imaging, biomarkers and lifestyle (AIBL) study of aging: methodology and baseline characteristics of 1112 individuals recruited for a longitudinal study of Alzheimer's disease. *Int Psychogeriatrics 21*(4), 672–87.

Gerber, S., T. Tasdizen, P.T. Fletcher, S. Joshi, and R. Whitaker (2010). Manifold modeling for brain population analysis. *Medical Image Analysis 14*(5), 643–653.

Lorenzen, P., B.C. Davis, and S. Joshi (2005). Unbiased atlas formation via large deformations metric mapping. In *MICCAI 2005.*

Raniga, P., P. Bourgeat, J. Fripp, O. Acosta, V.L. Villemagne, C. Rowe, C.L. Masters, G. Jones, G. O'Keefe, O. Salvado, and S. Ourselin (2008, Nov). Automated 11C-PiB standardized uptake value ratio. *Acad Radiol 15*(11), 1376–1389.

Sabuncu, M.R., S.K. Balci, M.E. Shenton, and P. Golland (2009, Sep). Image-driven population analysis through mixture modeling. *IEEE Trans Med Imaging 28*(9), 1473–1487.

van der Maaten, L., E. Postma, and H. van den Herik (2007). Dimensionality reduction: A comparative review. *10*(February), 1–35.

Wittman, T. (2005). MANIfold learning matlab demo. http://www.math.ucla.edu/~wittman/mani. Version 2.5.

Wolz, R., P. Aljabar, J.V. Hajnal, A. Hammers, D. Rueckert, and the Alzheimer's Disease Neuroimaging Initiative (2009). LEAP: learning embeddings for atlas propagation. *NeuroImage.*

Computational Vision and Medical Image Processing – Tavares & Natal Jorge (eds)
© *2012 Taylor & Francis Group, London, ISBN 978-0-415-68395-1*

2D MRI brain segmentation by using feasibility constraints

Valentina Pedoia & Elisabetta Binaghi
Dipartimento di Informatica e Comunicazione Insubria University, Varese, Italy

Sergio Balbi, Alessandro De Benedictis & Emanuele Monti
Dipartimento di Scienze Chirugiche Insubria University, Varese, Italy

Renzo Minotto
Ospedale di Circolo e Fondazione Macchi, Varese, Italy

ABSTRACT: Perform a robust MRI brain segmentation is an hard task, specially in presence of tumor that affect the normal brain tissue texture and intensity features. The brain tumors can take various shape, position and intensity level. For these reasons perform an accurate and general brain tumor segmentation is very difficult. The brain segmentation is an essential pre processing task for develop a good tumor detection and segmentation algorithm. In this paper we propose a new 2D brain segmentation algorithm that use graph searching principles. The aim of our work is to translate the segmentation problem in a constrained optimization easily solvable with a graph. To achieve this goal the brain boundary must be described by a feasible function and a setof constrains easily describable through the connections of a graph. Trough a preprocessing phase that "unwrup" the image in polar coordinates the brain boundary is a feasible function that can be found looking for the minimal path of a weighted graph with the dynamic programming. The brain segmentation algorithm proposed in this paper is a fully automatic and non-supervised method and don't consider a priori condition. The algorithm is validated on a set of volumetric FLAIR MR image, it appears robust in the presence of tumors different in terms of shape and position.

Keywords: MRI, Brain Segmentation, Polar Conversion, Feasibility Constraints, Graph Optimization

1 INTRODUCTION

Brain segmentation is an essential step for the solution of many problems of neuroimaging, especially in the study regarding segmentation of the brain tumor in Magnetic Resonance Imaging (MRI). Several methods have been proposed and experimentally evaluated, working on both 2D slice images or the entire 3D brain volume (Shattuck, Sandor-Leahy, Schaper, Rottenberg, and Leahy 2001), (Mikheev, Nevsky, Govindan, Grossman, and Rusinek 2008).

Well known approaches are based on histogram analysis (Mangin, Coulon, and Frouin 1998). Other methods use a deformable model which evolves to fit the brains surface. This method is for example implemented in FEAT FSL BET (Brain Extraction Tool) which is one of the most used brain segmentation tool (Smith 2002). Despite the sizable achievement obtained, the strong deformation of the normal tissue caused to the tumor presence may strongly affect the performances of the most promising methods.

To overcome this limitation, Khotanloua et al. (Khotanlou, Colliot, Atif, and Bloch 2009) have proposed a segmentation method based on the asymmetry analysis, considering that tumors are generally not symmetrically placed in both hemispheres, while the whole brain is approximately symmetrical respect the Mid Sagittal Plane. Proceeding from the assumption that in the normal brain the symmetry plane of the head in MRI is approximately equal to the symmetry plane of the segmented brain, Khotanloua developed a robust brain segmentation algorithm in presence of tumor. The applicability of this approach is limited by the validity of the symmetry assumption.

Our goal is to propose a novel fully automatic MRI brain segmentation method able to cope with critical cases in which tumors cause strong brain deformation. The method, free of any symmetry assumption, is inspired to the optimal surface segmentation based on graph optimization (Li, Wu, Chen, and Sonka 2006).

2D boundary-based segmentation utilizing graph searching principles has become one of the most frequently utilized in medical image segmentation tool. It has been especially applied to ultrasound images (Olszewski, Wahle, Mitchell, and Sonka 2004), but never to MRI brain segmentation. For this application we designed a preprocessing phase, that 'unwrap' the MRI head in polar coordinates, in such a way that it is possible to describe the brain edge like a feasible function with a set of constrains and then to represent the segmentation problem in terms of constrained optimization.

2 MINIMAL COST FEASIBLE BOUNDARY DETECTION

In this section the application of general 2D segmentation algorithm that uses graph searching is described.

Let be $I_{cart}(x, y)$ an image described on a square cartesian discrete grid $[x, y]$ (Fig. 1a). The image can be 'unwrapped' converting it in polar coordinates, obtaining $I_{pol}(\rho, \theta)$ with

$$\rho = \sqrt{(x - x_c)^2 + (y - y_c)^2}; \theta = arctan\left(\frac{y - y_c}{x - x_c}\right) \quad (1)$$

where (x_c, y_c) is the centroid of the object computed with the mean of the coordinates of the non-zero voxel. The polar sampling is a topic much discussed in literature (Dincic, Peric, and Jovanovic 2011) in this work we have chosen to consider a square grid for the description of the polar space for this reason an interpolation algorithm using an average filter is applied for the representation of radial coordinates in the discrete grid $[\rho, \theta]$ (Fig. 1b).

Working on polar image, the boundary of a circular object can be represented by a function $f(x)$ and it can described by a set of feasibility constrains. The feasible edge is defined as follows:

• in each column exist the edge and it has a single value so that it can be represented by a function $f(x)$;

• $|f(x+1) - f(x)| \leq 1$ for $1 \leq x \leq N - 1$ where N is the number of columns of the image.

Each feasible function $f(x)$ can be the object boundary. The goal is then to find the minimum cost edge subject to the feasibility constraints. The boundary cost is defined as follows:

$$B_{cost} = \sum_{x=1}^{N} c(x, f(x)) \quad (2)$$

where $c(x, y)$ is a cost image, that is, in our application the vertical gradient image (Fig. 2b).

In this context, the segmentation goal can be formulated as the search of the edge that minimizes the boundary cost. Segmentation becomes then an optimization problem whose solution can be represented in terms of a graph.

Graph nodes are cost image pixels whose values are node weights. The feasibility constraints become the edges of the graph as shown in Figure 3. Minimal cost feasibility boundary is the minimum cost path in weighted node graph. Dijkstra or Dynamic Programming algorithms can be applied to solve the optimization problem.

In this work we use the second technique.

The recursive solution is implemented by a bottom-up scheme: the solution of the whole problem is built from the solutions of the sub-

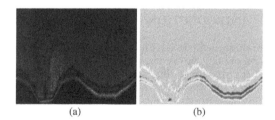

(a)   (b)

Figure 2. Cost image a) polar image b) vertical gradient.

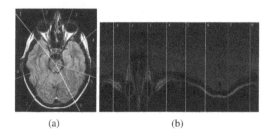

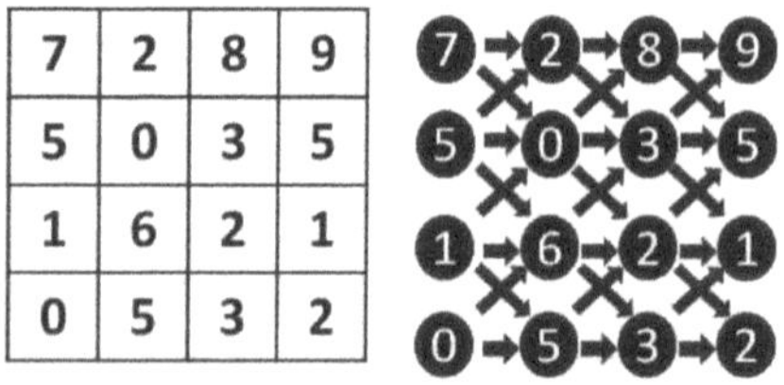

(a)   (b)

Figure 1. Polar conversion of a Brain MRI image, a) original image b) polar converted image.

7	2	8	9
5	0	3	5
1	6	2	1
0	5	3	2

(a)   (b)

Figure 3. a) cost image b) graph representation.

Algorithm 1.   Algorithm for computeing the Path Cost Image

---

for $j = 0$ to M-1 **do**
  $pImg(j,1) \leftarrow cImg(j,1)$
end for
for $i = 1$ to N-1 **do**
  for $j = 0$ to M-1 **do**
    if $i = 0$ **then**
      $pImg(j,i) \leftarrow cImg(j,i) + min(pImg(j,i-1), pImg(j+1,i-1))$
    else
      if $i = N-1$ **then**
        $pImg(j,i) \leftarrow cImg(j,i) + min(pImg(j,i-1), pImg(j-1,i-1))$
      else
        $pImg(j,i) \leftarrow cImg(j,i) + min(pImg(j-1,i-1), pImg(j,i-1), pImg(j+1,i-1))$
      end if
    end if
  end for
end for

Figure 4.   a) path cost image b) in red minimal path $B_{cost} = 4$ c) minimal path on the original graph.

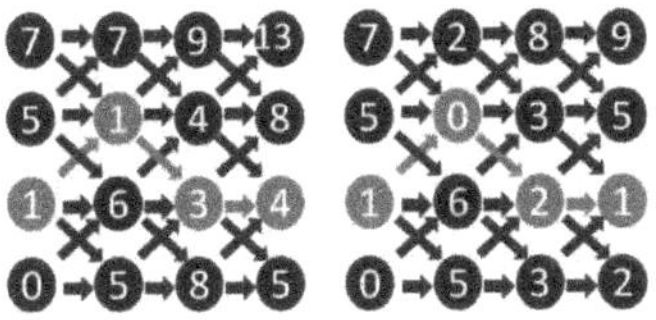

problems. The cost of the solution is equal to the cost of solving subproblems plus the cost attributable to the choice. The path cost image collects the intermediate information useful for defining the global optimal solution (Bellman 2003). The cumulative path cost image is computed with the Algorithm 1 where N is the number of column in the cost image, M is the number of rows, $pImg$ is the path cost image and $cImg$ is the cost image. In the path cost image the minimum value of the last column is the cost of the minimal path Figure 4a. Starting from this point and passing through the graph up to the first column, the minimal path is found choosing for each visited point the least of the adjacent nodes (Fig. 4). By this way the feasible function that minimizes the cost is detected. Working on polar image another constraints should be taken into account: converting the boundary found in cartesian coordinates that must be closed, than must be true the relationship $f(1) = f(N)$.

In the proposed algorithm this constraints is not considered in the minimization process but its validity is checked in the results.

3   BRAIN BOUNDARY ESTIMATION BY FEASIBILITY CONSTRAINTS

In this section the application of the technique illustrated above, to the 2D MRI brain segmentation, is presented. The algorithm is composed of two phases, conceived after the preprocessing polar conversion.

In the first phase the skull boundary is detected and in the second the brain is segmented. The edge points are then converted in cartesian coordinates.

As between the brain and the skull there is a layer of liquor, in the gradient MR image in the transition from the brain and this 'liquor cushion' and from the skull and the external air are similar and can be confused. Considering that in the FLAIR image, the bone is more intense than the brain tissue, the minimum cost feasible boundary on a polar 'unwrapped' head MR image coincides with the skull edge.

The 2D brain segmentation is accomplished in two phases as shown in Figure 5.

Phase 1: Sobel filter is used to compute the vertical gradient on the polar unwrapped image. The description of the cost through the vertical gradient of polar image is a particulary successful technique if the boundary is a circle in cartesian coordinates therefore is an horizontal line in the θ, ρ plan. In assial images of the brain this feature is very strong, especially by changing the aspect ratio of the image to emphasize the spherical shape of the brain volume. Is easy to identify the ellipse that contains all pixels brain image that are higher than the average of the intensity value, the relationship

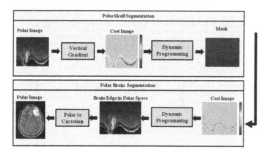

Figure 5. Brain segmentation.

between the major axis and minor axis of this ellipse gives the brain image aspect ratio, which can be made uniform changing the image size. Experiments have shown that this preprocessing phase emphasizes the boundary in the cost image but is not strictly necessary for the success of the segmentation algorithm. Every pixel of this cost function are the weights of thegraph nodes and using the feasibility constraints the graph connections are identified. The minimal path in the graph is computed using the dynamic programming algorithm illustrated above and skull boundary is found. A binary mask is computed distinguishing between pixels with ρ less and greater than the edge. This mask is applied to cost function and it is inverted for finding a new cost function for the second step: the actual brain segmentation.

Phase 2: The dynamic programming algorithm for the extraction of the minimal path is applied on this new cost function. The minimal path in the graph is the brain edge in the polar space. The last step is the conversion in cartesian coordinate of the detected boundary.

The algorithm is iterated on all the volume slices for finding the 3D brain segmentation.

4   EXPERIMENTAL RESULTS

Many experiments are performed for assess the good performance of the algorithm. In Figures 6(a)(b) some examples of brain segmentation are shows. The images shown are obtained with a FLAIR sequence, the slice thickness is 5 mm, the sequence is characterized by a long repetition times and by a reversal of the spin pulse at 180 degrees, the measurement is performed when the value of the liquid is close to 0. This allows the removal of the signal of liquid normally hyperintense in sequences with long repetition time. In the first row of the images the original slices are displayed, in the second the boundary detected by the

algorithm is superimposed on the original image and in the last row only the brain is extracted. The presence of the tumor don't affect the good performance of the algorithm. Is important to note that the algorithm performance remain good even in slices at eye level, in the follow will be shown how these situations are not so well managed to the FSL Brain Extraction Tool.

In Figure 6(b) some brain segmentation examples on different patients are shown. The results were qualitatively assessed by a panel of experts, all the experiment have been well evaluated by the experts. In Figure 7 two example of postoperative MRI are shown, is very important that the algorithm, as shown, is robust even in this cases that have high clinical relevance. The morphological and signal alterations detectable in the examination are due to the aftermath of the removal of the expansive mass. One of the goal of the postoperative control is to identify any tumor residual. For this reason, assuming the brain segmentation algorithm as a preprocessing phase for tumor detection segmentation and analysis, the goodness of the algorithm both in these cases is essential, for asses the robustness and the actual usability of the system. Both the cases are FLAIR sequences, in the first (Fig. 7(a)) the slices are continues with thickness is 5 mm, the second (Fig. 7(b)) is a volumetric sequence with isotropic voxel (0.6 mm); this allows a good anatomical detail and the possibility of a reconstruction on different orthogonal planes (assial, sagittal, coronal), however, at the expense of signal to noise ratio. In the first case, it is noted uneven area at the site of intervention due to the surgical cavity in which cerebrospinal fluid is observed, traces of blood and air bubbles. It's detectable a rim of perilesional edema (hyperintense) and into the deepest parts, in the vicinity of the lateral ventricle, the signal hyperintensity is consistent with a small tumor residual. Among the brain and the opercolum, which has been repositioned at the end of the intervention, there is a small flap hyperintense, consistent with a subdural flap, located in the meningeal subdural space between the brain and the skull, with a maximum thickness of 5 mm. Outside of the cranial theca there is an important thickening of the subcutaneous tissues overlying the operculum, clearly uneven, due to edematous imbibition. In the more external part there are the stitches with a typical signal distortion. Again in Figure 7(b) an MRI after surgical removal od right frontal expansive mass is shown. Contrary to the previous case here the operculum was removed to allow decompression of the brain. Near the lesion you can see a hyperintense edematous gliolitico

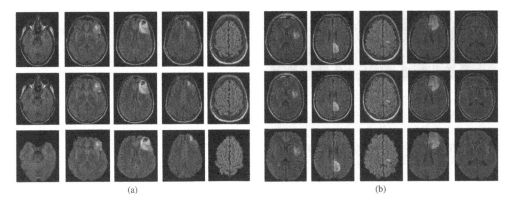

(a)

(b)

Figure 6.   Example of brain segmentation.

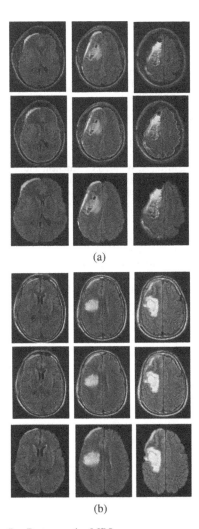

(a)

(b)

Figure 7.   Postoperative MRI.

halo; small right frontal subdural flap with a maximum thickness of 3 mm. All these anomalies compared to the structure of a standard brain MRI, make the automatic brain segmentation an hard task. Moreover, the big difference between the cases highlight the inadequacy of a knowledge based approaches to solve effective the segmentation problem. In both cases the segmentation algorithm results have been well evaluated by the experts. The presence or absence of the operculum, the asymmetries and large deformations seems don't effect the performance goodness. Our algorithm is compared with a well known and more used segmentation algorithm: FEAT FSL Brain Extraction Tool (BET) (Smith 2002) that use a deformable model which evolves to fit the brains surface.The results of the comparative analysis has shown similar behavior of the two algorithms in the standard situation, where the tumor does not alter the statistical distribution of gray image, the overlap of the results is almost perfect, considering the central slices of the MRI volumes. In Figure 8 some example of the comparison are shown, the red boundary is found by using the Brain Extraction Tool and the green one with our method. This good overlap is not keeps when considering slices at the eyeball level. In these cases, our algorithm seems better-detect the profile of the brain. In Figure 9 some example are shown with the same convention of the previous figure. Errors like those shown in Figure 9 may not be as serious if the brain segmentation is used only for the extraction of the image portion that is brain for example in fMRI analysis for detect the voxel that may be affected by the activation, instead become unacceptable errors if the brain segmentation if a preprocessing phase for a more complex analysis like tumor detection.

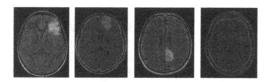

Figure 8. Performance comparison of our Algorithm vs FSL BET: central slice, good overlap.

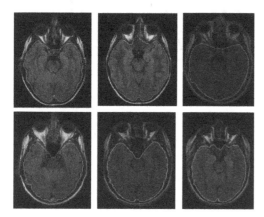

Figure 9. Performance comparison of our Algorithm vs FSL BET: slices at the eyeball level, bad overlapp.

5 CONCLUSION

In this paper a fully automatic and non-supervised method for the brain segmentation in MRI images is presented. The algorithm is tested on a large set of image and the results are qualitative evaluate by a pool of experts. The algorithm seems robust to presence of tumor that alters the standard distribution of the gray value of the image.

The aim of this work is to represent the segmentation problem in terms of constrained optimization and solve it finding the minimal path in a graph. The algorithm works separately on each slice of the MRI volumes, therefore without considering the topological constraints in z direction. The 3D version of this algorithm is certainly an interesting future work.

REFERENCES

Bellman, R.E. (2003). *Dynamic Programming*. Dover Pubn Inc.

Dincic, M., Z. Peric, and A. Jovanovic (2011). Optimal polar image sampling. *Opto-Electronics Review 19*, 249–255. 10.2478/s11772-011-0013-7.

Khotanlou, H., O. Colliot, J. Atif, and I. Bloch (2009, May). 3d brain tumor segmentation in mri using fuzzy classification, symmetry analysis and spatially constrained deformable models. *Fuzzy Sets Syst. 160*, 1457–1473.

Li, K., X. Wu, D.Z. Chen, and M. Sonka (2006, January). Optimal surface segmentation in volumetric images-a graph-theoretic approach. *IEEE Trans. Pattern Anal. Mach. In-tell. 28*, 119–134.

Mangin, J., O. Coulon, and V. Frouin (1998). Robust brain segmentation using histogram scale-space analysis and mathematical morphology. *1496*, 1230–1241. 10.1007/BFb0056313.

Mikheev, A., G. Nevsky, S. Govindan, R. Grossman, and H. Rusinek (2008, June). Fully automatic segmentation of the brain from T1-weighted MRI using ¡I¿Bridge Burner¡/I¿ algorithm. *Journal of Magnetic Resonance Imaging 27*(6), 1235–1241.

Olszewski, M.E., A. Wahle, S.C. Mitchell, and M. Sonka (2004). Segmentation of intravascular ultrasound images: a machine learning approach mimicking human vision. *International Congress Series 1268*, 1045–1049. CARS 2004—Computer Assisted Radiology and Surgery. Proceedings of the 18th International Congress and Exhibition.

Shattuck, D.W., S.R. Sandor-Leahy, K.A. Schaper, D.A. Rottenberg, and R.M. Leahy (2001, May). Magnetic resonance image tissue classification using a partial volume model. *Neuro Image 13*(5), 856–876.

Smith, S.M. (2002, November). Fast robust automated brain extraction. *Human brain mapping 17*(3), 143–155.

Computational Vision and Medical Image Processing – Tavares & Natal Jorge (eds)
© 2012 Taylor & Francis Group, London, ISBN 978-0-415-68395-1

Stochastic bone remodeling process: From isotropy to anisotropy

Nedra Mellouli & Anne Ricordeau

MAP5—Paris Descartes University—Paris, Rue des Saints-Pères, Paris Cedex, France
IUT de Montreuil, Université Paris, France

ABSTRACT: The present study proposes simulations of the bone remodeling process adapted to anisotropic trabecular bone structure. Anisotropy is related to bone mechanical properties which are complex. Many studies have been concerned with this biological process using voxel-level finite element models. As the remodeling process is known to take place in Bone Multicellular Units (*BMUs*), a stochastic germ-grain model seems well-adapted. Inspired from this random model where grains correspond to *BMU* area, we propose a *BMU*-level model. Driven by a few parameters matching biological ones, our model is more to be seen as a black-box model. First we present an isotropic version of this spatial point process, meaning that all its characteristics are homogeneous with respect to direction. This first step allows validation on 2D and 3D images. To take into account anisotropy, a variant of the previous model is proposed. Anisotropic structure of trabecular bone is known to reflect bone adaptation to directional stress. Many recent works focus on a better comprehension of anisotropic impact on the biological process. Integrating these results, we have modified the first model and obtained preliminary images. Simulating the process on more complex realistic images will allow bone quality descriptive parameters to be evaluated.

1 INTRODUCTION

The purpose of the current study is to propose a simulation process which mimics trabecular bone surface remodeling. This type of bone is a porous tissue made up of a mesh-like network of tiny pieces of bone called trabeculae. Trabecular bone is known to have a highly anisotropic structure reflecting bone adaptation to main directional stress, thus depending on skeleton sites [1]. During remodeling, cellular activity is both regulated by mechanical factors and chemical factors. Modification of some of these factors may induce trabeculae thinning or perforation, even trabeculae disappearance as can be seen in some osteoporotic contexts.

Let's now recall some of the main knowledge concerning the biological process. This process is a cyclical continuous one aiming at repairing damage and replacing old bone. Remodeling activity takes place in compact surface areas where two main types of cells, osteoclasts and osteoblasts, have a coordinated action in what is called basic multicellular units (*BMUs*) [13]. The life cycle of a *BMU* consists essentially of three successive phases: activation, resorption and formation. Activation involves recruitment of osteoclast precursors and their fusion into osteoclast cells. After activation, the resorption phase is carried out by these osteoclasts that attach to the surface and progress along it. The formation phase is carried out by osteblasts

which deposit osteoid and mineralize it, thus actually forming new bone. The reason a particular site is chosen for a *BMU* origination is not yet totally clear, but osteocytes are known to be involved in such an activation. Osteocytes are cells present throughout the mineralized bone matrix. They reside in lacunae and communicate with each other and probably with other surface bone cells through a canalicular network. These cells are known to act as mechanical sensors. They are sensitive to local stress orchestrating osteoclast and osteoblast activity [2,4,12]. Osteocyte apoptosis and mechanical induced microcracks may also stimulate the remodeling process [16,7]. In the following sections, we first present a random point process which is isotropic, meaning that all its characteristics are homogeneous with respect to direction. As there is now more evidence that directional stress is felt during remodeling activity, a variant of the isotropic model is then proposed including directional factors. It is worth noting that these random models, which are driven by a few parameters matching biological ones are more to be seen as black-box models aiming to generate synthetic images.

2 ISOTROPIC PROCESS

Remodeling is simulated as a temporal process where *BMUs* are principal objects (a *BMU*-level model). Our aim has been to propose a random description for number, location and shape of such objects driven with a few parameters matching as possible biological classic ones. Let's recall that the main parameters that are commonly used to describe the biological remodeling process are activation frequency (*AF*), related to number of *BMUs* activated by unit of time, and balance between formation and resorption known as bone balance (Δ*B*), where a negative bone balance corresponds to bone loss as observed in osteoporosis. With *BMU* shapes corresponding to saucer-shaped cavities resorbed by osteoclasts, Δ*B* represents the lack of volume reformed with new bone. To measure *BMU* activity in trabecular bone, the following formulae have been proposed in [13] to describe the relationship between *AF*, origination frequency (*OF*), total bone surface area (| *S* |) and number of *BMUs* created per unit of surface and per unit of time (*N*):

$$N = \frac{AF \cdot |S|}{W \cdot R} = OF \cdot |S| \cdot \sigma$$

(*W* is the mean width of BMU_S, *R* the mean rate of progression across the surface and σ the mean lifespan of *BMUs*).

A stochastic process can be used to simulate *BMU*-locations with *N* points or germs taking place randomly on the surface *S*, hence a set of random locations $\{X_1, .., X_N\}$. As the number of *BMU* is proportional to | *S* |, it can be expressed as realizations of a Poisson distribution with intensity λ, thus with mean $\lambda |S|$. With a point (germ) X_i considered as a *BMU* origination site and ε_i its shape (grain), this can be formulated as a germ-grain model [10]:

$$U \quad (X_i \oplus \varepsilon_i)$$

More precisely, each ε corresponds to the volume to be resorbed, where length (*L*), width (*W*) and depth (*D*) are taken randomly taking into account realistic values. However, locations for germs can't be chosen purely randomly, meaning uniformly on *S*. As previously mentioned osteocytes, encapsulated in the bone matrix, play a prevalent role in the biological process [3]. They are known to initiate osteoclast recruitment, inhibit osteoblast formation. Even without taking into account anisotropy, their signal or lack of signal is likely to ensure that surface areas which have been just remodeled are not of primary importance. Hence, the process has to be targeted. To this purpose, what can be seen here as an activation energy, is calculated at a *BMU*-level. We note $M(x_i, \varepsilon_i)$ the

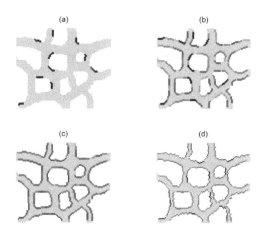

Figure 1. Example of a 2, *D* simulation, where the constraint is applied with a percentile τ corresponding to $\kappa = 85\%$. Images (*a*), (*b*) and (*c*) without resorption ($\alpha = 100\%$); image (*d*) with $\alpha = 50\%$.

state of the mineralized bone matrix for a given *BMU*. It is a set of voxel values simply expressed as the age from last formation, as the most plausible purpose for bone remodeling is to prevent excessive bone ageing, which can cause osteocyte death and increase susceptibility to fatigue micro-damage [11]. To this purpose, a constraint is introduced to validate each new proposed *BMU*. Average of values in $M(x_i, \varepsilon_i)$ (noted $\overline{M}$) is compared to a threshold τ. This threshold corresponds to a percentile evaluated from an estimated version of $\overline{M}$ distribution and a percentage κ. Taken as a global parameter κ is related to the fact that the process is more or less targeted.

3 ANISOTROPIC PROCESS

Trabecular bone is mainly found in different skeleton sites as vertebral, femoral and calcaneum bones. In such sites bones are subjected to different forces, such as compressive, tensile and shearing. According to Wolff's law, the trabecular bone structure is adapted to sustain the load by aligning the direction of the trabeculae to the direction of the stress trajectories [9]. This results in trabecular networks being highly anisotropic depending on anatomical sites. Such a network can correspond to an arrangement of vertical columns reinforced with horizontal struts in a vertebra looking like a plate-rod like structure, while in calcaneum a rod-rod like structure can be associated to compressive and tensile trabeculae.

Moreover, mechanical stress occurring during normal activities produces microscopic cracks of

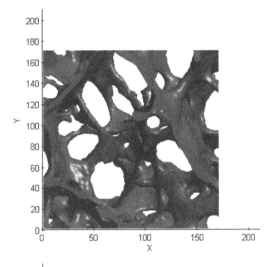

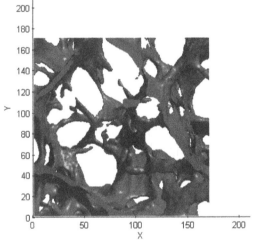

network which, likely to be sensitive to fluid flow, can also be damaged by microcracks. Stress and induced damage being supposedly dependent on trabecular orientation, a variant of the first isotropic model is now proposed.

To avoid having to modify mineralized bone-matrix status at a voxel-level, as it is done in finite element models, inhomogeneity is taken into account based solely on the directional labels. It is supposed that trabeculae have been labeled on the basis of their main orientations related to main stress. A initial study has consisted of supposing that BMU shape parameters are dependent on label L. Moreover, validation for a new L-labeled BMU is done on the basis of a threshold τ_L calculated on conditioned density $\overline{M}_L$. This conditioned constraint ensures that all the surface is taken into account. As can be seen in figure3, a global thinning is observed, depending on the label.

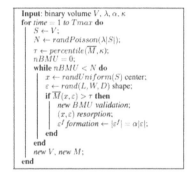

Figure 2. Initial volume with a resolution of $20\,\mu m$ corresponding to femoral head bone (Thanks to J.C. Souplet from INSERM U658 Orleans). Isotropic 3D simulation applied with a percentile τ corresponding to $\kappa = 85\%$ and resorption $\alpha = 50\%$. We observed plate and rod thinning, perforation of thin plates and disconnection or disappearance of rods.

different types: linear microcracks, small localized cracks in a cross-hatched pattern, diffuse damage and fully fractured struts. Studies have shown that such damage is dependent on the mode of loading [8]. Roughly speaking a compressive stress yields to linear microcracks while a tensile stress initiates diffuse damage [7]. Osteocytes are known to play an important role in the targeted bone remodeling process aimed to repair damage. They act as mechano-sensory receptors for stress and mechanical load through their canalacunar

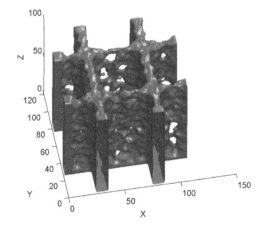

Figure 3. Example of an anisotropic 3D simulation where two labels L_1 and L_2 are assigned to a plate-plate like structure. $\varepsilon_{L_1} = (L,W,D)$, $\varepsilon_{L_2} = (L,W,2D)$ and formation parameter $\alpha = 50\%$. Thinning and perforations are more important on L_2-labeled plate.

4 CONCLUSIONS

The preceding results, more particularly concerning the anisotropic version of the model, are preliminary. Segmentation of real trabecular structure aiming to give directional labels remains to be done. A recent study given by [6] proposes a good approach of volume segmentation into plates and rods. Based on these results, it will be possible to calculate orientation of each trabeculae individually [5,17].

Inspired by random germ-grain models, we have proposed BMU-level models which are more to be seen as black-boxes driven with a few parameters. These can't be compared to much more precise voxel-level models using finite element analysis to calculate local mechanical strains resulting from external loads [2,3]. Such models have been able to explain essential features of the remodeling process, such as progression of osteoclast, BMU shapes and possible bone directional adaptation. But their main limitation is that they have a high computing cost.

Simulating our random process on more complex realistic images will enable bone quality descriptive parameters to be evaluated. Their robustness could be tested, as well as correlation between $3D$ parameters and corresponding $2D$ parameters obtained from simulated radiographic images. Temporal evolution scenarios could also be generated. The model being driven by a few realistic parameters correlated to physiological observed ones, a time parameter might be possible. Then relevant temporal scenarios might also be generated, such as young healthy bone remodeling and increasing remodeling rate in menopause due to estrogen deficiency and targeted failure.

ACKNOWLEDGEMENT

This work is a research topic of the MATAIM (Modèles Anisotropiques de Textures. Applications à l'Imagerie Médicale) project ANR-09-BLAN-0029-01 supported by a Research National Agency (ANR).

REFERENCES

[1] D. Chappard, M-F. Baslé, E. Legrand, M. Audran. *Trabecular bone microarchitecture: a review.* Morphologie, 92:162–170 (2008).

[2] J.C. Souplet, R. Hambli, C.L. Benhamou. *Anisotropy and mechano-transduction.* Osteoporos Int, 21, (2010).

[3] R. van Oers, B. van Rietbergen, K. Ito, P. Hilbers, R. Huiskes. *3D simulation of remodeling at the level of the cell and its deregulation in disuse* Osteoporos Int, 21, (2010)

[4] F. Peyrin, A. Larrue. Micro-ct imaging at the cellular scale: a new tool for the 3D visualisation of bone microcracks and osteocyte lacuna. Osteoporos Int, 21, (2010).

[5] A. Bonnassie, F. Peyrin, D. Attali. *Classification topologique locale d'images 3D.* Proc.18ème colloque GRETSI sur le traitement du signal et des images. Toulouse, France, (2001).

[6] G. Aufort, R. Jennane, R. Harba, A. Gasser, D. Soulat, C.L. Benhamou. Mechanical assessment of porous media using hybrid skeleton graph analysis and finite elements. Application to trabecular bone. ICASSP2006 Proceedings 2: 14–19, (2006).

[7] A. Robling, A.B. Castillo, C. Turner. *Biomecanical and molecular regulation of bone remodeling.* Ann Rev Biomed Eng. 8, 455–498, (2006).

[8] A. Badiei, Non invasive assessment of trabecular bone structural anisotropy -relevance to mecanical anisotropy. Thesis at Adelaide University, (2008).

[9] H.M. Frost, *Skeletal structural adaptations to mechanical usage* Anatomical Record 226, 403–422, (1990).

[10] D. Stoyan, W.S. Kendall, J. Mecke, *Stochastic geometry and its applications, 2nd edition* Wiley ed. (1995).

[11] A.M. Parfitt, Implications of architecture for the pathogenesis and prevention of vertebral fracture. Bone 13, 41–47, (1992).

[12] A.M. Parfitt, *Bone age, mineral density, and fatigue damage* Calcif Tissue Int. 53, (1993).

[13] C.J. Hernandez, S.J. Hazelwood, R.B. Martin, The relationship between basic multicellular unit activation and origination in cancellous bone., Bone 25(5), 585–587, (1999).

[14] C.J. Hernandez, G.S. Beaupré, D.R. Carter. *A model of mechanobiologic and metabolic influences on bone adaptation.*, JRRD 37(2), 235–244, (2000).

[15] C.J. Hernandez, G.S. Beaupré, D.R. Carter. A theoretical analysis of the relative influences of peak BMD, age-related bone loss and menopause on the development of osteoporosis., Osteoporos. Int. 14, 843–847, (2003).

[16] R. Ruimerman, B. van Rietbergen, P. Hilbers, R. Huiskes, The effects of trabecular-bone loading variables on the surface signaling potential for bone remodeling and adaption, Annals of Biomed. Eng., 33(1), 71–78, (2005).

[17] L. Pothiaud, P. Levitz, L. Benhamou. *Simulation of osteoporosis bone changes: effect on the degree of anisotropy* Int Noninvasive assessment of trabecular bone architecture and the competence of bone., Kluwer, New York, 496:111–121.

Computational Vision and Medical Image Processing – Tavares & Natal Jorge (eds)
© 2012 Taylor & Francis Group, London, ISBN 978-0-415-68395-1

Carotid artery atherosclerosis plaque analysis using CT and histology

F. Santos
CBQF/Escola Superior de Biotecnologia—Universidade Católica Portuguesa, Porto, Portugal
Department of Biomedical Engineering, Tampere University of Technology, Tampere, Finland

A. Joutsen
Department of Biomedical Engineering, Tampere University of Technology, Tampere, Finland

J. Salenius
Department of Surgery, Tampere University Hospital, Tampere, Finland

H. Eskola
Department of Biomedical Engineering, Tampere University of Technology, Tampere, Finland

ABSTRACT: This research had its focus in the creation of a protocol able to diagnose atherosclerosis and to segment the atherosclerotic plaques into different tissue components. The protocol compared *in vivo* and *in vitro* Multidetector Computed Tomography (MDCT) with histology studies. Four patients composed the data set. After the plaque samples were extracted in carotid artery endarterectomy, they were cast in paraffin, imaged, sliced and stained for the histology study. ImageJ was used to draw by hand regions of interest around the plaque, and to obtain an auto-segmentation of the plaques and their components. The final results showed a correct correlation and representation of the atherosclerotic plaque between the different modalities. The protocol and methods used in this study were confirmed as a viable way of diagnostic and follow-up of the patients suffering from atherosclerosis in the carotid arteries.

1 INTRODUCTION

Vascular disorders are becoming a great peril to the western world by being one of the most common reasons of mortality or morbidity in the last century and also named the disease of the XXI century (McKinney et al., 2005). When talking specifically of atherosclerosis usually the most known are the coronary and the carotid atherosclerosis but in fact it is a systemic disease (Shinohara et al., 2008). Being present from a very tender age and developing with the years by reasons also not fully understood, there has been the need to evolve the current diagnostic methods and protocols.

The risk of stroke is related to the severity of stenosis, plaque composition and morphology. (de Weert et al., 2009; Kwee et al., 2009; Miralles, 2006) Certain symptoms allow an early study of the evolution of atherosclerosis facilitating a correct decision on the steps to take to prevent or treat, if it has already reached an advanced stage of the disease. (Vukadinovic et al., 2010; Enterline et al., 2006) MDCT has been accepted in previous studies as a viable way of assessment of the atherosclerotic plaque and plaque components in carotid arteries and a tool for the classification of the plaque surface. (de Weert et al., 2008; de Weert et al., 2009; Enterline et al., 2006; Randoux B. et al., 2001) Wintermark has also determined that there is a correspondence between the *in vivo* CT and the *in vitro* histology analysis as representing correctly the plaque composition. (Wintermark M. et al., 2008)

The goal of this study was to study a viable way to improve and help the diagnostic of atherosclerosis using different methods of analysis as MDCT (*in vivo* and *in vitro*) and histology, this one as a comparison, and the ability to evaluate the presence of each plaque component.

2 MATERIALS AND METHODS

2.1 *Patients*

Four male patients (age 66.3 ± 15.9) undergoing carotid artery endarterectomy were recruited from the Tampere University Hospital, Tampere,

Finland. Before the patients went to endarterectomy a Computed Tomography Angiography (CTA) exam was made between the aorta arch and the vertex of the skull for the study of probable thrombosis in the brain and to study the anatomy of the vessels.

Endarterectomy of the internal carotid artery was executed with the extraction of the plaques, followed by the storage of the plaques in 10% formalin for 24 hours. After this were moved to another container with ethanol 70%.

Only one of the patients (Patient n° 1) underwent the three types of imaging: *in vivo* MDCT, *in vitro* MDCT and histology. Patient n° 4 underwent *in vivo* and *in vitro* MDCT, and Patients n° 2 and n° 3 only *in vivo* MDCT.

2.2 *Imaging*

For the *in vivo* CTA two different MDCT machines were used: a General Electric LightSpeed (helical scanning, slice thickness of 0.5 mm, slice increment of 0.5 mm, 120 kVp and a current ranging from 157 mAs to 653 mAs) and a Phillips Brilliance (helical scanning, slice thickness of 1 mm, slice increment of 0.5 mm, 120 kV and a current ranging from 310 mAs to 461 mAs). The resulting transverse image matrixes were 512×512 pixels in size.

For the *in vitro* study the plaques were cast in paraffin and after that sliced with a microtome and stained. Only one of the patient's sliced plaques (Patient n° 1) was imaged using MDCT (Philips Brilliance 64, Helix protocol, 0.55 mm slice thickness with spacing between slices of 0.27 mm, 120 kVp, and 300 mAs).

This same patient was used for the histology study, stained with Hematoxylin and Eosin (HE). The histology images were in a stored in the serve of Institute of Medical Technology of University of Tampere and downloaded using JVSview (Isola J. et al., 2010).

Patient n°4 had his plaque imaged using MDCT with the same parameters as of the Patient n° 1 to obtain a reconstruction of the whole plaque.

2.3 *Segmentation, quantification and mapping*

For the segmentation of the *in vivo* CT images the Hounsfield Units (HU) intervals for each plaque component (lipid, fibrous and calcified) had to be searched within the existent literature. Also, for the differentiation between surrounding tissues and the vessel, the Intima-Media Thickness (IMT) had to be determined.

The resultant images from the *in vivo* MDCT, *in vitro* MDCT and histology were exported to ImageJ (Rasband; National Institute of Mental Health, Bethesda, Md., USA), with custom made plugins (CT Window & Level, ROI Manager, DICOM Sort) and the PolyMeasure package made by Erik Meijering of the Erasmus University (de Weert et al., 2006). After locating the atherosclerotic plaque in the vessel using the presence of calcified tissue as a differentiating factor, ten Regions of Interest (ROI) were created proximal and distal to the atherosclerotic plaque in the carotid artery. The purpose was to determine the attenuation of the blood/contrast agent in each patient. In CT images the stenosis is usually visible as a narrowing of the vessel lumen, which has a higher attenuation because of the contrast agent. This allows determining the lumen HU interval so a correct segmentation and separation between lumen and atherosclerotic plaque is produced.

After this preliminary study the *in vivo* plaques were segmented using two sets of ROIs, one for the lumen and another one for the total area of the vessel. IMT was used to expand the vessel ROI to include also the vessel wall. The final step was to use the ImageJ plugin PolyROI with the HU intervals for each component for the auto-segmentation of the plaques using the two ROI sets (Fig. 1).

The resultant data was inserted into an Excel sheet for statistical analysis and to create the plaque profile. ImageJ exported a TIFF file than was imported to a custom-made Matlab routine to obtain a 3D rendering of the plaques.

For the *in vitro* segmentation the PolyROI was used with the plaque outline ROIs. For the *in vitro* histological segmentation ImageJ's ROI Manager plugin, was used, which allowed creating ROIs by hand in each component's outline- Figure 2. The criterion used for the separation between tissues

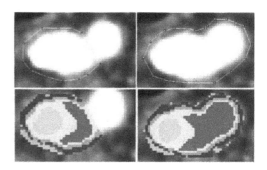

Figure 1. Segmentation of the *in vivo* samples (carotid bifurcation) (top to bottom; left to right). Panel 1 and 2: ROI definition of the entire vessel. Panel 3 and 4: Segmentation result after processing. Coloring: Red: Blood (344–390 HU); Yellow: Calcified tissue (210–771 HU); Darker yellow: Calcified tissue (over 771 HU); other colors are fibrotic and lipid tissue.

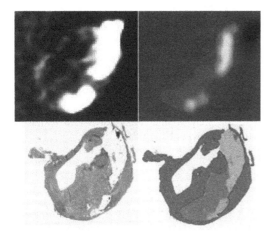

Figure 2. Segmentation of the *in vitro*. Panel 1 and 2: Paraffin casted plaque and segmentation. Panel 3 and 4: Plaque isolated and segmentation. Coloring: Red: Red: Fibrotic tissue (63–122 HU); Purple: Lipid tissue (30–57 HU) Cyan: Calcified tissue (210—∞ HU).

was the outline of each component using the pre-segmented *in vitro* and *in vivo* CT images to separate the different tissues.

As a final step the HU intervals of each hand-segmented component was assessed to see if the segmentation of histological plaque could be a viable path to study.

3 RESULTS

3.1 *IMT*

The resultant IMT values obtained from the article analysis (78 articles used) are represented in Table 1.

The increase seen was 34% in men and 36% in women, with no difference between sexes.

The thickness of the vessel wall (IMT) used was 1.0 mm to be sure to include all the vessel structures in the *in vivo* segmentation.

3.2 *HU intervals*

From the literature review of 40 articles the resultant HU intervals for each component of the atherosclerotic plaque were as seen in Table 2.

The difference between the maximum of the soft tissue and the minimum of the fibrous is minimal, possibly leading to errors in the segmentation and differentiation between these two components. The calcified interval had to have an open higher value because it often surpasses the attenuation of bone.

Table 1. IMT values for normal and atherosclerotic vessel in men and women (mm).

	Healthy		Atherosclerosis	
	Men	Women	Men	Women
Average	0.72	0.69	0.97	0.94
Standard deviation	0.16	0.14	0.24	0.23

Table 2. HU interval for the different atherosclerotic components.

HU values	Soft	Fibrous	Calcified
Minimum	30	63	21
Maximum	57	122	∞

Table 3. Patient's stenosis measured by the physician and by the methodology.

Patients	Physician	Segmentation	Error
1	95%	100%	5%
2	70%	98%	28%
3	75%	100%	25%
4	80%	100%	20%

3.3 *Maximum stenosis*

As can be seen in Table 3 the correspondence between physician and protocol measurement is not the best.

The discrepancy can be explained by the problems in the analysis protocol and in the differences between both measurement methods.

3.4 *Components*

The error calculation in patient n° 1 is between *in vitro* and histology as these are the only modalities that can be compared because of the existence of slices instead of a whole plaque, case of the patient n° 4 which error calculation is between *in vivo* and *in vitro*.

From this data we can say that the worst correspondence happens within the lipid tissue and between *in vivo* and *in vitro* studies, in our case the CT images in these two modalities.

The low correlation between the *in vivo* and *in vitro* CT can be attributed to the effect of the paraffin on the soft tissues, lipid and fibrotic. The merging of this substance with the tissues decreases this last ones HU values altering their HU interval. The HU intervals can be seen in Table 5, with the comparison between the literature review HU intervals and the ones from the *in vitro* study.

Table 4. Results of the segmentation of the data for each modality giving the percentage of each plaque component and lumen.

Patient		1	2	3	4
Lipid	*In vivo*	7.3%	3.9%	7.9%	6.0%
	In vitro	26.0%			21.1%
	Histology	24.3%			
Error		1.7%			15%
Fibrous	*In vivo*	18.0%	12.0%	17.4%	15.7%
	In vitro	68.8%			12.8%
	Histology	71.2%			
Error		2.4%			2.9%
Calcified	*In vivo*	19.8%	41.3%	41.0%	53.8%
	In vitro	5.2%			46.2%
	Histology	4.5%			
Error		0.7%			7.5%
Lumen		32.5%	25.3%	12.8%	5.2%

Table 5. Comparison between HU component intervals for the literature review and the *in vitro* study.

		Minimum	Maximum
Literature	Lipid	30	57
	Fibrous	63	122
	Calcified	210	771
Experimental	Lipid	−180	−7
	Fibrous	−204	136
	Calcified	−22	520

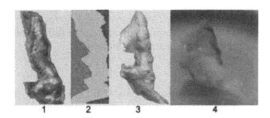

Figure 3. Atherosclerotic plaque for Patient n° 4. Panel 1: *In vivo* CT. Panel 2: Plaque profile for percentage of each component. Panel 3: *In vitro* CT—whole plaque. Panel 4: Photo after endarterectomy Coloring in the panels 1, 2 and 3. Red: Blood (344–390 HU); Yellow: Calcified tissue (210–771 HU); Green: Calcified tissue (over 771 HU).

And as a last observation that can be made is the similar comparison between the *in vitro* modalities, proving that the segmentation was correctly done.

Figure 3 represents all the imaging modalities and the different studies after the Matlab rendering with a photo of the plaque for Patient n° 4.

4 DISCUSSION

The major problems found in this study were from the image definition of the acquired data. The work-stations the doctors use in the diagnostic apply a smoothing algorithm when representing the vessel. The smoothing alters the contours and shape of the vessel diverting from the true stenosis. Also the image planes are reformatted to have a transversal view of the vessel.

The doctors use the NASCET criteria to evaluate the level of stenosis (visual measurement and defined as one minus the result of the quotient between the smallest vessel internal diameter at the stenosis and the internal diameter of the normal sized vessel). In the case of our semi-automatic segmentation the stenosis level is the percentage occupied by the plaque inside artery wall. We could use the NAS-CET criteria but as we cannot define with certainty the inner and outer vessel walls in the CT images because of the lack of definition, the measurement of two diameters would possibly introduce more significant errors in the measurement and calculation.

Partial-volume effect, usual in all the imaging studies, which is defined by the reconstruction algorithms of the CT machine by merging and averaging neighborhood pixel values to create a new pixel, was also seen in the image sets with a loss of the edge definition. The result is a higher difficulty to separate and differentiate the tissues present in the plaque. This effect was seen both in the *in vivo* and in the *in vitro* images. This could be also the effect of two different factors: the differences between dense and sparse material (abrupt changes of the HU values in the component borders cause errors in the reconstruction algorithm) and because of the data acquisition format. This last topic comes from the way that the CT scanning was done. The imaging of the vessel wasn't made perpendicular to the vessel but oblique, giving wrong wall thickness and making it not the most suitable to the segmentation. As a result the component percentage study can be undervaluing or overvaluing the true tissue volumes.

5 CONCLUSIONS

The first conclusion that we can apprehend from this study is that atherosclerosis in the carotid arteries increases significantly the IMT without much difference between sexes. As in the references the most prevalent tissue inside the lesion was the calcified. It was easy to identify and differentiate with a large variability between patients. The most viable way of conducting an *in vitro* study of the plaque after endarterectomy is to image the plaque as a whole and without casting to prevent any distortions of the tissues HU value intervals.

The results obtained meet the same conclusions of the previous studies, that MDCT and histology are viable tools to study, define and characterize the atherosclerotic plaques in *in vivo* and *in vitro* situations. One difference is that we conclude that histological studies alter the plaque morphology in a way that becomes practically impossible to relate with the in vivo correspondence and should only be done when studying cell population and plaque evolution instead of diagnostic and morphology analysis.

The choice of the methods of analysis was made by the fact that MDCT studies had been already done and the equipment was available in the Tampere University Hospital (TUH). ImageJ was chosen because it is a freeware tool that has already many plugins available online and represented an easy tool for the early study that is this work. A future approach to this theme may be the inclusion of different methods of diagnostic as ultra-sounds and magnetic resonance imaging and with an improved protocol with a more specific programming tool, as Matlab to be able to create a more specific algorithm of analysis and rendering of the plaques.

As a final conclusion we can say that the developed protocol was confirmed to be a viable way of diagnosis and follow-up of the patients suffering from atherosclerotic plaque in the carotid arteries.

REFERENCES

de Weert T.T., Cretier S. 2009. Atherosclerotic plaque surface morphology in the carotid bifurcation assessed with multidetector computed tomography angiography. *Stroke* 40(4): 1334–1340.

de Weert T.T., Ouhlous M. 2006. *In vivo* characterization and quantification of atherosclerotic carotid plaque components with multidetector computed tomography and histopathological correlation. *Arteriosclerosis, Thrombosis and Vascular Biology* 26(10):2366–2372.

de Weert T.T., Monyé C. 2008. Assessment of atherosclerotic carotid plaque volume with multidetector computed tomography angiography. *International Journal of Cardiovascular Imaging* 24(7):751–759.

Enterline D.S., Kapoor G. 2006. A practical approach to CT angiography of the neck and brain. *Technical Vascular Interventional Radiology* 9(4):192–204.

Isola J., Tuominen V.J. 2010. Linking Whole-Slide Microscope Images with DICOM by Using JPEG2000 Interactive Protocol. *Journal of Digital Imaging* 23(4): 454–62.

Kwee R., Teule G. 2009. Multimodality Imaging of Carotid Artery Plaques. *Stroke* 40(12): 3718–3724.

McKinney A.M., Casey S.O. 2005. Carotid bifurcation calcium and correlation with percent stenosis of the internal carotid artery on CT angiography. *Neuroradiology* 47(1):1–9.

Miralles M., Merino J. 2006. Quantification and characterization of carotid calcium with multi-detector CT angiography. *European Journal of Endovascular Surgery* 32 (5): 561–567.

Randoux B., Marro B. 2001. Carotid artery stenosis: prospective comparison of CT, 3D gadolinium-enhanced MR and conventional angiography *Radiology* 220(1):179–185.

Shinohara M., Yamashita T. 2008. Atherosclerotic plaque imaging using phase-contrast X-ray computed tomography. *American Journal of Physiology and Heart Circulation Physiology* 294(2): 1094–1100.

Vukadinovic D., van Walsum T. 2010. Segmentation of the outer vessel wall of the common carotid artery in CTA. *IEEE Transactions on Medical Imaging* 29(1):65–76.

Wintermark M., Jawadi S.S. 2008. High-resolution CT imaging of carotid artery atherosclerotic plaques. *American Journal of Neuroradiology* 29(5): 875–882.

Computational Vision and Medical Image Processing – Tavares & Natal Jorge (eds)
© 2012 Taylor & Francis Group, London, ISBN 978-0-415-68395-1

Level set framework for detecting arterial lumen in ultrasound images

Amr R. Abdel-Dayem

Department of Mathematics and Computer Science, Laurentian University, Sudbury, ON, Canada

ABSTRACT: This paper presents a scheme for extracting arterial lumen from ultrasound images using Level Sets. The scheme uses a single seed point as an input. A level set framework, based on Chan and Vese model, is employed. The scheme produces accurate results compared to the gold standard images. Moreover, the proposed scheme was compared to various edge-based snake models found in literature. Experimental results over a set of 40 images showed that the proposed scheme generally outperforms edge-based snakes. Finally, sensitivity analysis over the entire set of test images revealed that the scheme is insensitive to the seed point location, as long as it is located inside the artery area.

1 INRODUCTION

Vascular plaque, a consequence of atherosclerosis, results in an accumulation of lipids, cholesterol, smooth muscle cells, calcifications and other tissues within the arterial wall. It reduces the blood flow within the artery and may completely block it. As plaque layers build up, it can become either stable or unstable. Unstable plaque layers in a carotid artery can be a life-threatening condition. If a plaque ruptures, small solid components (emboli) from the plaque may drift with the blood stream into the brain. This may cause a stroke. Early detection of unstable plaque plays an important role in preventing serious strokes.

Currently, carotid angiography is the standard diagnostic technique to detect carotid artery stenosis and the plaque morphology on artery walls. This technique involves injecting patients with an X-ray dye. Then, the carotid artery is examined using X-ray imaging. However, carotid angiography is an invasive technique. It is uncomfortable for patients and has some risk factors, including allergic reaction to the injected dye, renal failure, the exposure to ionic radiation, as well as arterial puncture site complications, e.g., pseudoaneurysm and arteriovenous fistula formation.

Ultrasound imaging provides an attractive tool for carotid artery examination. The main drawback of ultrasound imaging is the poor quality of the produced images. It takes considerable effort from clinicians to assess plaque build-up accurately. Furthermore, manual extraction of carotid artery contours generates a result that is not reproducible. Hence, a computer aided diagnostic (*CAD*) technique for segmenting carotid artery contours is highly needed.

(Hamou *et al.* 2004) proposed a segmentation scheme for carotid artery ultrasound images

based on Canny edge detector. This scheme has shortcomings dealing with noisy images, leading to contour bleeding in such cases.

(Da-chuan *et al.* 2008) introduced a dual dynamic programming method to detect arterial wall in ultrasound images. Some progress has been achieved in reducing the sensitivity to speckle noise. However, the computational complexity of the proposed method is questionable. Moreover, it requires the user to manually select the region of interest for further processing.

Abdel-Dayem *et al.* proposed many schemes for segmenting carotid artery ultrasound images, including the watershed based segmentation (Abdel-Dayem *et al.* 2005a,b), fuzzy region growing based segmentation (Abdel-Dayem *et al.* 2005c), fuzzy c-means based segmentation (Abdel-Dayem *et al.* 2006), graph-based segmentation (Abdel-Dayem *et al.* 2007), and complex diffusion based segmentation (Abdel-Dayem *et al.* 2009). These schemes provide satisfactory performance (overlap with the clinician-segmented images) in most cases.

All methods, described so far, may fail to produce accurate contours in some challenging cases (images with shadowing effects, high noise levels, partially occluded or incomplete contours). This performance pitfall hinders the applicability of the proposed schemes in real clinical trials. Active contours (snakes) are good candidates, if properly tuned, to overcome some of these shortcomings particularly, the incomplete contour problem.

Active contours are widely used in various computer vision applications to locate object boundaries. They are divided into two main categories: edge-based (Kass *et al.* 1988, Malladi *et al.* 1995 & Caselles *et al.* 1997) and region-based (level set active contour) models (Mumford *et al.* 1989, Osher *et al.* 1988 & Chan *et al.* 2001).

(Mao *et al.* 2000) proposed a scheme for extracting carotid artery walls from ultrasound images using a deformable model. The model's external force is defined in terms of the gradient image, which is highly influenced by the noise level within the original image. As a result, this scheme is susceptible to poor convergence to artery boundaries.

(Da-chuan *et al.* 1999) proposed a modified snake model for automatic detection of intimal and adventitial layers of the common carotid artery wall in ultrasound images using a snake model. The proposed model modified the Cohen's snake (Cohen *et al.* 1991) by adding spatial criteria to obtain the contour with a global minimum cost function. However, this scheme has the same pitfall as (Mao *et al.* 2000), where the gradient image is used to calculate the model's external energy. Moreover, the computational time for the proposed model was significantly high.

Based on their initial contribution in (Hamou *et al.* 2004), (Hamou *et al.* 2007) used Canny edge detector to provide a more robust estimation of the image's edge map. Then, a parametric active contour model is used to extract the artery boundaries. Due to the higher accuracy of Canny edge detector, compared to simply using the gradient image as in (Mao *et al.* 2000) and (Da-chuan *et al.* 1999), some improvements have been achieved. Similar to (Hamou *et al.* 2004), Canny edge detector generates lots of false edges which influence the progression of the active contour. Moreover, the scheme requires the user to provide an accurate initial contour, which limits the use of the proposed scheme in clinical trials.

Abdel-Dayem (Abdel-Dayem 2010) proposed a modified snake to extract carotid artery contours from ultrasound images. The snake's energy functions are designed to force the snake to converge to a robust edge map, which is produced by employing complex diffusion-based filtering scheme.

The above-mentioned studies (Mao *et al.* 2000, Da-chuan *et al.* 1999, Hamou *et al.* 2007 & Abdel-Dayem 2010) employ edge-based active contour models, with some variations in the driving forces, to accomplish the segmentation task. As edge-based active contours depend on the image gradient to detect boundaries and to stop the contour's evolution, they are generally sensitive to both noise and to the location of the initial contours. These limiting factors are significant in the application under consideration, since ultrasound images have poor quality with high noise levels. Moreover, minimal user interaction is an essential requirement in our application since generating accurate initial contours are tedious and time consuming for clinicians.

Region-based active contours are good candidates to overcome the drawbacks of edge-based models.

(Mumford *et al.* 1989) introduced their basic region-based model to extract the boundaries of distinct regions while smoothing the image within these regions. Considered as one of the most popular region-based models in recent years, (Chan *et al.* 2001) proposed their pioneer model as a piece-wise constant Mumford and Shah model and solved it into a level set frame work. In Chan and Vese model, the stopping term does not depend on the gradient of the image. It shows superior performance in detecting objects with very smooth boundaries or even with discontinuous boundaries. These two types of objects are typical examples of objects that exist in ultrasound images.

This paper proposes a scheme, based on Chan and Vese model (Chan *et al.* 2001), to extract carotid artery contours from ultrasound images. The proposed scheme overcomes most of the shortcomings of the previous work in (Mao *et al.* 2000, Da-chuan *et al.* 1999, Hamou *et al.* 2007 & Abdel-Dayem 2010). First, a single seed point is needed to initialize the snake. This saves considerable clinician time and effort, making the system more attractive for real clinical applications. Second, Chan and Vese model (Chan *et al.* 2001) is employed to extract the artery contours. As a result, the influence of noise, shadowing effects, and objects with incomplete contours is diminished.

The rest of this paper is organized as follows. Section 2 presents a summary of the Chan and Vese model. Section 3 describes the proposed scheme in details. Section 4 and Section 5 present the experimental setup and the obtained results, respectively. Then, Section 6 offers the conclusions of this paper. Finally, Section 7 highlights the major directions to extend this research in future.

2 CHAN AND VESE MODEL

This section presents a brief description of Chan and Vese model. Readers interested in more details are advised to consult (Chan *et al.* 2001).

Let Ω be a two-dimensional area, with $\partial\Omega$ its boundary. Let $u(x,y)$ be the input image, defined over the area Ω. Assume that the image is formed by two regions (object and background) of approximately piecewise-constant intensities, denoted by c_o and c_b, respectively. Let C denotes the collection of evolving curves in Ω that separates the objects from the background. Chan and Vese model minimizes the following energy function:

$$F(c_o,c_b,C) = \mu \cdot \text{Length}(C) + \nu \cdot \text{Area}(inside(C))$$
$$+ \lambda_o \int_{inside(C)} |u(x,y) - c_o|^2 \, dx\, dy \quad (1)$$
$$+ \lambda_b \int_{outside(C)} |u(x,y) - c_b|^2 \, dx\, dy$$

where $\mu, \nu \geq 0$, and λ_o, $\lambda_b > 0$ are parameters to be tuned by the user.

Let ϕ be the level set function defining the evolving curve C such that:

$$\begin{cases} C = \{(x,y) \in \Omega : \phi(x,y) = 0\}, \\ inside(C) = \{(x,y) \in \Omega : \phi(x,y) > 0\} \\ outside(C) = \{(x,y) \in \Omega : \phi(x,y) < 0\}. \end{cases} \quad (2)$$

Figure 1 illustrates the definition of the level set function ϕ. Using the Heaviside function H, and the Dirac measure δ_0 defined by

$$H(z) = \begin{cases} 1, & \text{if } z \geq 0 \\ 0, & \text{if } z < 0, \end{cases} \qquad \delta_0(z) = \frac{d}{dz} H(z) \quad (3)$$

The energy function (defined in Equation 1) can be expressed as (the arguments x and y of u and ϕ will be omitted for simplicity from now on):

$$\begin{aligned} F(c_o, c_b, C) = {} & \mu \cdot \int_\Omega \delta(\phi) |\nabla \phi| \, dx \, dy \\ & + \nu \cdot \int_\Omega H(\phi) \, dx \, dy \\ & + \lambda_o \int_\Omega |u - c_o|^2 \, H(\phi) dx \, dy \\ & + \lambda_b \int_\Omega |u - c_b|^2 \, (1 - H(\phi)) dx \, dy \end{aligned} \quad (4)$$

Keeping ϕ fixed and minimizing the energy function $F(c_o, c_b, C)$ with respect to the constants c_o, c_b, it is easy to express these constants as

$$c_o(\phi) = \frac{\int_\Omega u H(\phi) dx \, dy}{\int_\Omega H(\phi) dx \, dy} \quad (5)$$

$$c_b(\phi) = \frac{\int_\Omega u(1 - H(\phi)) dx \, dy}{\int_\Omega (1 - H(\phi)) dx \, dy} \quad (6)$$

It can be easily seen that the values of $c_o(\phi)$ and $c_b(\phi)$ represent the average intensities of the original image over the objects ($\phi \geq 0$) and the background ($\phi < 0$), respectively.

Keeping c_o, c_b fixed and minimizing $F(c_o, c_b, C)$ with respect to ϕ, the associated Euler-Lagrange equation for ϕ takes the form of

$$\begin{aligned} \frac{\partial \varphi}{\partial t} = {} & \delta_\varepsilon(\varphi) \left[\mu \operatorname{div} \left(\frac{\nabla \varphi}{|\nabla \varphi|} \right) - \nu \right. \\ & \left. - \lambda_o (u - c_o)^2 + \lambda_b (u - c_b)^2 \right] = 0 \text{ in } \Omega, \\ & \varphi(0, x, y) = \varphi_0(x, y) \text{ in } \Omega, \quad \text{(initial contour)} \\ & \frac{\delta_\varepsilon(\varphi)}{|\nabla \varphi|} \frac{\partial \varphi}{\partial \vec{n}} = 0 \quad \text{on} \quad \partial \Omega \end{aligned}$$
$$(7)$$

where δ_ε denotes a regularized version of δ as $\varepsilon \to 0$, $\vec{n}$ denotes the exterior normal to the boundary $\partial \Omega$, and $\partial \phi / \partial \vec{n}$ denotes the normal derivative of ϕ at the boundary. The initial value of the level set function ϕ_0 is computed as the distance from an initial boundary curve placed onto the image. The detailed mathematical derivations and the numerical approximation of the model (Equations 5, 6 and 7) are outside the scope if this paper. Interested readers may consult (Chan *et al.* 2001) for more details.

3 THE PROPOSED SOLUTION

This paper presents a *two-stage* scheme to extract carotid artery boundaries using ultrasound images. The former stage is a pre-processing stage, which aims at enhancing the input image for further processing. Then, the latter stage utilizes the Chan and Vese active contour model to extract the artery boundaries. In the following subsections, a detailed description of each stage is introduced.

3.1 *The pre-processing stage*

Ultrasound images suffer from several drawbacks. One of these drawbacks is the presence of random speckle noises, caused by the interference of the reflected ultrasound waves. Another sever problem is that ultrasound images have relatively low contrast. These factors severely degrade any automated processing and analysis of the images. Hence, it is crucial to enhance the image quality prior to any further processing. In this stage, we try to overcome these problems by performing two preprocessing steps. The first is a histogram equalization step to increase the dynamic range of the image gray levels. In the second step, the histogram-equalized image is filtered using a median filter to reduce the amount of the speckle noise in the image. It was empirically found that a 3×3 median filter is suitable for the

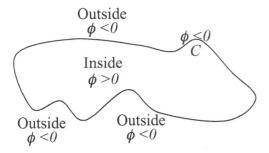

Figure 1. Definition of the level set function $\phi(x, y)$.

removal of most of the speckle noise without affecting the quality of the edges in the image.

3.2 *Segmentation stage*

In this stage, Chan and Vese Model (Section 2) is used to extract the artery boundaries from the pre-processed image from the previous stage. As discussed in the introduction section, introducing a system with minimal clinician interaction is a major design decision in this scheme. As a result, only a single seed point is required from the user. From this seed point, a circle with radius r is automatically generated and used as an initial contour ($\phi(0,x,y)$ in Equation 7). Then, this initial contour evolves, according to Equation 7, to minimize the energy function defined in Equation 1. The value of r was set to 30 pixels, which is believed to represent a close approximation of the size of a typical carotid artery. The scheme's sensitivity to the seed point selection was experimentally studied, and the results are reported in Section 5.1.

4 EXPERIMENTAL SETUP

Our proposed scheme was tested using a set of 40 B-mode ultrasound images. These images were obtained using ultrasound acquisition system (Ultramark 9 HDI US machine and L10-5 linear array transducer) and were digitized with a video frame grabber. These images were carefully inspected by an experienced clinician and artery contours were manually highlighted to represent gold standard images. These gold standard images are used to validate the results produced by our proposed scheme.

4.1 *Objective analysis metric*

To compare the output of the proposed scheme to the gold standard images, we define the overlap ratio as:

$$Overlap\,ratio = \frac{TP}{FN + TP + FP} \qquad (8)$$

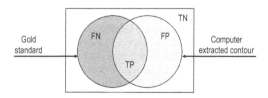

Figure 2. The definition of the *True Positive* (TP), *False Positive* (FP), *True Negative* (TN) and *False Negative* (FN) terms, used to calculate the *overlap ratio*.

Figure 2 shows the definition of the *True Positive* (*TP*), *False Positive* (*FP*), *True Negative* (*TN*) and *False Negative* (*FN*) terms.

5 RESULTS

We used the image shown in Figure 3 to demonstrate the output produced by one of our experiments. This image is a typical carotid artery ultrasound image.

Figure 4 shows the pre-processed image with the initial snake, defined as a circle, where a single seed point is required to represent the centre of the circle. Figure 5 shows the final output of the proposed scheme after the contour's convergence. Comparing Figure 5 to the gold standard image (Fig. 6) shows that the proposed scheme accurately highlights the artery lumen.

The performance of the proposed system over the entire set of 40 images was objectively compared to the gold standard images, using the *overlap ratio* (Equation 8) as a performance metric. On average, the proposed scheme produces an *overlap ratio* of 0.795.

Further experiments were conducted to evaluate the improvement achieved by employing a region-based active contour model (Chan and Vese Model) over the traditional edge-based models. Three different edge-based models were considered. In the first model, the energy function is designed to force the contour to converge to a robust edge

Figure 3. Original carotid artery ultrasound image.

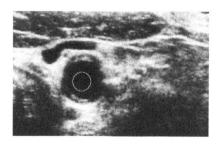

Figure 4. The initial contour superimposed over the pre-processed image.

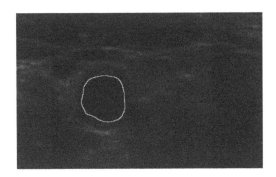

Figure 5. The final output of the proposed scheme.

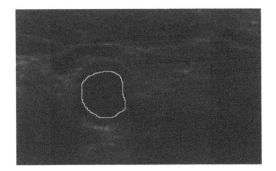

Figure 6. Gold standard image, where the artery contour is highlighted by an experienced clinician.

map, which is produced by employing complex diffusion-based filtering scheme (Abdel-Dayem 2010). Whereas, the second and third schemes use Canny edge detector and Sobel operator, respectively, to calculate the image's edge map. All experiments used the entire 40 test images (same data set), the same seed point and contour initialization. The three experiments produces overlap ratios of 0.766, 0.654 and 0.578, respectively; see Table 1 and Figure 7 for detailed comparison results. This comparison shows that region-based active contour models are promising candidates to extract artery boundaries, as the proposed scheme surpasses the edge-based active contour models, under the same testing conditions.

5.1 Sensitivity analysis

Since, the seed point represents the only input from the user, it is crucial to analyze the proposed scheme sensitivity to the seed point selection. For this analysis, we used the entire 40 test images. For each image, four seed points were randomly selected *inside the artery*. The artery region was segmented for each selected seed point. Then, these segmented binary images were added up to

Table 1. The performance measure of our experiments over the entire set of images.

	Proposed scheme	Snake with diffusion filters	Snake with canny	Snake with sobel
Average overlap ratio	0.795	0.766	0.654	0.578
Standard deviation	0.124	0.113	0.179	0.217
95% confidence interval	[0.761, 0.830]	[0.735, 0.797]	[0.605, 0.704]	[0.517, 0.638]

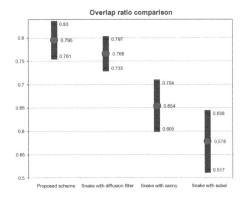

Figure 7. The 95% confidence interval of the overlap produced by the proposed scheme, edge-based active contour models with edge map extracted by diffusion-based filters, Canny edge detector, Sobel operator, respectively.

produce a grayscale image that demonstrates the overlapping areas between segmented regions generated by the four seed points. Finally, the *percentage overlap* between segmented areas (the number of pixels having a value of 4 over all non-zero pixels) was calculated.

The statistical analysis over the entire 40 test images revealed that, on average, the proposed scheme achieved a *percentage overlap* equal to 93.3%. Hence, we can conclude that the proposed scheme is insensitive to the selected seed point, as long as it is located inside the artery area. Note that, selecting a seed point within the artery area is a trivial process even for ordinary user. Hence, the proposed scheme provides accurate results, which are independent of the clinician's level of expertise.

6 CONCLUSION

In this paper, a segmentation scheme is introduced to extract carotid artery contours from ultrasound images. The proposed scheme employs the well know Chan and Vese active contour model, as a representative of the class of region-based active contours. The proposed scheme was experimentally compared to three different edge-based active contour models, found in literature. The three models force the contour to converge to the image's edge map, which is produced by complex diffusion filter, Canny edge detector, or Sobel operator. Comparative studies, using identical testing conditions, showed that region-based active contours are promising direction for highlighting carotid artery contours from ultrasound images. Finally, sensitivity analysis over the entire set of test images revealed that the scheme is insensitive to the seed point location, as long as it is located inside the artery area.

7 FUTURE WORK

During the experiments presented in this paper, the parameters ν, λ_o, and λ_b of Equation 4 were set to the default values (0, 1, and 1, respectively) set by (Chan *et al.* 2001). The parameter μ was empirically set to three. While the results obtained by these default settings are satisfactory, we believe that better results can be obtains by parameter tuning. We are currently conducting more experiments with different parameter settings, and preliminary results are encouraging. We plan to employ discrete optimization techniques to find *nearly optimal* parameter settings. Upon successful completion of this optimization step, the effect of changing the size of the initial contour on the final segmentation output will be thoroughly investigated to estimate the sensitivity of the proposed scheme to initial contour size.

REFERENCES

Abdel-Dayem, A., El-Sakka, M. & Fenster, A. 2005a. Watershed segmentation for carotid artery ultrasound images. Proc. of the IEEE Int. Conf. on Computer Systems and Applications: 131–138.

Abdel-Dayem, A. & El-Sakka, M. 2005b. Carotid Artery Contour Extraction from Ultrasound Images Using Multi-Resolution-Analysis and Watershed Segmentation Scheme. ICGST International Journal on Graphics, Vision and Image Processing 5(9): 1–10.

Abdel-Dayem, A. & El-Sakka, M. 2005c. Carotid Artery Ultrasound Image Segmentation Using Fuzzy Region Growing. Proc. of the Int. Conf. on Image Analysis and Recognition, ICIAR 2005, Springer-Verlag Berlin Heidelberg, LNCS 3656: 869–878.

Abdel-Dayem, A. & El-Sakka, M. 2006. Multi-Resolution Segmentation Using Fuzzy Region Growing for Carotid Artery Ultrasound Images. Proc. of the IEEE Int. Computer Engineering Conf., 8 pages.

Abdel-Dayem, A. & El-Sakka, M. 2007. Fuzzy c-means clustering for segmenting Carotid Artery Ultrasound Images. Proc. of the Int. Conf. on Image Analysis and Recognition, ICIAR 2007, Springer-Verlag Berlin Heidelberg, LNCS 4633: 933–948.

Abdel-Dayem, A. & El-Sakka, M. 2009. Diffusion-based Detection of Carotid Artery Lumen from Ultrasound Images. Proc. of the Int. Conf. on Image Analysis and Recognition, ICIAR 2009, Springer-Verlag Berlin Heidelberg, LNCS 5627: 782–791.

Abdel-Dayem, A. & El-Sakka, M. 2010. Segmentation of Carotid Artery Ultrasound Images Using Graph Cuts", Int. Journal for Computational Vision and Biomechanics, Vol. 3, No. 1, pp. 61–71, 2010.

Abdel-Dayem, A. 2010. Detection of Arterial Lumen in Sonographic Images Based on Active Contours and Diffusion Filters. Proc. of the Int. Conf. on Image Analysis and Recognition, ICIAR 2010, Springer-Verlag Berlin Heidelberg, LNCS 6112: 120–130.

Caselles, V., Kimmel, R. & Sapiro, G. 1997. On geodesic active contours. Int. Journal of Comp. Vision 22(1): 61–79.

Chan, T. & Vese, L. 2001. Active Contours Without Edges. IEEE Trans. Image Processing 10(2): 266–277.

Cohen, L. 1991. On active contour models and balloons. Computer Vision, Graphics, and Image Processing: Image Understanding 53(2): 211–218.

Dachuan, C., Schmidt-Trucksass, A., Kuo-Sheng, C., Sandrock, M., Qin, P. & Burkhardt, H. 1999. Automatic detection of the intimal and the adventitial layers of the common carotid artery wall in ultrasound B-mode images using snakes. Proceedings of the International Conference on Image Analysis and Processing 452–457.

Dachuan, C. & Xiaoyi, J. 2008. Detections of Arterial Wall in Sonographic Artery Images Using Dual Dynamic Programming. IEEE Trans. Information Tech. in Biomedicine 12(6): 792–799.

Hamou, A. & El-Sakka, M. 2004. A novel segmentation technique for carotid ultrasound images. Proc. of the IEEE Int. Conf. on Acoustics, Speech and Signal Processing 3: 521–424.

Hamou, A., Osman, S. & El-Sakka, M. 2007. Carotid Ultrasound Segmentation Using DP Active Contours. Proc. of the Int. Conf. on Image Analysis and Recognition, ICIAR 2007, Springer-Verlag Berlin Heidelberg, LNCS 4633: 961–971.

Kass, M., Witkin, A. & Terzopoulos, D. 1988. Snakes: Active contour models. Int. Journal of Comp. Vision 1: 321–331.

Malladi, R., Sethian, J. & Vemuri, B. 1995. Shape modeling with front propagation: A level set approach. IEEE Trans. Pattern Anal. and Machine Intell. 17: 158–175.

Mao, F., Gill, J., Downey, D. & Fenster, A. 2000. Segmentation of carotid artery in ultrasound images. Proc. of the 22nd IEEE Annual Int. Conf. on Engineering in Medicine and Biology Society 3: 1734–1737.

Mumford, D. & Shah, J. 1989. Optimal approximations by piecewise smooth functions and associated variational problems. Communications on Pure and Applied Mathematics 42: 577–685.

Osher, S. & Sethian, J. 1988. Fronts propagating with curvature-dependent speed: Algorithms based on Hamilton-Jacobi formulations. Journal of Computational Physics 79(1): 12–49.

Computational Vision and Medical Image Processing – Tavares & Natal Jorge (eds)
© 2012 Taylor & Francis Group, London, ISBN 978-0-415-68395-1

Micromovement measurements of endosseous dental implants with 3D Digital Image Correlation (DIC) method

A.T. Rodrigues
Department of Dentistry, Faculty of Medicine, University of Coimbra, Portugal

B.A. Neto
Departament of Mechanical Engenaire, University of Coimbra, Portugal

C.P. Nicolau
Department of Dentistry, Faculty of Medicine, University of Coimbra, Portugal

ABSTRACT: Dental implants are largely used due to their excellent prognosis and longevity, which is related to osseointegration. One of the first causes for not occurring osseointegration is the excessive micromovements between the implant and perimplant bone. However, that we know of, there is no clinical method available to directly measure micromovements. Resonance Frequency Analysis (RFA), method largely used, quantifies implant stability indirectly without measuring displacements. 3D Digital Image Correlation method (3D DIC) is a non-contact optical measurement technique that tracks the surface displacement field of an object. The primary objective of this work is to validate 3D DIC with the RFA method, by quantitatively measuring the displacement of 30 dental implants placed in fresh porcine mandibles under a vertical compressive load of 100 N. Results were compared with ISQ values (Implant-StabilityQuotient) obtained previously by RFA. The data obtained suggest correlation between 3D DIC method and ISQ values obtained by RFA.

1 INTRODUCTION

Dental implants are largely used to replace missing teeth due to their excellent prognosis and longevity (Nicolau, 2007). This longevity is related to the concept of osseointegration—direct union between bone and implant surface (Bränemark, 1977).

Investigation has shown that one of the first causes for not occurring osseointegration is the excessive micromovements between the implant and perimplant bone (Brunsky, 1993). When excessive, these micromovements are one of the first causes for perimplant bone loss and consequently implant failure. However, within a controlled range, these can be very useful and positively influence dental implant osseointegration (Vandamme, 2007). In a study recently published (Kimura, 2010) the conclusions presented indicate the level of micromovements as a numerical index of osseointegration.

Different methods to objectively evaluate implant stability have been proposed, but until our days, there is no clinical method available to directly measure dental implants micromovements. Resonance Frequency Analysis (RFA) is one of the most used in the literature (Degidi, 2010), with high reproducibility of results for the same implant in the same clinical conditions. RFA is measured by an electronic device Osstell® (Osstell, Gothenburg, Sweeden) using a magnetic abutment that is tightened to the implant by a screw. Despite being one of the most trusted methods to evaluate implant stability, it doesn't give direct objective information about dental implant displacement.

3D Digital Image Correlation method (3D DIC) is a non-contact optical measurement technique that can determine the three dimensional contour of an object's surface and track the surface displacement field of the object in a series of images, using digital images from two cameras and the principles of optics to stereo-triangulate the surface contour of the object. The technique 3D DIC, despite not being a clinical method, gives direct objective information about displacement. This technique has already been used in experimental studies with human teeth (Göllner, 2009; Goellner, 2010) and in one study with dental implants placed in a resin mandible (Sutton, 2009), but the method itself, has never been validated for measuring dental implants micromovements.

The primary objective of this work is to validate 3D DIC with the RFA method. Secondarily, we pretend to understand if the change of prosthetic abutments from Standard (SD) to Platform-Switching (PS) influences dental implant micromovements and if the 3D DIC technique has potential to be applied in the future as a clinical method in implantology for measuring implants micromovements.

2 MATERIAL AND METHODS

In this study we used an experimental model *in vitro* with isolated fresh porcine mandibles where were placed 30 endosseous implants Ø4,3 mm × 13 mm *Screw-line Implant, Promote® plus* (Camlog Biotechnologies®, Wimsheim, Germany), using always the same surgical protocol for implant placement, following the instructions of the fabricant. After each implant placement, randomization of the cylindrical healing abutment Ø4,3 mm × 4 mm was performed by raffle (SD and PS, n = 15 for each group) (Camlog Biotechnologies®, Wimsheim, Germany). The system implant-abutment-bone was submitted to a punctual vertical compressive load of 100 N with a metallic sphere of Ø5 mm installed in a universal forces tests machine (Shimadzu, Tokyo, Japan). Simultaneously, micromovements measurements were performed by the optical method of image correlation with two high speed photographic cameras (Point Grey GRAS-20S4M-C, 1624 × 1224 pixels) and the video correlation system Vic-3D 2010 (CorrelatedSolutions®, Columbia, USA) (Fig. 1).

Results from the video correlation program Vic-3D 2010 were compared with ISQ values (Implant Stability Quotient) obtained previously by RFA (Osstell, IntegrationDiagnostic, Sweden).

2.1 Resonance Frequency Analysis (RFA)

RFA system consists in an electronic device, the Osstell® (Osstell®, Gothenburg, Sweden), composed by a frequency detector and a small

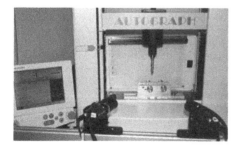

Figure 1. Universal forces tests machine (Shimadzu, Tokyo, Japan) with the metallic sphere of Ø5 mm installed for load application. Equipment of CID 3D system placed for images capture.

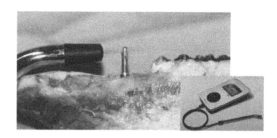

Figure 2. ISQ (Implant Stability Quotient) measuring with the RFA system Osstell® (Osstell®, Gothenburg, Sweden).

metallic magnetized abutment, wireless, and named smartpeg, which is tightened to the implant by a screw (Fig. 2).

When excited by an electromagnetic pulse, the smartpeg emits a sinusoidal wave produced by its vibration. This vibration frequency is received by the frequencies detector which performs the Resonance Frequency Analysis (RFA). The smartpeg has a vibration frequency between 1 and 10 kHz, which means a considerable sensibility for detection of lower dental implants stability values.

2.2 3D Digital Image Correlation (3D DIC)

CID 3D DIC method is an optical measurement technique that can determine the three dimensional contour of small object's surfaces, obtaining displacement fields without contact and with high resolution (MJ, 2011). This system uses the digital image of two high speed photographic cameras (Point Grey GRAS-20S4M-C, 1624x1224 pixels) and the video correlation software Vic-3D 2010 (CorrelatedSolutions®, Columbia, EUA), to track the surface displacement field of an object. For this technique, its needed a pattern with heterogeneous distribution, which image is initially taken for calibration (Fig. 3). The pattern used in this work was handmade throw the heterogeneous deposition with an airbrush of paint spots with appropriate size for the measuring surface, which is a critical step in this technique because influences measuring exactitude (MJ, 2011).

Several images are then taken while load is being applied. 3D DIC uses the digital images from the two cameras and the principles of optics to stereo-triangulate the surface contour of the object. An algorithm defines a field of "subsets" on the object's surface using the digital images. These subsets are N by N pixel boxes that contain an array of pixel gray-scale values. An advanced tracking algorithm can determine the translation, rotation and deformation of these subsets in

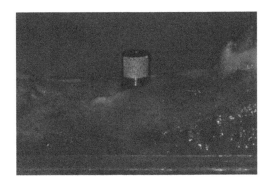

Figure 3. Heterogeneous pattern on the surface of the healing abutment screwed to the dental implant.

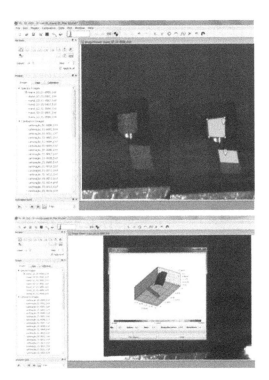

Figure 4. Images of the Vic-3D 2010 software running for determine the displacement field of the object surface with the pattern.

loaded images with respect to a reference frame. The result is a time history of the specimen's surface displacement field. The determination of the displacement field results from the video correlation between the heterogeneous pattern in the initial image (reference) and in the final image (loaded) (Fig. 4).

3 RESULTS

Results obtained are presented in Tables 1 and 2.

3.1 Statistical analysis

For the statistical analysis, a 5% significance level ($\alpha = 5\%$) was considered.

In order to verify the existence of significant statistical differences between implants with healing abutments PS and SD, it was applied a test for independent samples. Kolmogorov-Smirnov test (with Lilliefors correction) was applied to verify if the variable distribution is normal.

For implants with platform-switching (PS) healing abutment, mean and standard deviation values are: U Direction (0,0474 ± 0,0004); W Direction (0,0611 ± 0,0150); Mesio-Distal Direction (70,6333 ± 0,2000); Bucal-Lingual Direction (67,1000 ± 0,0260). For implants with standard (SD) healing abutment, mean and standard deviation values are: U Direction (0,0562 ± 0,0020); W Direction (0,0740 ± 0,2000); Mesio-Distal Direction (69,5667 ± 0,2000); Bucal-Lingual Direction (66,6333 ± 0,0810). Micromovements measured for V Direction were not considered neither for implants with PS or SD abutments, because it is not possible to obtain the correspondent ISQ values.

The tests for independent samples applied to verify the existence of significant statistical differences between the two groups of healing abutments were: Mann-Whitney test for Directions U (p = 0,602), W (p = 0,690) and Bucal-Lingual (p = 0,734); and t-Student test for Mesio-Distal Direction (p = 0,523). The results obtained show that the values for implants with different healing abutments (PS and SD) do not present significant statistical differences (p>α), neither for micromovements measured in Directions U and W, or for the ISQ values obtained by RFA for the Directions Bucal-Lingual and Mesio-Distal.

Spearman correlation coefficient was used to verify correlation between micromovements values measured by 3D DIC for U and W Direction, and the ISQ correspondent values obtained by RFA for Mesio-Distal and Bucal-Lingual Direction. Analysing correlation without dividing the two groups of healing abutments (PS and SD), the results show significant statistical inverse correlation (p<α) for the correspondent ISQ and micromovements values in the Direction U-Mesio-Distal, with a Spearman correlation coefficient of –0,407. For the correspondent ISQ and micromovements values in the Direction W-Bucal-Lingual, there is no significant statistical correlation (p>α).

Table 1. Maximum displacement values (μm) measured with 3D DIC and mean ISQ values obtained by AFR for implants with platform-switching (PS) healing abutment.

Micromovements (μm)			ISQ values	
U direction	V direction	W direction	Mesio-Distal direction	Bucal-Lingual direction
5,4	65,1	38,8	74	75
21,4	73,2	12,2	72	68
19	109,3	24,6	74	74
26,6	95,4	37,7	71	67,5
11,5	2,5	19,2	70	67
6,4	38,6	96	73	71,5
14,6	18,7	24,8	75	71
55,8	28,6	130	69	63
113,5	91	52,9	60	49
16,2	40,5	14,2	68	67
36,2	54,1	27,7	64,5	65,5
16,5	51,4	76,2	75	67
30,3	54,6	45,2	75	67
134	170,6	138,5	72	68
204	134,4	254	67	66

Table 2. Maximum displacement values (μm) measured with 3D DIC and mean ISQ values obtained by AFR for implants with standard (SD) healing abutment.

Micromovements (μm)			ISQ values	
U direction	V direction	W direction	Mesio-Distal direction	Bucal-Lingual direction
1	75,1	37,4	74	75
20,1	105,1	12	74	74
23	99,3	37,7	72	72
7,3	9,7	56	69	64
25,6	58	90,8	75	67
48	49,1	151,5	68	61,5
13	48,5	1,4	68	67,5
20,7	51,1	16,15	63	64
58,2	70,4	82	75	67
186	98,5	43,1	60	49
165	33,3	20,8	74,5	71,5
191	211	113,3	72	68
143	176,3	93,7	67	66
63,4	140,5	173	66	65
26	138,6	180,5	66	68

4 DISCUSSION

RFA system, being one of the most trusted for implant stability measurements, is largely used in clinical studies with high reproducibility of the results for the same implant in the same clinical conditions (Fischer, 2009; Rodrigo, 2009; Song, 2009; Turkyilmaz, 2008; Cannizzaro, 2009), reason for selecting this method to validate the Three Dimen-sional Digital Image Correlation (3D DIC) optical technique. Despite being one of the most referred in literature, RFA does not measure dental implant displacements directly. This system presents other limitations. Even with reproducible results for the same implant in the same clinical conditions, however, it is not possible to compare stability values between different implants, with different lengths or diameters, or placed in different types of bone. Other limitation is that, after definitive fixed prosthesis placement, it is no longer possible to measure implant stability by this method without removing the prosthesis, which is, in some clinical situations, not very practical or even impossible without destroying it. Another limitation of this system is related to the impossibility of measuring implant stability in the Apical Direction, reason by which the statistical analysis was not made for micromovements values obtained in V Direction, because ISQ correspondent values cannot be measured.

The 3D DIC technique, has become more used in the last years because of its versatility and high resolution (MJ, 2011). However, until our days, the method has not been validated for dental implants micromovements measuring. 3D DIC has potential to become very useful in implantology because it allows to examine in detail the mechanical behavior of a dental implant in contact with bone tissue. This might contribute to improve dental implants geometry, prosthetic rehabilitation and even the surgical technique. Micromovements measurements with this system may provide the clinician with more significant information about dental implants rehabilitation prognosis, complementing the other existing methods. Besides, this technique might be useful in the limitations of the other existent systems, and be used to measure displacements when definitive fixed prosthesis are placed or when implants are being loaded. For all these reasons, 3D DIC was considered of interest for the performance of this study.

The results show that the measurements obtained for the implants with the two different healing abutments (PS and SD) do not present significant statistical differences (p>α), neither for micromovements measured in U and W Directions, or for the ISQ values obtained by RFA for Bucal-Lingual or Mesio-Distal Directions.

However, displacement mean values for implants with healing abutments SD and PS, were always higher for PS abutments, independently of the Direction measured or of the technique used (3D DIC or RFA).

Analysing correlation between micromovements values measured with 3D DIC and ISQ values obtained by RFA without dividing the two groups of healing abutments (PS and SD), the results show significant statistical inverse correlation (p<α) in the Direction U-Mesio-Distal. In the Direction W-Bucal-Lingual, the correspondent ISQ and micromovements values do not show significant statistical correlation (p>α).

5 CONCLUSIONS

Within the limitations of this study, 3D DIC seems to be capable of measuring dental implants micromovements. The results obtained seem to be correlated with the values measured by RFA. Implants with healing abutments PS presented lower mean values of micromovements.

REFERENCES

Bränemark, PI; Hansson, BO; Adell, R; Breine, U.; Lindstrom, J.; Hallen, O.; et al. 1977. *Osseointegrated implants in the treatment of the edentulous jaw. Experience from a 10-year period. Scand J Plast Reconstr Surg* 16:1–132.

Brunski, JB. 1993. *Avoid pitfalls of overloading and micromotion of intraosseous implants. Dental implantology update* 4:77–81.

Cannizzaro, G.; Felice, P.; Leone, M.; Viola, P.; Esposito, M. 2009. *Early loading of implants in the atrophic posterior maxilla: lateral sinus lift with autogenous bone and Bio-Oss versus crestal mini sinus lift and 8-mm hydroxyapatite-coated implants. A randomised controlled clinical trial. Eur J Oral Implantol* 2: 25–38.

Degidi, M.; Daprile, G.; Piattelli, A. 2010. *Determination of primary stability: A comparison of the surgeon's perception and objective measurements. Int J Oral Maxillofac Implants* 25(3):558–561.

Fischer, K.; Backstrom, M.; Sennerby, L. 2009. *Immediate and early loading of oxidized tapered implants in the partially edentulous maxilla: a 1-year prospective clinical, radiographic, and resonance frequency analysis study. Clin Implant Dent Relat Res* 11: 69–80.

Goellner, M.; Schmitt, J.; Karl, M.; Wichmann, M.; Holst, S. 2010. *Photogrammetric measurement of initial tooth displacement under tensil force. Medical Engineering & Physics* 32:883–888.

Göllner, M.; Holst, A.; Berthold, C.; Schmitt, J.; Wichmann M; Holst, S. 2009. *Noncontact intraoral measurement of force-related tooth mobility. Clin Oral Investigations.*

Kimura, K.; Fukase, Y.; Makino, M.; Masaki, C.; Nakamoto, T.; Hosokawa, R. 2010. *Preoperative assessment of treatment planning on minimization of micromovement during healing period of immediate-loaded implants using X-ray CT data-based simulation. J Oral Implantol.*

MJ; Lopes, HM; Vaz, M.; Campos, LM; Vasconcelos, M.; Campos, JCR. Sociedade Portuguesa de Biomecânica (ed) 2011. *Estudo do comportamento mecânico dos compósitos de restauro dentário utilizando técnicas ópticas—4° Congresso nacional de biomecânica.* 5:275–278.

Nicolau, P. Coimbra (ed): Faculdade de Medicina, Universidade de Coimbra 2007. *A randomized clinical study between immediate and early loading. Immediate loading of endosseous implants—clinical and biomechanical evaluation.*

Rodrigo, D.; Aracil, L.; Martin, C.; Sanz, M. 2009. *Diagnosis of implant stability and its impact on survival: a prospective case series study. Clin Oral Implants Res* 21:255–261.

Song, YD; Jun, SH; Kwon, JJ. 2009. *Correlation between bone quality evaluated by cone-beam computerized tomography and implant primary stability. Int J Oral Maxillofac Implants* 24:59–64.

Sutton, MA; Orteu, JJ. Schreider, HW. New York: Springer, 2009. *Image correlation for shape, motion and deformation measurements.*

Turkyilmaz, I.; Aksoy, U.; McGlumphy, EA. 2008. *Two alternative surgical techniques for enhancing primary implant stability in the posterior maxilla: a clinical study including bone density, insertion torque, and resonance frequency analysis data. Clin Implant Dent Relat Res* 10:231–237.

Vandamme, K.; Naert, I.; Geris, L.; Vander, SJ.; Puers, R.; Duyck, J. 2007. *Influence of controlled immediate loading and implant design on peri-implant bone formation. J Clin Periodontol* 34:172–181.

Computational Vision and Medical Image Processing – Tavares & Natal Jorge (eds)
© 2012 Taylor & Francis Group, London, ISBN 978-0-415-68395-1

Monte Carlo simulation of PET images for injection dose optimization

Jiří Boldyš & Jiří Dvořák
Institute of Information Theory and Automation of the ASCR, Prague, Czech Republic

Otakar Bělohlávek & Magdaléna Skopalová
Na Homolce Hospital, PET Center, Prague, Czech Republic

ABSTRACT: When a patient is examined by positron emission tomography, radiotracer dose amount has to be determined. However, the rules used nowadays do not correspond with practical experience. Slim patients are given unnecessary amount of radiotracer and obese patients would need more activity to produce images of sufficient quality. We have built a model of a particular PET scanner and approximated human trunk, which is our region of interest, by a cylindrical model with segments of liver, outer adipose tissue and the rest. We have performed Monte Carlo simulations of PET imaging using the GATE simulation package. Under reasonably simplifying assumptions and for special parameters, we have developed curves, which recommend amount of injected activity based on body parameters to give PET images of constant quality. The dependence qualitatively differs from the rulesused in clinical practice nowadays and the results indicate potential for improvement.

Keywords: positron emission tomography, Monte Carlo simulation, biological system modeling, image quality

1 INTRODUCTION

Positron Emission Tomography (PET) is a functional imaging modality. Resulting images do not show anatomical objects. They rather display functional processes in a patient body, e.g. glucose metabolism or blood flow. These examinations allow us to monitor tumor treatment, examine epilepsy seizure foci, etc. For a detailed discussion on PET see e.g. Powsner & Powsner (2007).

PET imaging is based on injecting radioactive tracer. For small activities, resulting image quality grows with injected activity amount. However, the dose amount recommendation used nowadays (see Jacobs et al. (2005)) does not sufficiently normalize for image quality in daily routine. Slim patients are given unnecessary amount of radiotracer and obese patients would need more activity to produce images of sufficient quality. Figure 1 shows examples of CT and PET images of slim and obese patients.

Previous studies published in literature aimed at achieving maximum quality of the resulting image for each patient. This approach might lead to unnecessary radiation exposure of light patients, especially children. A brief overview of these studies, together with different metrics of image quality they use, is presented in Section 2.

The goal of this paper is different—to qualitatively determine, based on significant patient body parameters, the amount of injected radiotracer needed to achieve constant quality of the resulting PET images, even for patients with different body habitus. This would help improve consistency of the diagnostic process.

This paper describes first results of our initial study in this direction. At the beginning of our research, we have adopted several justifiable simplifications explained further on. We limit ourselves to examination of liver and body segment surrounding it.

To achieve our objectives, we have performed Monte Carlo simulations of PET imaging using GATE simulation package. Details, including description of PET scanner and body model, will follow in relevant sections. We will also explain the adopted image quality measure. Finally we come to the desired curves which we call curves of constant quality.

2 MAXIMIZING IMAGE QUALITY

Previous studies concerning the dependence of image quality on the amount of the injected radiotracer aimed at maximizing the image quality for each patient. This section provides a brief (and certainly not complete) overview of these studies.

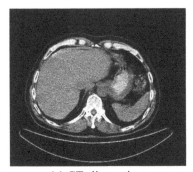

(a) CT-slim patient

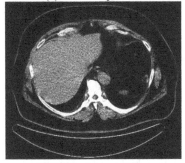

(b) CT-obese patient

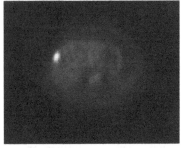

(c) PET-slim patient

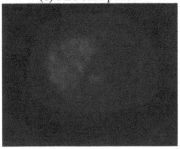

(d) PET-obese patient

Figure 1. CT images of similar transverse plane containing liver—gray homogeneous region on the left. Reader can observe different thickness of the subcutaneous adipose tissue for a slim (a) and an obese (b) patient. Images (c) and (d), resp., show corresponding sections of PET images. Notice lower intensity of the (d) image.

A popular tool for describing quality of PET images is the noise equivalent count, NEC (see Section 7). It quantifies the statistical quality of the raw data and is not affected by the choice of reconstruction algorithm. Studies using NEC to describe PET image quality or modeling the dependence of NEC on the amount of injected activity include Accorsi et al. (2010), Danna et al. (2006), Mizuta et al. (2009) and Watson et al. (2005).

Quality of reconstructed images can be expressed e.g. in terms of signal-to-noise ratio. Relevant references include Mizuta et al. (2009) and Watson (2004).

Other possibility is to assess the subjective visual quality of the images using a numeric scale or verbal description (rating the quality e.g. from excellent to non-diagnostic). This type of psychophysical measurement is usually very time-consuming sincethe set of analyzed images has to be assessed by one or more experienced practitioners. See e.g. Everaert et al. (2003) or Halpern et al. (2005).

The ultimate measure of PET image quality, from the medical point of view, is performance of a human observer in a given diagnostic task. The most common task is the detection of small foci of increased activity indicating the presence of a tumour. Again, human observer studies are time-consuming and so mathematical model observers were developed to mimic the performance of human observers in a specific task. The most important of these observers are Hotelling and channelized Hotelling observer and their variants. Relevant references include Abbey & Barrett (2001), Gifford et al. (2000) and Halpern et al. (2005).

3 RADIOTRACER DOSE IN PET IMAGING

PET examination is useful for example for tumor imaging. Tumors accumulate glucose more than surrounding tissues. Therefore, patient is in advance injected a dose of ^{18}F-FDG , what is radioactive analogue of glucose. ^{18}F-FDG is accumulated into tumor and it is emitting positrons. Positrons almost immediately annihilate, resulting into two photons moving in opposite directions and detected approx. at the same time. Reconstructed image is based on number of detected photon pairs and their lines of response (LORs—lines joining two detector segments which detected the photons in coincidence)—see Figure 2 presenting PET scanner scheme.

There are rules what amount of activity A should be injected into patient. A depends on patient's weight. More weight means more fat, less probability to detect incidences of photon pairs and finally image of worse quality.

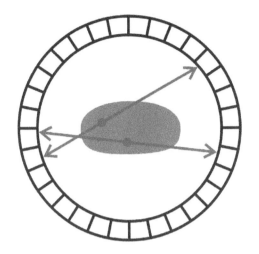

Figure 2. PET modality scheme showing the detector ring, annihilation events (dots) and pairs of photons moving in opposite directions (with their respective LORs).

It has already been mentioned that todays rules prescribe too much activity to slim patients and insufficient activity to obese patients. There is historical justification for these rules, but everyday clinical practice calls rather for different approach. It would be desirable to produce the same image quality for patients with different body parameters. It is our objective to find prescription for this activity.

PET scanner detectors register not only true coincidences, where the photons travel from the annihilation point to the detectors without any interaction. It also happens that photons interact with the tissue and deflect. More tissue causes more photon deflections and finally wrong LOR attributions—they are called scattered coincidences. Furthermore, so called random coincidences happen when two photons from two different annihilations are detected at the same time.

Scattered and random coincidences have undesired effect on the resulting image. They introduce blurring and noise to the data.

Numbers of all coincidences grow with increasing activity. However, random coincidence count grows the fastest, causing image quality to deteriorate above some injected activity. This means that for obese patients with high amounts of injected activity we might not be able to get image of sufficient quality.

4 MONTE CARLO SIMULATIONS

Process of PET imaging can be modeled by Monte Carlo methods. There are several simulation packages available for this purpose. We have chosen the GATE simulation package, see Jan et al. (2004). GATE is an open-source software and currently it is able to simulate PET, SPECT and CT imaging. GATE is developed by Open GATE collaboration.

The main GATE component is the Geant4 toolkit for the simulation of the passage of particles through matter. It allows us to model usual particle physics interactions, like Compton or Rayleigh scattering, etc.

GATE performs PET imaging simulation after specifying the following: PET scanner model, phantom model (in our case body model), source model, time of examination, and eventually other data. In the next sections body and scanner models are commented in detail.

5 PATIENT MODEL

For general PET imaging simulations, an elaborate full body model would find its use. Our first objectives are rather qualitative and thus we can afford a very simplified body model at this stage. In this paper we choose liver as our main region of interest. Thus we confine ourselves to the trunk area surrounding liver with some overlap.

We further attempt to simplify model of a transverse section through a body in liver area from the point of view of PET imaging. We segment the section into three areas: subcutaneous adipose tissue SA (underskin fat), liver LI, and everything inside SA, what we call inner segment IS, see Figure 3. We have a database of 18 CT images, where we have localized one reference transverse section based on liver shape. The three defined segments were then manually segmented and areas of segments SA and IS were measured. These areas were then recalculated into effective radii R_{SA} and R_{IS} of corresponding cylinder bases.

On our limited set of CT images, radii R_{SA} and R_{IS} can be statistically explained using linear regression by patient's weight m and height h only. Other parameters such as age or BMI were found insignificant (in statistical sense). We initially focus only on male patients due to different way of fat deposition. To further simplify the simulations we set $h = 180$ cm and we vary only the weight m.

Cylindrical model of patient's trunk is then constructed as follows, see Figure 3(b). Cylinder with height 25 cm and radius R_{IS} models the inner segment. It is surrounded by another cylindrical layer with radius R_{SA} which models the SA segment. Liver is modeled by a sphere with radius $R_{IS}/2$ touching the far left point of the IS segment. The radii R_{SA} and R_{IS} depend on the parameter m and are determined according to the linear regression model mentioned above.

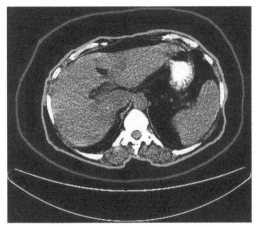

(a) Segmentation of SA and IS

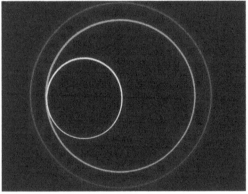

(b) Cylindrical body model

Figure 3. (a) CT images were segmented to get the SA and IS segments. Their areas are basis of the equivalent cylindrical model (b).

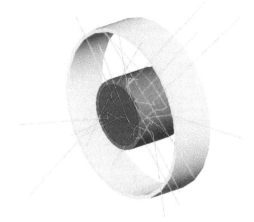

(a) Detectorring,bodymodel

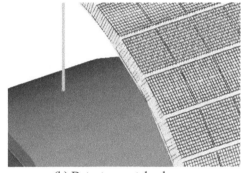

(b) Detectorcrystals-closeup

Figure 4. Model of our studied PET scanner together with the body region of interest used in GATE simulations. (a)—the whole setup, (b)—closeup. In the body model, adipose tissue and the inner segment are visible. Liver is hidden inside and it is not visible.

Materials for all the segments were appropriately chosen from the GATE material database. As for the distribution of activity in the model of patient's trunk, we chose homogeneous distribution in all the segments SA, LI and IS. The ratios of unit activity (activity per cubic centimeter) in different segments correspond to average ratios determined from PET images of real patients. Such kind of a simple model filled with specified materials was found sufficient to approximate body region of interest for PET imaging simulations.

6 SCANNER MODEL

Siemens Biograph40 TruePoint TrueV HD PET scanner is modeled in this contribution. It is a cylindrical type of scanner, see Figure 4. Necessary technical data were kindly provided by technicians of both the PET Center of Na Homolce Hospital in Prague and Siemens company. Simulated acquisition time was 60 s.

7 IMAGE QUALITY ASSESSMENT

There are many image quality measures available in the field of image analysis. Overview of such measures suitable for PET imaging was given in Section 1. For the purpose of this paper so called Noise Equivalent Count (NEC) was chosen. It is a very simple and right sufficient measure for our objectives. At the same time it is widely used in nuclear medicine community. Moreover, it is not affected by the choice of reconstruction algorithm, so in fact no reconstruction was needed for this study.

It is based on the total numbers of true coincidences T, scattered coincidences S and random coincidences R. Data for NEC calculation are available from outputs of our simulations and there is no need for tomographic reconstruction.

$$NEC = \frac{T^2}{T + S + R}$$

NEC equals T times the ratio of true coincidences to the number of all coincidences. Thus it can be intuitively interpreted as an effective number of true coincidences with respect to the resulting image quality. Due to behavior of dependences of T, S and R on activity A mentioned earlier in this paper, dependence NEC(A) is first growing and then decreasing.

8 SIMULATION RESULTS

We have performed PET imaging simulations with the PET scanner model and patient body model described above. For simplicity and as mentioned above, we were varying only the weight parameter m. Simulated activities are far covering the range examined in practice.

We simulated 6 different weights evenly distributed in the range from 48 kg to 130 kg. From the given weight and default height 180 cm we calculated parameters R_{SA} and R_{IS} needed to specify the patient body model. For every patient (i.e. for every weight) we performed 15 PET imaging simulations with varying activity. NEC was then computed for every simulation based on T, S and R. Results for one particular weight are plotted in Figure 5.

One additional simulation with the activity determined according to Jacobs et al. (2005) was performed to provide a reference level of NEC for the given weight.

Resulting dependence NEC(A) can be fitted by a curve NEC(A) = $p_1 + p_2 A^{p_3}$, where p_i's are fitted parameters. The resulting curve can be used to propose activity A, which has to be used to achieve a reference NEC for particular patient weight.

Such activities are plotted in Figure 6. Different symbols correspond to different levels of reference image quality NEC. Solid line shows the prescription used today in clinical practice.

It is evident that the dependence of injected activity on body parameters is qualitatively different from the prescription used nowadays. The resulting curves of constant quality (interpolated through the marks) show rather convex tendency on the contrary to todays standard.

The results support observations from clinical practice. It seems that there is potential to save slimmer patients from radiation load, what is

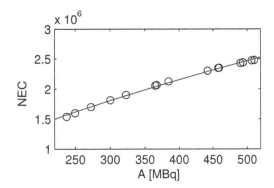

Figure 5. Dependence of NEC image quality measure on simulated activity for a particular patient model ($m = 81$ kg).

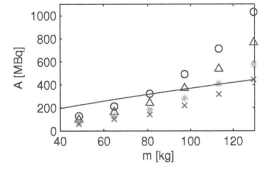

Figure 6. Prescription for applied activity based on patient weight. Different symbols correspond to different reference image quality NEC. For example, circles determine the amount of activity that would produce images with the same NEC as was achieved in simulation of patient with $m = 81$ kg. Solid line—activity injected according to the rule currently used in medical practice.

crucial for reducing the potential risk of radiation induced cancer by PET investigation. On the other hand, wehave a methodology how to find suitable activities for simulated obese patients to get clinically informative PET image.

9 CONCLUSIONS

In this paper we describe our PET imaging simulations using the GATE package. We provide details about the body region of interest and about the PET scanner. We use the NEC global image quality measure to derive curves of constant quality. We show how image quality depends on injected activity for particular body parameters.

We have achieved the main goal of this study—we have derived curves of constant quality, which qualitatively predict the amount of injected radiotracer to produce resulting PET image of constant quality, for particular body parameters. The results support clinical experience of physicians performing PET examinations. Based on these results, the PET Center of Na Homolce Hospital in Prague has started a clinical study.

Our plans for the future include elaboration of more realistic body model. We will investigate also other image quality measures.

ACKNOWLEDGMENTS

We are very grateful to Filip Šroubek, Pavel Máca and Radek Matějka for fundamental technical help. Also many thanks to the OpenGATE Collaboration for GATE development.

This work has been supported by the Czech Ministry of Education under the project No. 1M0572 (Research Center DAR).

REFERENCES

Abbey, C.K. & Barrett, H.H. 2001. Human- and Model-Observer Performance in Ramp-Spectrum Noise: Effects of Regularization and Object Variability. *The Journal of the Optical Society of America A* 18 (3): 473–488.

Accorsi, R., Karp, J.S. & Surti, S. 2010. Improved Dose Regimen in Pediatric PET. *The Journal of Nuclear Medicine* 51 (2): 293–300.

Danna, M., Lecchi, M., Bettinardi, V., Gilardi, M.C. & Stearns, C.W. 2005. Generation of the Acquisition-Specific NEC (AS-NEC) Curves to Optimize the Injected Dose in 3D ^{18}F-FDG Whole Body PET Studies. *IEEE Transactions on Nuclear Science* 53 (1): 86–92.

Everaert, H., Vanhove, C., Lahoutte, T., Muylle, K., Caveliers, V., Bossuyt, A. & Franken P.R. 2003. Optimal Dose of ^{18}F-FDG Required for Whole-Body PET Using an LSO PET Camera. *European Journal of Nuclear Medicine and Molecular Imaging* 30 (12): 1615–1619.

Gifford, H.C., King, M.A., de Vries, D.J. & Soares, E.J. 2000. Channelized Hotelling and Human Observer Correlation for Lesion Detection in Hepatic SPECT Imaging. *The Journal of Nuclear Medicine* 41 (3): 514–521.

Halpern, B.S., Dahlbom, M., Auerbach, M.A., Schiepers, C., Fueger, B.J., Wolfgang A. Weber, W.A., Daniel H.S., Silverman, D.H.S., Ratib, O. & Czernin, J. 2005. Optimizing Imaging Protocols for Overweight and Obese Patients: A Lutetium Orthosilicate PET/CT Study. *The Journal of Nuclear Medicine* 46 (4): 603–607.

Jacobs, F., Thierens, H., Piepsz, A., Bacher, K., Van de Wiele, C., Ham, H. & Dierckx, R.A. 2005. Optimised tracer-dependent dosage cards to obtain weight-independent effective doses. *European Journal of Nuclear Medicine and Molecular Imaging* 32 (5): 581–588.

Jan, S., Santin, G., Strul, D., Staelens, S., Assie, K., Autret, D., Avner, S., Barbier, R., Bardies, M., Bloomfield, P.M., Brasse, D., Breton, V., Bruyndonckx, P., Buvat, I., Chatziioannou, A.F., Choi, Y., Chung, Y.H., Comtat, C., Donnarieix, D., Ferrer, L., Glick, S.J., Groiselle, C.J., Guez, D., Honore, P.F., Kerhoas-Cavata, S., Kirov, A.S., Kohli, V., Koole, M., Krieguer, M., van der Laan, D.J., Lamare, F., Largeron, G., Lartizien, C., Lazaro, D., Maas, M.C., Maigne, L., Mayet, F., Melot, F., Merheb, C., Pennacchio, E., Perez, J., Pietrzyk, U., Rannou, F.R., Rey, M., Schaart, D.R., Schmidtlein, C.R., Simon, L., Song, T.Y., Vieira, J.M., Visvikis, D., Van de Walle, R., Wieers, E. & Morel, C. 2004. GATE: a simulation toolkit for PET and SPECT. *Physics in Medicine & Biology* 49 (19): 4543–61.

Mizuta, T., Senda, M., Okamura, T., Kitamura, K., Inaoka, Y., Takahashi, M., Matsumoto, K., Abe, M., Shimonishi, Y. & Shiomi, S. 2009. NEC Density and Liver ROI S/N Ration for Image Quality Control of Whole-Body FDG-PET Scans: Comparison with Visual Assessment. *Molecular Imaging and Biology* 11 (6): 480–486.

Powsner, R.A. & Powsner, E.R. 2007. *Essential nuclear medicine physics.* Wiley-Blackwell.

Watson, C.C. 2004. Count Rate Dependence of Local Signal-to-Noise Ratio in Positron Emission Tomography. *IEEE Transactions on Nuclear Science* 51 (5): 2670–2680.

Watson, C.C., Casey, M.E., Bendriem, B., Carney, J.P., Townsend, D.W., Eberl, S., Meikle, S. & DiFilippo, F.P. 2005. Optimizing Injected Dose in Clinical PET by Accurately Modeling the Counting-Rate Response Functions Specific to Individual Patient Scans. *The Journal of Nuclear Medicine* 46 (11): 1825–1834.

Computational Vision and Medical Image Processing – Tavares & Natal Jorge (eds)
© *2012 Taylor & Francis Group, London, ISBN 978-0-415-68395-1*

The use of medical thermal imaging in obstetrics

Ricardo Simões
Institute for Polymers and Composites IPC/I3N, University of Minho, Campus de Azurem, Braga, Guimarães, Portugal
Polytechnic Institute of Cávado and Ave, Campus do IPCA, Barcelos, Portugal

Cristina Nogueira-Silva
Life and Health Sciences Research Institute (ICVS), School of Health Sciences, University of Minho,
Campus de Gualtar, Portugal
ICVS/3B's—PT Government Associate Laboratory, Braga/Guimarães, Portugal
Department of Obstetrics and Gynecology, Hospital de Braga, Sete Fontes, S. Victor, Braga, Portugal

ABSTRACT: Digital thermography has been employed in the medical field for several years. However, its use has been clearly focused on breast cancer diagnosis, while other applications having been much less explored. The aim of this prospective study was to assess the feasibility of employing thermal imaging in obstetrics, namely as an additional diagnosis tool available for physicians to use synergically with other techniques in their standard practice.

Keywords: medical imaging, thermal imaging, thermography, obstetrics, pregnancy

1 INTRODUCTION

1.1 *Medical digital thermal imaging*

Medical digital thermal imaging (DTI) is a passive, noninvasive, diagnostic technique that enables visualizing and quantifying changes in skin surface temperature [1]. The key advantage of this technique is that the device does not need to get in physical contact with patients. The imaging device interprets infrared radiation emitted from the skin, which depends on the temperature and emissivity of the skin, and converts them into a digital image that can be seen and analyzed through dedicated software. The visual thermal image that maps body temperature is usually termed a thermogram and features a color spectrum. The color spectrum is matched to a temperature range and changes in color indicate an increase or decrease of infrared radiation emitted from the body surface, and thus, an increase or decrease of skin temperature.

Skin blood flow is controlled by the sympathetic nervous system. The human body usually exhibits a high degree of thermal symmetry, and the dermal pattern in a healthy individual is fairly consistent and reproducible [2]. Medical DTI can register these patterns to a sensitivity of circa 0.1–0.01°C. Any deviations from this symmetry, such as those resulting from the development of a tumor, can be identified, through medical DTI [3]. Even very subtle changes can be identified and measured through analysis software.

Medical DTI is particularly valuable due to its capability to show physiological change and its high sensitivity to certain pathologies in the vascular, muscular, neural and skeletal systems [4]. Thus, it can contribute significantly to the pathogenesis and diagnosis made by the physician. Medical DTI has been extensively used in human medicine in the U.S.A., Europe and Asia for the past 20 years. However, the required equipment was excessively expensive and extremely cumbersome until recent years. These facts have hampered its pervasive use and its usefulness in a variety of cases. Current state-of-the-art equipment designed specifically for clinical application, and specialized computer software to aid the analysis, have facilitated the use of the technique.

The clinical uses for DTI include:

- Identifying the extent of a lesion for which a diagnosis has been previously made;
- Localizing an abnormal area not previously identified, so that additional diagnostic tests can be performed;
- Detecting early lesions before they are clinically evident;
- Monitoring post-surgical healing or the effectiveness of specific treatments.

1.2 *Applications of Medical DTI*

Thermal imaging was originally developed for military use in night vision, but it has since found several applications in medicine.

The most common application of Medical DTI is oncology, namely the detection of breast cancer in women [5,6]. Its use in this field derives from the fact that tumors typically result in increased blood supply and angiogenesis, in addition to increased metabolic rate, which results into higher temperature gradients compared to surrounding normal tissue [3]. It is particularly effective as an adjunct to mammograms. Medical DTI has been approved since 1982 by the US FDA (United States Food and Drug Administration), for uses such as breast cancer screening, as an adjunctive medical imaging modality.

Other applications in the clinical field include rheumatology, neurology, physiotherapy, sports medicine, pediatrics, orthopedics, chiropractic, dentistry, and vascular medicine/cardiology. It can be successfully applied to the diagnostic of a number of disorders in human body including, respiratory dysfunctions, urinary diseases, cardiovascular disorders, circulatory disorders, lymphatic dysfunctions, nervous dysfunctions, endocrine problems, locomotors disorders, skin problems, and many others. Infrared thermography has also been applied, to a much small degree, to the study of reproductive disorders [7], such as polycystic ovaries, endometriosis, or uterine fibroids.

2 MOTIVATION

2.1 *Gestation and labor*

Pregnancy is a very particular situation and thus demands extreme care. Conditions which normally would not affect the woman's physical health can affect her pregnancy. An important advantage of thermography, in early detection of potential problems, is the fact that during pregnancy, the woman's body is changing very rapidly. Some of these modifications might be symptomatic but pass unnoticed. The woman might not even consider reporting them to her obstetrician.

Thermography is also interesting in this context to indicate abnormal muscle strain, which might be troubling the pregnant woman but discarded as a natural occurrence, and could indicate to the attending obstetrician the need for additional support of the breasts, abdomen or the use of different sleep positions.

In the case of breast tumors, the growth and shape modification of breasts during pregnancy, and in the months subsequent to labor, particularly for first-time mothers, will make self-examination much more difficult. Also, during this period, most concern is focused on the baby, and the mother is prone to pay less attention to her own health.

2.2 *Application of DTI in obstetric practice*

The main goal of this study was to assess the feasibility of employing DTI in obstetrics, namely examine the evolution of the skin temperature profile of different body regions and compare them to the expected patterns, in order to identify characteristics of the pregnancy.

As a secondary goal we explored the possibility of early identification of potential complications arising along the pregnancy.

3 METHOD

3.1 *Participants*

The study subjects were pregnant women, between 30 and 39 weeks of gestation, who consented to having their vital signals and thermal body image collected. Informed consent forms have been collected from all subjects.

3.2 *Equipment*

We employed a FLIR® SC640 infrared camera with software package (FLIR Systems AB, Sweden; Fig. 1). The camera is factory calibrated within 0.2°C and features a precision of 0.1°C. Accuracy of temperature measurement is randomly checked on a regular basis for this equipment. The resolution of the camera is 640 × 480 pixels.

This camera allows the use of a memory card to record multiple thermal images, but it can also be directly connected to a computer in order to obtain video thermal imaging (up to 30 frames per second). It has an adjustable viewfinder and also an external LCD viewer that can rotate to facilitate operation. Multiple options can be controlled; some in the camera itself, while some others can still be adjusted with the analysis software afterwards. The camera must be manually focused, either through a button or by rotating the lens.

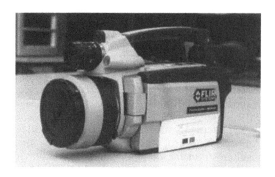

Figure 1. FLIR SC640 infrared camera.

After the camera is focused, one must wait for it to perform auto-calibration before a snapshot can be taken. Although extremely more advanced than models of the past decade, there are still improvements to look forward in the future of this type of infrared cameras.

3.3 Data collection procedure

Tests took place between April and July of 2011, at the School of Health Sciences, University of Minho, Braga, Portugal. The sampling room is permanently maintained at 18°C. Subjects were requested to remove their clothes from the waist up, and to stand near a white wall with the palms resting on their hips. The camera remained stationary, and the subject was requested to turn 90° for each subsequent image. In this way, images were collected for each perspective quadrant (front, left, back, right). This procedure was then repeated with the subjects crossing their palms behind their head, so that the arms were essentially absent from the scan.

Several problems were detected in preliminary tests, which required modifications to the protocol in subsequent tests. A total of 11 trial runs, with 8 different subjects, were used until the collection process was considered stable enough for the study to begin.

These preliminary validation tests indicated the following:

– Indications must be given for the subject to avoid resting her palms on her waist or her abdomen area while waiting for the tests to start or between scans (this can be a problem due to the calibration time even for the current best commercial equipment). The same applies in terms of the subject covering her breasts with her palms in those periods. These first aspects have to do with the fact that the palms are typically one of the hottest regions and will effectively appear in the thermal scan and interfere with the collected data. If this is not prevented, there will be not only ghost images of palms on her skin, but also surrounding areas will heat up, influencing the temperature readout.

– The subject should have removed her clothing around the torso and abdomen at least a couple of minutes before the thermal scan is performed. Typical pregnancy support strips, sometimes worn around the abdomen, must also be removed preemptively, both because they contribute to heating up that region but also because they may block imaging of a significant part of the abdomen. In order to minimize the total time required from the evaluation of each subject and, simultaneously, prevent periods of total inactivity, if the study protocol includes other data collection procedures, it may be possible to implement one of those procedures during this period of thermal equilibration.

– In addition, all the traditional concerns in thermal imaging must also be applied. These include removal of jewelry from all locations where they may interfere with the analysis. Last, long hair (quite common in the population of interest for this study), interferes with the analysis, and it must be displaced at every thermal scan (namely when the subject is facing the camera and later facing away from the camera.

3.4 Data analysis procedure

All data analysis was performed using the software package provided with the thermal camera, namely: ThermaCAM Researcher Professional 2.8 SR-2, FLIR Systems AB, Sweden.

The scanned image includes the temperature map, the temperature range, and the color code/temperature scale. As a thermal image actually corresponds to a pictographic representation of a temperature map, it is important to understand that the image itself is not sufficient for analysis. Temperature analyses from standard computer images that were created based on thermograms are not possible. Typical colored images from thermography provide at best an estimation of temperature distribution, but are not able to provide measurements.

The temperature information must also be available, together with the image. This creates the need for particular care in handling the image (such as editing it with general image editing software, trimming, resizing, and other operations). It is best that the image created by the equipment is kept in its original form.

In the case of our system, the infrared camera creates JPEG images, but which also contain the temperature information embedded in the JPEG image file.

4 RESULTS

4.1 Normal features—anterior

Some features were present in the majority of the scans, and can be identified as "normal" or "typical" profiles. In the front, the breasts and the axilla exhibit the highest temperatures, almost invariantly. Such a profile, of the breast region, is shown in Figure 2 for a subject exhibiting the typical features.

The increased vascular activity in the breasts was expected, and should increase along the pregnancy. In the subject shown in Figure 2, the

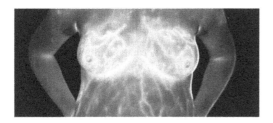

Figure 2. Normal thermal profile of the breast region at 39 weeks of gestation (anterior view). Note the mapping symmetry and also the high vascular activity on the breasts.

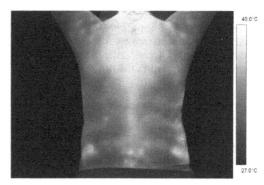

Figure 3. Normal thermal profile at 39 weeks of gestation (posterior view). Note the symmetric pattern of the thermal map. On the waist line there is some effect from the subject having rested her palms on her waist rather than on her hips previously to the scan being taken.

temperature on the surface of the breasts ranges from circa 34.5 to 37.5°C, which is about 3 to 4°C higher than the abdominal region. Also, the temperature just under the breast fold in this patient was around 38 to 39°C; this slight increase depends significantly on the breast shape and size. We have observed this increased local temperature effect in cases where the breast lays over the abdominal region. However, deeper investigation is clearly warranted to clarify which factors affect this localized temperature increase.

When analyzing anterior thermal scans such as that in Figure 2, any deviations from symmetry should be further investigated by the obstetrician. These may result from minimum and non-threatening malformations, from muscle strain (as will be discussed in later sections), or other causes.

Aside from asymmetries, any abnormally cold or hot spots should be identified and looked into by the obstetrician. Hot spots indicate a higher vascular activity in the region, which could be indicative of an infection or angiogenesis. In the case of cold spots, they may appear due to something as simple as a localized burn sometime in the past, but they can also pinpoint scar tissue from previous surgical procedures.

4.2 Normal features—posterior

The majority of scans have also enabled identifying "normal" or "typical" profiles for the back. In this case, the spinal region invariantly exhibits the highest temperatures.

Such as profile is shown in Figure 3, for the same subject of Figure 2. The cervical and thoracic spine regions exhibit higher temperatures by about 3°C compared to other back regions.

In this Figure, the temperature range of the thermal map has been fixed between 27°C and 40°C, thus exceeding the maximum value captured by the camera. Tweaking the minimum and maximum of the visualization scale has no effect on the measurements themselves, and facilitate visual interpretation

of the image. Adjusting the scale minimum allows removing the background and focusing only on the subject. Adjusting the scale maximum to above the highest measured value prevents the appearance of absolute white in the image (which we have found to be visually preferable).

It should be noticed, as previously explained, that patients were requested to cross their palms behind their heads. Thus, this effectively removed their palms from the thermal scans. However, the various measurements made with different arm positions have clearly indicated that the hands usually exhibit high temperatures.

In Figure 3, it should be pointed out that the higher temperatures in the cervical and thoracic region likely result also from the muscle strain (on the trapezius) resulting from the abdominal region weight and the change in posture that pregnant women adopt along the later stages of pregnancy. Since this subject was at a little over 39 weeks of gestation, the fetus is near its maximum weight before delivery.

4.3 Abnormal back profile

In another subject, the back thermal map features significant asymmetry, with higher temperature profiles on the right upper back side; see Figure 4. This analysis was performed with the subject at 36 weeks of gestation. The neck and spinal regions exhibited high temperature values, but this is typical for all subjects. Although these are just preliminary results, we believe that this localized temperature increase on the right upper back are indicative of muscle strain resulting from the fetus being located to the right.

In this figure, the left and right sides of the upper back region differ by up to 3°C when comparing

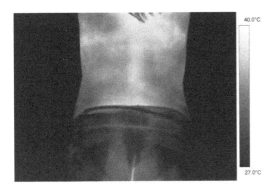

Figure 4. Abnormal thermal profile at 36 weeks of gestation (posterior view). Note the asymmetric pattern of the thermal map.

single points, and by a little over 1°C if a larger sampling area is considered for calculation.

The fetal position and size, depending on the daily activities of the subject and many other factors, may force the subject to compensate fetal weight by shifting her normal posture. We intend to confirm this on other subjects, since it could provide interesting information regarding fetal position.

For this particular subject, the strain caused by the fetus' weight on the back might justify the use of an abdominal support waist band. This is a decision that the obstetrician should consider, depending on multiple other factors. The same applies to the need for potential additional breast support.

It should be noted that this type of thermal map with asymmetry between the two upper back sides has been identified in other subjects, also at late stages of pregnancy. The common features between subjects in this group are i) a large fetus; and ii) the fetus being positioned towards the side corresponding to the higher temperatures on the upper back.

4.4 Further considerations

The abdominal region exhibits a wide range of features and seems to depend on: fetus location, fetus size, gestation week, placenta location, and other variables. This preliminary assessment has provided us with notions of what can be studied and some data for analysis, but clearly further work is required and will be sought after by the authors.

To facilitate the comparison between different readings and between different subjects, the same scale should always be employed (in as far as possible, considering possible exceptions for the study of particular features).

5 CONCLUSIONS AND FUTURE WORK

5.1 Concluding remarks

Obtaining useful digital thermal images for medical use is not trivial. The conducted study enabled pinpointing a series of obstacles and potential problems to the practical application of this technology. While the use of thermography has been extensively studied and documented for breast cancer diagnostics, other applications are much less covered in the literature. Clearly, much more work is warranted to enable this technology to fulfill its full potential.

In the case of obstetrics, before digital thermal imaging can become a viable tool to aid in diagnostic, several aspects require considerable attention:

– A database of "typical" profiles for different types of pregnancies (e.g. single vs. multiple), for different body types, and for different fetal characteristics, must be created.
– The thermal map evolution of pregnancies along the full term must be documented.
– Relations must be established between specific features of the thermal map and pathologies / problems arising during pregnancy.
– Since it is very difficult to obtain thermal maps from before pregnancy for comparison, it might be possible to get pertinent data from thermal scans conducted sufficiently long after delivery.

5.2 Future work

Having identified potential avenues for research in this area, we will continue the tests in order to establish statistical significance to some of the features we have observed and to support some trends which we believe are indicate of particular physiological processes that could be extremely valuable as additional diagnostic support tools.

A very useful data would be a temperature profile for the subjects taken before they became pregnant (or at the earlier possible week), as this would enable comparisons which were not possible in this study.

ACKNOWLEDGEMENTS

Foundation for Science and Technology, Lisbon, through the 3° Quadro Comunitário de Apoio, and the POCTI and FEDER programs. Thermal equipment provided under the REEQ/1033/CTM/2005 POCI 2010 program. Project "Do-IT", co-financed by FEDER, Programa Operacional Factores de Competitividade.

REFERENCES

[1] Gershon-Cohen J, Haberman JA, Brueschke EE, Medical thermography: a summary of current status, Radiol Clin North Am (1965) 3, 403.

[2] Uematsu S, et al, Quantification of thermal asymmetry. Part 1: Normal values and reproducibility, J Neurosurgery (1988) 69, 552–555.

[3] Carmeliet P, Jain RK, Angiogenesis in cancer and other diseases, Nature (2000) 407, 249–57.

[4] Jones BF, A reappraisal of the use of infrared thermal image analysis in medicine, IEEE Trans Med Imaging (1998) 17, 1019–27.

[5] Lawson R, Implications of surface temperature in the diagnosis of breast cancer, Canad MAJ (1956) 75, 309–310.

[6] Nimmi A, et al, Effectiveness of a noninvasive digital infrared thermal imaging system in the detection of breast cancer, The American Journal of Surgery (2008) 196, 523–526.

[7] Birnbaum SJ, Kliot D, Thermography—obstetrical applications, Annals of the New York Academy of Sciences (1964) 121, 209–222.

Computational Vision and Medical Image Processing – Tavares & Natal Jorge (eds)
© 2012 Taylor & Francis Group, London, ISBN 978-0-415-68395-1

Analysis system of sudomotor function using digital image processing

J.L. Quintero, E. Nava & M.S. Dawid
*CIMES—Autonomic Nervous System Unit, Department of Communications Engineering,
University of Malaga, Spain*

ABSTRACT

Objective: To design and develop a system that assesses sudomotor function with spatial and temporal resolution, through digital image processing techniques.

Background: The current methods to evaluate post-ganglionic sudomotor function are not very successful because they are too expensive or they do not give enough information. It will be desirable to achieve useful results with a low cost approach. Inorder to this, it can be used a pH indicator on the skin of the patient that changes colour when it comes in contact with sweat and a digital image processing algorithm to quantify it.

Methods: Sweating has been stimulated chemically by iontophoresis of pilocarpine. Then the pH indicator was applied and a video sequence of 10 minutes was recorded. These pictures were converted to an appropriate colour space specifically designed for our system. The movements of the patient and lighting variations were corrected, and segmentation was carried on using optimal thresholds to get sudomotor response information. Finally, a quantification of the percent surface area and virtual volume affected by sweating was performed.

Results: The sudomotor function in 8 patients, 2 of them hyperhidrotic, 3 normohidrotic and 3 hypohidrotic has been tested. There was a high correlation between our results and those of others kinds of sweat tests. Hyperhidrotic patients presented around 60% marked surface area, while hypohidrotic hardly reached 5%.

Conclusions: It is possible to implement an evaluation system for sudomotor function using digital image processing with a low cost solution. The specific colour space is a key concept because it simplifies the analysis system and its design enablesus to obtain the required information, with the minimum probability of error.

Keywords: sudomotor function, neurophysiology, colour space, image processing

1 INTRODUCTION

Assessment of sudomotor function has increased in importance in the evaluation of several diseases and disorders, specially those associated with peripheral nerve disease. It is useful as a diagnostic tool for the following disorders: amyloid neuropathy, diabetic autonomic neuropathy, distal small fiber neuropathy, idiopatic neuropathy, multiple system atrophy, pure autonomic failure, reflex sympathetic dystrophy and Sjogren's syndrome (of Neurology 1996). But high cost and complex equipment have prevented its widespread use (Low et al. 2006).

There are several techniques to characterize sudomotor function: silicone impressions, thermoregulatory sweat test (TST), sympathetic skin responses (SSR), acetylcholine sweat-spot test. There are also quantitative techniques: quantitative sudomotor axonreflex test (QSART) and quantitative direct and indirect axon reflex testing (QDIRT) which offer numerical data that can be useful in the assesment of disease progression or degree of recovery. A good review of these techniques, with a detailed description of testing methodology and limitations, is presented in (Illigens and Gibbons 2009).

As a brief summary, to evaluate post-ganglionic sudomotor function with spatial and temporal resolution, QSART (Riedel et al. 1999) measures changes in relative humidity inside a sweat capsule over a restricted area. The steps to be followed are: first, a sudomotor response is induced by iontophoresis of a cholinergic antagonist, then this area is covered with a hermetic capsule that carries a hygrometer, and data are collected for 15 minutes. The equipment, particularly the capsule, is very expensive, andtherefore QSART is not used frequently. There are other qualitative techniques, like the Silicone Imprint Method or Skin Sympathetic Response, but these do not provide as much information as QSART.

A good technique would be an application allowing a dynamic and real-time quantification of sudomotor function, and computerized image analysis would be a natural choice. In addition, three more objectives can be addressed: process time should be satisfactorily short, the whole system should be economical, and it should insure the health and well-being of the patients (Gibbons et al. 2008).

2 CONCEPTUAL MODEL

The basic performance of our system is based on detecting and quantifying the colour of a pH marker that changes when it comes in contact with sweat.

Applying modular design techniques, the whole task can be split into smaller subsystems, facing problems one by one, using a divide and conquer strategy. The structure of the proposed algorithm is presented in Figure 1.

These blocks are:

- Image Acquisition. A video sequence is obtained and selected digital images are chosen.
- Conversion to colour Space YC_xC_y. Using a specifically designed adaptive colour space for this application, the images are transformed to the new colour coordinates.
- Lighting Changes Correction. A subsystem to compensate temporal variations in the luminance of the images.
- Movements Correction. It compensates possible movements of the patients.
- Segmentation. Sweat area is detected, marked and quantified, using a simple two step thresholding technique.
- Results. Graphs of the dynamic evolution of sweat are computed and presented.

3 ANALYSIS

We have carried out up to 28 tests in eight selected patients with a wide range of sweat function

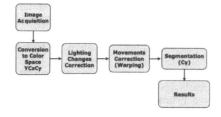

Figure 1. Block diagram of the system.

(hyperhidrotic, normohidrotic and hypohidrotic) with also a wide range of features (age, colour skin ...). In each case, the tested area was the right forearm.

The different tasks and subsystems that form the sweat test are detailed below. Some are not really technical works, but they have to do correctly by the medical staff.

Sweating stimulation and preparation of patients: It can be reduced the latency of sudomotor response by means of iontophoresis stimulation (1.5 mA, 10 minutes, Pilogel®). This technique consists in applying an electric field on the skin that injects a pharmacologic agent, i.e. pilocarpine, that stimulates sweating. In this way, the test duration can be reduced with a better response from the patient.

When iontophoresis has finished, a blue mark is applied around the stimulated area, and the skin is covered with a pH indicator (in this case, alizarin red, cornstarch and sodium pyruvate). This indicator changes its colour, from light brown into red, asmuch change as much sweat is diluted in it.

The blue mark has standard dimensions (4 × 4 cm²), and we have manufacture a rubber stamp of this size. This stamp enables an easy and fast procedure and the mark also can be used as a calibration reference to relate pixels with centimetres.

Images acquisition: In order to meet the low-cost requirements of the system, a video sequence of ten minutes was recorded at standard rate (25 fps) with a conventional web-cam camera for each test, which meets the resolution and quality required by our application. This video sequence started just after the stimulation of sweat and images with sizes of 1200 × 768 pixels (probably, it can be used a lower resolution without sensible degradation of results) are extracted every ten seconds to obtain a set of 60 images per test. Atypical example of the obtained images is presented in Figure 2.

In this image, the red pixels correspond to the sweaty skin surface. All external elements (the background and the blue square mark) were blue because this colour is unusual in human skin. The choice of blue is important because, in that way, each part ofthe images could be clearly identified using colour information.

Additionally, the images are subjected to a preprocessing step that consists of decimate and filter operations, in order to reduce computational load, to keep safe the significant information, and to avoid some interference and aberration artefacts of theoriginal pictures.

Colour Space: Given that the important information of the images is related to colour, the

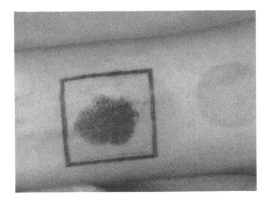

Figure 2. Forearm with the marked work area.

$$\begin{pmatrix} 0 \\ 100 \\ 255 \end{pmatrix} = \begin{pmatrix} B_{mark} & R_{mark} & 1 \\ B_{skin} & R_{skin} & 1 \\ B_{aliz} & R_{aliz} & 1 \end{pmatrix} \begin{pmatrix} c \\ d \\ f \end{pmatrix} \qquad (3)$$

where B_{mark} and R_{mark} are the C_b and C_r components of blue mark, B_{skin} and R_{skin} of skin of the patient, and B_{aliz} and R_{aliz} of red alizarine, respectively. It is important to have a fixed reference for alizarine colour, and so to be able to compare results of different patients. For this reason, it has been performed a study with patients who show a significant amount of sweat and the experimental values of 100 for B_{aliz} and 190 for R_{aliz} were selected as adequate.

Lighting change correction: In the clinical practice, illumination is spatially non-uniform when conventional lighting is used, but these changes were not found significant in our work because of the small area displayed in the images. In addition to spatial variation, there are also temporal changes, due to flicking and small changes in the ambient illumination, which are typical of a clinical environment (i.e. the opening of the door where the test is under realization produces small changes in the mean illumination of the scene). These changes not only modify the luminance but also the chromatic components.

In order to prevent errors in our measurements, it has been developed a method to compensate the average lighting variations for each sequence in the temporal domain. This algorithm compute the mean value of a small area which is not stimulated with pilocarpine and this value is used to normalize the overall image.

Movement correction: Even if our test is very short in time, compared with other sudomotor function assessment systems, it is not possible that the patient be completely still during ten minutes without immobilization techniques. To allow a certain degree of comfort for the patient, a motion compensation algorithm has been implemented.

Due to the position of the forearm, rested on a flat surface, the dominant movement is the torsion around its own arm axis. From the point of view of the camera, the images suffer not only linear translations but also non-linear deformations. This problemcan be addressed by applying warping techniques after finding the corners of the square that limits the work area and tracking them along the video sequence. This is the idea to use a blue square mark during the tests.

In order to find the four corners of the square, Harris & Stephens detector was used (Harris and Stephens 1988), but in the thresholding phase, a set with more than four points were chosen as corner candidates. To decide which quadruple of points

choice of the correct colour space is crucial. After trying several options with standard colour spaces, we have decided to design a specific one to this system, based on colourspace YC_bC_r (ITU-R BT.601). We named the new colour space as YC_xC_y and it has three components: Y, the luminance component; Cx, a component with higher values for blue elements and skin; and Cy, the component with high values for red pixels, optimized for sweat response.

The new colour space is adaptive and the values of the transformation matrix are calculated for each particular test or patient. Images are recorded and saved in RGB format and converted to YC_bC_r colour space using a standard methodology. Then, a simple segmentation of blue background and free-sweat small areas is performed to compute C_b and C_r average values of the skin of the patient and background of the image. The values of red alizarin in the YC_bC_r colour space have been calculated only once time like the average of multiple realizations. The advantage of this approach is that the system can adapt to different skins and situations.

The new YC_xC_y coordinate system is defined as

$$\begin{pmatrix} Y \\ C_x \\ C_y \end{pmatrix} = \begin{pmatrix} 1 & 0 & 0 \\ 0 & a & b \\ 0 & c & d \end{pmatrix} \begin{pmatrix} Y \\ C_b \\ C_r \end{pmatrix} + \begin{pmatrix} 0 \\ e \\ f \end{pmatrix} \qquad (1)$$

where the parameters $\{a,b,c,d,e,f\}$ model the skin of the patient and environmental conditions. To compute these parameters, the following two linear equations are solved

$$\begin{pmatrix} 255 \\ 0 \\ 0 \end{pmatrix} = \begin{pmatrix} B_{mark} & R_{mark} & 1 \\ B_{skin} & R_{skin} & 1 \\ B_{aliz} & R_{aliz} & 1 \end{pmatrix} \begin{pmatrix} a \\ b \\ e \end{pmatrix} \qquad (2)$$

in the set arethe best ones, the following similarity measure $R = R_1R_2$ is computed, where R_1 and R_2 are defined as

$$R_1 = |h^2 - a^2 - b^2| \qquad (4)$$

$$R_2 = \sum_{i=1}^{4} |L_i - \overline{L}| \qquad (5)$$

where R_1 is the Pythagoras theorem for the triangle defined by three of the points in the quadruple and R_2 is the L1-norm of the lengths of the four edges of the polygon L_i and $\overline{L}$ is its mean value

$$\overline{L} = \frac{1}{4}\sum_{i=1}^{4} L_i$$

The point quadruple with a minimum value of R is selected as the best four edge polygon. To compensate deformation, an affine transfomation is used

$$\begin{pmatrix} x_f \\ y_f \end{pmatrix} = \begin{pmatrix} a & b \\ c & d \end{pmatrix}\begin{pmatrix} x_i \\ y_i \end{pmatrix} + \begin{pmatrix} e \\ f \end{pmatrix} \qquad (6)$$

where (x_i,y_i) and (x_f,y_f) are the Cartesian coordinates of the corresponding pixels of the previous and actual images, respectively, a,b,c,d,e,f are a set of unknowns that can be solved using the equation 6 with the vertices of the four-points polygon and the diagonals cross point.

Figure 3 shows the superposition of the first image and the most displaced image in a sequence, concretely the Y luminance component of these, before and after warping. It can be seen how the squared mark remains in the same place when movement correction is applied. The goal of these geometrical corrections is to preserve the pixels inside the blue square, where important information is contained, allowing a simple tracking of the polygon.

Other methods and techniques for motion compensation (Jain and Jain 1981) has been tested but the results are better using our warping technique. Figure 4 shows a comparative between some of them applied to a sequence: the original displacement of the image, normalize cross-correlation technique (Barjatya 2004), block-matching with exhaustive search (Barjatya 2004), block-matching with 3 steps search (Barjatya 2004), and our warping technique. A detailed comparison and discussion can be found in (Quintero 2011)

Segmentation: After the correction of lighting temporal variations and movements of the arm, the sweat area is segmented using the proposed C_x and C_y components. To do that, the optimal

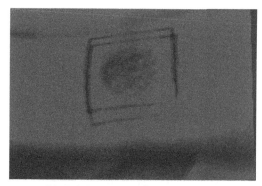

(a) Original images-not corrected

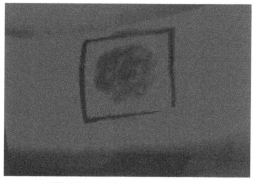

(b) Warped images-corrected

Figure 3. Superposition of worst case owing to movement.

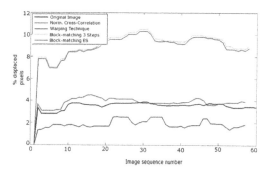

Figure 4. Comparative between different displacement correction techniques.

thresholding method with minimum probability error proposed by Otsu (Otsu 1979) is used with both chromatic components. Using the C_x component, pixels are classified as skin or blue, and with C_y component, the skin pixels are classified as sweat and non sweat. The thresholding values T_x and T_y, respectively, were found using the whole set of patient cases to optimize the best value for the T_x value and using the set of patients with high levels of sweat to determine the T_y value. In our work, obtained values were $T_x = 119$ and $T_y = 153$.

Sweat quantification (results): To assess the dynamics of sweating, the final results are shown on two ten minutes time graphs, one of them giving the percentage of area which is affected by sweating, computed as the sum of pixels classified as sweat, and the other is a virtual volume which is obtained by the product of this area and the red colour intensity using the C_y chromatic component. All final values has been normalized to the dimensions of the blue square, which encloses the work zone.

Figure 5 shows a typical result for a normohidrotic patient, who presented a noticeable amount of sweat at the end, as it can be qualitatively seen in images 5a) and 5b), which correspond to the the initial and final images of the sequence, respectively. The pair of graphs presented in Figure 5c) are the dynamics of sweat area and virtual volume. In both cases, there is an initial steep slope, that levels off at the end. A measure of this gradient could be useful to define sweating response.

Sometimes, the sweat accumulation can lead to some errors and interferences that it can be seen at the end of the graphs presented in Figure 5c), where a fall in the sweat area and virtual volume can be seen. This is due because a drop of sweat rolled down around the skin and fell on the non visible background.

When the movement of the patient is not significant and lighting variations are small, the

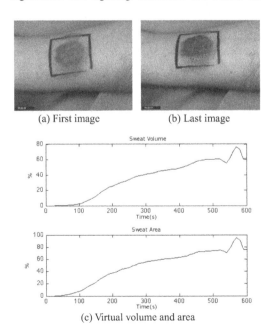

(a) First image   (b) Last image

(c) Virtual volume and area

Figure 5.   Response of an normohidrotic patient.

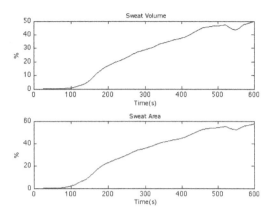

Figure 6.   Response of an normohidrotic patient using only color space and segmentation subprocesses.

corrections subsystems can be omitted, as it's shown if Figure 6, where the final result, in this case, is similar to the result of the complete system. It can be easily seen that the use of the specific colour space is the key block of our system.

4   RESULTS

Using a training set of 28 patients to improve different algorithms for our system, it has been arrived at the final version that is described in this paper. The sudomotor function of 8 subjects (2 hyperhidrotic, 3 normohidrotic and 3 hypohidrotic) was assessed by this test. The response of hyperhidrotic patients reached around 60% sweat production area, its gradient moved higher to low till to get saturation status. In the case of normohidrotic subjects, final values were similar, but the slope was nearly constant in the course of the test. The response of hypohidrotic patients hardly reached 5%. Sweat response, measured with our system, was consistent with the results seen by other testing techniques.

Figure 7 shows the sweat area percentage of the three typical behaviours. The top one corresponds to a hyperhidrotic patient, thus the graph increases fast from the beginning until it reaches saturation state. The intermediate plot is a normohidrotic profile, its graph has almost linear performance during the experiment. Last, we can see a hypohidrotic result in the lower curve, whose graph presents very low values all the time because the patient produces very little sweat.

The computational cost of the algorithm is less than five minutes in a typical PC computer (2.4 GHz Intel Core 2 Duo and 4GB of memory). Because the adquisition of images needs ten minutes, results could be ready a few seconds after the sudomotor

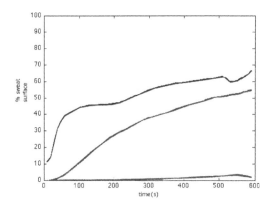

Figure 7. Example of hyperhidrotic (dashed), normo-hidrotic (dot line) and hypohidrotic (solid) results.

test is finished. This good performance is due to an optimal code for warping process, more efficient that other techniques, and to the reduced image resolution, enough to get good results, preserving the sweat information.

5 CONCLUSIONS

In general, qualitative results obtained with the proposed system correlate well with silicone impression and other sweating tests, and they are complied with clinical predictions, quantitative results seem to be similar to QSART and QDIRT techniques, buta rigorous comparison has not been done.

One of the main goals was to obtain a low cost system to assess the sudomotor function without specialized equipment, the only equipment needed is an inexpensive computer, an ordinary web cam, an iontophoresis system, the rubber stamp and washable blue ink and some chemicals.

Also the comfort and well-being of patients are respected. They only have to keep as still as possible for 10 minutes and wash their forearms when the experiment have finished.

In summary, sweat response can be assessed with spatial and temporal resolution using digital image processing, and this solution does not need complicated equipment or a large economic investment. In this way, it has been developed a simple and inexpensive tool for the research of the sudomotor function that can be used in neurophysiology diagnosis and other disciplines.

REFERENCES

AAN, A.A.o.N. (1996). Assessment: Clinical autonomic testing report of the therapeutics and technology assessment subcommittee of the american academy of neurology. *Neurology 46*(3), 873–880.

Barjatya, A. (2004). Block matching algorithms for motion estimation. *DIP 6620 Spring 2004 Final Project Paper (Utah State University, USA)*, 1–6.

Gibbons, C.H., B.M.W. Illigens, J. Centi, and R. Freeman (2008, June 10). Quantitative direct and indirect test of sudomotor function. *Neurology* (24), 2299–2304.

Harris, C. and M. Stephens (1988). A combined corner and edge detector. In *Proceedings of The Fourth Alvey Vision Conference*, pp. 147–151.

Illigens, B.M.W. and C.H. Gibbons (2009, April). Sweat testing to evaluate autonomic function. *Clinical Autonomic Research 19*(2), 79–87.

Jain, J. and A. Jain (1981, December). Displacement measurement and its application in interframe image coding. *IEEE Transactions on Communications 29*(12), 1799–1808.

Low, V.A., P. Sandroni, R.D. Fealey, and P.A. Low (2006, July). Detection of small-fiber neuropathy by sudomotor testing. *Muscle and Nerve 34*(1), 57–61.

Otsu, N. (1979, January). A threshold selection method from gray–level histograms. *IEEE Transactions on Systems, Man and Cybernetics 9*(1), 62–66.

Quintero, J.L. (2011). *Sistema de análisis de la funcin sudomotora mediante la aplicación del tratamiento digital de imágenes*. Universidad de Málaga (Master thesis, in spanish).

Riedel, A., S. Braune, G. Kerum, J. Schulte-Mnting, and C. Lcking (1999, September). Quantitative sudomotor axon reflex test (qsart): a new approach for testing distal sites. *Muscle and Nerve 22*(9), 1257–1264.

Computational Vision and Medical Image Processing – Tavares & Natal Jorge (eds)
© 2012 Taylor & Francis Group, London, ISBN 978-0-415-68395-1

3D geometry reconstruction from gray and RGB medical images

P. Talaia, M. Parente, A. Fernandes & R. Natal Jorge
IDMEC—pólo FEUP, Universidade do Porto, Porto, Portugal

ABSTRACT: This work presents the modeling of human organs by means of 3D geometry reconstruction using medical images. The base images were obtained from the "Visible Human Project" (VHP) database. The first part of the work consists in image reconversion, color optimization and alignment. For process optimization, each organ is delimited in a box volume, for image cropping. The feature recognition is then performed for the organ in the selected volume. After features recognition, the aligned contours are extracted and a cloud point is generated for the organ in analysis. The geometry can then be generated from the obtained cloud points.

1 INTRODUCTION

1.1 Motivation

Representations of the human body are one of the very first's forms of art. Such representations of the human body are being done as art portraits of the human quotidian or sacred deities.

Modeling parts of the human body in a schematic way, with medicine proposes, was found in ancient civilizations such as the Egyptian or the Babylonian civilization.

Nowadays the concept of model has gained a new dimension with the advent of the computing technologies. Such technologies can mimic in projected 3D environment human actions and mimic in real time our emotions and expressions. If we look around, from the 3D games, crossing the 3D animation, until reaching the virtual crash dummies, all these human models share the same principle as back-ground, the computer science.

The work presented explores the reconstruction of the human body organs geometries, having in mind detailed models for of the human body for trauma and crash simulation proposes, orthopedics or other medical science proposes.

1.2 Some existing models

Some similar models (Fig. 1) have been already done, as the THUMS (Iwamoto *et al.*, 2002) or the HUMOS (Arnaux *et al.*,). In the HUMOS model, a cadaver was frozen in t he car driver position, sliced and with the images from the slices it was reconstructed, including the major organ features in the human body: bones, flesh, skin, lungs, heart, etc. A stand version of HUMOS was also done, moving the model slowly and gently from the seated to the stand version.

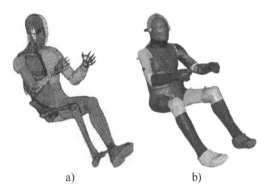

Figure 1. FEM human models: a) THUMS (Iwamoto *et al.*, 2002); b) HUMOS.

These models are validated and are an important tool in complement to the dummies used for example in the automobile industry, like the HYBRID III or the EUROSID. But models such as the THUMS or HUMOS remain with some limitations. These limitations arise from several reasons, poor laws for the soft tissues, the lack of activeness in the muscles, or poor joint definitions in regions not critical in typical car scenarios accidents (Haug *et al.*, 2004).

2 IMAGE PROCESSING

In all cases, the starting point in the models was the geometry reconstruction from images obtained on humans. In such task, the use of images for reconstruction is usual as in other medical needs, simulation or evaluation (Tavares *et al.*, 2009). The recreation of anatomical geometries is more and more a tool for engineers and medical doctors (Barneva *et al.*, 2010). Gray scale images from the typical CT scans or MRI are the usual supports, but when the study object is the entire person, and physiology and anatomy is a must, it is necessary to use other type of images, as used on the THUMS or HUMOS models.

One example of such images is the database "Visible Human Project" (VHP) from the U.S. National Library of Medicine, pre-processed by Talaia *et al.*, 2011a and 2011b for this study.

2.1 *Geometry reconstruction*

From the pre-processed images from the VHP, the starting point is the geometry reconstruction of the bones, moving later-on to the soft tissues. From Talaia *et al.,* 2010a and 2010b it is easy to obtain in Matlab a point cloud that is then exported in ASCII to any commercial software for CAD reverse-engineering. Our goal is to perform the point filtering, triangulation, triangulation optimization and/or reduction using Matlab. Such inclusion will improve the first stage of feature recognition on the image level, giving to the user a faster and reliable feed-back, and support-ready to any CAE software.

The initial approach for the algorithms explored is based on the "The Natural Neighbor Radial Point Interpolation Method" (Belinha, 2010), allowing the reduction of points of interest for triangulation (the reduction can be from millions of points to less than one hundred). After that, the triangulation algorithm follows the principle of the marching triangle (Hilton *et al.*, 1996) or ball-pivoting algorithm (Bernardini *et al.*, 1999), both feasible to handle complex surfaces and multi-surfaces in the same point cloud.

One example of the geometries obtained with such methods are presented in the Figure 2.

2.2 *Reconstruction from medical images*

The first biological structures that are needed to assemble the proposed model are the bones, and the description of the major contours: skin, soft tissues, layer, etc.

For such tasks, the traditional medical images are able to give enough information to a good quality shape for the structures being acquired.

The algorithm follows is described in the load of the original image (Fig. 3.a) and transform it to a false image with optimized colors (Fig. 3.b).

The transformation follows several steps according to the level of contrast on the image relatively to the biological structures and the area of the body, which in the example presented is the head (and part of the neck). For the head, and from the

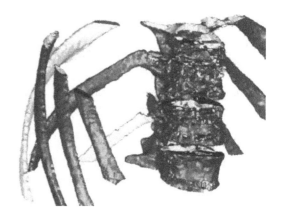

Figure 2. Section of the rib cage, before any filtering or resampling.

images, we can easily separate 3 areas: the skin, the bones and the soft tissues (excluding parts of it as adipose tissue).

The skin (Fig. 3.c) selects the external contours of the body, including internal features, as hearing cavities, nasal cavities and others.

The soft tissues (Fig. 3.d) includes muscles, brain, spinal cord, tong, eyes and other tissues that come in similar grays tones in the medical image.

The bones (Fig. 3.e) that includes in our case: skull, and some cervical vertebras.

Conjugating the Figure 3.c, b and c we can obtain a false image (Fig. 3.b) where a forth feature is notorious, appearing as dark gray. The dark gray no is notorious and shows the other physiological structures, like the adipose tissue, meninges, etc.

2.3 *3D reconstruction*

The acquired medical images have been taken in different values of amplification, on the transverse plane, with several increments. To get a collection of images on the sagittal or dorsal plane, it was added transversal images by means of cubic interpolation, taken from the features already extracted.

In the 3D geometries presented in this work, it was used the dorsal plane (Fig. 4.a) to get the contours from the respective features. The same approach gives a better distribution in terms of point clouds, making easier the process to obtain the cloud points for the respective feature being reconstructed (something that can be seen in the plan itself, Fig. 4.b).

The user has a 3D structure that allows him to work in the images in any of the main planes. The generation of the point cloud is so ready to be used according to the user needs. From the previous extract structures, skin and bone

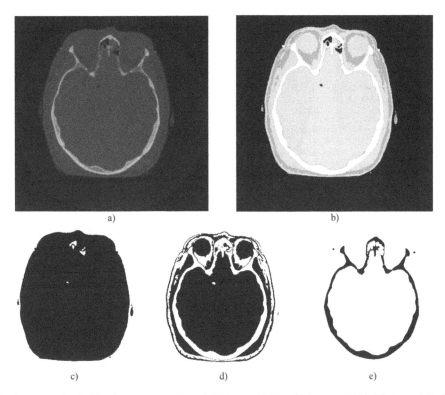

Figure 3. Images to the skull in the transverse plan: a) CT image; b) false CT image; c) "skin" feature; d) "soft tissues" feature; f) "bone" feature.

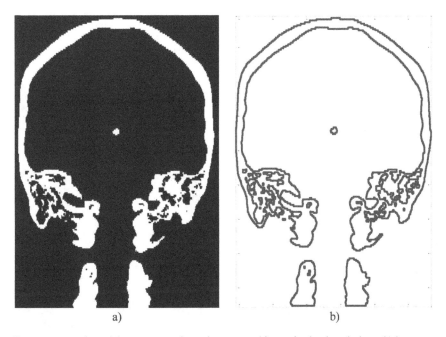

Figure 4. Bone segmentation: a) bone extracted, on the corrected image in the dorsal plane; b) bone contour in the respective plane.

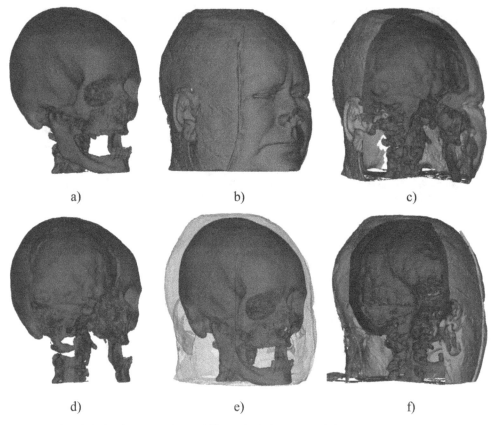

a)　　　　　　　　b)　　　　　　　　c)

d)　　　　　　　　e)　　　　　　　　f)

Figure 5.　Render of the head geometry from stl file: a) skull (fronto-lateral view); b) head skin (fronto-lateral view); c) skin and skull with section in the quadrant fronto-lateral (view from same direction); d) skull with section in the quadrant fronto-lateral (view from same direction); d) translucent head skin with skull (fronto-lateral view); e) skin and skull with section in the quadrant anterio-lateral (view from same direction).

have been selected to rendering as illustrated in Figure 5. The main parameter for the rendering has been triangle reduction to a maximum of 250,000, with point space of 0.4 mm. The obtained geometries are almost without surface errors, with expectation where a number of small details with internal cavities appear, like the zone of the orbits. Improvements must be done in the feature extraction concerning the small details and small holes in the structures.

2.4　Current work and color images

Actually, more advanced algorithms are being applied to solve some of the issues found on the traditional medical images.

Associated to the gray images, the capabilities to distinguish structures on the color images (Fig. 6) is enormous.

One of the current tasks is the use the previous data from CT as masks on the color images, since

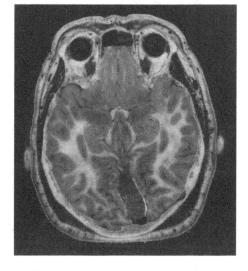

Figure 6.　Head section from the cadaver slice.

some of the color ambiguities found in color images are solved in the CT images. One example is the similar color in color images between cortical bone and adipose tissue, something that was already segregated in the CT images handling.

3 CONCLUSIONS

The presented work presents a simple and effective way to extract three-dimensional anatomic features from usual and no aural medical images.

The use of CT images have proven to give good results in terms of the bone structures, and body skin, and give a potential toll segregating the soft tissues in two or more group (the handled body part gives a segregation in two groups).

The possibility to have multi-direction images was implemented, and used to acquire a better point distribution in terms of contour.

Improvements must be done in the feature extraction concerning the small details and small holes in the structures. Such improvements will allow to sped-up the triangulation process, and giving less probability to get erratic surfaces.

ACKNOWLEDGMENTS

The authors are thankful to the Fundação para a Ciência e a Tecnologia for the researcher grant SFRH/BI/33924/2009, and the projects "Methodologies to Analyze Organs from Complex Medical Images—Applications to the Female Pelvic Cavity" and "Cardiovascular Imaging Modeling and Simulation—SIMCARD", with references PTDC/EEA-CRO/103320/2008 e UTAustin/CA/0047/2008.

The author acknowledge the U.S. National Library of Medicine, for the images from the project "Visible Human Project".

REFERENCES

Arnaux, P., Kayvantash, K., Thollon, L., The RADIOSS Human Model for Safety (HUMOS)—Validation of the Radioss HUMOS model; Definition of a model evaluation procedure—Model Version 14D.

Barneva, R.P., Brimkov, V.E., Hauptman, H.A., Natal Jorge, R.M., Tavares, 2010, J.M.R.S. (Editors), Computational Modeling of Objects Represented in Images, LNCS Series, ISBN 978-3-642-12711-3.

Belinha, J., 2010, "The Natural Neighbour Radial Point Interpolation Method", PhD thesis, feup, Porto, Portugal.

Bernardini, F., Mittleman, J., Rushmeier, H., Taubin, G., 1999, "The Ball-Pivoting Algorithm for Surface Reconstruction", IEEE Transactions of Visualization & Graphics.

Haug, E., Choi, H.-Y., Robin, S., Beaugonin, M., 2004, "Human Models for Crash and Impact Simulation", in "Handbook of Numerical Analysis, Vol. XII—Computational Models for the Human Body", Eds. Ayache, N., Ciarlet, P.G., Elsevier Ltd., pp. 231–452.

Hilton, A., Stoddart, A.J., Illingworth, J., Windeatt, T., 1996, "Marching Triangles: Range Image Fusion for Complex Object Modeling. Image Processing", Vol. 1., pp. 381–384. Sep 1996.

Iwamoto, M., Kisanuki, Y., Watenabe, I., Furusu, K., Miki, K., Hasegawa, J., 2002, "Development of a finite element model of the total human model for safety (THUMS) and application to injury reconstruction", 2002 International IRCOBI Conference, pp. 31–42.

Talaia, P., Parente, M., Fernandes, A., Natal, R., 2011a, "Criação de geometrias anatómicas recorrendo a imagens RGB", 4° Congresso Nacional de Biomecânica, February 4–5, Coimbra, Portugal.

Talaia, P., Parente, M., Fernandes, A., Natal, R., 2011b, "Manipulação de imagens RGB e reconstrução de geometrias anatómicas", CMNE2011—Congress on Numerical Methods in Engineering, June 14–7, Coimbra, Portugal (accepted).

Tavares, J.M.R.S., Natal Jorge, (2009), R.M. (Editors), Advances in Computational Vision and Medical Image Processing, Computational Methods in Applied Sciences Series, Vol.13, Springer, ISBN 978-1-4020-9085-1.

Computational Vision and Medical Image Processing – Tavares & Natal Jorge (eds)
© *2012 Taylor & Francis Group, London, ISBN 978-0-415-68395-1*

The breast phantom construction for a research purpose

M. Ribeiro
Escola Superior de Tecnologia da Saúde de Lisboa—Área Científica de Radiologia, Departamento de Anatomia da Faculdade de Ciências Médicas da Universidade Nova de Lisboa, Portugal

J. O'Neill
Departamento de Anatomia da Faculdade de Ciências Médicas da Universidade Nova de Lisboa/CEFITEC, Portugal

J. Mauricio
Universidade da Beira Interior/DIAMECON Tomar, Portugal

ABSTRACT: The purpose was to perform a breast phantom to test in a Magnetic Resonance system 1,5 T, the effectiveness of the fat suppression techniques. Based on the literature available, previous to select the best phantom components, were performed some trials mixing different ingredients. The Gel Carrageenan (CAGN) phantom is highly useful and practical for experiments such as in MRI. Carrageenan, unlike agarose, has little effect on T1 and T2 relaxation times. CAGN is a linear sulfated polyssacharide, which is extracted from red seaweeds, and therefore expensive and very difficult to find available. For this reason, the carrageenan was replaced by another jelly agent, the agarose, which was mixed with water and gelatin and heated in a microwave till boiled. The mixture was then cooled to get solidification. The final result was an internal model with a breast shape, filled with a mix by agarose, gelatin, distilled water, pork fat and breast turkey. The mold in which the final composition was introduced was built by a human model to mimic the best as possible the breasts of a woman with middle morphometric characteristics. The proportion of the pork fat/breast turkey was different between the left and the right breast to simulate two different breast compositions—the fibroglandular and the adipose breast tissue. The complete phantom was after submitted to a Magnetic Resonance system to analyze the performance of STIR, SPIR and SPAIR weighted sequences in the breast fat saturation.

1 INTRODUCTION

Magnetic Resonance Imaging (MRI) combines some of the most interesting principles of physics and some of today's most sophisticated technology to make medical images of amazing clarity and surprisingly high diagnostic accuracy. MRI today is more revolutionary than x-ray imaging was a century ago. Twenty-five years ago, when MRI was first introduced to clinical practice, its richness of application to medical imaging could not have been imagined. It quickly was demonstrated that MRI is useful in the diagnosis of diseases[1]. The richness of MRI is continuing to unfold. Breast imaging is one more example of the unexpected versatility of MRI[1,2].

In 1986, MRI was used for the first time in the study of the breast and, since then, this diagnostic method has undergone significant advances, revealing that it is promising in the investigation of breast cancer.

MRI of the breast is a non-invasive technique with high tissue differentiation. This technique has been widely discussed and evaluated, mainly because it provides additional data not obtained by conventional imaging methods, such as mammograms and breast ultrasound. Breast MRI is particularly useful in the evaluation of newly diagnosed breast cancer, in women whose breast tissue is very dense and not suitable for screening, to the follow-up after therapy or quimioteraphy, to study the breast implants and in women with a high lifetime risk of breast cancer due to their family history or genetic disposition[1,3].

Is known that the uniformity and inhomogeneity of the breast MR images are due to the amount of the fat tissue, present in the different breast composition.

The purpose was to perform a breast phantom to test in a Magnetic Resonance system 1,5 T, the effectiveness of the fat suppression techniques. After this study aims to indicate between STIR, SPAIR and SPIR the most effective technique to decrease uniformity and inhomogeneity and improve image quality.

Based on the literature available, previous to select the best phantom composition, were performed some trials mixing different ingredients which was result in seven different samples composition. All these composition procedures were rigorously carried out in collaboration with the laboratory of the Chemistry Department of and its experts. (Fig. 1)

According to Kato et al. (2005), a gel carrageenan (CAGN) phantom is equivalent to most human tissues for electrical conductivity and relaxation times by Magnetic Resonance (MRI) detection. The CAGN phantom is highly useful and practical for experiments such as in MRI. Carrageenan, unlike agarose, has little effect on T1 and T2 relaxation times. CAGN is a linear sulfated polyssacharide, which is extracted from red seaweeds, and therefore expensive and very difficult to find available. For this reason, in this study, the carrageenan was replaced by another jelly agent, the agarose, which was mixed with water and gelatin and heated in a microwave till boiled. The mixtures were then cooled to solidify it.

These mixes were introduced in sterilized packages (Fig. 1) and submitted to a Magnetic Resonance system to determine which one was more similar with the breast tissue.

The samples were after observed by 5 experts to choose which one was the most similar to a breast tissue. The final result was a model with a breast shape, filled with a mix by agarose, gelatin, distilled water, pork fat and breast turkey. (Samples 1 and 7 from Table 1.

The proportion of the pork fat/breast turkey was different between the left and the right breast to simulate two different breast compositions—the predominance of the fibroglandular or the adipose breast tissue.

To the phantom looks similar to the anatomical region studied was designed a cast of traditional plaster Biplastrix®, which was rubberized with a polyethylene bag and coated with the sample 1 and then filled with the sample 7, according to the Table 1. The mold in which the final composition of the study was introduced, to be studied by the breast dedicated coil, was built by a human model in the Prosthesis laboratories (Figs. 3–6), to mimic the best as possible the breasts of a woman with morphometric characteristics measured by the BRA with

Table 1. Description and composition of phantom samples.

Samples	Ingredients
1	Agarose; Gelatin; distilled water
2	Agarose; Gelatin; distilled water; Gadoliniun Chloride (GdCl3)
3	Agarose; Gelatin; Gadoliniun Chloride (GdCl3); distilled water; Olive oil
4	Agarose; Gelatin; Gadoliniun Chloride (GdCl3); distilled water; Corn oil
5	Agarose; Gelatin; Gadoliniun Chloride (GdCl3); distilled water; pork fat
6	Turkey breast; Agarose; Gelatin; distilled water; pork fat (small geometry)
7	Turkey breast; Agarose; Gelatin; distilled water; pork fat (large geometry)

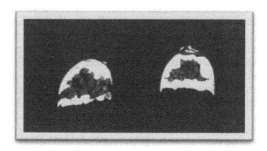

Figure 2. MRI of the Breast phantom in STIR-transversal weighted sequence.

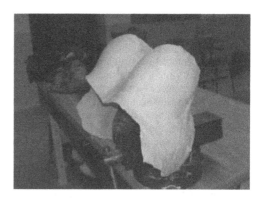

Figure 3. Construction of the Phantom outside (Phase 1).

D cup and 35 cm width. The phantom ingredients were used in the proportions shown in Table 2.

In a second phase, not covered by this text, this phantom was submitted to a MR system and were applied the weighted sequences SPIR, STIR and SPAIR, and assessed the corresponding images, to

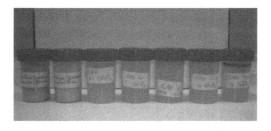

Figure 1. Samples contained in sterilized packages.

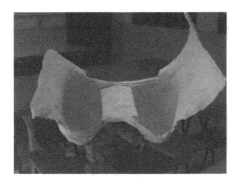

Figure 4. Construction of the Phantom outside (Phase 2).

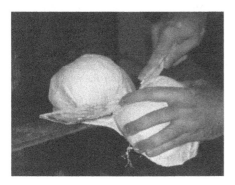

Figure 5. Construction of the Phantom outside (Phase 3).

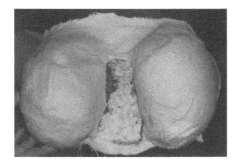

Figure 6. Construction of the Phantom outside (Phase 4).

conclude the fat suppression technique most effective that must be applied in each case.

2 METHOD S AND MATERIALS

2.1 *Phantom Construction—Phases (Figs.3–6)*

After the evaluation of the images obtained, the selected sample was the most consistent with the proposed target, this mean, according to the breast

Table 2. Summary of the composition ingredients and respectively proportions in the breast phantom.

Ingredients	Composition (/100 g)	Proportions
Agarose		17.35 g
Gelatine		29.7 g
Distilled water		990 ml
Turkey breast (RB*)	Protein 15.5 g Lipids 0.8 g	150 g
Pork fat (RB*)	Saturated fats 38–43% Unsaturated fats 56–62%	55.56 g

anatomy. Thus, as phantom content the sample chosen was the seven, and as a coating the sample one.

In this study, the agarose and the gelatin (gelling agents) were used to provide the phantom sufficient strength and long enough T1 and T2 values to mimic the human breast tissue.[9-11]

In order to simulate the heterogeneity of fat and parenchyma that occurs within breasts, the pork fat representing the breast adipose tissue and the turkey breast representing the breast parenchyma were put in different quantities on each breast. The left breast has less 20% of turkey breast and more 20% of pork fat than the right breast (Fig. 2).

It was used small cubes of turkey breast in equal size mixed with cooking pork fat by means of a glass rod. The volume of turkey breast added to the phantom was determined by water displacement, while the volume for liquefied cooking pork fat was measured.

3 CONCLUSIONS

Fat suppression is a generic term that includes various techniques, each with specific advantages, disadvantages and pitfalls.

The suppression of fat signal from breast tissue is often inconsistent and non-uniform. There has been no published evaluation of different breast fat suppression techniques to guide the optimization for clinical imaging[22].

MRI Radiographers have access to a range of fat suppression methods, which work by exploiting particular characteristics of the MR (magnetic resonance) signals from fat and water. Understanding the mechanisms of each method provides insight into appropriate applications and situations where artifacts can be anticipated. Controlling the fat suppression can enhance the sensitivity and specificity of an MRI breast examination in many clinical settings[22], so the MR Radiographer must be familiar with the available fat suppression techniques and know when to apply them.

According to the guidelines and the ethical procedures is not acceptable to undergo one female to a radiofrequency in MR more than 30 minutes. Thus, to find another possibilities and alternatives, such as phantom construction, with a research purpose combine with a low cost, is today a challenge in the University departments.

REFERENCES

American College of Radiology. ACR Practice Guideline for the Performance of Contrast-Enhanced MRI of the Breast. 2008; 25: 561–567.

Boston, Raymond C. [et al]. Estimation of the content of fat and parenchyma in breast tissue using MRI T1 histograms and phantoms. Elsevier 2005; 23: 591–599.

Genson, Charles C. [et al]. Effects on Breast MRI of Artifacts caused by metallic tissue marker clips. American Journal of Radiology 2007; 188: 372–376.

Greatrex, Kathleen V. [et al]. Current Role of Magnetic Resonance Imaging in Breast Imaging: A primer for the primary care physician. The Journal of the American Board of Family Practice 2005; 18: 478–490.

Hendrick, Edward R. Breast MRI: fundamentals and technical aspects. Springer 2008; USA; 1–145.

Kopans, Daniel B. Magnetic Resonance Imaging. In: Lippincott—Raven, Second Edition. Breast Imaging. New York: 1998; James Ryan, 1997; 617–634.

Kato, Hirokazu. [et al]. Composition of MRI phantom equivalent to human tissues. Am. Assoc. Phys. Med. 2005; 32(10): 3199–3208.

Lauenstein, Thomas C. Spectral Adiabatic Inversion Recovery (SPAIR) MR Imaging of the Abdomen. Magnetom Flash 2008; 2: 16–20.

Lee, Nancy A. [et al]. Fatty and Fibroglandular Tissue Volumes in the Breasts of Women 20–83 Years Old: Comparison of X-Ray Mammography and Computer-Assisted MR Imaging. American Journal of Radiology 1997; 168: 501–506.

Lin, C. [et al]. Quantitative Evaluation of Fat Suppression Techniques for Breast MRI at 3.0T.

Medved, Milica. [et al]. High Spectral and Spatial Resolution MRI of Breast Lesions: Preliminary Clinical Experience. American Journal of Radiology 2006; 186: 30–37.

Madsen, Ernest L. [et al]. Anthropomorphic Breast Phantoms for Qualification of Investigators for ACRIN Protocol 6666. Radiology 2006; 239: 869–874.

Niitsu, Mamoru. [et al]. Fat Suppression Strategies in Enhanced MR Imaging of the Breast: Comparison of SPIR and Water Excitation Sequences. Journal of Magnetic Resonance Imaging 2003; 18: 310–314.

Ribeiro, Margarida. [et al]. Técnicas de Supressão de Gordura: Estudo Comparativo em Ressonância Magnética Mamária. Acta Radiológica Portuguesa, Vol. XXII 2010; 85: 21–22.

Riedl, E. [et al]. The role of STIR MRI sequence in the evaluation of the breast following conservative surgery and radiotherapy. Neoplasma 2001; 48(1): 7–114.

Computational Vision and Medical Image Processing – Tavares & Natal Jorge (eds)
© 2012 Taylor & Francis Group, London, ISBN 978-0-415-68395-1

Engineer methods of assistance of toraco-chirurgical operation

B. Gzik-Zroska, W. Wolański & M. Gzik
Silesian University of Technology, Gliwice, Silesia, Poland

J. Dzielicki
Medical University of Silesia, Katowice, Poland

ABSTRACT: In this work the application of new visualization technologies in correction of funnel chest is presented. The virtual model of chest worked out in MIMICS program was designed to determine state of load after correction of deformation by stabilizing plate. From biomechanical point of view the knowledge of load value affecting stabilizer is necessary to select optimal parameters of the plate. The force value affecting plate used in correction of deformation of chest by Nuss method was evaluated on the base of funnel chest skeleton model formulated in ANSYS. Research works which aim was selection of optimal thickness of the plate were carried out in next stage. In this work a parametrical model of the plate was formulated, where thickness, length, width and flexion size of the plate are parameters of the model. Calculations were conducted for three alternative constraints.

1 INTRODUCTION

In recent decade new visualization technologies along with systems of computer assistance of engineer works find more and more application in medicine. The most often used to model bones and to plan the operation. Introduction of three-dimensional displaying technique enable to generate 3D models that make possible more precise medical diagnosis and detailed planning of operation. The history of surgical treatment on funnel chest dates back to 1949 and shows that bad outlook of the cage and low self-esteem were sufficient to undertake the surgical treatment. Funnel chest is a congenital deformation, result of rickets or family inheritance where sternum is displaced to the back of chest. In consequence the frontal—rear size is to a large degree reduced and cause displacement of heart with possibility of its compression. Because of the respiration is limited the person get tired quicker and have limited abilities of activeness. Surgical treatment with various technique becomes a requirement then. Surgical procedure is associated however with quite extensive preparation in the front wall area of the chest what in a consequence leads to generating large after-surgical scars.

Method of correction of deformation proposed in 1987 by doctor Donald Nuss [1] is less invasive and doesn't require resection of rib cartilages and extensive cutting of front wall of the chest. For that purpose we use a stabilizing plate that push out deformed sternum and hold it in a right position for a period of 12 to 24 months [4].

Sometimes it comes to complications due to displacement, permanent deformation or fracture of some type of implants in result of fatigue. Damaged implant may lead to reverse deformation of the chest but also may cause real danger for human life. To avoid such problems it becomes necessary to work out a suitable method of selection of implant with regards to existing in correction of deformation state of load. The attempt to determine optimal process of selection of the plate used in Nuss method was made in this work.

2 MODELLING OF FUNEL CHEST

2.1 *The study of geometry of model in MIMICS*

In order to determine state of load of funnel chest after its correction by Nuss method it was necessary to formulate model of funnel chest. For analyzed case a virtual model was worked out through utilization of MIMICS program. The reconstruction process has begun with import of data from computer scanning making the full three-dimensional reconstruction of shape of structures of the chest possible. Model generated automatically very often includes some impurities or artefacts due to for example the inaccuracy of output picture. Therefore received body should be in next stage analyzed in order to remove unnecessary elements. Off course doctor's hints who defines which fragments refclect reality and which are artefacts are crucial here (especially in case of complicated pathologies). At last we obtain solid body taking into account geometry of bone.

Table 1. Mechanical properties of structure of the chest [2,3].

Element	Young's modulus [MPa]	Poisson ratio
Ribs	5000	0,3
Cartilage ribs	200	0,4
Sternum	11500	0,3
Vertebrae	11500	0,3
Intervertebral discs	110	0,4
Cartilage elements	150	0,4

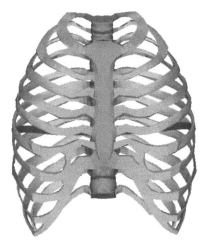

Figure 1. Model of funnel chest with stabilizing plate.

Received in this way model is fully functional and can be modified depending on needs.

2.2 *The study of numerical model in ANSYS*

In next stage the geometry of chest worked out in MIMICS was imported into ANSYS in order to carry out numerical calculations.

In modelling process the following assumptions were accepted:

- vertebrae, ribs, cartilage connections and sternum are treated as homogeneous bodies with isotropic properties reflecting real geometry,
- the model consider discs, intervertebral joints and joints that connects ribs with vertebras of linear-elastic characteristic,
- the pressure inside chest and the influence of internal organs were skipped,
- the model was restrained and loaded in accordance with conditions of research.

For modelled chest an isotropic and linear mechanical properties of structures were on the ground of literature data [2,3] accepted and collected in Table 1.

In order to analyze loads and strains in chest after conducted operation the stabilizing plate complying with geometry of the plate used in Nuss method were added to the model of funnel chest.

Interaction between plate and chest (Fig. 1) was modelled through common knots. The mesh of finite elements forming model with stabilizing plate consist of 11 516 elements. In total 23 900 knots were received what resulted in 71 700 degrees of freedom.

3 STATE OF LOAD OF THE CHEST

In order to analyze loads and strains in chest the deformation was corrected by stabilizing plate.

A displacement equal the size of deformation was given in knots of the plate and deformed fragments of chest were pushed out. On the contrary the rear wall of chest were supported through taking away all degrees of freedom in konts of vertebras.

Below we present examples of following simulation results: displacement (Fig. 2), strain (Fig. 3) and stress (Fig. 4). On its basis the analysis of influence of correction of deformation on chest's properties was carried out.

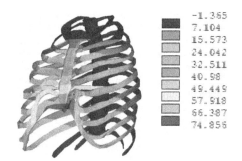

Figure 2. Displacements obtained in the chest during correction of deformation.

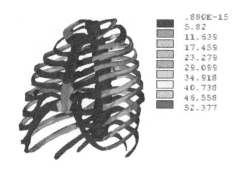

Figure 3. Stress obtained in the chest during correction of deformation.

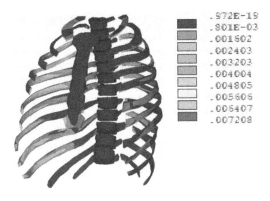

Figure 4.   Main strain ε1 obtained in the chest's skeleton during correction of deformation.

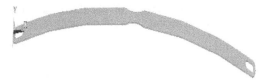

Figure 5.   Numerical model of stabilizing plate.

Table 2.   Mechanical properties of stabilizing plate.

Steel grade	Young's modulus [MPa]	Poisson ratio
Cr-Ni-Mo	210	0,3

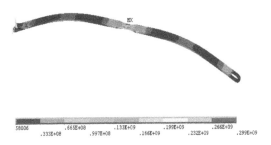

Figure 6.   Reduced stress for optimal thickness of the plate for second variant of calculations.

The force value required for correction of deformation was estimated from numeric calculations. In analysed case obtained value amounts to 296 N.

4   OPTIMIZATION OF GEOMETRIC CHARACTERISTICS OF STABILIZING PLATE

Selection of optimum thickness of stabilizing plate has begun from study of parametrical model of the plate. In APDL language a batch file for ANSYS was formulated. Numerical model complies with geometry of produced by MIKROMED plate used in correction of deformation by Nuss method. In the model of stabilizing plate the following parametrical data were accepted: thickness, length, width and size of the flexion (Fig. 5). It was also introduced the variable of load derived from pressure of front wall of the chest after funnel chest correction.

The geometrical model model of plate was split into finite elements with the same parameters and type (SOLID 95) what the model of chest. Afterwards mechanical properties presented in Table 2 were given to the plate.

The following criteria were taken into consideration during selection of optimum thickness:

- assurance of minimum dislocation of plate,
- assurance of suitable stamina conditions of plate that is not exceeding a limit of plastic strain.

In the selection process of optimum constructional features of stabilizing plate an optimization module available in ANSYS was used. Optimization problem was formulated as minimization problem of stabilizing plate volume with following contraints:

- thickness of plate,
- dislocation of plate along axis Oy,
- stress.

Numerical calculations were conducted for three variants of limitations. Following figures shows stress received for optimum thickness value of plate.

5   RESULTS, ANALYSIS AND CONCLUSIONS

Computer assistance of operation procedure determine innovatory method of quality assurance of treatment and contributes to increase patient's safety during the operation. Obtained results of numerical calculations made possible the analysis of loads and deformations formed in funnel chest after its correction with Nuss method. Model made possible determination of the force value required for correction of deformation. Obtained information was base for definition of influence of correction on stress and strain pattern and for specification of areas where unexpected injuries might occur. In analyzed case loads are uniformly transmitted mostly through osseous ribs and lower part of sternum. Obtained force value required for correction of deformation amounts to 296 N. In next studies this force was used for optimization of geometrical parameters of stabilizing plate and the same for determination of optimal treatment conditions.

In this work the selection of optimum constructional features of stabilizing plate was conducted, using its formulated parametrical model and taking into consideration interaction of skeletal system—implant.

ACKNOWLEDGMENT

This work is supported by Polish Ministry of Science and High Education from project no NN501 236139.

REFERENCES

1. Correira de Matos, Bernardo E.J., Fernandese E.J (1997) Surgery of chest wall deformities. European Journal of Cardio-thoracic Surgery, 12.

2. Forbes P.A., Development of a Human Body Model for the Analysis of Side Impact Automotive Thoracic Trauma, Waterloo, Ontario.

3. Furusu K., Watanabe I., Kato Ch., Miki K., Hasegawa J., Fundamental study of side impast analysis using the finite element model of the human thorax, JSAE, 22, 195–199, 2001.

4. Jacobs P.J., Quintessenze J.A., Morell V.O., Botero L.M., van Gelder H.M., Tchervenkov C.I., (2002) Minimally invasive endoscopic repair of pectus excavatum. European Journal of Cardio-thoracic Surgery 21.

5. Nackenhorst, U., Numerical simulation of stress stimulated bone remodeling, Technische Mechanic 17 (1): 31–40, 1997.

Computational Vision and Medical Image Processing – Tavares & Natal Jorge (eds)
© 2012 Taylor & Francis Group, London, ISBN 978-0-415-68395-1

Stress analysis of the tympanic membrane through image

C. Garbe, M. Parente, P. Martins & R. Natal Jorge
IDMEC—Faculdade de Engenharia da Universidade do Porto, Porto, Portugal

F. Gentil
IDMEC-FEUP, ESTSP, Clínica ORL—Dr. Eurico Almeida, Widex, Portugal

J. Paço
Hospital CUF, Faculdade de Medicina da Universidade de Lisboa, Lisbon, Portugal

ABSTRACT: To better understand the ear functioning, a biomechanical study of the tympanic ossicular chain of the middle ear was made. This chain consists of the tympanic membrane (which has 3 layers), three ossicles (malleus, incus and stapes), six ligaments, tendons and respective two muscles. The objective of this study was to analyze the stresses of the tympanic membrane through images, allowing a comparison of the different frequencies used. A geometric model of the tympanic membrane and ossicles was built through images of Computerized Axial Tomography (CAT). The discretization of this model was done using the finite element method, based on the ABAQUS software. The mechanical properties were obtained from previous work. The results were compared in the dynamic analysis of the tympanic ossicular chain for a frequency range between 100 Hz and 10 kHz, for a sound pressure level of 105 dB SPL, applied on the tympanic membrane. We can observe differences for each frequency in the tympanic membrane.

1 INTRODUCTION

1.1 *Auditory system*

The human ear is the organ that allows us to perceive and interpret sound waves in a frequency range between 16 Hz and 20 kHz and intensities between 0 dB and 130 dB (Henrique, 2002).

The sound energy is driven by the external auditory canal to the tympanic membrane, where it is transformed into mechanical energy, which in turn is communicated to the middle ear ossicles. The tympanic membrane separates the external ear and the middle ear and it is divided into two parts: *pars tensa* and *pars flaccida*.

The tympanic membrane is like a mirror of what goes on inside of the middle ear, and knowledge of this structure is fundamental to the understanding of many diseases (Paço, 2003).

The purpose of this study was to analyze the stresses of tympanic membrane through images. For this purpose, some specific objectives were established: the study of the sound transmission by the middle ear; creating a model that simulates the tympanic ossicular chain; discretization of this model based on finite element method; simulation of vibro-acoustic tympanic ossicular chain; collection of the results in the form of image.

1.2 *Finite element method*

In simple terms, it can be noted that the application of the method involves dividing the area into parts, called finite elements, which bind to each other at certain points, called nodes.

Thus, it works on simple elements, even if they belong to the geometric areas of complex shapes. These elements can have characteristics of one, two and three-dimensional. In the case of two-dimensional applications, the most used are a triangular or quadrangular, while problems in three-dimensional are tetrahedral or hexahedral elements.

Through images of CAT, a 3D digital model of the tympanic ossicular chain was constructed (Gentil, 2009). The discretization of the model was done using the finite element method. The mechanical properties were obtained from previous work (Prendergast, 1999). The stresses of tympanic membrane for a frequency range between 100 Hz and 10 kHz, for a sound pressure level of 105 dB SPL, applied on the tympanic membrane, were obtained.

2 MATERIALS AND METHODS

2.1 *Construction of model*

A digital model of the tympanic membrane and ossicles of the middle ear, based on images taken from CAT belonging to a woman of 65 years old, with normal hearing (Fig. 1).

Using the software ABAQUS (ABAQUS, 2007) the discretization of the tympanic ossicular chain, was made generating thus the finite element mesh. Figure 2 shows a representation of the geometric model used in the tympanic ossicular chain together with the finite element mesh.

The tympanic membrane was seen with three layers, (Garbe, 2009) with the use of hexahedral elements 11,165 of the type C3D8, totaling 15,295 nodes. The tympanic membrane is also divided into 2 parts (Fig. 3): the *pars flaccida* (located at the top and slightly fibrous) and *pars tensa* (membrane itself and is responsible for its vibration).

Referring to the ossicles, tetrahedral elements of the type C3D4 are chosen, due to highly irregular geometries. The malleus is composed of 18,841 elements, the incus 39,228 elements and the stapes by 9,218 elements.

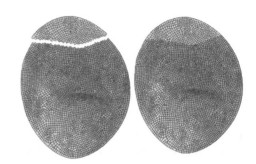

Figure 3. Model of the tympanic membrane: *pars tensa* and *pars flaccida*.

2.2 Material properties

Relevant material properties for the various components of the model, such as Young's modulus, Poisson's ratio, densities and damping coefficients, are applied, being based on previously published work (Prendergast, 1999), where E is the Young's modulus, with the index θ indicating the tangential direction and r radial direction (Table 1).

The *pars flaccida* is considered elastic isotropic and the *pars tensa* is considered with three layers, where the middle one is orthotropic and the others isotropic.

The tympanic membrane was assigned as a Poisson's ratio of 0.3, based on literature (Prendergast, 1999). The density of this component was set at $1.20E+03$ Kg/m³.

The properties used for the bones are set out in Table 2.

Based on the model Yeoh, the ligaments were considered as a nonlinear hyperelastic behavior. The energy function of deformation ψ for this material model is given by equation (1):

$$\psi = c_1(I_1-3) + c_2(I_1-3)^2 + c_3(I_1-3)^3 \qquad (1)$$

where I_1 is the first invariant of Cauchy-Green tensor on the right, and c_1, c_2 and c_3 are the material constants (Martins, 2006).

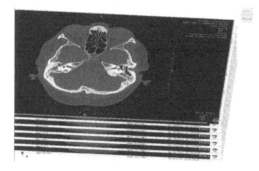

Figure 1. Axial 2D image obtained by CAT of the tympanic ossicular chain.

2.3 Boundary conditions

Regarding the boundary conditions, the tympanic membrane was fixed according to Figure 4, simulating the tympanic sulcus.

The stapes was fixed on its periphery, simulating the annular ligament.

The malleus has the anterior, superior and lateral ligaments, and incus, superior and posterior ligaments.

The links between the ossicles malleus/incus and incus/stapes were made by contact formulations, with a friction rate equal to 0.7 (Gentil et al., 2007).

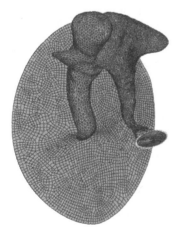

Figure 2. Model of the tympanic ossicular chain with the finite element mesh.

Table 1. Properties of the tympanic membrane.

Model			Poisson's ratio	Young's modulus (N/m²)	
Tympanic membrane				E	
Pars flaccida	Elastic	Iso	0.3	1.00E + 07	
				E(θ)	E(r)
Pars tensa	Layer 1	Elastic	Iso	0.3	1.00E + 07	1.00E + 07
	Layer 2		Ort		2.00E + 07	3.20E + 07
	Layer 3		Iso		1.00E + 07	1.00E + 07

Table 2. Properties of the ossicles.

Density (Kg/m³)			Model		Poisson's ratio	Young's modulus (N/m²)
Ossicles						E
Malleus	Head	2.55E + 03	Elastic	Isotrópic	0.3	1.41E + 10
	Neck	4.53E + 03				
	Manubrium	3.70E + 03				
Incus	Body	2.36E + 03				
	Short	2.26E + 03				
	Long	5.08E + 03				
Stapes		2.20E + 03				

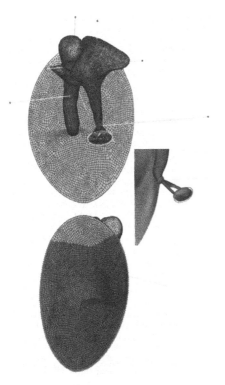

Figure 4. Representation of the boundary conditions.

2.4 Simulation

In order to understand the behavior of the tympanic ossicular chain of the middle ear, along a frequency range between 100 Hz and 10 kHz, simulations were carried out applying a uniform sound pressure level corresponding to 105 dB SPL.

The Sound Pressure Level (SPL) is the level corresponding to the pressure caused by the vibration of sound, measured at a certain point. The scale decibels SPL defines sound levels by comparing the sound pressure levels, p, with a reference sound pressure, p_0, that is given by equation (2):

$$SPL = 20\log\left(\frac{p}{p_0}\right) \tag{2}$$

which $p_0 = 20$ µPa is called reference sound pressure, corresponding to the threshold of audibility. Results of the tympanic membrane stress were obtained for an application of pressure of 3.56 Pa (105 dB SPL).

3 RESULTS

This work investigated the application of the finite element method in the biomechanical study of tympanic ossicular chain, concerned of tensions obtained on tympanic membrane.

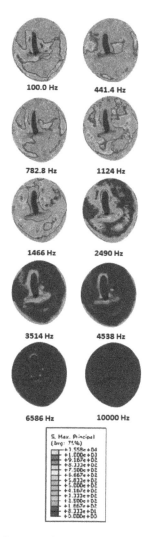

Figure 5. Stresses of the tympanic membrane for different frequencies.

To this end, a computer model to simulate the biomechanics of the tympanic ossicular chain was used.

An excitation in the tympanic membrane of sound pressure level of 105 dB SPL was induced.

We can observe that for low frequencies the stresses obtained are greater than for high frequencies.

We can see that the higher level of tension has been observed for frequency of 441.4 Hz, where it is shown the highest incidence of gray (representing the highest levels of tension in Fig. 5).

It was also noted that the second highest level of stress occurs for the frequency of 782.8 Hz.

We also observed that higher levels of stress are located in the region that focus on the boundary conditions for the tympanic sulcus, which is located almost entirely around of the *pars tensa*.

For frequencies greater than 1 kHz, we can observe that the highest stress occurs around the manubrium of the malleus.

4 CONCLUSIONS

We can conclude from the images presented that the highest level of tension occurs for low frequencies, being the greater observed for frequency of 441.4 Hz and then for 782.8 Hz.

The highest stress levels are located in the region that focus boundary conditions for the tympanic sulcus.

This work may lead to other studies, notably the inclusion of the outer ear and inner ear, tympanic cavity, simulating conditions such as tympanic perforation, ear infections, otosclerosis, myringosclerosis, tympanosclerosis, as well as application of prosthesis of the middle ear, thus contributing to well for future studies related to rehabilitation.

AGRADECIMENTOS

Thanks to funding provided by the Ministry of Science and Higher Education (FCT—Portugal) through project "Estudo bio-computacional do zumbido" (PTDC/SAU-BEB/104992/2008).

REFERENCES

ABAQUS. (2007). Analyses User's Manual, Version 6.5.
Garbe, Carolina. (2010). Estudo biomecânico para reabilitação do ouvido médio humano. Tese de Mestrado. Mestrado em Engenharia Biomédica. Faculdade de Engenharia da Universidade do Porto. *Portugal.*
Garbe, C., Gentil, F., Parente, M., Martins, P., Natal Jorge, R. (2009). *Aplicação Do Método Dos Elementos Finitos No Estudo Da Membrana Timpânica.* Audiologia Em Revista. Volume II, Número 3, 99–106.
Gentil, F., Jorge, R.M.N., Ferreira, A.J.M., Parente, M.P.L., Moreira, M., Almeida, E. (2007). Estudo do efeito do atrito no contacto entre os ossículos do ouvido médio, *Revista Internacional de Métodos Numéricos para Cálculo y Diseño en Ingeniería.* Vol. 23, 2, 177–187.
Gentil, F., Jorge, R.N., Parente, M.P.L., Martins, P.A.L.S., Ferreira, A.J.M. (2009). Estudo biomecânico do ouvido médio, *Clínica e Investigação em Otorrinolaringologia,* 3 (1), 24–30.
Henrique, L. (2002). *Acústica Musical.* Fundação Calouste Gulbenkian.
Martins, P.A.L.S., Jorge, R.M.N., Ferreira, A.J.M. (2006). A Comparative Study of Several Material Models for Prediction of Hyperelastic Properties: Application to Silicone-Rubber and Soft Tissues. Strain. 42, 135–147.
Paço, J. (2003). *Doenças do timpano.* Lisboa. Portugal: Lidel.
Prendergast, P.J., Ferris, P., Rice, H.J., Blayney, A.W. (1999). Vibro-acoustic modelling of the outer and middle ear using the finite element method, *Audiol Neurootol.* 4, 185–191.

Computational Vision and Medical Image Processing – Tavares & Natal Jorge (eds)
© 2012 Taylor & Francis Group, London, ISBN 978-0-415-68395-1

Simulation and modeling the thermal behaviour of textile structures

M.J. Geraldes
Beira Interior University, Covilhã, Portugal

L. Hes
Technical University of Liberec, Liberec, Chzec Republic

M. Araújo
Minho University, Guimarães, Portugal

ABSTRACT: The total comfort of a garment comprises, not only, the sensorial and thermophysiological comfort, but also aesthetic, colour and size aspects, wich make up the so called psychological comfort. But, it is the thermophysiological comfort, wich historically justifies the existence of clothes themselves, that is characterised by two important properties: thermal properties (heat transfer) and physiological properties (mass transfer). The mathematical modelization of the principal thermal properties in functional knit structures was done, and founded good correlations between the theoretical and experimental values of the refered properties.

1 INTRODUCTION

From the results achieved by some researchers, the following equation, for the total comfort, was derived:

$$K_{Total} = \frac{1}{3} K_{Sensorial} + \frac{2}{3} K_{Termophysiological}$$

Where,

K_{Total} = Total comfort;
$K_{Sensorial}$ = Sensorial comfort;
$K_{Thermophysiological\ comfort}$ = Thermophysiological comfort.

The main thermophysiological properties of textile materials are heat transfer, moisture transfer and air transfer resulting from basic physiological activities of skin and needs while wearing a clothing product.

The heat permeability throught textile layer is in accordance with resistance of heat transfer by conducting, connecting and radiating. Intensity of thermal characteristics is mainly determined by air volume caught in macromorphological structural unit. It is caused by the fact that the thermal conductivity of air is considerable lower compared to the thermal conductivity of fibre and lower as well compared to the thermal conductivity of a two dimensional textile structure.

The moisture permeability throught textile layer is well determined by resistance of moisture transfer

through textile layer. Regarding the physiology, it is important for this quantity to reach the lowest values and at the same time it is important to consider the resistance of heat transfer through the textile layer. The resistance of moisture transfer and resistance of heat transfer through textile layer are not always in conformance. The resistance of heat and moisture transfer ratio is expressed by index of moisture transfer.

Regarding the phenomenon of underclothing microclimate, situated between skin and contact textile layer, the textiles must be constructed in a way to suck the maximum of humidity from skin to outside layers. Such textile guaranties a dry underclothing microclimate and comfort while wearing. They are the called "Functional Textiles", with at least, two different layers: an hydrophilic layer or outside layer (Absorption layer) and an hydrophobic layer or inside layer (Separation layer).

The development of the mathematical model of thermal properties in functional knits structures was based in the following theoretical conditions:

- The knit structure is in the wet state and is completely saturated (what is not completly true);
- We are considering only the static state, because in the dynamic state we have the influence a lot of parameter, like the contact pression;
- In the static state, the conditions are well defined and we intend to found a relation between the principal thermal properties.

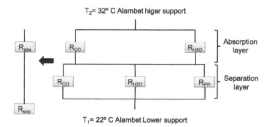

T₂= 32° C Alambet higer support

T₁= 22° C Alambet Lower support

Where:
R_{co}: Cotton thermal resistance;
R_{H_2O}: Water thermal resistance;
R_{pp}: Polypropylene thermal resistance;
R_{abs}: Absorption layer thermal resistance;
R_{sep}: Separation layer thermal resistance.

Figure 1. Electrical scheme of a functional knit structure, wich separation layer is composed by cotton and polypropylene (with suction channels).

Using an electrothermal analogy, it is possible to represent the knit structures, like electrical schemes, where the thermal resistances are equivalent to the electric resistances, as illustrated in Figure 1.

Since the equivalent thermal resistance of the absorption layer is a combination of two resistances in parallel, it is possible to calculate from the relation:

$$R_{abs} = \frac{R_{co} \times R_{H_2O}}{R_{co} + R_{H_2O}} [m^2 \cdot K/W] \tag{1}$$

For the separation layer, we have a parallel combination of three resistances: R_{co}, R_{H_2O}, R_{pp}.

Once we know the thickness of the absorption and separation layer, it is possible to calculate a thermal resistance for the same layers through the equation:

$$R = \frac{h}{\lambda} [m^2 \cdot K/W]$$

The total thermal resistance R_T of a functional knit structure will be:

$$R_T = R_{abs} + R_{sep} = \frac{R_{co} \times R_{H_2O}}{R_{co} + R_{H_2O}} + \frac{h_{sep}}{\lambda_{sep}}$$

$$= \frac{R_{co} \times R_{H_2O}}{R_{co} + R_{H_2O}} + \frac{h_{sep}}{\lambda_{pp} \times \frac{p}{100} + \lambda_{abs}\left(1 - \frac{b}{100}\right)} \tag{2}$$

Since R_T is affected by the structure thickness, the conductivity of the diferents structure will be calculated from the following relation:

$$\lambda_T = \frac{h_T}{R_T} = \frac{h_T}{R_{abs} + R_{sep}} [W/m \cdot K] \tag{3}$$

Where:
λ_T: Total thermal conductivity;
h_T: Total knit structure thickness;
R_T: Total thermal resistance.

About thermal absorptivity, we used the relation:

$$b = \sqrt{\lambda \rho c} \, [W \cdot s^{1/2}/m^2 \cdot K]$$

Where:
b: Thermal absorptivity;
λ: Thermal conductivity;
c: Specific heat;
ρ: Density.

If, when measuring the knit absorptivity, there is an ideal contact between the sample and the Alambeta measuring head, it is possible to define the next relation:

$$b_W = b_S \times Coef$$

Where:
b_w: Thermal absorptivity in the wet state;
b_S: Thermal absorptivity in the dry state;
$Coef$: Increase of the thermal conductivity (λ) and the thermal mass (ρc), in the wet state.

In the wet state, the thermal absorptivity will be:

$$b_W = \sqrt{(\lambda \rho c)_W}$$
$$\Rightarrow b_W^2 = (\lambda \rho c)_W$$

Considering:
ρ: Knit specific mass in the wet state;
m: Knit water mass, in the wet state;
$\rho(1+m)$: Knit density in the wet state;
C: Specific heat (to the water is 4200);
C_{result}: Final specific heat $= c_{initial} + (m_{H_2O} \times 4200)$

And developing the last absorptivity equation, we obtained a first approximation to the absorptivity, when the structure is in the wet state:

$$b_W = \sqrt{\lambda_W \left[\frac{b^2}{\lambda} + m\frac{b^2}{\lambda} + 4200\rho m(1+m)\right]} \tag{4}$$

To validate these three new equations (A, B, and C), the experimental values of the thermal properties

Table 1. Experimental and theoretical values of thermal properties.

Knit (Refª.)	Absorptivity (b) [Ws$^{1/2}$/m²K]		Conductivity (λ) [W/m · K] × 10^{-3}		Resistance (r) [m²K/W] × 10^{-3}	
	Teórica	Exp.	Teórica	Exp.	Teórica	Exp.
1	501,4	662,0	184,0	184,0	5,6	7,7
2	480,7	543,0	142,3	141,0	5,9	5,5
3	407,0	586,0	136,4	145,0	14,0	13,7
4	409,4	618,0	113,7	119,0	13,4	12,8
5A	426,9	563,0	168,2	158,0	8,5	12,0
5B	430,0	434,0	134,3	124,0	7,52	8,3
5C	500,0	460,0	146,9	140,0	9,05	9,7
6A	424,0	496,0	127,4	131,0	11,1	10,6
6B	343,9	493,0	142,7	141,0	10,3	10,7
6C	415,8	545,0	124,6	146,0	11,8	11,6
7A	462,0	473,0	114,5	153,0	15,9	12,0
7B	425,3	479,0	128,0	136,0	11,8	9,3
7C	460,6	508,0	148,3	138,0	9,3	10,2
8	418,5	532,0	126,1	147,0	11,5	9,7

have been evaluated and a comparative study between the experimental and theoretical values was done.

3 RESULTS AND DISCUSSION

3.1 Thermal properties

Data summarizing measured and evaluated properties related to thermal absorptivity, thermal conductivity and thermal resistance are given in Table 1.

3.2 Results analysis

The comparative study between the experimental and theoretical values, give us the followings graphic representations:

3.2.1 Thermal absorptivity

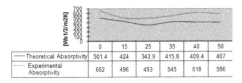

Figure 2. Comparation between the experimental and theoretical thermal absorptivity values.

3.2.2 Thermal conductivity

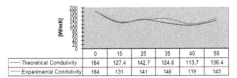

Figure 3. Comparation between the experimental and theoretical thermal conductivity values.

3.2.3 Thermal resistance

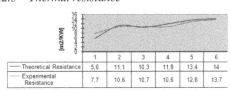

Figure 4. Comparation between experimental and theoretical thermal resistance values.

4 CONCLUSIONS

The theoretical modelization of the principal thermal properties in functional knits, give us three new equations which translate in a very similar way the behaviour of these properties. Through the comparative study, it was possible to verify a good concordance between the experimental values and the values obtained with these new equations. So, it is possible to conclude that the application of this model to the development of new functional products, has a very high level scientific precision.

REFERENCES

Brownless, N., Anand, S.C., Holmes, D.A., Rowe, T., "The Dynamics of Moisture Transportation", Journal of The Textile Institute, 87, Part 1, nº. 1, 1996.
Geraldes, M.J., "Experimental Analysis of the Thermal Comfort of Functional Knits in the Wet State", Doctoral Dissertation, Minho University, Portugal, 2000.
Holmer, I., "Protective Clothing for the Extrme Cold". In: Proceedings of the 2nd International Symposium on Clothing Comfort, Japon, 1991.

Computational Vision and Medical Image Processing – Tavares & Natal Jorge (eds)
© 2012 Taylor & Francis Group, London, ISBN 978-0-415-68395-1

Reaction force produced in the coccyx in different degrees of prolapse

T.H. Da Roza, R. Natal Jorge & M. Parente
IDMEC—Faculty of Engineering, University of Porto, Porto, Portugal

T. Mascarenhas, J. Loureiro & S. Duarte
Faculty of Medicine, University of Porto, São João Hospital, Porto, Portugal

ABSTRACT: The Pelvic Floor (PF) is a supporter structure of the pelvic organs and their functions are to support and suspend the pelvic organs, maintaining urinary and fecal continence, sensory and emptying abnormalities of the gastrointestinal tract and lower urinary tract. Dysfunctions of PF include a group of disorders affecting the adult woman and cover the organ prolapse and urinary incontinence. The aim of this study is to determine the reaction force that occurs at the coccyx when a woman performs the increase of intra-abdominal pressure. We have a 3D model of muscle pubovisceral was created through magnetic resonance imaging. A finite element model was then generated and the intra-abdominal pressure was simulated. It was found that the tested women had different behaviors with increasing intra-abdominal pressure.

1 INTRODUCTION

Pelvic floor is formed by a group of muscles that are called Pelvic Floor Muscles (PFM) which refers to the plate of different muscular layers extending from the pubic symphysis along the sidewalls of the os ilium towars the coccyx [1, 2]. This musculature is required to provide multiple functions, requiring adjustments which may give rise to problems, called Pelvic Floor Disorders (PFD).

The female pelvic floor can be divided into three compartments: the anterior containing the urethra and bladder, the medium containing the vagina and the posterior containing the rectum [3]. Each of these compartments is supported by the endopelvic fascia and the levator ani muscle [4].

PFD are a prevalence condition in women especially among older age group. It includes a wide variety of clinical conditions, which is urinary incontinence and fecal incontinence, pelvic pain and pelvic organ prolapsed [5]. A way to evaluate the female pelvic floor is through Magnetic Resonance Imaging (MRI). This technique has been used increasingly to assess pelvic anatomy in women with pelvic floor disorders, where its image produces detailed pictures of the soft tissues of the pelvic floor [6]. This technique holds great promise because of its potential for identifying injuries to the muscles and fascia of the pelvic floor [7].

Pelvic Organ Prolapsed (POP) is a common gynecological problem [8], being defined as the protrusion of pelvic organs into or out of the vaginal canal. As life expectancy increase, significantly greater number of women will present with POP requiring surgical intervention. Currently, the lifetime risk of undergoing prolapsed or continence surgery in the USA is one in 11 and up to 30% of patients will require repeat prolapsed surgery [9].

All the muscles surrounding the abdominopelvic cavity have a potential influence on pelvic floor position [10]. When the Intra-Abdominal Pressure (IAP) increases, for example due to coughing or sneezing, the pelvic floor is pushed down. This produces a reaction force at the back where the muscle is inserted, in the coccyx.

MR images can contribute to generate Three-Dimensional (3D) solids of pelvic floor muscles through manual segmentation. To study the biomechanical behavior of pelvic floor muscles contributing to analyze this complex musculature structure [11], these 3D solids are discretezed to apply the Finite Element Method (FEM) [12].

The aim of this study is to determine the reaction force that occurs at the coccyx when a woman performs the increase of IAP, in different levels of prolapsed.

2 MATERIALS AND METHODS

2.1 Subjects

For this study five women were selected, all underwent a clinical and gynecological. Information was collected about the clinical history, gynecological, obstetric, urinary symptoms and prolapsed. To quantify, describe and stage pelvic support was used the Pop-Q (pelvic organ prolapsed quantification) exam.

Two women had prolapse in the posterior compartment, one of them had prolapse in posterior and anterior compartment, and the two last had prolapse in three compartments. Women had a mean age of 59.6 (±8.3), all were multiparous and underwent magnetic resonance.

2.2 *Magnetic Resonance Images (MRI)*

The MR images were acquired from the subject supine position, with half-bent legs and were asked to not perform pelvic floor contraction or valsalva maneuver. The images were acquired in the axial plane in a system of 3.0 T, 2 mm thick with 2 mm gap. This study used twenty consecutive images for the model construction.

2.3 *Building procedure*

Each model was built, from a set of MR images obtained in DICOM—Digital Imaging and Communications in Medicine—format and subsequently converted to jpeg format, with all the same image size. These images were imported into CAD—Computer Aided Design—software, where the images are located in parallel planes, separated according to the value at which the MR images were obtained.

Images are included in the plans where manual segmentation can be performed. This segmentation is to circumvent the pubovisceral muscle (a part form the pelvic floor muscles) using background images.

The method is performed in each slide, and then all contours are connected, forming the Three-Dimensional (3D) model (Fig. 1). The first slide shows anterior compartment and the last show the posterior compartment (coccyx).

2.4 *Simulation*

Before starting the simulation process is necessary to export the 3D model to the software of numerical simulation "ABAQUS" to create the numerical model. For the model was created a mesh of tetrahedron solid elements type C3D4.

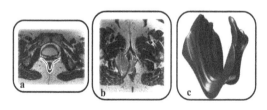

Figure 1. Process of building the 3D model.

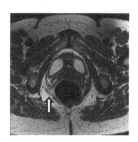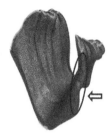

Figure 2. On the left we see the MRI where the tendinous arch no makes connection with the muscles and on the right finite element model without BC in that region.

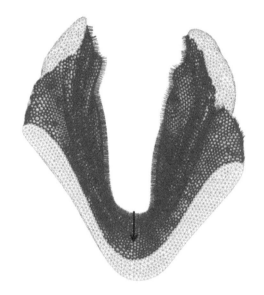

Figure 3. Region of intra-abdominal pressure.

The next step is the diffraction of the Boundary Conditions (BC). In all women were placed BC in the region of the coccyx and the upper side of the muscle. In the region where the upper side on the MR images could be seen that did not have connection with the tendinous arch, due to prolapse, let it "loose" this region (Fig. 2).

Then the model is completely ready, intra-abdominal pressure is applies, this pressure was considered to act perpendicular to the ventral surface (Fig. 3). Each pelvic floor underwent to a value of pressure 173 cm h_2o, and thus analyzed the values of reaction in the coccyx.

3 RESULTS

The results of analysis of the Reaction Force (RF) of each woman can be seen in Table 1.

Table 1. Reaction force in coccyx for each women.

Woman	Degree of prolapse	RF (N)
POP—CP	II	224
POP—CP	III	328
POP—CA/CP	I/I	376
POP—CA/CM/CP*	I/I/I	519
POP—CA/CM/CP*	II/I/II	595

*CA (compartment anterior); CM (compartment medium); CP (compartment posterior).

It may be noted that the relationship of the reaction force produced in the coccyx is proportional to the number of compartments prolapsed, and the degree of prolapse is a factor to increase the strength of reaction.

4 CONCLUSIONS

This work shows that one can use the finite element method to better understand the biomechanics of the pelvic floor. We can conclude that the degree of prolapse and the amount of compartments affected are directly related to the reaction force that produces the tailbone when increasing the IAP. This may indicate that a woman with prolapse, should be treated as soon as possible so that the coccyx not subject to large forces, thus avoiding further damage the pelvic floor.

REFERENCES

[1] Messeling B. Benson T. Berghmans B. Bo K. Corcos J. Fowler C. Laycock J. et al. 2005. Standardisation of terminology of pelvic floor muscle function and dysfunction: report from the pelvic floor clinical assessment group of the international continence society. *Neurourol Urodyn* 24:374–380.

[2] Ashton-Miller J.A. DeLancey J.O.L. 2007, Functional anatomy of the female pelvic floor. *Ann N Y Acad Sci.* 1101:266–296.

[3] Law Y.M. Fielding J.R. 2008, MRI of pelvic floor dysfunction: review. *AJR Am J Roentgenol.* 191: S45–53.

[4] Di Benedetto P. Coidessa A. Floris S. 2008. Rationale of pelvic floor muscles training in women with urinary incontinence. *Minerva Ginecol.* 60: 529–534.

[5] Weber, A, M.; Buchsbaum, G,M.; et al. 2004. Basic science and translational research in female pelvic floor disorders: Proceeedings of an NIH-Sponsored meeting. *Neurourology and Urodynamics*, 23: 288–301.

[6] Klutke, C.G. Siegel, C.L. 1995. Functional female pelvic anatomy. *Urol Clin North Am* 22:487–498.

[7] Strohbehn K. Ellis J.H. Strohbehn J.A. DeLancey J.O.L. 1996, Magnetic resonance imaging of the levator ani with anatomic correlation. *Obstet Gynecol* 87:277–285.

[8] Koduri S. Sand P.K. 2000. Recent developments in pelvic organ prolapsed. *Curr Opin Obstet Gynecol* 12:399–404.

[9] Olsen A.L. Smith V.J. Bergstrom J.O. Colling J.C. Clark A.L. 1997. Epidemiology of surgically managed pelvic organ prolapsed and urinary incontinence. *Obstet Gynecol* 89:501–506.

[10] Thompson J.A., O'Sullivan P.B. Briffa N.K. Neumann P. 2006. Differences in muscle activation patterns during pelvic floor muscle contraction and valsalva manouver, *Neuro and Urody* 25:148–155.

[11] S. Van der Helm J. Blok S.B.F.C.T. 2003. Mensuring morphological parameters of the pelvic floor for finite elements modeling purpose. *J Biomech* 36: 749–757.

[12] Parente M.P.L. Natal Jorge R.M. Mascarenhas T. Fernandes A.A. Martins J.A.C. 2008. Deformation of the pelvic floor muscles during a vaginal delivery. *Int Urogynecol J* 19:65–71.

Computational Vision and Medical Image Processing – Tavares & Natal Jorge (eds)
© 2012 Taylor & Francis Group, London, ISBN 978-0-415-68395-1

Texture analysis and pattern recognition in X-band SAR images for urban forestry

S. Canale, A. De Santis, D. Iacoviello, F. Pirri & S. Sagratella
Department of Computer and System Sciences Antonio Ruberti, Sapienza University of Rome, Italy

ABSTRACT: In this paper Synthetic Aperture Radar (SAR) images in X-band are analyzed in order to infer ground properties from data. The aim is to classify different zones of urban forestry integrating information from different sources. In particular the X-band is sensitive to the moisture content of the ground that can be therefore put into relation with the gray level of the image. A segmentation with respect to the texture content of the image is provided and integrated with a pattern recognition method in order to identify interesting zones, such as lawns, water pounds, trees canopies, roads and so on. Results are shown on the area of Castel Fusano, a large urban forest near Rome.

Keywords: SAR images, segmentation, texture analysis, classification, fire susceptibility map

1 INTRODUCTION

The use of Synthetic Aperture Radar (SAR) images is well established for environment monitoring. As a matter of fact, in this last decade, more than 15 SAR satellites have successfully been launched for scientific, commercial, and security-related applications. Various methods (Tanase et al. 2010, Anguela et al. 2010) have been devised to recognize areas of different soil and vegetation types, by meanly exploiting regression analysis of backscattering models relating the measured signal to some parameters characterizing the soil conditions. In this context the use of the X band is quite recent and its capability in environmental monitoring is yet to be fully evaluated.

A crucial scientific contribution to urban management in European metropolis, where large urban forests and parks form a beautiful interface with the metropolitan settlement, is to provide a strategic view of vulnerability to fire. From several studies on European fires (e.g. (Martinez, Chuvieco, and Martin 2004; Reineking, Weibel, Conedera, and Bugmann 2010)) anthropic factors have been proved to be determinant in the fire impact on land. Numerous fires usually start by careless human actions such as sparks from equipment, arced power lines, campfires, burning debris, discarded smoking products, and also because of pyromaniacs. The main difficulty in these studies is to conceal different data sources providing a suitable integration methodology that can face such a complex data structure. In fact,

higher resolution datasets usually suffer a loss in favor of the lowest common resolution available.

In this paper we consider a different approach in the analysis of X-SAR images to infer ground properties from data: an integration of image segmentation and machine learning methods is studied to classify different zones of urban forestries, such as trees canopies, lawns, water pounds, roads, etc., directly from the gray level signal properties. The X-band is known to be sensitive to the ground roughness and moisture content, therefore the signal value and its texture account for the different appearance of different areas.

We use as area test the Castel Fusano area, a large urban forest near Rome (Italy), see Figure 1. This choice relies on a large ground truth data base made available by the Italian Civil Protection. It contains a quite complete set of urban forestry items, such as canopies, brushwood, Mediterranean maquis, roads, buildings, rivers, burned areas, sea shore and so on.

The paper is organized as follows. In Section 2 the characteristics of X-band SAR images are described along with the adopted method for their processing. In Section 3 an example of moisture feature extraction procedure is presented on the target zone of Castel Fusano. In Sections 4 we show how features of X-SAR images can be extracted using correlation with coregistered optical images obtained from Google Earth. In Section 5 data integration and classification procedure are outlined and in Section 6 some conclusions and future development are illustrated.

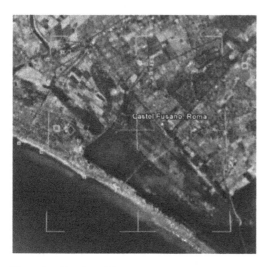

Figure 1. The Castel Fusano area.

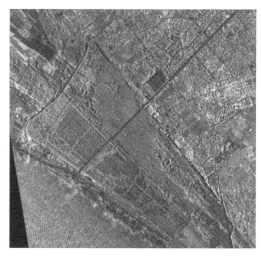

Figure 2. X-band SAR image of the Castel Fusano area.

2 SAR IMAGES AND ANALYSIS

Synthetic Aperture Radar (SAR) data have a great potential as a source of relevant and near real time information for change detection, early warning, mitigation, and forecast and management of natural disasters. That is because of its observation capability regardless climate conditions and sun illumination. Indeed, SAR is an active form of remote sensing. The surface is illuminated by a beam of energy with a fixed wavelength that can be anywhere from 1 cm (K band) to approximately 70 cm (P-band). These long wavelengths penetrate clouds and atmospheric interferences common to optical imagery and therefore are not limited spatially or temporally because of solar illumination or atmospheric interferences. The images available for the present paper are Cosmo-SkyMed products delivered by the Italian Space Agency (ASI). They are high quality and high spatial definition, with resolution ranging from 0.6 to 1 m in the SpotLight mode, level 1C-GEC, speckle filtered, only obtained in the X-band (wave length ranging from 2.4 to 3.8 cm). Smooth surfaces have a darker response to X-band than ragged ones. Indeed, the X-band is known to be sensitive to changes in the target moisture content, namely the response is lighter on increasing humidity. On the other hand different patterns on X-SAR images, corresponding to regions with different characteristics, are distinguishable by the gray level spatial distribution (texture) only. In Figure 2 an example of X-SAR image of the chosen area is shown.

A first step in the interpretation of SAR images is achieved by a segmentation procedure based on a discrete level set method, see (De Santis

et al. 2007), applied to a suitable transformation of the data, aiming at the enhancement of the texture properties that better describe the characteristics of the zones to be identified. The regions with different characteristics have different textures and therefore are distinguishable by some properties of the gray level spatial distribution. The most effective transformations we found so far are uniformity and local contrast. Uniformity is obtained as the sum of the square of the local image histogram bins value, while the local contrast is based on the local signal variance, both evaluated on square neighbor of size 30. Furthermore the contrast image is processed by a bank of rank filters obtained by varying kernel size and rank order. In order to identify the larger area of Castel Fusano burned in the fire event of year 2000, the uniformity transformation is well suited, allowing the discrimination between the burned area and the neighboring regions, see Figure 3. A four levels discrete level set segmentation of the region of interest applied to the transformed data provides a simplified representation of the original image preserving the information to be retrieved. A four levels segmentation is obtained by successive image binarizations: first the image I is partitioned into two distinct subregions (not necessarily simply connected) A_1, A_2 and represented, for any pixel (i, j) of the domain D, as follows:

$$I_b(i,j) = c_1 \chi_{A_1}(i,j) + c_2 \chi_{A_2}(i,j)$$

The constants c_1, c_2 are the signal mean values within the sets A_1, A_2 respectively. Function χ_A is the characteristic function of a set A. The sets

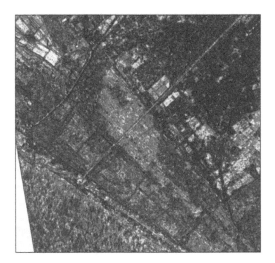

Figure 3.   Uniformity image.

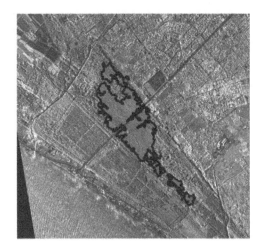

Figure 4.   The burned area.

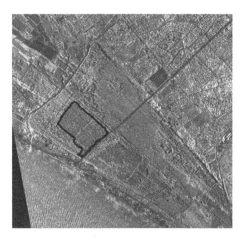

Figure 5.   Contour of the canopy subregion in the Castel Fusano area.

A_1, A_2 are described by the level set function ϕ : $D \rightarrow R$ as follows:

$$A_1 = \left\{(i,j) \in D : \phi(i,j) \geq 0\right\}$$
$$A_2 = \left\{(i,j) \in D : \phi(i,j) < 0\right\}$$

To obtain the binarization elements $(c_1, c_2, \{\phi(i,j)\})$ a cost function is minimized: it contains the fit error between the image and its binary representation and a regularization term for the level set function:

$$F\left(c_1, c_2, \phi\right) = \lambda \sum_{(i,j)} \left(I(i,j) - c_1\right)^2 \chi_{A_1}(i,j)$$
$$+ \lambda \sum_{(i,j)} \left(I(i,j) - c_2\right)^2 \chi_{A_2}(i,j) + \sum_{(i,j)} \phi(i,j)^2$$

Parameter λ is chosen to enhance the fit error influence over the optimal solution. In (De Santis et al. 2007) it has been shown that the problem has a unique optimal solution.

Once the first level optimal binarization is obtained, the regions A_1, A_2 are further binarized with the same procedure. Thus a four levels optimal segmentation is finally obtained.

In Figure 4 the burned area obtained by segmenting the uniformity image is represented, whereas the measure of the local contrast allows in the chosen zone of Castel Fusano the identification of subregions like the typical canopy of the old oak forest, planted in rows, see Figure 5.

About ten different subregions can be identified in the above defined zone, using as data to be segmented different rank filters of the contrast image. For each of the identified zone an accurate

determination of the contour and extension is provided; the gray level mean value is correlated with the local moisture content, one of the relevant physical parameter in the fire susceptibility model.

In the next section, by exploiting the zones identified by the segmentation, an example of moisture feature extraction procedure is presented. In this way the local humidity level can be sensed on the base of a global meteorological data acquired over a larger area containing the test zone.

3   MOISTURE INFORMATION

The homogeneous zones identified can be monitored by a periodical acquisition of X-SAR images: their average gray level value can be correlated with ground truth data obtained by the meteorological stations. In particular, the Aviation Digital Data Service (http://www.aviationweather.gov) provides the daily temperature and dew point values (24 hours) of Castel Fusano. The dew point value represents the temperature to which a given parcel of air or, more precisely, water vapor, must be cooled down to condense into water at constant barometric pressure. It is strictly related to the humidity value RH. To retrieve this value we can consider a psychrometric chart or a look-up table, or by means of empirical relations such as the following:

$$RH = \frac{E}{E_s}100$$

where E is the actual water vapor pressure and E_s is the saturated water vapor pressure, in units of millibar. These quantities can be evaluated using the dew point values T_d and the temperature values T, both in Celsius scale:

$$E_s = 6.11 \cdot 10^{(7.5 \cdot T/(237.7+T))}$$
$$E = 6.11 \cdot 10^{(7.5 \cdot T_d/(237.7+T_d))}$$

From the above relations the average relative humidity of the considered target area is obtained, and the values correlated with the identified subregions can be found by a simple proportion, using their average gray level value, evaluated over the segmented zones identified according to the procedure of Section 2.

Periodical image acquisition provides a time series RH moisture values for every subregion. The moisture content of each zone is strictly related with the weather conditions but also on the soil and vegetation characteristics.

4 X-SAR FEATURES

To identify X-SAR features in the absence of other bands, a very first problem is to register the image so as to compute the cross correlation between different intensity and color channels. Here in Figure 6 the registration of a cell of a Spot-Light image over Google Earth is illustrated. Registration is achieved automatically, even with cell reduction. In fact the original image is of size 25856×25856 and it is represented in uint16. Using the rich information provided by Cosmo-SkyMed products in xml, the image can be suitably cropped in order to study correlation with optical images.

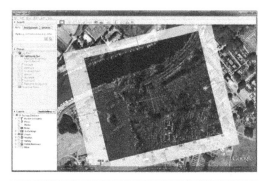
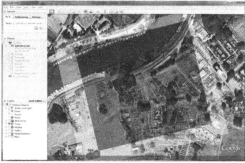

Figure 6. Registration of a cropped cell from a spotlight XSAR image on Google Earth.

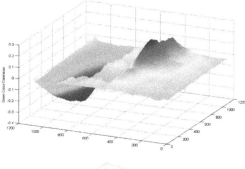
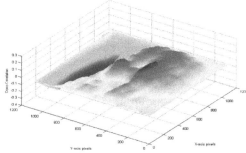

Figure 7. Cross correlation between the RGB and XSAR coregistered images.

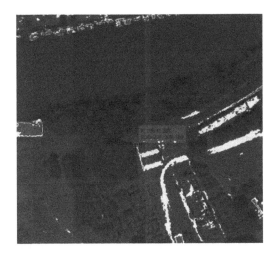

Figure 8. Roads and covers highlighted by cross local entropy using the 4 channels.

Although no rotation is provided, clearly a similarity transformation needs to be done, in order to register the image with a view of Google Earth taken according to the computed coordinates. For a similarity transformation four pairs of control points are needed. The process can be repeated producing a whole tessellation of the original SpotLight image, with each cell very well manageable. A first analysis of features can be done by considering the cross correlation between the backscattering and the color image; here we provide the normalized cross correlation between the X-SAR cropped image and each of the channel of the corresponding Google image, see Figure 7.

We can see that there is an inverse correlation with respect to the water, in this case the river, while there is a strong correlation with respect to the green. This implies that the 4 channels can be used for early texture analysis.

In Figure 8 it is shown feature extraction of the roads and the covers, obtained by local entropy filtering. Further analysis have exploited Markov Random Fields.

5 AREA CLASSIFICATION BY PATTERN RECOGNITION

In this section we present the data model and the machine learning based approach for data analysis. The goal of data analysis is that of defining an accurate area classification on the base of information extracted directly from X-SAR images provided by Cosmo-SkyMed.

Once different areas have been identified by the segmentation algorithm described in Section 2, our aim is that of identifying accurate classification rules in order to recognize the structure of particular kinds of areas in an urban forestry, e.g. burned areas, lakes, roads, and so on. These classification rules will be then used to recognize automatically the areas of interest in different images.

The data integration model we consider allows to describe each pixel by a set of quantitative features based on the gray level in the X-SAR image. These features define the spatial cross correlations among the closest pixels in terms of gray level. In particular, the features of interest in this work are characteristics of the image texture: there is a former set of differential features, computed by image convolution with the derivatives of a Gaussian kernel, and a latter set of textural features consisting of contrast, uniformity and entropy.

An automatic classification of the areas of interested by training a Support Vector Machine over collected sample images is provided. We define an input space where each record of quantitative attributes describes an atomic area of the image. For each segmentation level we define a pattern recognition problem. Then we assign to each record x a binary label y according to the segmentation level. The set of these records and their labels represents the training set $\{(x^1,y_1), ..., (x^m,y_m)\}$. Our aim is that of identifying the classification rule defined over the training set and using this rule to assign the correct class to areas that have not classified yet (test set).

In order to define the classification rule we train a Support Vector Machine (Schölkopf et al. 2001) over the training set and test the resulting classifier over the test set. In this case, for each atomic area x of the image the classification function f will assign the label represented by the value

$$f(x) = \text{sgn}\left(\sum_{i=1}^{m} y_i k(x,x^i)\alpha_i + \beta\right)$$

The kernel function k used for the feature map has been accurately chosen on the base of the kind of attributes in the input space while the kernel parameter values were selected by standard cross validation procedure. The best classification rules have been obtained by adopting a Radial Basis Function kernel. The values of the parameters α and β in f have been estimated by training a Support Vector Machine.

Experimental results on the classification of oak tree areas in Castel Fusano show that the classification rule has a good accuracy on both the training set (around 90%) and the test set: the

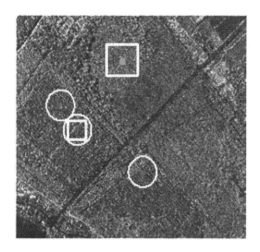

Figure 9. Around areas represent the oak tree zones (accuracy 90.03%); squares ones represent areas being outside the oak tree forest (accuracy 89.4%).

accuracy of the classification of oak tress areas has been more than 90% while a test area different from oak tree has been classified with an accuracy of 89.4%, see Figure 9. As mentioned in Section 2, because of uniformity, the oak tree areas can be easily recognized by adopting our data model. These encouraging classification results prove that the adopted data model yields useful information about the different kinds of areas of interest and that an accurate pattern recognition method can play a fundamental role for extracting useful information from X-SAR images.

6 FURTHER DEVELOPMENT AND CONCLUSION

The integration of image segmentation and machine learning methods provides a finite partition of the target zone in areas of different characteristics. This is obtained by a suitable characterization of the signal properties that constitute a SAR label for each area. It is of great interest to evaluate if such a set of features easily generalizes to different urban forestries in the world. In this case the X-SAR databases could be endowed with semantic queries utilities, searching directly for "canopies", "roads", "ponds", etc. As a further application the problem of forests fires can be addressed by studying the fire susceptibility of a zone of interest by classifying the fuel characteristics within each subarea. In this case the segmentation/classification is just one of the layer of a database that includes land use data, meteorological data, human intervention and anthropic factors, including past fires histories. This could help land management authorities in defining fire susceptibility maps taking into account changing conditions that determines a vulnerability to fire ignition, either spontaneous or not.

ACKNOWLEDGMENTS

The work reported in this paper has been supported by the Italian Space Agency (ASI) within the Cosmo-SkyMed Announcement of Opportunity (DCOST-2009-116). Data have been provided by ASI Cosmo-SkyMed constellation.

REFERENCES

Anguela, T.P., Zribi, M. Baghdadi N. and Loumagne, C. 2010. Analysis of Local Variation of Soil Surface Parameters With TerraSAR-X Radar Data Over Bare Agricultural Fields, *IEEE Trans. On Geoscience and Remote Sensing*, 48(2): 874–881.

De Santis, A. and Iacoviello, D. 2007. Discrete level set approach to image segmentation, *Signal, Image and Video Processing*, 1(4): 303–320.

Martinez, J., Chuvieco, E. and Martin, P. 2004. Estimation of risk factors of human ignition of fires in Spain by means of logistic regression. *In Proc. of the Second International Symposium on Fire Economics, Planning, and Policy*.

Reineking, B., Weibel, P., Conedera, M. and Bugmann, H. 2010. Environmental determinants of lightning—v. human-induced forest fire ignitions differ in a temperate mountain region of switzerland. *International Journal of Wildland Fire*, 19(5): 541–557.

Schölkopf, B. and Smola, A. 2001. Learning with Kernels. *Support Vector Machines, Regularization, Optimization, and Beyond*. MIT Press.

Tanase, M.A., Pérez-Cabello, F., Juan de la Riva and Santoro, M. 2010. TerraSAR-X Data for Burn Severity Evaluation in Mediterranean Forests on Sloped Terrain, *IEEE Trans. On Geoscience and Remote Sensing*, 48(2): 917–928.

Computational Vision and Medical Image Processing – Tavares & Natal Jorge (eds)
© 2012 Taylor & Francis Group, London, ISBN 978-0-415-68395-1

Cosmo-Skymed SAR data for urgency situations-study of a real case

R.L. Paes, E.H. Shiguemori & M. Habermann
Institute for Advanced Studies, São José dos Campos, Brazil

A.M.R. Neto & R.M. Andrade
Paulista University, São José dos Campos, Brazil

ABSTRACT: Air France flight 447 shocked the world and it was one of the largest aerial accidents involving the Brazilian air traffic control management. On such work, we will discuss some difficulties of having accurate data and about the methodology for extract information with the available data. Wavelets techniques algorithms were tested and we got interesting resulting leading us to detect unexpected objects and features, collaborating for search and rescue operations over the sea.

1 INTRODUCTION

Air France flight 447 shocked the world and it was one of the largest aerial accidents involving the Brazilian air traffic control management. On such work, we will discuss some difficulties of having accurate data and about the methodology for extract information with the available data. Present work objective is to present to decision makers people a factual schema for helping on search and rescue situations, especially on the ocean environment (Figs. 1, 2).

2 COSMO-SKYMED SATELLITE

Italian satellite Cosmo-Skymed has a high temporal resolution, too much necessary for surveillance

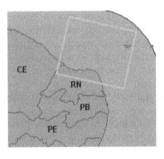

Figure 2. Imagery representation area where the Cosmo-Skymed satellites were achieved to get useful information.

applications. Four SAR sensors satellites compound such constellation and the acquired data follows this brief description:

- strip of ScanSAR Wide Region mode images (20° to 60° incident angle range; 100 × 100 km swath) were acquired, covering a 100 × 500 km oceanic area—related to five scenes, according to Cosmo-Skymed *System Description & User Guide* and Cosmo-Skymed *SAR Products Handbook* [1].

3 METHODOLOGY

We started applying some wavelet techniques because their capabilities of detecting signal patterns not detectable for human eyes. Thus, we choose two common wavelets: Haar and Cohen-Daubechies-Feauveau 9/7—CDF97. Our intentions is not to compare their results, but explore

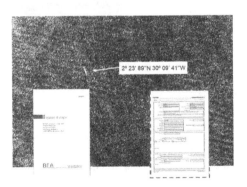

Figure 1. Cosmo-Skymed Scansar Wide Region (100 × 100 km) multilook image. After processing this multilook image only merchant vessels and black stripes could be detected. However, some bright cluster were noticed and they have correspondence with official reports.

the different aspects that they can detect. Haar wavelet is a symmetric and orthogonal and it has two coefficients to low-pass and high pass synthesis and analysis. The latter, CDF97 (biorthogonal and symmetric), has seven low-pass and nine high-pass synthesis coefficients, and with others nine low-pass and seven high-pass analysis coefficients [2–4]. Thus, we applied them onto accident. After it, we compared the results with the ground truth [5].

4 FIRST RESULTS AND CONSIDERATIONS

Despite this data be acquired on real situation, we have to handle with a ground truth fragmented information. Recently we obtained the official reports [5] and it was possible to verify our work performance, however, it still more studies. Once such imageries were acquired on real situation, no scientific care was taken by the ground truth providers. Thus, we just expect to improve our level of confidence. Then, as way to continue the research to find small metallic objects on medium to small SAR images resolution, we will request other series of imageries, but onto controlled environments, lake and ocean.

We got the first results (Fig. 3) from the area which has high probability of containing the reported wreckages. After images processing, we analyzed such patterns and we can conclude that such methodology is quite useful, but we need to invest on technologies to process faster the incoming data, which leads to co-processing with General Purpose Graphic Processor Unit (GPGPU). Almost all of the employed algorithms are adaptative, involving looping structures and increasing the computational burden. We had to handle with more than 10 GB of data and the processing time is crucial for helping in real operations.

SAR Remote sensing resources showed are very useful once the atmosphere is almost ever

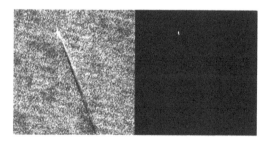

Figure 3. Cosmo-Skymed subset image over Atlantic Ocean—Brazilian waters domain. Merchant ship detected was engaged temporally supporting the operations. Original image (left); CDF97 output (rigth).

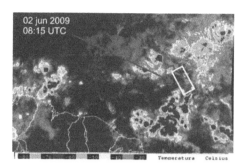

Figure 4. GOES-12 image acquired on June, 2nd 2009, 08:15 UTC, close to the first image acquisition time. The scale above are in Celsius degrees.

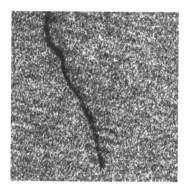

Figure 5. Suspect oil slick close to the first wreckage site.

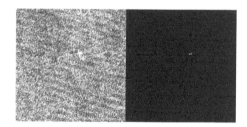

Figure 6. Undefined object: Original image (left); Haar wavelet (right).

transparent for radar microwaves and it is independent of Sun illumination. On that occasion, sky was overcastted (Fig. 4) and the visibility was harmful reduced, limiting the aerial operations. Another example of SAR application is the situational awareness improvement: Figure 5 shows a suspect oil slick close to the site where found the first wreckages; Figure 6 shows a detection of a metallic object onto the first wreckage spot.

But, is early to affirm what it is, because there are reports of large extensions garbage floating on the sea surface. It also looks like a vessel, but there is no information about on such position. BEA's official report [5] points to that place as the first wreckage spot, nevertheless, based on visual sighting and consequently with no fine precision.

Finally, we continue our research on this operational approach and we are testing different techniques based on statistical threshold [6], decision tree [7], physical properties [8] and other wavelets schema [9]. We can conclude the present work summarizing the importance of a satellite constellation for fast subsequent images acquisitions; and the development of faster processors, noticing the potentiality of GPGPU architectures for rapid responses. At last but not least, despite such promising techniques discussed here which their development is highly recommended; we state that a simple visual analysis of a SAR image can be very useful on real emergency situation, improving the situational awareness for the rescue teams, due to its all-weather imaging capability.

ACKNOWLEDGEMENTS

Our special thanks to Telespazio Brasil S.A./ Italian Spatial Agency (ASI) for provide us the Cosmo-Skymed SAR data. We also thank to the Brazilian Navy and to the PETROBRAS Brazilian Oil Company Research Center (Cenpes) for provide the ground truth.

REFERENCES

[1] Telespazio—A Fiomeccania/Thales Company. TELESPAZIO/COSMO-SKYMED. Available in: <http://www.telespazio.it/cosmo.html>. Last access in: December 18th, 2009.

[2] Mallat, S.G., *A Theory for Multiresolution Signal Decomposition: The Wavelet representation.* IEEE Transactions On Pattern Analysis And Machine Intelligence Vol. 2, N. 7. 1989.

[3] Daubechies, I., *Ten lectures on wavelets.* CBMS conference on wavelets, university of lowell, ma, June 1990—Philadelphia, PA: Society for Industrial and Applied Mathematics, (1992).

[4] Cohen, A., Daubechies, I., Feauveau, J.C., *Biorthogonal bases of compactly supported wavelets,* Comm. Pure & Appl. Math 45, pp. 485–560, 1992.

[5] Interim Report 1 on the accident on 1st June 2009 to the Airbus A330-203 registered F-GZCP operated by Air France flight AF 447 Rio de Janeiro—Paris. Bureau d'Enquêtes et d'Analyses pour la sécurité de l'aviation civile—BEA. Available in: <http://www.bea.aero/fr/publications/rapports/liste.php?annee=2009>.

[6] Paes, R.L., Lorenzzetti, J.A., Gherardi, D.F.M., *Ship Detection Using TerraSAR-X Images in the Campos Basin (Brazil),* Geoscience and Remote Sensing Letters, IEEE. July 2010, Vol. 7, Issue 3, pg 545–548.

[7] Yildiz, O.T., Alpaydin, E., *Linear discriminant trees.* International Journal of Pattern Recognition and Artificial Intelligence. Vol 19, No. 3 (2005).

[8] Gambardella, A., Nunziata, F., Migliaccio, M., *A Physical Full-Resolution SAR Ship Detection Filter.* Geoscience and Remote Sensing Letters, IEEE. Oct. 2008, vol. 5, Issue 4, pg. 760–763.

[9] Tello, M., Lopez-Martinez. C, Mallorqui, J.J., "A novel approach for the automatic detection of punctual isolated targets in a noisy background in SAR imagery". *Radar Conference,* 2005. EURAD 2005. European. p. 41–44. Paris (2005).

Computational Vision and Medical Image Processing – Tavares & Natal Jorge (eds)
© 2012 Taylor & Francis Group, London, ISBN 978-0-415-68395-1

Using satellite imagery to develop a detailed and updated map of imperviousness to improve flood risk management in the city of Lisbon

T. Santos, S. Freire & J.A. Tenedório
e-GEO—Research Centre for Geography and Regional Planning, Faculdade de Ciências Sociais e Humanas, FCSH, Universidade Nova de Lisboa, Lisboa, Portugal

Ana Fonseca
LNEC—Laboratório de Engenharia Civil de Lisboa, Lisboa, Portugal

ABSTRACT: The present paper describes the generation of a Land Cover Map for the city of Lisbon, Portugal. The data source is an IKONOS pansharp image, from 2008, with a spatial resolution of 1 m, and a normalized Digital Surface Model (nDSM) from 2006. The methodology was based on the extraction of features of interest, namely: vegetation, soil and impervious surfaces. It is demonstrated that using a methodology based on Very-High Resolution (VHR) images, quick updating of detailed land cover information is possible and can be used to support decisions in a crisis situation where official maps are generally outdated. Urban flood risk is the case study presented, where the spatial distribution and extent of the pervious and impervious areas in the city are important variables for planning, mitigate, prepare and respond to potential events.

Keywords: Urban flood risk, impervious mapping, soil sealing, Lisbon

1   INTRODUCTION

Natural disasters like urban floods are a major problem, often resulting in extensive damage to private and public property and sometimes claiming people's lives. Urban floods are a good example of a 'natural hazard' compounded by human action, thus more appropriately classified as a 'semi-natural' disaster. In fact, the urbanization process results in the impermeability of land surfaces, thus increasing the soil sealing, which contributes to elevate the risk of flooding. Sealing surfaces generate intense rainwater run-off which the drainage network cannot accommodate, thus promoting flooding events. The availability of appropriate flood risk maps is imp ortant to support decisions in most phases of the emergency management cycle:

– Planning: flood risk maps are essential to locate, assess and rank areas at risk of flooding;
– Mitigation: flood risk maps should be used to implement mitigation measures in areas of higher risk in order to decrease severity of potential outcomes;
– Preparation: flood risk maps can be used to locate response means and resources close to areas at higher risk and to monitor those areas before and during events;

– Response: flood risk maps can assist response after events of heavy rainfall by giving indication on the areas that were worst hit and possible water depth and thus help to tailor means and resources.

Some areas in the city of Lisbon, Portugal, are subject to cyclical flooding due to a combination of factors: intense rainfall, inappropriate draining infrastructure, and other geographic conditions (e.g., effect of ocean tide). Also the human activity (including slope cutting, artificial fills and river channel diversion) as a consequence of urban development, contributes to the flooding phenomenon.

Efficient management of urban flooding is based on mapping its risk, for which maps of ground imperviousness are essential. Highly permeable landscapes reduce erosion and flood risk, recharge groundwater and stabilize stream flows over time. However, when soil permeability is reduced, surface runoff, erosion and flood risk increase, groundwater recharge is reduced, and stream flows fluctuate more over time. Frequently, cadastral information on land cover is not available with sufficient spatial resolution. This information is difficult to obtain and rapidly becomes outdated in cities having a dynamic development. Instead, satellite data can be used for mapping and quantifying sealed surfaces in a quick way and at low costs. Furthermore, continuous acquisition of satellite data allows updating already existing land cover maps, contributing to a more accurate estimate of the actual proportion of sealing ground within city areas.

Remote sensing imagery due to its spectral, temporal and geographic characteristics, can be used in flood risk analysis, as a source for related information like land use and land cover, surface roughness, terrain relief or soil moisture. Ebert et al. (2009) modeled the influence of land use types and their spatial pattern on the flood hazard, using satellite data (Landsat, SPOT and ASTER). Chormanski et al. (2008) and Canters et al. (2006) examined the impact of different methods for estimating impervious surface cover from satellite data (IKONOS and Landsat), on the outcome of a distributed rainfall-runoff model. Aponte (2007) used a QuickBird image in order to detect different types of impervious surfaces, and studied the relationship between the rainfall-infiltration-runoff rates, the land cover and the geomorphologic susceptibility. Shamaoma et al. (2006) extracted building footprints and boundaries of informal settlements from QuickBird imagery and laser scanning data, and tested its potential in providing the information required to run flood risk models.

The present work details the development of an updated and detailed map of imperviousness for the city of Lisbon using IKONOS-2 satellite imagery, and a nDSM from 2006. The Vegetation-Impervious-Soil (VIS) model, developed by Ridd (1995), was used as the basis for extracting land cover information at the city-scale. It is a conceptual representation that allows simplifying the analysis of urban surfaces by decomposing it in three basic land cover components: vegetation, impervious surface and soil.

After collecting data on land cover from remote sensing data, several applications can be assessed. Indicators on land sealing area, quantification of green area, or the available soil in the city, are ecological measures that can be used for monitoring and analyzing trends over the territory. Studies on impacts of urbanization, responses to natural and man-made disasters, vulnerability analysis or housing conditions, all require updated land cover information.

2 DATA SET AND STUDY AREA

The dataset explored in this paper includes spectral data, acquired by the IKONOS-2 satellite. The IKONOS image was acquired in June, 30, 2008, and has a spatial resolution of 4 m in the multispectral mode (visible and near-infrared bands) and 1 m in the panchromatic mode, and a radiometric resolution of 11 bits.

The study area is the city of Lisbon (Fig. 1). The municipality occupies an area of 84 Km²,

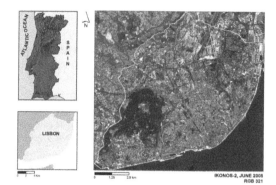

Figure 1. Study area and data set used for building lisbon's impervious surface map.

and is a typical European capital city, with a very diverse land use dynamics, varying from historical neighborhoods where the street-network is dense and the most of the area is built-up, to modern residential ones, with on-going construction of roads and multi-family buildings. Between these two situations, there are more heterogeneous places with land uses such as residential, parks, agriculture, vacant land, industrial, utilities, and schools.

3 METHODOLOGY

The cartographic workflow based on remote sensing data, begins with the pre-processing stage where the images are orthorectified. Afterwards, the digital processing takes place to produce a map with the location of the land cover features.

The nomenclature is organized in two levels of detail, following the VIS model. The 1st level includes the classes "Vegetation", "Impervious Surfaces", and "Soil". On the 2nd level, seven classes were defined: "Trees", "Low Vegetation", "Buildings", "Roads", "Other impervious surfaces", "Soil", and "Shadows and Water" (Table 1).

Table 1. Land cover nomenclature.

Level 1	Level 2
Vegetation	Trees
	Low vegetation
Impervious surface	Buildings
	Roads
	Other impervious surfaces
Soil	Soil
Shadow and water	Shadow and water

3.1 Pre-processing

The IKONOS-2 image was orthorectified in order to reduce the geometric distortions introduced by the relief and to attribute a national coordinate system (ETRS89). Previously, a pansharp image of the visible and panchromatic bands was produced, using the method available at PCI Geomatica.

Afterwards, a Normalized Difference Vegetation Index (NDVI) (Rouse et al. 1973) image was produced to integrate the dataset for feature extraction.

3.2 Feature extraction

Current and future VHR satellite imagery provides an advantageous alternative to detect and map urban features. However, their effective use requires the development of novel approaches that enable a timely and consistent discrimination, classification and delineation of these specific land uses with quality indices that match the corresponding map scale. In this context, Geographic Object Based Image Analysis (GEOBIA) approaches are the recent response to this emerged sophisticated user needs and expectations on geographic information products (Hay & Castilla, 2008).

All feature extraction was performed in Feature Analyst (FA) v4.2 (by VLS) for ArcGIS (ESRI). The classification is based on a supervised approach and aims at extracting the three main components of land cover: "Vegetation", "Impervious Surfaces" and "Soil".

The first class to be extracted was "Shadow and Water". Dark objects, that include both water and shadows, were extracted with a histogram thresholding method. A synthetic brightness image was initially computed though the mean value of the near-infrared, red and green bands and then a pixel-based histogram of brightness was analyzed to determine an optimum threshold value for shadows and non-shadows (a threshold value of 170 was set). As mentioned by Zhou et al. (2009), this histogram is bimodal, with the lower part being occupied by the darker features (shadows and water). In our case study, the selected threshold included shadows and deep water bodies.

After extracting shadows and water elements, the next steps explored the possibility of classifying the study area in two major classes—"Vegetation", "No-vegetation"—and in the subsequent stages, each individual class of the nomenclature was extracted independently.

The vegetation extraction was conducted for the unclassified areas (i.e., no shadow or water elements). In order to separate vegetated from non-vegetated surfaces in the urban environment, the NDVI was used, based on the pansharp image. A threshold of 0.22 was determined depending on the intensity values to mask the vegetated regions. This layer stands for the level 1 class "Vegetation" and includes the city's green surface. In the 2nd level of the nomenclature, two classes were distinguished: "Trees" and "Low Vegetation". The first class identifies trees and tall bushes, whereas the other identifies lawns and other herbaceous vegetation. The "Trees" were extracted with FA using 8 training areas, the pansharp and the NDVI image, Bull Eye's 3 for the input representation, width 5, masking in the level 1 class "Vegetation", and 5 pixels of aggregation. After training the classifier, the final map was obtained after one 'add missing areas' process. The low vegetation class was the remaining vegetation.

The next major class to be extracted was "Soil", and was applied in the unclassified areas (i.e., no shadow, no water, and no vegetation). The dataset included the pansharp image and the nDSM. The classifiers' learning was done in two independent extractions, considering two types of soil classes: bare land with some earth, and thin soil. Bare land was extracted with the Manhattan algorithm, width 3, and 100 pixels of aggregation, and the other class with the same algorithm, but considering 50 pixels for aggregation. The bare soil was subject to an iteration of removing clutter. The final step was the generalization of the soil polygons using the aggregate polygons tool from ArcGIS.

The map of impervious areas includes a wide range of materials, some of which have very different spectral properties (e.g., pavement, concrete, roof tiles, etc.). The 1st level class "Impervious Surface" corresponds to the land surface after masking out the "Vegetation", "Soil", "Shadow", and "Water" classes. In the 2nd level of the nomenclature, three classes were distinguished: "Buildings", "Roads" and "Others", based on the pansharp image and the nDSM.

"Buildings" were extracted in three stages, considering different roof materials. For the red tiles, the parameters used were Manhattan representation, width 7, and 75 pixels of aggregation. For the darker roof materials and for the brighter ones, Manhattan representation, width 7, and 100 pixels of aggregation were the selected parameters. All learning's were followed by remove clutter or add missing data iterations to reach the final "Buildings" class. The last step included generalize the building polygons using the same parameters as for the "Soil" class.

The class "Roads" was extracted in three independent processes, using different parameters. For the larger roads, Bull's Eye 2, width 25, and 1100 pixels of aggregation were considered. For the narrow roads, Bull's Eye 2, width 19, and 500 pixels of aggregation were considered. The remaining

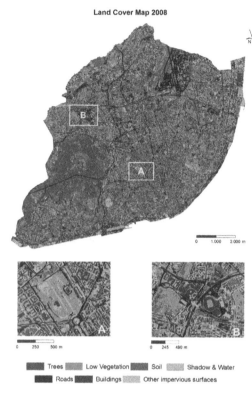

Land Cover Map 2008

Trees | Low Vegetation | Soil | Shadow & Water
Roads | Buildings | Other impervious surfaces

Figure 2. Land cover map of 2008 derived from IKONOS imagery for the city of Lisbon.

asphalt pavement was extracted with Bull's Eye 2, width 25, and 500 pixels of aggregation. These three layers were then merged to produce the "Roads" class. The final layer was obtained by generalization.

The "Other impervious surfaces" (like sidewalks or railroads), were the remaining areas within the "Impervious surface" class, after masking out the "Buildings" and "Roads" classes.

Figure 2 shows the final Land Cover Map produced for 2008, for the city of Lisbon, using satellite data.

4 CONCLUSIONS

A methodology for mapping impervious surfaces in the riverside city of Lisbon, with high-resolution optical satellite imagery was presented. The land cover map is the most detailed and updated dataset for the city. It is expected that such a dataset will aid in improving all phases of flood risk management at the municipal level, from planning to response and rehabilitation. Furthermore, all land cover layers produced in this work are eminently suitable for

diverse urban information and planning functions due to its very high geometric resolution. They can be used, for example, to update the land use plan inventory as well as biotope mapping.

ACKNOWLEDGEMENTS

This work was conducted in the framework of project GeoSat—Methodologies to extract large scale GEOgraphical information from very high resolution SATellite images, funded by the Portuguese Foundation for Science and Technology (PTDC/GEO/64826/2006).

The authors would like to thank Logica for the opportunity of using the LiDAR data set.

REFERENCES

Aponte, A.G.P. 2007. Runoff coefficients using a quickbird image for mapping flood hazard in a Tropical Coastal City, Campeche, Mexico. *Geoscience and Remote Sensing Symposium, 2007. IGARSS 2007. IEEE International*, 4702–4706.

Canters, F., Chormanski, J., van de Voorde, T., Batelaan, O. 2009. Effects of different methods for estimating impervious surface cover on runoff estimation at catchment level. *7th International Symposium on Spatial Accuracy Assessment in Natural Resources and Environmental Sciences.*

Chormanski, J., van de Voorde, T., Batelaan, O., Canters, F. 2008. Improving Distributed Runoff Prediction in Urbanized Catchments with Remote Sensing based Estimates of Impervious Surface Cover. *Sensors 2008*, 8: 910–932.

Ebert, A., Banzhaf, E., McPhee, J. 2009. The influence of urban expansion on the flood hazard in Santiago de Chile, *2009 Urban Remote Sensing Joint Event.*

Hay, G.J., Castilla, G. 2008. Geographic Object-Based Image Analysis (GEOBIA): A new name for a new discipline? In T. Blaschke, S. Lang, G.J. Hay (eds), *Object-Based Image Analysis—spatial concepts for knowledge-driven remote sensing applications*, 75–89, Springer-Verlag.

Nichol, J.E., Wong, M.S. 2007. Assessing urban environmental quality using multiple parameters. In Q. weng and D.A. Quattrochi (ed.) *Urban Remote Sensing*, 253–266, CRC Press.

Shamaoma, H., Kerle, N., Alkema, D. 2006. Extraction of flood-modelling related base-data from multi-source remote sensing imagery, *ISPRS Mid-term Symposium 2006, Remote Sensing: From Pixels to Processes.*

Yan, M., Ren, L., He, X., Sang, W. 2008. Evaluation of Urban Environmental Quality with High Resolution Satellite Images, *Geoscience and Remote Sensing Symposium, 2008. IGARSS 2008. IEEE International*, 3: 1280–1283.

Rouse, J.W., Hass, R.H., Schell, J.A., Deering, D.W. 1973. Monitoring vegetation systems in the great plains with ERTS. *Third NASA ERTS Symposium*, 1: 309–317.

Computational Vision and Medical Image Processing – Tavares & Natal Jorge (eds)
© 2012 Taylor & Francis Group, London, ISBN 978-0-415-68395-1

Feature extraction from satellite imagery and LiDAR to update exposure to tsunami and improve risk assessment in dynamic urban areas

S. Freire, T. Santos & J.A. Tenedório
e-GEO—Research Centre for Geography and Regional Planning, Faculdade de Ciências Sociais e Humanas (FCSH), Universidade Nova de Lisboa, Lisboa, Portugal

ABSTRACT: Mapping of human and structural exposure to hazards is a fundamental risk assessment undertaking, which should be based on detailed and up-to-date geo-information. However, the dynamics of land change in large cities cause base maps and censuses to rapidly become outdated, possibly resulting in inaccurate assessment of risk. Using tsunami hazard in Lisbon as the case study, this paper presents an approach to improve the mapping and analysis of exposure and risk by updating the municipal cartography and creating 3D urban models having functional information. The methodology is based on the updating of building features using LiDAR data and Very-High Resolution (VHR) satellite imagery and their further characterization using ancillary spatial data sets. Results include more up-to-date structural and socioeconomic geographic information that can benefit Emergency Management activities as well as other urban planning tasks.

Keywords: Tsunami, exposure, municipal maps, Lisbon

1 INTRODUCTION

Mapping and quantifying exposure to potential or actual hazards is a fundamental risk assessment task that is increasingly included in the roster of emergency management activities (Balk et al. 2006; Comenetz, 2009). Disaster risk is a function of hazard combined with population exposure and its vulnerability (UNDP, 2004). However, until recently, mapping and assessing human exposure and vulnerability has been overlooked in favor of hazard analysis efforts (Pelling, 2004). Also, accurate exposure analysis (of people and their assets) requires detailed and updated geo-information (Aubrecht et al. 2009).

The city of Lisbon, Portugal, has suffered the occurrence of several tsunami events in the past, including the well-known 1755 disaster (Baptista & Miranda 2009). Currently, due to the large number of people and activities present along the coastal zone and river banks, a large tsunami could have devastating effects in the city, especially if taking place in the daytime period (Freire & Aubrecht 2011). The Regional Plan for Territorial Management for the Lisbon Metropolitan Area (PRO-TAML) includes a detailed Tsunami Inundation Susceptibility map for the area, showing that significant coastal areas are at risk in case of an event (CCDR-LVT 2010). However, the last

comprehensive large-scale mapping effort for the city dates from 1998. Due to the numerous spatial changes taking place in the last decade or so, with continued urbanization along the river front, this geo-information is becoming outdated, preventing accurate analysis of exposure and a rigorous assessment of risk. The high frequency and scope of spatial changes in dynamic cities demands ways of expediting the production and updating of large-scale geographic information. For that purpose, current and future Very High Spatial Resolution Satellite Imagery (VHR), due to their availability, wide coverage, and cost, may be an advantageous alternative to classical data sources and methods, i.e., aerial photography and photogrammetry (Ehlers 2007). For urban mapping and modeling, its value is especially increased when used in combination with LiDAR (Light Detection And Ranging) data.

The present work aims at demonstrating an approach to improve modeling and analysis of exposure to tsunami hazard by automatically updating the city's building map, in order to benefit urban risk assessment. First, the city's base map of buildings was updated using LIDAR data and QuickBird imagery. Then, updated buildings were characterized using ancillary data sets, to create a 3D urban model having functional information. Finally, residential population is estimated, and this updated exposure is combined with the tsunami inundation susceptibility to re-assess risk.

2 STUDY AREA AND DATA

For this study, a dynamic area subject to potential inundation by tsunami, located to the northeast of the downtown of the city of Lisbon, Portugal, was selected (Fig. 1).

This area occupies approximately 24 ha in the former grounds of the 1998 Lisbon World Fair (*Expo '98*), and has been suffering intense development and land use changes since then. The updating of buildings and exposure for risk reassessment takes place within the tsunami hazard zone, given the need to prioritize areas of high risk.

Several types of digital spatial data sets were combined for building extraction, map updating, and urban modeling: altimetric data was provided by a normalized Digital Surface Model (nDSM), biophysical data was obtained from a QuickBird image, land use information was provided by the Urban Atlas, topographic information was obtained from the Municipal cartography, and socioeconomic (population) information from the 2001 Census (Table 1).

The QuickBird imagery was acquired in March 11 2007, with a sun azimuth and elevation of 161°.4 and 46°, respectively. The imagery was orthorectified in order to reduce the geometric distortions introduced by the relief and to attribute a national projected coordinate system (ETRS89-PT-TM06).

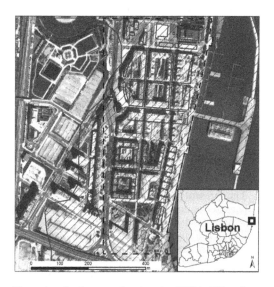

Figure 1. Study area, showing the 1998 building footprints and the tsunami inundation zone overlaid on the 2007 pansharpened QuickBird image.

Table 1. Main input data sets used.

Data set	Date	Data type	Resolution (m)/Scale
QuickBird image	2007	Raster	2.4
LiDAR (nDSM)	2006	Raster	1
Urban Atlas	2007	Vector	1:10,000
Resident population	2001	Vector	–
Municipal map	1998	Vector	1:1000

The orthorectification was performed using the Rational Polynomial Coefficients (RPCs) with 29 GCP's retrieved from the 1:1000 planimetric and altimetric cartography of 1998 and validated with 22 checkpoints. The RMSE (Root Mean Square Error) of the transformation was less than one pixel. A pansharpened image was also created for reference.

The nDSM stores for every pixel its height relative to the terrain plane, and was obtained from combining a LiDAR-derived DSM with a Digital Terrain Model, both having 1 m resolution.

The Urban Atlas project maps land use for selected European cities, including Lisbon, using 19 thematic classes and has a MMU of 0.25 ha (for 'Artificial surfaces'). Data for Lisbon was downloaded from http://www.eea.europa.eu/data-and-maps/data/urban-atlas.

Spatial information on Tsunami hazard was obtained in the form of a detailed Tsunami Inundation Susceptibility map (vector), included in the Regional Plan for Territorial Management for the Lisbon Metropolitan Area (PROTAML). This map depicts areas susceptible to inundation by tsunami using two classes or levels, *High* and *Moderate*. All of the study area is highly susceptible in the event of a tsunami.

3 METHODOLOGY

The methodology includes two main stages, namely: a) the updating of the 1998 municipal building map for 2006, and b) functional characterization and subsequent modeling and analysis of exposure and risk assessment. Figure 2 shows the main steps of the complete modeling approach.

3.1 *Updating of Buildings map*

The updating of the Municipal 1998 Buildings map is based on a change detection procedure. Using the nDSM, the 1998 building map is assessed for the detection of changes occurring between that year and 2006. This process corresponds to the modeling steps inside the dashed line in Figure 2 which are detailed in Figure 3.

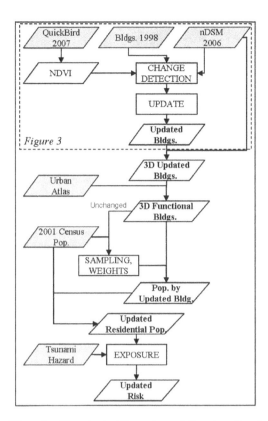

Figure 2. Flowchart of the main modeling steps (input data sets in light gray, outputs in bold).

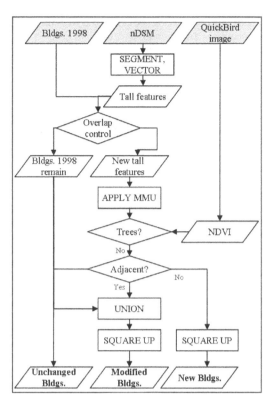

Figure 3. Flowchart of the modeling steps to obtain the Updated Buildings map (input data sets in light gray, outputs in bold).

The process is initiated with the segmentation and vectorization of the nDSM grid into features having at least a height of 1 floor (i.e., 3 meters). These 'tall features' are overlaid with the 1998 buildings to evaluate and detect those buildings that disappeared, those that remain, and the 'tall features' that are new in 2006. After retaining only those features wider than 5 meters, those that correspond to trees are dismissed. Identification of trees is performed using the NDVI (Normalized Difference Vegetation Index), computed using the Red and Near-Infrared bands of the 2007 QuickBird multispectral image (Rouse et al. 1973). The NDVI is a robust, widely-used indicator of vegetation presence and its greenness. The mean NDVI value was computed for all features, and a value of 0.1 was used to discard features above that threshold.

The obtained buildings are subject to an 'adjacency test' with the remaining 1998 buildings from the initial assessment, in order to identify the 1998 buildings that are adjacent to new buildings, and the new buildings that are isolated structures.

The remaining 1998 buildings which are not adjacent to new ones are deemed "Unchanged

Buildings". Those that are adjacent are merged with their contiguous new buildings and are squared up, resulting in "Modified Buildings". The new isolated buildings are squared up and labeled as 'New Buildings' on the Updated Buildings map. The squaring up of building features (polygons) was performed using Feature Analyst 4.2 (Overwatch Systems), as an extension for ArcGIS (Esri).

3.2 Characterization of Updated Buildings map and assessment of exposure and risk

The modeling and analysis of exposure and risk assessment is initiated by the creation of a 3D urban model of the buildings in the study area (see Fig. 2). This 3D model is created by combining the updated 2D map of buildings with height information from the LiDAR.

Land use information from the Urban Atlas is used to infer the main function of each updated building block (e.g. residential or commercial) in 2006. Areas classified as 'Urban fabric' are assumed to have a residential function.

This information can be combined with the 2001 Census data to estimate the resident population for the updated buildings map. This can only be done for those enumeration areas (census blocks) which are completely contained in the study area, and whose buildings were therefore subject to assessment and updating. The updating of resident population is performed by extrapolating the population density based on residential building volume obtained from Unchanged Buildings in unchanged census blocks. Residential buildings in unchanged census blocks are sampled to derive population density weights that are combined with the building volume of residential 'Modified' and 'New' Buildings to estimate their resident population. This estimated resident population for Updated Buildings can be aggregated to their respective census enumeration areas in order to update the census' resident population.

Finally, changes in exposure of residents to tsunami hazard in those census blocks can be analyzed and compared, and risk re-assessed to reflect transformations due to urban development.

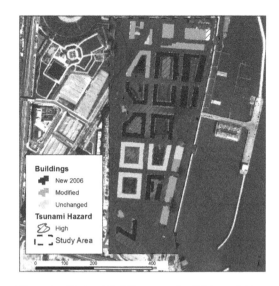

Figure 4. Updated Buildings map for 2006, overlaid on the nDSM and the 2007 pansharpened QuickBird image.

4 RESULTS AND DISCUSSION

The proposed methodology outputs the following results for the study area:

a. Updated map (2D) of building blocks for 2006;
b. A 3D urban model having functional information;
c. Updated model of population exposure to tsunami;
d. Improved risk assessment of tsunami hazard.

Figure 4 shows the 2D Updated Buildings map for the study area. Without additional information (e.g. cadastral plots), buildings can only be extracted and updated at the building block level (Freire et al. 2010). A building block may correspond to one isolated building or several buildings when these are contiguous.

The initial 1998 Municipal map included 95 individual building structures in 32 building blocks in the study area. The Updated Buildings map includes 34 building blocks, of which 6 are 'Unchanged' from 1998, 11 were 'Modified', and 17 are considered 'New' in 2006. Although a formal validation of results was not yet conducted, it can be observed that some problems are caused by the on-going construction taking place in the study area at the time of data acquisition.

Compared to producing a building map for 2006 using simple direct extraction of buildings from the LIDAR data, this approach to updating the 1998 Building's map based on change detection has the advantage of preserving the original footprint of unchanged buildings while assessing changes. Such a procedure can be used to quickly obtain an updated map for urban analysis and management before another, more costly, topographic database is available (Santos et al. 2010).

From the 3D Updated Buildings model the number of storeys above ground can be derived. This reveals that the new buildings vary from 1 to 6 floors, with the largest blocks having 6 floors.

The 3D Functional Buildings model is presented in Figure 5.

The functional analysis based on the Urban Atlas information shows that most of the building blocks, including all the new buildings, have a residential use, while three blocks, in the north of the study area, correspond to "Industrial, commercial, public, military and private units".

The combination of the 3D Functional Buildings model with the Census 2001 data allowed the estimation of densities and the updating of resident population for 10 'Modified' and 'New' building blocks, based on their size and function in 2006.

Figure 6 shows the estimated resident population for residential 'Modified' and 'New' building blocks whose respective census enumeration areas are completely within the study area.

Table 2 shows, for those updated census blocks identified in Figure 6, the resident population figures from the 2001 census and those estimated for 2006.

Results show that there is a striking change in resident population in these census enumeration zones, from 0 residents in 2001 to a total of 1011.

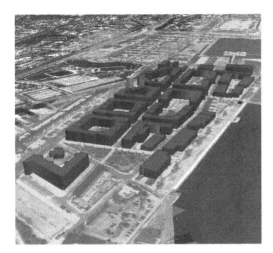

Figure 5. Perspective view to the northwest of the 3D Functional Buildings model for 2006, overlaid on the Tsunami Inundation Zone and the 2007 pansharpened QuickBird image.

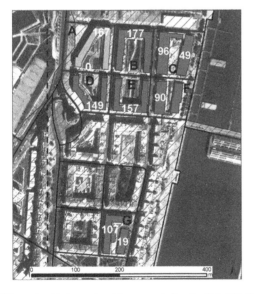

Figure 6. Estimated resident population for 'Modified' and 'New' Building blocks, overlaid on the 2007 pansharpened QuickBird image.

The fact that there wasn't yet any resident population in 2001 suggests that either a) the former existing structures were not residential, or b) the buildings were not yet completed and inhabited. The definitive figures from the 2011 Census, due to be released in 2012, will allow to validate these estimates and the model' assumptions.

Table 2. Resident population by updated census block.

Census block ID	Census pop. 2001	Pop. estimate 2006
A	0	167
B	0	177
C	0	145
D	0	149
E	0	157
F	0	90
G	0	126
Total	0	1011

The updated exposure of resident population to potential Tsunami hazard (by living in a zone highly susceptible to inundation) indicates that there may be an increase in risk from 1998 to 2006, in the area under analysis. Taking into account the fact that the study area is predominantly residential in 2006, exposure and risk might have especially increased in the nighttime period, when more residents are expected to be at home. Availability of data on inundation depth would allow for a more accurate assessment of potential tsunami impact.

5 CONCLUSIONS AND OUTLOOK

This study presented an approach to improve advanced modeling and analysis of potential population exposure to tsunami hazard by updating a municipal buildings map, in a dynamic urban area. The methodology was mostly automatic, benefiting from the high temporal consistency of the different spatial input data sets used for modeling. This effort constitutes a first approach at evaluating the effects of urban planning decisions on the risk of natural hazards, and can be applied to other study areas.

Results show that the study area suffered significant changes within a few years, becoming increasingly built-up and residential. This development process has likely increased the population exposure to tsunami hazard and therefore amplified the risk. The analysis highlighted the importance of keeping base maps and spatial databases up to date, especially in known hazard zones, in order to benefit risk assessment and planning. We believe this approach can generate valuable information both for urban planning and management, as well as for all phases of Emergency Management.

Future work includes conducting a quality assessment procedure to validate results, and the temporal disaggregation of population exposure, by estimating the population by building block in the daytime period.

ACKNOWLEDGEMENTS

This work was conducted in the framework of project GeoSat—Methodologies to extract large scale GEOgraphical information from very high resolution SATellite images, funded by the Portuguese Foundation for Science and Technology (PTDC/GEO/64826/2006). The authors acknowledge *Logica* for providing the LiDAR data set.

REFERENCES

Aubrecht, C., M. Köstl, K. Steinnocher 2009. High-level geospatial modeling of population patterns for exposure and impact assessment. In: Tavares J.M.R.S., Natal Jorge R.M. (Eds.): *Computational Vision and Medical Image Processing: VipIMAGE 2009*. Taylor & Francis, CCR Press. 379–384.

Balk, D.L., U. Deichmann, G. Yetman, F. Pozzi, S.I. Hay, A. Nelson 2006. Global mapping of infectious diseases: methods, examples and emerging applications. In Hay, S.I., Graham, A.J. & Rogers, D.J. (eds), *Advances in Parasitology*, vol. 62. London: Academic Press, pp. 119–156.

Baptista, M.A. and Miranda, J.M. 2009. Revision of the Portuguese catalog of tsunamis, *Natural Hazards and Earth System Sciences*, 9, 25–42.

CCDR-LVT 2010. PROTAML: Diagnóstico Sectorial—Riscos e Protecção Civil, Lisbon. Available at http://consulta-protaml.inescporto.pt/plano-regional.

Comenetz, J. 2009. Building a global demographic map database for disaster relief and crisis management. *Proceedings of the International Cartography Conference—ICC 2009*, Santiago (Chile), 15–21 November 2009.

Ehlers M. 2007. New developments and trends for Urban Remote Sensing. In *Urban Remote Sensing*: 357–375. CRC Press.

Freire, S., Santos T., Gomes N., Fonseca A., Tenedório J.A. 2010. Extraction of buildings from QuickBird imagery—what is the relevance of urban context and heterogeneity? *Proceedings of ASPRS/CaGIS/ISPRS Fall Conference*. Orlando, USA, November 15–18, 2010.

Freire, S. & Aubrecht, C. 2011. Assessing Spatio-Temporal Population Exposure to Tsunami Hazard in the Lisbon Metropolitan Area. Mendonça & Dugdale (Eds.): *ISCRAM 2011, 8th International Conference on Information Systems for Crisis Response and Management*. Proceedings. Lisbon, Portugal, May 8–11, 2011.

Pelling, M. 2004. Visions of risk: a review of international indicators of disaster risk and its management. UNDP Bureau for Crisis Prevention and Recovery, Geneva.

Rouse, J.W., Haas, R.H., Schell, J.A., Deering, D.W. 1973. Monitoring vegetation systems in the Great Plains with ERTS, *Third ERTS Symposium*, NASA SP-351 I: 309–317.

Santos, T., Freire S., Fonseca A., Tenedório J.A. 2010. Producing a building change map for urban management purposes. *Proceedings of 30th EARSeL Symosium*. Paris, France, 31 May—June 3, 2010.

UNDP (United Nations Development Programme) 2004. *Reducing Disaster Risk: A challenge for development*. New York: UNDP Bureau for Crisis Prevention and Recovery, 146 pp.

Computational Vision and Medical Image Processing – Tavares & Natal Jorge (eds)
© *2012 Taylor & Francis Group, London, ISBN 978-0-415-68395-1*

Situational awareness on Rio de Janeiro's terrain sliding using Cosmo-Skymed data-study of a real case

R.L. Paes, O.D. Zaloti Jr., F.M. Barros & C.H.L. Ribeiro
Institute for Advanced Studies, São José dos Campos, Brazil

ABSTRACT: Summer storms frequently affect Brazilian cities. When they localized onto peculiar geographical terrains, the risk of a disaster is then empowered. As an attempt for collaborating with the civilians authorities, we followed this work with an approach of detecting access ways and plane terrains for the rescue choppers landing. We, then, applied wavelet techniques and decision trees algorithm to extract descriptors and to classify interest areas, respectively. The imageries were acquired from Cosmo-Skymed SAR sensor and we got a confident ground truth.

1 INTRODUCTION

On the Rio de Janeiro's hills, specifically on the cities of Teresópolis, Petrópolis, Nova Friburgo and their respective counties suffered, on the last 2011 summer, a very intensive terrain sliding and floods caused by the torrential rains. Risk areas area are usually known, but the potential real disaster magnitude is unknown. Such cities' region is characterized by a chain of cliffs and valleys. The human presence is noticed disorganized even onto the cliffs as on the valleys, what probably contributed to weaken the vegetation soil protection. Preliminary studies from the local governments noticed that such situation is intrinsic to that geology and environment, what lead us to understand that it will happen sooner.

Anyway, our approach is not to understand or to point out what or why it happened, but, yes, for helping the authorities responsible by the search and rescue operations and by the natural disaster protection team. Thus, we worked with available data and many times it is not sufficiently enough to follow a usual methodology of remote sensing of the environment. It means that we tried to accomplish tasks like finding access ways and plane terrain for choppers landing.

Despite there's no available optical image from such region, once it was fully covered by clouds for many days. On the critical areas, the access was possible just by helicopters and by offroad trucks. Then, the ground truth applied here was firstly obtained joint to the citizens and through the local news. After that, with the clearance for visiting that places, our team went there got precise data.

Cosmo-Skymed satellite images covered that area, once only SAR images could have some information about what was really happening. Some optical images were presented on the media, but any of its sources were available for sharing such data. We described our imagery data on the following topic.

2 COSMO-SKYMED SATELLITE

Cosmo-Skymed is four satellites SAR sensor from the Italian Spatial Agency, carrying each one an X-band multimode SAR. It has the capability to acquire different polarizations (HH, VV, HV, VH) and its main imageries modes are: Spotlight; Stripmap; and ScanSAR. It flies on a sun-synchronous dusk-dawn near-polar orbit platform at an altitude of 620 km.

In the present work, images from the Stripmap mode were acquired, covering a 50 × 50 km from each city. There are images with Level 1A of processing (full resolution Single Look Complex (SLC) images, with ground range resolution ~5.0 m and azimuth resolution ~56 m, according to Cosmo-Skymed *System Description & User Guide* and Cosmo-Skymed *SAR Products Handbook*) [1]. However, we will initially show the first results with multilook data, which we have HH polarization and ascending and descending satellites path passes.

3 METHODOLOGY

Our first step, due to lack of precise data, was trying to recognize reported affected areas on the Google Earth software. It allowed us to understand that regions and to establish our main approach.

We also got topographic charts that confirmed our visual observations.

Thus, we isolated through masks some interest points/areas as an attempt to extract good descriptors (Fig. 1). We did not have notion about how such places could be mixed with mud and wreckage (Fig. 2). So, we selected some samples empirically and we applied different wavelet techniques as descriptors [2–5].

The next step was to put such data onto an oblique Decision Tree (DT) for classifying that region [6]. SAR images have an intrinsic peculiarity named speckle. SLC SAR images have too much noise; despite has better resolution compared to other processing possibilities. Hence, we processed the data on decision tree, classifying into three regions: a) mountain top; b) cliffs; c) flat regions.

4 FIRST RESULTS AND CONSIDERATIONS

SLC image have strong speckle occurrence, thus it was the strongest obstacle to handle. There are many preprocessing steps proposed on the literature and we still exploring them. DT showed a very good capability to discriminate features instances. However, it is strongly necessary to extract the appropriate descriptors.

Then, to handle with that, we initially applied Kuan filter due to deal with the image texture, reducing speckle. It was chosen empirically, comparing with other similar filters. Wavelets were achieved as features descriptor extractor. Among them, we chosen Db2 and Haar, even so we do not found large difference. However, it still research approach. After DT processing, we filtered again with ISODATA algorithm, even that an unsupervised classifier, was achieved for visually improves DT output (Fig. 3).

Our first results are yet prototypes from our methodology. We got responses from cliff terrain; from mountain tops; and from concentrated urban area (flat region). Such results showed that our approach is doing fine the indirect detection approach. Once the decision tree is feed with precise descriptors, it responds fast and accurately.

Now, we work to improve the classification output, but also interested on finding manmade structures likewise soccer or golf fields and roads, highlighting helicopters landing places and access via for ground civilian defense forces. We are compared and verified image processing results with

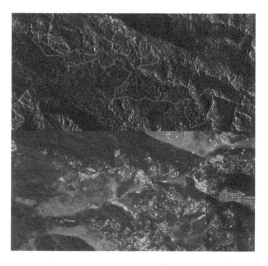

Figure 1. Cosmo-Skymed subset image over Teresopoils city—Brazil. Red line marks the surveyed sub-area. At top, it shows the Cosmo-Skymed image. Bellow, our first optical source: Google Earth software resources.

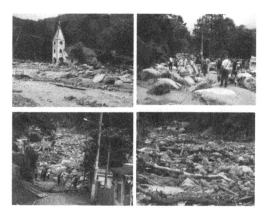

Figure 2. Photographs from such previously red line marked area, showing the disaster impact onto that neighborhood.

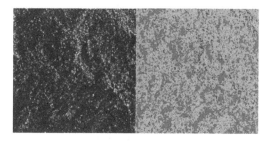

Figure 3. Cosmo-Skymed Kuan filtered image (left) and classification output, after DT and ISODATA processing, respectively. Blue spots are the mountain tops; Green is the slope terrain; and in Red, plane terrains (urban area concentration. Teresopoils city—Brazil is represented on this figure.

topological charts and with the team ground truth. Image processing scheme showed that is possible to obtain indirectly the desired information.

SAR technology operates in all-weather conditions, providing users to have information independent of Sunlight and rainy day. On this case, the first optical images were acquired more than two weeks later. The fast response of a satellite constellation, as Cosmo-Skymed, helps the improvement of situational awareness and scenario update for decision makers and operational teams.

ACKNOWLEDGEMENTS

Our special thanks to Telespazio Brasil S.A./ Italian Spatial Agency (ASI) for provide us the Cosmo-Skymed SAR data. We also thank to that volunteers civilians that helped us for obtaining our ground truth.

REFERENCES

[1] Telespazio—A Fiomeccania/Thales Company. TEL-ESPAZIO/COSMO-SKYMED. Available in: <http:// www. telespazio.it/cosmo.html>. Last access in: December 18th, 2009.
[2] M, Tello, C. Lopez-Martinez, J.J. Mallorqui, "A novel approach for the automatic detection of punctual isolated targets in a noisy background in SAR imagery". *Radar Conference*, 2005. EURAD 2005. European. p. 41–44. Paris, 2005.
[3] Mallat, S.G., *A Theory for Multiresolution Signal Decomposition: The Wavelet representation.* IEEE Transactions On Pattern Analysis And Machine Intelligence Vol. 2, N. 7. 1989.
[4] Daubechies, I., *Ten lectures on wavelets.* CBMS conference on wavelets, university of lowell, ma, June 1990—Philadelphia, PA: Society for Industrial and Applied Mathematics, (1992).
[5] Cohen, A., Daubechies, I., Feauveau, J.C., *Biorthogonal bases of compactly supported wavelets,* Comm. Pure & Appl. Math 45, pp. 485–560, 1992.
[6] Yildiz, O.T., Alpaydin, E., *Linear discriminant trees.* International Journal of Pattern Recognition and Artificial Intelligence. Vol 19, No. 3 (2005).

Computational Vision and Medical Image Processing – Tavares & Natal Jorge (eds)
© 2012 Taylor & Francis Group, London, ISBN 978-0-415-68395-1

Identification of wildfire precursor conditions: Linking satellite based fire and soil moisture data

C. Aubrecht
AIT Austrian Institute of Technology, Vienna, Austria

C.D. Elvidge & K.E. Baugh
National Geophysical Data Center, National Oceanic & Atmospheric Administration, Boulder CO, USA

S. Hahn
Institute of Photogrammetry and Remote Sensing, Vienna University of Technology, Vienna, Austria

ABSTRACT: Since satellite remote sensing of fires started in the 1970s, fire monitoring has become increasingly important, particularly in the context of mitigating social impacts. Light from fires can be identified in nighttime satellite imagery featuring the visible part of the electromagnetic spectrum. A procedure for detection of fire lights and near real-time monitoring of spatial patterns of fire occurrence has been successfully implemented based on low-light imaging data from the Defense Meteorological Satellite Program, Operational Linescan System (DMSP-OLS). Satellite based soil moisture data can be used to investigate potential correlations between soil conditions and water related hazards such as floods and droughts, the latter often closely associated with wildfire incidence. It is envisaged that regional monitoring of soil moisture can help to identify changes in the conditions of an ecological system before major impacts take place. Information on current and previous soil conditions enable identification of potentially hazardous situations.

Keywords: DMSP-OLS, nighttime lights, fire detection, ASCAT, soil moisture anomaly, time series

1 INTRODUCTION

Fire has been a regulating environmental factor for thousands of years shaping landscape structure, pattern, and ultimately the species composition and biological diversity of ecosystems. Forest and wildland fire is a vital and natural process initiating natural cycles of vegetation succession and maintaining ecosystem viability. However, uncontrolled or misused fires can cause tremendous adverse impacts on the environment and human society, affecting land cover/land use patterns and having huge implications on human health and socio-economic system structures. The majority of wildland fire outbreaks result from a combination of location-specific climatic characteristics and human activity. The contribution of natural fires (e.g., caused by lightning) is insignificant compared to the number of human-induced fires. Most fires are intentionally set in forests, savannas, grasslands and other wildland areas for timber harvesting, land conversion, slash-and-burn agriculture, and socio-economic conflicts over questions of property and land use rights (Levine et al., 1999).

Satellite based observation of nocturnal lighting opens up a variety of research and application fields dealing with certain relations of light with and associated impacts on the environment, for both artificial lighting types (e.g., human settlements) and natural forms (e.g., wildfires). It has been known since the early 1970's (Croft, 1973) that fires can be detected at night using remotely sensed low light imaging data, as recorded by the U.S. Air Force Defense Meteorological Satellite Program (DMSP).

To date there have been few direct comparisons of DMSP-based fire detection and results obtained through the use of other satellite systems. Elvidge et al. (1999a) highlighted that DMSP fire detection was comparable to the results obtained from AVHRR (Advanced Very High Resolution Radiometer) and GOES (Geostationary Operational Environmental Satellite) analyzing a set of known fires in New Mexico during 1996. Fuller and Fulk (2000) found a strong spatial and temporal correspondence between DMSP and AVHRR fire detection patterns in Kalimantan, Indonesia during 1997.

In recent studies, MODIS (Moderate Resolution Imaging Spectroradiometer) data has been used successfully to detect active forest fires (Giglio et al., 2006). It is anticipated that a multi-sensor approach to fire monitoring would provide a better overall depiction of fire events than reliance on data from a single satellite system. However, DMSP data have the unique capability of detecting nighttime lights even in dim light and (moderate) cloud cover, thus providing options for near-real-time fire monitoring.

Particularly in the context of mitigating social impacts, contextual fire monitoring has recently become increasingly important. In the framework of the ongoing GMSM project ('Global Monitoring of Soil Moisture for Water Hazards Assessment') we investigate potential correlations of satellite derived soil moisture anomalies with water related hazards such as floods and droughts, the latter often closely associated with wildfire incidence.

In this study a set of fire composite products for Africa for the year 2009 are compared with microwave remote sensing soil moisture data for the same period. 2009 was recorded as an especially extreme year in terms of low cumulative rainfall. Low seasonal rains, which would usually come between the months of March and June, resulted in severe droughts, with the Northern Sahel region and Eastern Africa particularly affected. It is envisaged that regional monitoring of soil moisture can help to identify changes in the conditions of an ecological system before major impacts take place. Information on current and previous soil conditions enable time series analyses and anomaly assessments for identification of potentially hazardous situations.

2 INPUT DATA

2.1 *DMSP nighttime lights*

The National Oceanic and Atmospheric Administration's National Geophysical Data Center (NOAA-NGDC) processes and archives nighttime lights data acquired by the U.S. Air Force Defense Meteorological Satellite Program (DMSP) Operational Linescan System (OLS). This sensor—an oscillating scan radiometer—was initially designed for global observation of cloud cover using a pair of visible (near infrared included, 0.5–0.9 μm) and thermal (10.5–12.5 μm) spectral bands. With the DMSP satellites flying in sun-synchronous, low altitude polar orbits and with a swath width of 3,000 km each OLS collects a complete set of imagery of the earth twice a day. At night a photomultiplier tube (PMT) intensifies

the visible band signal, basically in order to enable the detection of moonlit clouds. The boost in gain additionally allows the observation of faint sources of visible near-infrared emissions present at the surface of the Earth, i.e. permitting the measurement of radiances down to 10^{-9} watts/cm^2/sr/μm. Most of these light detections can be linked to human settlements (Elvidge et al., 1997) and ephemeral fires (Elvidge et al., 1999a/b, 2001), but also gas flares and offshore platforms (Elvidge et al., 2009) as well as heavily lit fishing boats can be identified.

Nighttime image data from individual orbits meeting pre-defined quality criteria (i.e. referring to geolocation, sunlight, moonlight, cloudiness conditions) form the basis for global latitude-longitude grids (e.g., annual/monthly composites) with 30 arc second resolution cells corresponding to approximately 1 km^2 at the equator. Aubrecht et al. (2008) provide more detailed explanations in the context of data selection criteria and data composition.

NOAA's NGDC stores and maintains the long-term digital DMSP archive (Table 1), and has built up comprehensive experience in nighttime image processing and algorithm development related to feature identification (e.g., lights and clouds) and data quality assessment (Elvidge et al., 1997). Dating back to 1992 the data archive enables the production of a time series of inter-comparable single-year data sets, e.g. for assessing temporal trends in human activity (Aubrecht et al., 2009).

2.2 *ASCAT Soil moisture soil water index data*

The Soil Water Index (SWI) is calculated from temporally irregular METOP ASCAT level 2 surface soil moisture measurements. The Advanced Scatterometer (ASCAT) is a C-Band Scatterometer flown on EUMETSAT's Meteorological Operational Satellite (METOP) series featuring a spatial resolution of about 25–34 km.

The SWI is a level 3 product and represents the profile soil moisture content obtained by filtering the Surface Soil Moisture (SSM) time series with an exponential function. The model is based on the assumption that moisture contained within a soil profile is basically due to precipitation and the

Table 1. DMSP digital archive 1992–2009 showing the satellites F-10-16 and their respective covered time span.

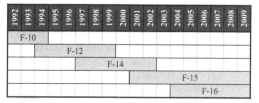

associated process of infiltration. The SWI retrieval algorithm (Wagner et al., 1999) is based on integrating surface soil moisture data over a preceding time period T (characteristic time length) using the following equation (1):

$$SWI(t_n) = \frac{\sum\limits_{i}^{n} SSM(t_i)e^{-\frac{t_n-t_i}{T}}}{\sum\limits_{i}^{n} e^{-\frac{t_n-t_i}{T}}} \quad for\, t_i \leq t_n \qquad (1)$$

The objective of this formulation is to describe a simple two-layer water balance model, where the first layer is accessible to the C-band scatterometer and the second layer is the part of the profile which extends downwards from the bottom of the soil surface layer.

The second layer is supposed to act as a reservoir which is connected to the atmosphere via the first layer. Thus, the highly temporal dynamic moisture conditions, which are predominant in the first layer, decrease with increasing profile depth in the second layer. The amount of water stored in the reservoir depends on the infiltration of water added to the first layer during precipitation events. Therefore the water content is solely controlled by past dynamics. Furthermore, it is obvious that more recent events have a stronger impact on the moisture conditions in the second layer, which is reflected in the exponential weighting function in the equation.

3 METHODS

3.1 *Fire detection in DMSP nighttime lights*

Time series analysis of nighttime DMSP-OLS observations allows the definition of reference data sets of "stable" lights, which are present consistently in the same location. The basic procedures used to generate the stable lights are described by Elvidge et al. (1997). Fires are identified as visible near-infrared emission sources detected on the land surface outside the reference set of stable lights and also not associated with lightning features (Elvidge et al., 1999b). As outlined by Elvidge et al. (2001) a set of algorithms is used to generate DMSP-OLS fire products. The processing steps can be grouped into two subsequent sections: (1) processing on the raw scanline format OLS data and (2) processing on georeferenced OLS data. Processing steps applied to the raw data include: orbit assembly and suborbiting, cloud identification, glare and sunlit data removal, light detection, geolocation and gridding. Steps performed on the georeferenced data include the removal of

lights associated with stable lights (i.e., lit pixels which occur in or directly adjacent to the known stable light locations), removal of lights over water surfaces, and final editing. The remaining pixels, which contain ephemeral visible band emission sources, are considered to be fires. Publications describing the use of digital DMSP data for fire detection include Kihn (1996), Elvidge et al. (1999a/b, 2001), Fuller (2000), and Fuller & Fulk (2000). The only systematic use of analog OLS film data from the pre-digital era for fire analysis was the inventory of African fires by Cahoon et al. (1992, 1994). More recent contributions based on digitally archived DMSP data are provided by Badarinath et al. (2007a/b, 2011) and Chand et al. (2006, 2007).

3.2 *Soil moisture anomaly assessment*

In addition to analyzing dryness in general via the SWI, we wanted to check if particularly anomalous conditions relate to fire outbreaks. SWI T = 20 data have been used together with a daily long-term soil moisture mean in order to derive SWI anomalies for 2009 over Africa. T = 20 is an indicator for the temporal resolution of the SWI data used in this study, meaning that SSM measurements of the past 20 days are recognized in each SWI value.

The term anomaly in this context refers to the deviation of the actual SWI value at a certain spatial location with respect to the long term mean of soil moisture for the day in question. High anomaly values indicate abnormal SWI conditions.

4 RESULTS

For this study the African continent has been taken as test area and successful DMSP fire detections could be associated with fire seasons in both northern and southern hemisphere. Figures 1 and 2 compare monthly aggregated 30 arc sec DMSP-OLS fire products (2009) with coarser scale MODIS fire detections for two different parts of the year (January vs. August). On a regional and temporally aggregated level these two data sources match very well.

Figures 3 and 5 visualize the SWI for the entire African continent, showing the peak of the dry seasons in the northern hemisphere (in mid February) and in the southern hemisphere (in late August) respectively. Brown colors indicate areas with low SWI values (i.e., dry soil conditions) while blue colors show areas featuring high SWI values (i.e., wet soil conditions). Looking at the SWI 2009 time series, the movement of rather dry and rather wet regions over the seasons between north and south of the equator can be observed.

349

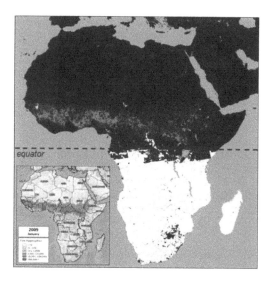

Figure 1. Aggregated DMSP-OLS fire detections in Africa for January 2009 (30 arc sec raster), compared to coarse scale (1 degree) MODIS fire detections of the same period.

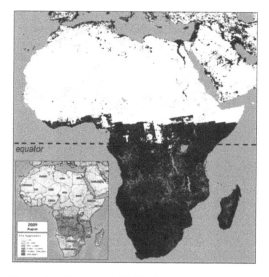

Figure 2. Aggregated DMSP-OLS fire detections in Africa for August 2009 (30 arc sec raster), compared to coarse scale (1 degree) MODIS fire detections of the same period.

The southern part of the Sahel zone is considered as first example (indicated in Fig. 3). Figure 4 presents a zoom detail of that area showing the SWI (a) and an overlay of the DMSP-based fire sources (b). A strong spatial correlation between detected fires and very dry soil conditions (i.e., very

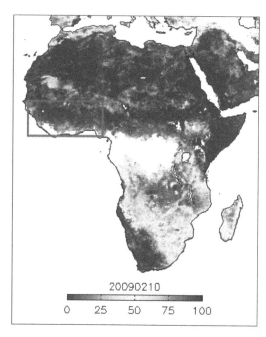

Figure 3. Soil water index (SWI) for Africa, showing the peak of the dry season in the northern hemisphere in mid February (brown colors indicate dry areas, blue colors show wet areas).

low SWI, dark brown color) can be observed. The same is noticed for the second example which is the central and southern part of Africa just south of the equator. The area is marked in Figure 5 and zoom details of SWI (a) and overlaid fires (b) are shown in Figure 6.

Coming to the basic conclusion that dry areas spatially correlate with fires seasonally (for the examined year of 2009) we wanted to check if in particular anomalously dry areas favor the fire development. SWI measurements were therefore compared to a long-term soil moisture mean with high deviations indicating abnormal SWI conditions, i.e. either unusually dry (negative values) or unusually wet (positive values). Figures 4 and 6 (c) show the calculated SWI anomalies for the two sample areas. In the southern Sahel zone just very low anomaly values can be observed, basically meaning that the conditions in the year 2009 were in line with the long-term trend. Also the second sample area in the southern central part of Africa shows a similar picture, with the exception of the southern part of the Democratic Republic of Congo where anomalously dry conditions could be detected (deviations of up to 35%). However, interestingly these areas do not seem to be particularly affected, i.e. there was no spatial correlation

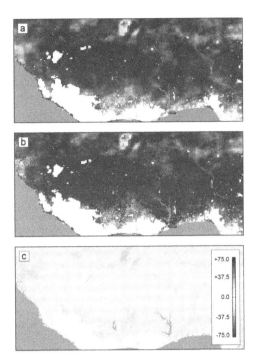

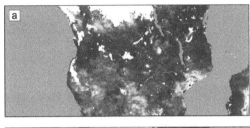

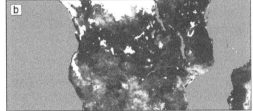

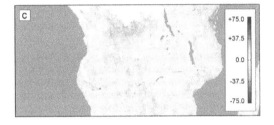

Figure 4.   Zoom detail indicated in figure 3: (a) SWI, (b) SWI with DMSP fires overlay (in purple), and (c) SWI anomaly (brown indicating unusual dry conditions, in contrast to blue).

Figure 6.   Zoom detail indicated in figure 5: (a) SWI, (b) SWI with DMSP fires overlay (in purple), and (c) SWI anomaly (brown indicating unusual dry conditions, in contrast to blue).

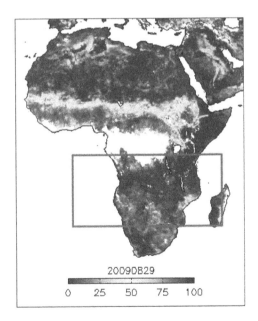

Figure 5.   Soil Water Index (SWI) for Africa, showing the peak of the dry season in the southern hemisphere in late August (brown colors indicate dry areas, blue colors show wet areas).

discovered between detected fire sources and high SWI anomalies.

5   DISCUSSION AND OUTLOOK

DMSP fire products can be generated (1) for single suborbits, (2) for mosaics from multiple suborbits to cover larger geographic regions, or (3) as temporal composites. Compositing fire detections from adjacent orbits over specific time intervals enables assembling continental-scale depictions of spatio-temporal pattern of biomass burning. In previous efforts, fires could be observed in the global nighttime lights product to latitudes of 60 degrees in the northern hemisphere. That indicates that fire detection capabilities of DMSP-OLS are not limited to tropical and temperate regions. One shortcoming of short-term temporal composites (e.g., monthly) is the shifting spatial coverage of nighttime data over the year. With an overpass time at 7:30 p.m. DMSP satellite F16 is only detecting nighttime data for the winter season in both hemispheres respectively.

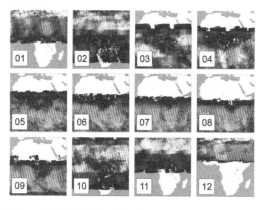

Figure 7. Monthly nighttime coverage of DMSP F16 data.

In terms of the applicability of the ASCAT-derived soil moisture information location specific measurement uncertainties have to be considered, such as problems with detection over tropical rainforest. A mask was therefore applied in order to block those areas from further integrative analyses and resulting misleading interpretations (see white areas in Fig. 3–6). The closer examination whether anomalously dry areas favor the fire development shows that it is not necessarily important to have exceptional dry conditions, since already the 'regular' dry periods are effectual in that sense.

Looking forward, next steps will include the addition of land cover (e.g., GLC 2000) and population data (e.g., African Population Database, AfriPop 2010). Eventually this will result in integrative vulnerability and risk assessments on various scales and dimensions. Given the global and frequent availability of the satellite based soil moisture information hazards thus not only comprise droughts and subsequent wildland fires, but also the other end of the spectrum, i.e. flooding events (Fleiss et al., 2011).

ACKNOWLEDGMENTS

Part of the presented research was performed within the GMSM (Global Monitoring of Soil Moisture for Water Hazards Assessment) project (http://www.ipf.tuwien.ac.at/gmsm/), funded by the Austrian Research Promotion Agency (FFG) in the frame of the Austrian Space Applications Programme (ASAP). Soil moisture data is processed and provided by the IPF, Vienna University of Technology. DMSP nighttime lights data is processed and provided by the Earth Observation Group of NOAA-NGDC.

REFERENCES

Aubrecht, C., Elvidge, C.D., Longcore, T., Rich, C., Safran, J., Strong, A.E., Eakin, C.M., Baugh, K.E., Tuttle, B.T., Howard, A.E., Erwin, E.H., 2008. A global inventory of coral reef stressors based on satellite observed nighttime lights. *Geocarto International*, 23(6), pp. 467–479.

Aubrecht, C., Elvidge, C.D., Eakin, C.M., Ziskin, D., Baugh, K.E., 2009. Coral reef risk assessment using DMSP nighttime lights—Temporal trends and global perspectives. Sustaining the Millennium Development Goals. 33rd International Symposium on Remote Sensing of Environment. Stresa, Lago Maggiore, Italy.

Badarinath, K., Kharol, S., Chand, T., 2007a. Use of Satellite Data to Study the Impact of Forest Fires Over the Northeast Region of India. *IEEE Geoscience and Remote Sensing Letters*, 4(3), pp. 485–489.

Badarinath, K.V.S., Kharol, S.K., Latha, K.M., Chand, T.R.K., Prasad, V.K., Jyothsna, A.N., Samatha, K., 2007b. Multiyear ground-based and satellite observations of aerosol properties over a tropical urban area in India. *Atmospheric Science Letters*, 8(1), pp. 7–13.

Badarinath, K.V.S., Sharma, A.R., Kharol, S.K., 2011. Forest fire monitoring and burnt area mapping using satellite data: a study over the forest region of Kerala State, India. *International Journal of Remote Sensing*, 32(1), pp. 85–102.

Cahoon, D.R., Stocks, B.J., Levine, J.S., Cofer, W.R., O'Neill, K.P., 1992. Seasonal distribution of African savanna fires. *Nature*, 359(6398), pp. 812–815.

Cahoon, D.R., Levine, J.S., Cofer, W.R., Stocks, B.J., 1994. The extent of burning in African savannas. *Advances in Space Research*, 14(11), pp. 447–454.

Chand, T.K., Badarinath, K.V.S., Krishna Prasad, V., Murthy, M.S.R., Elvidge, C.D., Tuttle, B.T., 2006. Monitoring forest fires over the Indian region using Defense Meteorological Satellite Program-Operational Linescan System nighttime satellite data. *Remote Sensing of Environment*, 103(2), pp. 165–178.

Chand, T.R.K., Badarinath, K.V.S., Murthy, M.S.R., Rajshekhar, G., Elvidge, C.D., Tuttle, B.T., 2007. Active forest fire monitoring in Uttaranchal State, India using multi-temporal DMSP-OLS—and MODIS-data. *International Journal of Remote Sensing*, 28(10), pp. 2123–2132.

Elvidge, C.D., Baugh, K.E., Kihn, E.A., Kroehl, H.W., Davis, E.R., 1997. Mapping of city lights using DMSP Operational Linescan System data. *Photogrammetric Engineering and Remote Sensing*, 63, pp. 727–734.

Elvidge, C.D. Pack, D.W., Prins, E., Kihn, E.A., Kendall, J., Baugh, K.E., 1999a, Wildfire Detection with Meteorological Satellite Data: Results from New Mexico During June of 1996 Using GOES, AVHRR, and DMSP-OLS. In: Lunetta, R.S., Elvidge, C.D., eds., *Remote Sensing Change Detection: Environmental Monitoring Methods and Applications*, London, UK: Taylor and Francis, pp. 74–122.

Elvidge, C.D., Baugh, K.E., Hobson, V.R., Kihn, E.A., Kroehl, H.W., 1999b. Detection of Fires and Power Outages Using DMSP-OLS Data. In: Lunetta, R.S., Elvidge, C.D., eds., *Remote Sensing Change Detection:*

Environmental Monitoring Methods and Applications, London: Taylor and Francis, pp. 123–135.

Elvidge, C.D., Nelson, I., Hobson, V.R., Safran, J., Baugh, K.E., 2001. Detection of fires at night using DMSP-OLS data. In: Ahern, F.J., Goldammer, J.G., Justice, C.O., eds., *Global and Regional Vegetation Fire Monitoring from Space: Planning a Coordinated International Effort*, The Hague: SPB Academic Publishing, pp. 125–144.

Elvidge, C.D., Ziskin, D., Baugh, K.E., Tuttle, B.T., Ghosh, T., Pack, D.W., Erwin, E.H., Zhizhin, M., 2009. A Fifteen Year Record of Global Natural Gas Flaring Derived from Satellite Data. *Energies*, 2(3), pp. 595–622.

Fleiss, M., Kienberger, S., Aubrecht, C., Kidd, R., Zeil, P., 2011. Mapping the 2010 Pakistan floods and its impact on human life: A post-disaster assessment of socio-economic indicators. Gi4DM 2011, GeoInformation for Disaster Management. Antalya, Turkey.

Fuller, D.O., 2000. Satellite remote sensing of biomass burning with optical and thermal sensors. *Progress in Physical Geography*, 24(4), pp. 543–561.

Fuller, D.O., Fulk, M., 2000. Comparison of NOAA-AVHRR—and DMSP-OLS—for operational fire monitoring in Kalimantan, Indonesia. *International Journal of Remote Sensing*, 21(1), pp. 181–187.

Giglio, L., Csiszar, I., Justice, C.O., 2006. Global distribution and seasonality of active fires as observed with the Terra and Aqua Moderate Resolution Imaging Spectroradiometer (MODIS) sensors. *Journal of Geophysical Research*, 111(G02016), 12 pp.

Levine, J.S., Bobbe, T., Ray, N., Witt, R.G., Singh, A., 1999. *Wildland Fires and the Environment: a Global Synthesis*. Nairobi, Kenya: United Nations Environment Programme (UNEP), Division of Environmental Information, Assessment and Early Warning (DEIA&EW), 46 pp.

Wagner, W., Lemoine, G., Rott, H., 1999. A method for estimating soil moisture from ERS scatterometer and soil data. *Remote Sensing of Environment*, 70(2), pp. 191–207.

Computational Vision and Medical Image Processing – Tavares & Natal Jorge (eds)
© 2012 Taylor & Francis Group, London, ISBN 978-0-415-68395-1

Development of an automated procedure for a patient specific segmentation of the human femur body from CT scan images

D. Almeida, J. Folgado & P.R. Fernandes
IDMEC—Instituto Superior Técnico, Technical University of Lisbon, Lisbon, Portugal

R.B. Ruben
ESTG, CDRSP, Polytechnic Institute of Leiria, Portugal

ABSTRACT: The present work presents an approach to a medical image segmentation problem. An automated computational procedure was developed which receives as input a stack of CT scan acquired images from a specific patient and returns a three dimensional representation of the body of the femur. This procedure uses a line following algorithm to obtain the bone region contour of each acquired image and 3D Delaunay triangulation to render the volume obtained.

Keywords: CT scan, threshold segmentation, Delaunay triangulation, Total Hip Arthroplasty

1 INTRODUCTION

Image segmentation techniques are based on the division of an image or a set of images in multiple regions or pixel sets according to some determined characteristic of the image or any of its computational properties, such as the intensities of the pixels in the color map or image gradient. Therewith, it is possible to obtain a more or less precise definition of the border between these regions and therefore proceed to its isolation for a more simple and precise analysis of the region of interest. A glimpse on the state of the art of this matter makes clear that, among the several different segmentation techniques developed, it is not obvious to state which one provides the best results for a generic use (Lakare, 2000; Unter et al., 2008). Depending on the image type, the segmentation approach must be previously studied in order to take full advantage of the image's specific characteristics. A common technique which leads to a relatively easy segmentation process is to photograph the object to segment with a phosphorescent background, making the object's frontiers easy to identify. However, even taking in account the most recent segmentation techniques developed, the user's experience is still a preponderate factor that clearly influences the obtained results. Therefore, it is still a work in progress the development of an algorithm that can perform a fully automatic segmentation without taking in account the images to segment and therefore constraining its use to a very specific application. In Medical Imaging this process is of

major interest because it allows the location and tracking of tumors or other pathologies as well as real time guidance for computer-aided surgery or the acquisition and computational representation of an organ or tissue, providing information about its properties and morphology. The fully automation of this process will save significant amount of time both in the identification of the pathology and in surgery preparation. In addition, the integration of such an algorithm in a commercial software package will allow less qualified users to perform such kind of analysis without having to fully comprehend the relying problems behind the graphic user interface.

Magnetic Resonance (MRI), x-ray Computed Tomography (CT) and ultrasounds are the most widely used methods to acquire in vivo medical images from the human body. These methods acquire a sequenced pile of images that are ideally parallel among them. This does not occur in most cases, due to the patient's movements during the exam or, in the case of ultrasonography, the force used to press the device against the patient's body. Therefore, the process of image segmentation and registration of a stack of medical images is slow and complex depending on the complexity of the anatomic structure and the quality of the images acquired. The better quality is desired, the more resolution per slice has to be taken in account as well as a reduction in the distance between the slices which will follow a larger number of slices for the same segmentation volume. There is also the probability of image artifacts to appear on the images, which increases the complexity of the process. These artifacts are generally related to the patient's natural movements during the acquisition process or even the functionality of the machine itself.

Image Segmentation techniques of medical volumes can be divided into three major groups: structural, stochastic and hybrids (Lakare, 2000). The structural segmentation techniques are essentially based in the structure and morphology of the region to segment while the stochastic approach takes in account a discrete analysis over every pixel characteristics or the characteristics of the pixel and the nearby region. The combination of both of these techniques gives rise to the hybrid approach which, in most cases, provides better results in an inferior computational time.

In this work, a computational procedure was implemented in order to select and map the region of each image which corresponds to the bone tissue which will define the shape of the three dimensional representation of the body (diaphysis) of the femur. This representation will allow the definition of a finite element mesh which can be used in several kinds of analysis to generate information about the femur morphology prior to the surgical intervention.

2 METHODS

2.1 Image acquisition

The stack of images used in the present work were acquired by X-ray computed tomography at the Orthopedics Department of São José Hospital, Lisbon, and gently given to us in the standard DICOM (Digital Imaging and Communications in Medicine) format by the Faculty of Medical Sciences of the New University of Lisbon. The patient was a middle aged male individual and presented a perfectly healthy femur. This acquisition method was chosen among the others for several more or less obvious reasons. It allows the acquisition of the anatomical structures in all three dimensions with no relative motion in the patient-machine system. In addition, different densities will result in different absorption rates by the tissues and consequently different intensity in the gray scale color map of the resulting acquired images. Therefore, different density values allow x-rays to clearly separate hard from soft tissues as shown in Figure 1. This fact will be become very useful in the segmentation process.

The usage of the DICOM image format has many advantages. Firstly, the image set may contain additional information related to the patient's details (e.g. age, gender), the acquisition process (e.g. date, place) or the image itself (e.g. resolution, distance between the slices). The image set contains

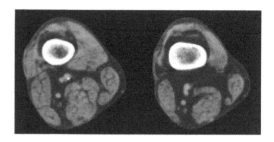

Figure 1.   Two examples of CT scan acquired images.

images equally spaced from each other. Every image has the same amount of pixels and the same color map. Each pixel has an intensity value of the gray scale color map according to the tissue's physical density. In the three dimensional model generation, the need to substitute the area unit (pixel) by a volume unite (voxel) is made very simple with the distance between the various image slices information contained in the DICOM file format.

2.2 Image processing

It was used the numerical simulation software MATLAB for the image processing. Firstly, it was developed a trivial procedure that will load the whole image set in a user specified directory, archiving all the relevant data in a matrix. At a first glimpse at Figure 1, it is notorious that the pixels corresponding to the bone tissue region have a characteristic intensity in the gray scale specter. Therefore, it was chosen to approach the problem through a pixel by pixel analysis in which a band-pass filter was implemented that sets the non-matching pixels' intensity to zero (black) graphically represented in Figure 2. The limits T_1 and T_2 of this filter are defined a priori by the user. The pixel by pixel pre-analysis of the image will provide important hints for the user to choose the most appropriate limits for the band-pass filter. This approach is called threshold segmentation (Weska, 2007).

This technique is very effective in getting segmentation done in volumes with a very good contrast between regions and has a low computational cost. On the other hand, it is a technique very sensitive to noise and intensity inhomogeneities. In order to avoid this last drawback, a stabilization algorithm was used to smooth the contours of the bone tissue regions (Sumengem et al., 2002). This algorithm takes in account the surrounding pixels and the image gradient to minimize the noise levels. There were slices where some major improvements were visible but the computational processing time was significantly higher. The region of interest is clearly identified at this stage, so a line following algorithm was implemented in order to

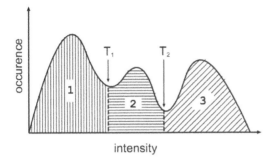

Figure 2.   Threshold segmentation filter.

return the position of each point that defines the contour on every slice. Storing the coordinates of the points that define each contour in a variable made the contour decimation implementation trivial. Allowing the user to define the number of points that will define the contour, it is possible to control the balance between the computational processing time and the level of detail of the structure 3D representation. The parameterization of the contour proved to be a very handy advantage when working with a very large set of images. The reduction of the number of points that define the contour will reduce the computational time of the process in a controlled way since the user will be aware of the detail level being lost in every step of decimation of the contour and vice versa.

2.3   *Three-dimensional representation*

The first step towards a three dimensional representation of the segmented volume was the plot in a Cartesian coordinate system of the points that define the contours of every slice. The distance between each slice of the stack is available in the DICOM file, in a field called *SliceThickness*. According to the position of the slice in the whole set, the third coordinate was added to each vector that previously defines a two-dimensional contour. The output was a set of points in the 3D Cartesian space which is the only necessary premise to the three-dimensional Delaunay Triangulation, shown in Figure 3.

Three-dimensional Delaunay triangulation for a set P of points in the plane is a triangulation dT(P) such that no point in P is inside the circumsphere of any tetrahedron in dT(P). This method maximizes the minimum angle of all the angles between the faces of the tetrahedrons in order to standardize the size of the tetrahedrons. The final output of this process is a three-dimensional representation of the body of the femur for any CT scan of this region.

The following chapter will present the results obtained through the methodology described. Firstly, results after the threshold filter. The contour

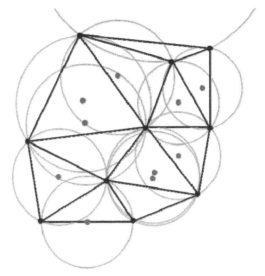

Figure 3.   Schematic representation of the three dimensional Delaunay triangulation.

parameterization and its influence on the three-dimensional representation will also be experimented and shown in chapter 3.

3   RESULTS

Figure 4 represents the two initial steps of the previously described method steps and proves the correct implementation of the band-pass filter limits. Each of the two image sets represented as a line on the figure correspond to a randomly chosen slice of the image set. On the left, we can observe the image as is after importation to the software. In the center, we have the output after the band-pass filter where only the pixels with intensity matching hard bone tissue are represented. The contour acquisition is shown on the right column of the image and, as we may confer, it proves to represent with authenticity the contour shown in the original images. Bone marrow presence is proven by the non-segmented hole in the center of the diaphysis of the femur. This occurs due to the similarity of its x-ray absorbance rate to the surrounding soft tissues. It is interesting to identify this region because it is of extreme importance when preparing a finite element analysis and defining the materials limits and properties.

At this stage, it was only been considered the outer contour of the femur simply because it is only intended to obtain a three-dimensional representation of its morphology. The procedure represented in Figure 4 was carried out for all the slices. The top

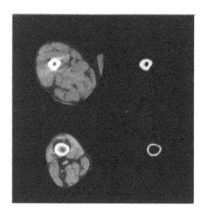

Figure 4. Two examples of CT scan acquired images: on the left the acquired image; on the center, the image after the process of filter segmentation; on the right, the obtained contour.

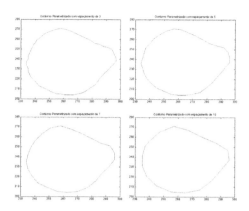

Figure 5. Various examples of the contour parameterizations obtained. From left to right and top to bottom, the numbers of points were reduced by factors of 3, 5, 7 and 10 respectively.

example corresponds to a slice in the medial zone of the diaphysis and therefore there is a predominance of the cortical bone over the trabecular bone. The bottom example is a slice closer to the knee joint and presents a larger section area and the predominance of trabecular bone as expected.

As said before, the bigger the spacing between the points that define the contour, the less detail we will observe in the segmented morphology of the diaphysis. Figure 5 has the representations of the parameterization of a certain contour. The chosen contour was obtained from a slice near the femoral neck. The less circular form of the contour is due to presence of the trochanter, with the protrusion on the right side. From left to right and top to bottom, we may notice the loss of detail level as we increase the number of the spacing between the points that define the contour, i.e., decrease the number of points by a factor of 3, 5, 7 or 10 respectively. However, this fact is inversely proportional to the computational time of the following procedures. It is the users decision whether to obtain a more detailed three-dimensional structure and study its morphology for example or a less detailed structure that will provide quicker results without compromising the quantitative results of the analysis.

The three-dimensional representation of the anatomical structure was achieved using 3D Delaunay triangulation, represented in Figures 6 and 7. In Figure 6, the respective three-dimensional models for the parameterization factors chosen before are shown. From top to bottom and from left to right, there is an increase in the size of the tetrahedrons due to the increase in the spacing between the points in the coordinate system. For the purpose, not all the slices in the image set were taken in

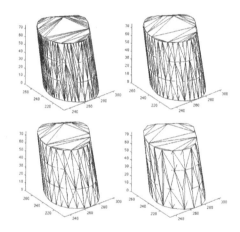

Figure 6. Various examples of the 3D representation of the parametrizations of body of the femur. From left to right and top to bottom, the numbers of points were reduced by factors of 3, 5, 7 and 10 respectively.

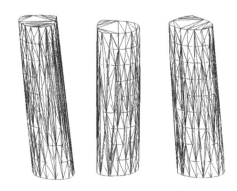

Figure 7. Three different views of the 3D representation of the body of the femur.

account. The correct segmentation of our region of interest on these examples is notorious. The parameterization of the contour shows that it is possible to obtain a less detailed structure resulting on a decrease of the computational time of the process.

A three-dimensional plot of the anatomical structure using the Delaunay triangulation with a larger number of slices is shown in Figure 7. The lines that define each tetrahedron are shown in the representation and some of the morphological characteristics of the body of the femur are identifiable, such as the non-circular section as it approaches the femoral head.

4 CONCLUSIONS AND FUTURE WORK

An automated, patient specific, segmentation approach was developed based in threshold segmentation. With this, it is possible to infer some information about the bone's morphology prior to the surgical intervention. The user inputs the image set acquired from the CT Scan and the threshold filter limits and obtains the contours corresponding to the femur diaphysis as well as a three dimensional representation that may constitute a starting point for the development of a finite element mesh. This approach revealed to be effective and the type of implementation of the contours very advantageous for the three-dimensional model generation. In a near future, this method will be available to totally segment the femur. Some difficulties were detected when segmenting articular areas which require a better formulation of this approach. The developed methodology will open doors to numerical experimentations and finite element analysis, which will hopefully provide a better preparation of the surgery from the physicians.

ACKNOWLEDGEMENTS

This work was supported by Portuguese Foundation for Science and Technology (FCT) through the project: PTDC/SAU-BEB/103408/2008. D. Almeida would, also, like to thank FCT for the scholarship SFRH/BD/71822/2010.

REFERENCES

B. Sumengem, B.S. Manjunath, C. Kenney, "Image Segmentation using Curve Evolution and Region Stability", Proc. IEEE (ICPR) 2002, Québec City, Canada, Aug. 2002.

M. Unter, T. Pock, H. Bischof, "Interactive Globally Optimal Image Segmentation", Institute for Graphics and Vision, Graz University of Technology, Graz, Austria, 2008.

S. Lakare, "3D Segmentation Techniques for Medical Volumes", Center of Visual Computing, New York, 2000.

S. Weszka, "A Survey of Thresholding Techniques. Computer Graphics and Image Processing", 259–265, 1997.

Computational Vision and Medical Image Processing – Tavares & Natal Jorge (eds)
© 2012 Taylor & Francis Group, London, ISBN 978-0-415-68395-1

Pseudo Fuzzy colour calibration for sport video segmentation

Catarina B. Santiago & Armando Sousa
Faculty of Engineering of the University of Porto, Porto, Portugal
Institute for Systems and Computer Engineering of Porto (INESC Porto), Porto, Portugal

Luis Paulo Reis
Faculty of Engineering of the University of Porto, Porto, Portugal
Artificial Intelligence and Computer Science Laboratory (LIACC), FEUP, Porto, Portugal

ABSTRACT: Video segmentation is one of the most important parts of a vision system which allows partitioning each frame into homogeneous regions that share a common property. This work proposes a new methodology that aggregates three different techniques: background subtraction, region growing and a pseudo Fuzzy colour model to define colour subspaces that characterize each class. In addition, the pseudo Fuzzy colour model allows a given colour to belong to more than one class and enables the expansion ofthe classes through a dynamic model based on belonging and persistence information. In case of shared colours among classes, regional features are searched in order to determine the object's class. Tests with test and real videos of sports footages show promising results.

Keywords: Computer Vision, Video Segmentation, Fuzzy Logic, Sports Videos

1 INTRODUCTION

Video and inherently image segmentation is the first step and probably the most critical step in any vision system. In fact, the quality of the final result is highly dependent on a good segmentation.

In this paper we present a methodology that combines colour region growing with a pseudo Fuzzy pixel labelling methodology to subdivide the colour space into colour classes, that may or may not be disjunctive depending on the objects to be segmented.

The methodology followed includes the identification of foreground pixels using background subtraction, the definition of colour classes for each object or groups of objects using a pseudo Fuzzy model, the labelling of foreground pixels into the corresponding object and a continuously update on the colour classes that characterize each object or group of objects. Preliminary results using test and real sport images show that this is a promising technique that may be used for sport video segmentation in order to take into account light variations among frame regions (due to shadows of other objects or non-uniform illumination) and between frames.

The paper structure is as follows. The next section presents some of the most used colour segmentation methodologies, Section 3 describes the algorithm implemented for performing the video segmentation. Section 4 presents the results achieved and finally section 5 concludes this paper presenting and draws some future work directions.

2 RELATED RESEARCH

Video segmentation can be seen of different perspectives, one may want to segment the video into meaningful temporal sequences which is known as temporal segmentation. Temporal segmentation usually corresponds to the first step of video annotation and tries to segment the video taking into account similarities/dissimilarities between successive frames (Koprinska and Carrato 2001).

On the other hand, one may be interested on analysing the content of each frame and extract information concerning the objects that are present in it, or in other words divide each frame content into homogeneous regions that correspond to independent objects and therefore perform a spatial segmentation. Despite the name, spatial segmentation, may be accomplished using temporal characteristics of the video as will be shown latter on this section.

The focus of this work is more on spatial segmentation, therefore for a detailed survey on temporal video segmentation please refer to (Koprinska and Carrato 2001).

Spatial video segmentation may be performed using the methodologies that are used for image segmentation and further enhanced using the temporal characteristics of video. In addition, when performing colour analysis there is also the need to choose a colour space.

Regarding colour image segmentation, a detailed survey is given by (Cheng et al. 2001). As they state, most of the existing colour image segmentation methodologies have their origins on grey scale image segmentation with the addition of a proper colour space choice.

There have been proposed several colour spaces. (Vandenbroucke et al. 2003) provide a taxonomical classification of colour spaces into primary colour spaces (RGB, XYZ) which result from the trichromatic theory, luminance-chrominance spaces (YIQ, YUV, L*a*b*), perceptual spaces (HSI, HSV, LCH) that try to mimic the human perception regarding to colour and independent axis spaces ($I_1I_2I_3$).

Additionally, they propose a new hybrid colour space that chooses the colour components of different colour spaces that best characterize each pixel class.

The main categories of image segmentation methodologies (Cheng et al. 2001) include:

- histogram thresholding by determining the peaks or modes of the multi-dimensional histogram of a colour image
- feature space clustering by grouping the image feature space into a set of meaningful groups or classes based on intensity, colour or texture characteristics of pixels and not on the spatial relation among them
- region based which include region growing, Watershed transform and region split and merge. These methods try to divide the image domain based on the fact that adjacent pixels in a same region have similar visual features (colour, intensity, texture or motion)
- edge detection methods that segment the image by finding the edges of each region using one of the well known edge detectors
- Fuzzy methods allow classes and regions to have a certain uncertainty and ambiguity which is general the case in image processing
- neural networks are very powerful tools that allow parallel processing and the incorporation of non-linearities. They can be used either to pattern recognition, classification or clustering.

Nowadays there is the tendency to aggregate techniques from different categories in order to achieve better results. A typical example of this case is the JSEG algorithm (Deng and Manjunath 2001) that initially clusters colours into several representative classes, afterwards replaces each pixel by their corresponding colour class label and only then a region growing process is applied directly to the class map.

On videos, contrary to static images, besides the two physical components and colour information there is also the time component. Using this property it is possible to segment images based on motion along time. In order to perform this task there are two main approaches, background subtraction and optical flow.

Background subtraction can be used in cases where a more or less fixed background can be assumed and in this case it is possible to subdivide the image into foreground and background. Several background subtraction techniques have been proposed in literature. The main issues on these methods is to obtain a good estimate of the background.

The simplest method to model the background is to use a single static image without objects. However this approach works rather poorly, because it does not take into account changes that may occur in the background (for example light effects). More robust methods include estimating the background model using a moving average (Heikkila and Silvén 1999), median or even a mixture of Gaussians (Grimson et al. 1998). Having the foreground regions detected it may still be necessary to perform their labelling orcategorization.

Optical flow (Barron and Thacker 2005) is based on the fact that when an object moves in front of a camera, there is a corresponding change in the image, however it assumes small displacements during time.

In this paper we propose a methodology that combines the ideas behind three of the described segmentation methods: background subtraction for detecting foreground regions, region growing and pseudo Fuzzy categorization for colour calibration.

3 PROPOSED VIDEO SEGMENTATION METHODOLOGY

The first step for the video segmentation to take place consists on a supervised calibration of the colours of each class which is achieved using a region growing method. The initial colour seeds for each class are set manually using the mouse to click on the objects that will be segmented, afterwards the surrounded pixels are agglomerate around these seeds using colour distance criteria. The colour expansion is performed on the HSL (Hue, Saturation and Luminance) colour space in order to minimize the effects of shadows and light variations.

The regions growth is performed in all directions in a recursive way until reaching a pixel that has a colour too far away from the seed or from the previous neighbour. During the colour expansion each pixel is attributed a given belonging degree to the class being calibrated (the number of classes is defined by the user). This degree is stored in a lookup table that contains for each colour triplet the belonging degree to each class. By using the lookup table it is possible to have a fast access to this information latter on the segmentation process.

The belonging degree can have four levels: no belong (by default and before the calibration takes place, all the colours are categorized with no belong degree to every class), low belong degree, full belong and additionally a full belong degree with the characteristic of also being a colour seed. The following heuristics (applied sequentially) are used to attribute the belonging degree to each colour during the region growing process:

- if the pixel was assigned to the class and physically is quite close to the initial seed pixel then it is also assumed to be a seed pixel with a full belonging degree
- if the Euclidean colour distance to the initial seed pixel is less than two thirds the maximum allowed distance for the growing then the pixel is categorized with a full belonging degree but without being a seed
- otherwise the pixel is categorized as belonging to the class with a low belong degree

By the end of the calibration process the colour space is subdivided into classes, which are not necessary disjoint since the same colour can belong to different classes with a given belonging degree.

The motivation behind having non-disjoint classes is related with the fact that objects may have different colours and also different objects may share a common colour, for example in the case of sport videos it is common that team have uniforms with white stripes.

Once the object classes have been calibrated, the image segmentation can take place. The first step consists on eliminating background regions. Since the background is more or less static on the images we want to deal with, the subtraction is performed using a blank image of the viewed scene and a dynamic threshold that is updated for each pixel in each frame. Only the pixels that are classified as background see their respective threshold updated, the pixels classified as foreground remain with the associated threshold unchanged. The update obeys to equation 1 and its value is never allowed to be below 4% of

the entire colour range (0–255). This value was obtained experimentally.

$$\sigma_{t+1}^c(\mathbf{x}, \mathbf{y}) = \begin{cases} \alpha(I_t^c(\mathbf{x}, \mathbf{y}) - B^c(\mathbf{x}, \mathbf{y})) + (1-\alpha)\sigma_t^c(\mathbf{x}, \mathbf{y}) \\ \qquad\qquad \text{if } I_t(\mathbf{x}, \mathbf{y}) \in B(\mathbf{x}, \mathbf{y}) \\ \sigma_t^c(\mathbf{x}, \mathbf{y}), \qquad \text{otherwise} \end{cases} \quad (1)$$

Where

- σ is the threshold of the pixel at position (x,y), time $t+1$ and colour component c,
- I is the colour intensity of the pixel at position (x,y), time $t+1$ and colour component c,
- B is the background colour intensity of the pixel at position (x,y), time $t+1$ and colour component c,
- α is a learning constant, that for our specific case was set to 0.02.

Pixels whose colour difference to the background image is less than the respective threshold are labelled as background, the others are labelled as foreground.

After the foreground pixels are identified, their colour is compared against the colour lookup table that resulted from the calibration process and classified into one of the classes. Since the same colour can belong to different classes it may occur that a pixel is classified into more than one class. To break this tie, information from adjacent pixels that have already been classified is used. The number of adjacent pixels that belong to each class are counted and those classes that have a count higher than one and a half times the minimum count are assigned two extra points in the belonging degree. This way, it is possible that, although the belonging degree of a pixel to a class based on the colour calibration information is lower than the belonging degree to another class it may be the winner due to the neighbourhood characteristics.

Additionally, if the winning class has a full belong to that colour triplet and corresponds to a seed colour then a region growing process is triggered and the colour lookup table that contains the information concerning the classes colours is updated. This auto expansion is more restrictive than the one performed during the manual initialization and is not performed at every frame, otherwise the processing would be too time consuming.

In order for this update to add not only colour triples to the classes but also to remove them (otherwise classes would grow too much), each colour triplet has associated a persistence to that class. Colours with lower belonging have lower persistence and colours with higher belonging have higher persistence. The initial persistence given to the colour is proportional to the time between auto expansions. This proportion factor is 1/8 for low belong colours and 1/4 for full belong colours.

The persistence is maximum when the colour is added to the class and diminishes whenever it is not "seen" in a frame, however seed colour have infinite persistence and will therefore always remain in the class. Whenever the persistence value reaches zero the colour triplet is removed from the class.

With the introduction of this dynamic it is possible to have mutable classes that adapt to light changes either occurring at different regions of the same frame or between frames.

At the same time the foreground pixels are classified, they are also aggregated horizontally to form run length encoding (RLE) structures that contain a label indicating the class they belong to, the y, x_{min} and x_{max} positions. Small RLEs are ignored in order to minimize noise. Finally the RLEs are merged vertically to form blobs. A full description of this pixel aggregation can be found in (Santiago et al. 2011).

4 RESULTS

In order to validate the proposed methodology a test video was made that consists on two colour squares with stripes as illustrated on Figure 1(a).

A few mouse clicks on the image resulted on the colour calibration of Figures 1(c) and 1(d), the different tones indicate different belonging degrees, also it is possible to verify (as expected) that the two colour classes superimpose on the green region of the global colour space.

On the final segmented image (Fig. 1(b)) the background is darkened and the pixels belonging to each object are identified by the respective colour class label. It is also possible to verify that

although the green colour is common to both objects the pixels are correctly labelled (due to the characteristics of the adjacent pixels).

In order to validate the continuously and automatic update of the colour classes, tests using a video of a sport match were performed. For the tests presented here the auto expansion process occurs at every 60th frame. It is important to highlight that videos with a more dynamic behaviour (which is the case of sport videos) require an update frequency higher than videos that are not so dynamic.

Initially the colour classes were calibrated using the mouse to click on the players which resulted on the colour classes of Figure 2(a) and the respective processed image of Figure 2(b).

After 900 frames (which correspond to 15 auto expansions) it is possible to verify that the colour classes have grown around the initial seeds (represented by the darker colours) which resulted on the updated colour classes of Figure 3(a). During this time players from both teams stayed on the area under analysis.

Afterwards, the players permanence on the area decreased during 2050 frames (34 auto expansions) which caused the colour classes to retract a little (Fig. 3(b)).

Table 1 provides an overview of the changes between these three cases. From the initial set 2(a)

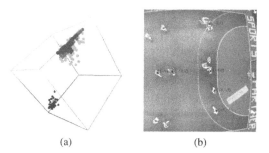

(a)   (b)

Figure 2.   Initial colour calibration. (a) colour classes being segmented and (b) segmented image.

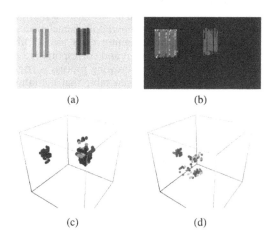

(a)   (b)

(c)   (d)

Figure 1.   (a) Frame from the test video, (b) segmented frame, (c, d) colour classes resulting from the initial calibration for the left and right objects (different colour tones indicate different belonging degrees).

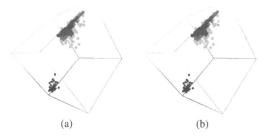

(a)   (b)

Figure 3.   Results of the colour auto expansion process. (a) Colours classes after 15 auto expansions. (b) Colour classes after more 34 auto expansions.

Table 1. Number of colour triples that belong to each class and the respective belonging degree for the initial set 2(a), set of Fig 3(a) and set of Fig 3(b).

Class	Belong	Init set	Fig 3(a)	Fig 3(b)
Green	Low	1	0	0
	Full	0	8	0
	Full + seed	33	34	34
Red	Low	43	27	26
	Full	16	18	16
	Full + seed	27	43	44

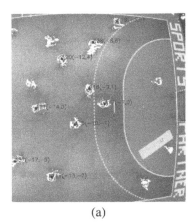

(a)

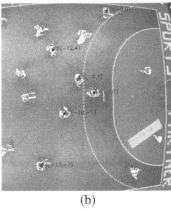

(b)

Figure 4. Result of the segmentation: (a) with colour auto expansion and (b) without colour auto expansion.

to Fig 3(a) set the number of colour triplets that fully belong to the two classes increases and the pixels that have a low belong degree decrease because the auto expansion process is more restrictive than the initial manual calibration.

Regarding the evolution to the colour classes of Fig 3(b), the number of triplets that belong to the red class decrease less (compared to the time of Fig 3(a)) then the ones of the green class because the players of the first class are the last to leave the area and the first to enter it again, since they are the defending team.

Comparing the results with and without the pseudo Fuzzy model of colour expansion it is possible to verify that the segmentation has better performance with the mutable colour classes as depicted on Fig 4. Fig 4(a) has more players from the green class detected and the players of the red class have more area detected.

5 CONCLUSIONS

In this paper we presented a methodology for segmenting sport video images. The main objectives were to develop a methodology that allowed not only the update of the background/foreground models but also of the object colour subspaces by continuously and automatically updating the colour classes in order to take into account different light conditions. The usage of a Pseudo Fuzzy technique allowed this update (increase or decrease the number of triplets to the classes) by taking into account the belonging degree of each colour triplet to the respective class. In addition, the Pseudo Fuzzy model enabled the same colour triplet to belong to different classes. The tie break was achieved by evaluating the characteristics of the adjacent pixels.

The proposed methodology was validated using a test video but also a real video from a sport match. Results are quite promising, but more tests with real videos must be performed not only with different teams but also with teams that share a common colour in their equipments. It would also be interesting to test this approach in videos where the objects to be segmented have higher areas, since the players are quite small in the video used.

ACKNOWLEDGMENTS

We would like to thank Fundacao Calouste Gulbenkian by the support given trough a PhD scholarship with ref. 104410.

REFERENCES

Barron, J. and N. Thacker (2005). Tutorial: Computing 2D and 3D optical flow. *Tina Memo Internal* (2004–12).

Cheng, H., X. Jiang, Y. Sun, and J. Wang (2001). Color image segmentation: advances and prospects. *Pattern recognition* 34(12), 2259–2281.

Deng, Y. and B. Manjunath (2001). Unsupervised segmentation of color-texture regions in images and video. *IEEE Transactions on Pattern Analysis and Machine Intelligence 23*(8), 800–810.

Grimson, W., C. Stauffer, R. Romano, and L. Lee (1998). Using adaptive tracking to classify and monitor activities in a site. In *Computer Vision and Pattern Recognition, 1998. Proceedings. 1998 IEEE Computer Society Conference on*, pp. 22–29. IEEE.

Heikkila, J. and O. Silvén (1999). A real-time system for monitoring of cyclists and pedestrians. In *Visual Surveillance, 1999. Second IEEE Workshop on,(VS'99)*, pp. 74–81. IEEE.

Koprinska, I. and S. Carrato (2001). Temporal video segmentation: A survey. *Signal processing: Image communication 16*(5), 477–500.

Santiago, C., A. Sousa, L. Reis, and M. Estriga (2011). Real Time Colour Based Player Tracking in Indoor Sports. *Computational Vision and Medical Image Processing*, 17–35.

Vandenbroucke, N., L. Macaire, and J. Postaire (2003). Color image segmentation by pixel classification in an adapted hybrid color space. Application to soccer image analysis. *Computer Vision and Image Understanding 90*(2), 190–216.

Computational Vision and Medical Image Processing – Tavares & Natal Jorge (eds)
© 2012 Taylor & Francis Group, London, ISBN 978-0-415-68395-1

Combining hierarchical watershed metrics and Normalized Cut for image segmentation

Tiago Willian Pinto & Marco Antonio Garcia de Carvalho
School of Technology—FT, University of Campinas—UNICAMP, Limeira—SP, Brazil

ABSTRACT: Combining partitioning techniques became a promising approach in order to implement image segmentation and has produced good results on different applications. Some works has studied the graph spectrum as a partitioning tool, by means of the so-called Normalized Cut method (NCut) as a final partitioning process for images modeled by different types of graphs. This work explores the Watershed Transform as a modeling tool, using different criteria of the hierarchical Watershed (Area, Volume and Dynamics), in order to convert an image into a graph, followed by the use of the NCut to perform the final segmentation. The main goal is to compare the image segmentation results obtained from graphs modeled by Watershed Transform with others relevant results, using images from Berkeley Database.

Keywords: image segmentation, watershed transform, graph partitioning, Normalized Cut

1 INTRODUCTION

The complexity of Image Segmentation makes it still in constant research for performance improvement and results enhancement, since there is not exists a general solution for every computational application. Some early publications made combinations of segmentation techniques to achieve better results and these hybrid approaches has brought promising results, i.e. (Monteiro & Campilho 2008), (Carvalho & Ferreira & Costa & Cesar Jr 2010). This paper will combine the Watershed Transform, a classic method used for image segmentation purposes, and the Normalized Cut (NCut), an early technique that explores linear algebra concepts and graph theory to segment an image into meaningful regions and take its semantic information, i.e. (Shi & Malik 2000). The Watershed Transform has the inconvenience of over-segmentation problems and NCut is known as a NP-hard complexity algorithm, but these weakness are treated naturally with the combination of both. The same process was done in (Monteiro & Campilho 2008) and (Bock & Smet & Philips 2005), but our approach will use different criteria of watershed and neighborhood structure for graph definition, in order to compare the results obtained with the original formula of NCut and another results in the benchmark found in (Ferreira, 2010). The next sections are organized as follows: In section 2 we give a general review of graph concepts that will be used in this work. Section 3 shows a review of the Watershed Transform and the criteria used for the graph modeling and section 4 shows the NCut theory basis.

Experiments and partial results are showed in section 5 and finally in section 6 the conclusions and perspectives for future works are exploited.

2 GRAPH REPRESENTATION

Assuming $G = (V, E)$ as an undirected graph where V is the set of nodes and E is the set of edges (i, j). Two nodes i, j are adjacent, represented by $i \sim j$, if there exist an edge linking i and j, and the weight associated to each edge (i, j) is represented by $w(i, j)$. The mathematical representation for this graph is given as follows:

- *Similarity matrix*: A similarity matrix A is a representation for a undirected weighted graph where each entry value $a(i, j)$ is an edge weight $w(i, j)$ linking a pair of nodes. The weights are given by a function that maximize the similarity between nodes i and j.
- *Weighted degree matrix*: Let $d(i) = \Sigma w(i, j)$ be the total connection from node i to all its neighbor nodes. Then the weighted degree matrix D is the diagonal matrix with d on its diagonal.
- *Laplacian matrix*: The laplacian matrix of a graph G is computed from $L(G) = (D - A)$, where D is the weighted degree matrix and A is the similarity matrix.

3 WATERSHED TRANSFORM

We consider the gradient image I as a topographic surface. In the watershed method, an image is segmented by constructing the catchment basins of its gradient image. The gradient image is flooded starting from selected sources (regional minima) until the whole image has been flooded. A dam is erected between lakes that meet with others lakes. At the end of flooding process, we obtain one region for each catchment basin of the gradient image.

Hierarchical watershed creates a set of nested partitions. A partition P of an image f is a set of disjoint regions R_i, $i = 1, 2, ..., n$, where the union of regions is the whole image. Let (P_k) be a sequence of partitions $P_1, P_2, ..., P_n$, of an image f. (P_k) is a hierarchy, also called *nested sequence of partitions*, if a partition at a fine level is obtained by merging regions of the coarse partition. Some criteria exploited in this paper are:

- Volume and Area: Geometric operators given for each region;
- Dynamics: Relationship between regional minima altitude, (Meyer 1996).

The watershed problem can be modeled using graphs. The gradient image is represented by a weighted neighborhood graph, where a node represents a catchment basin (region) of the topographic surface and two nodes are linked by an edge when its regions are neighbours. The use of Hierarchical Watershed can reduce the number of nodes (oversegmentation problem) in the correspondent graph enhancing the segmentation process performance.

4 NORMALIZED CUT

The Normalized Cut (Ncut) approach uses the algebraic properties of the laplacian matrix to separate the nodes according to the dissimilarity between them. In graph theoretic language, it is called cut and defined by:

$$Cut(S_1, S_2) = \sum w(u,v), u \in S_1, v \in S_2 \quad (1)$$

where S_1 and S_2 are two disjoint sets in a graph. Instead of using the total edge weight connection, this method computes the cut cost as a fraction of the total edge connections to all nodes in the graph:

$$NCut(S_1, S_2) = \frac{Cut(S_1, S_2)}{SumCon(S_1, V)} + \frac{Cut(S_1, S_2)}{SumCon(S_2, V)}$$

$$(2)$$

where $SumCon(S,V)$ is the total connection from nodes in the set S with all nodes in V. Expanding this equation the following equation can be found:

$$min_x NCut(x) = min_y \frac{y^T(D-A)y}{y^T Dy} \quad (3)$$

This equation, called *Rayleigh quotient*, has a property that it can be minimized by the smallest eigenvector x_0 of the Rayleigh quotients matrix (in this case, the Laplacian matrix) and its minimum value is the corresponding eigenvalue λ_0. So, the Normalized cut can be minimized solving a generalized eigenvalue system as shown below.

$$(D-A)y = \lambda Dy \quad (4)$$

Because of the first Laplacian's matrix smallest eigenvalue is 0, the second smallest eigenvalue is the real valued solution to the normalized cut problem. The corresponding eigenvector can tell exactly how to partition the graph only by separating the nodes represented by the positive values in the eigenvector from the negative ones for instance.

5 EXPERIMENTS

We obtained some partial results in our experiments using images for general purpuses from the Berkeley Database, in Figure 1 we show the original images; in Figure 2 is shown the segmentation using the original NCut method. The main goal

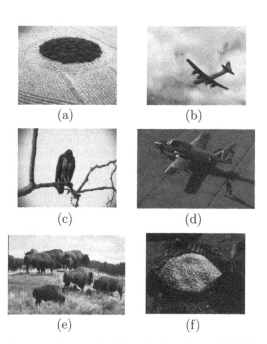

(a)

(b)

(c)

(d)

(e)

(f)

Figure 1. Images from Berkeley Database: (a) 86016; (b) 3096; (c) 42049; (d) 37073; (e) 38092; (f) 58060.

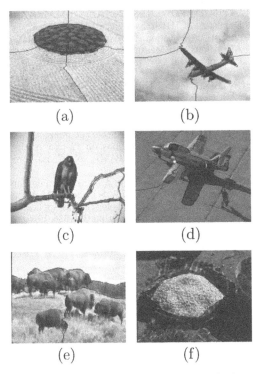

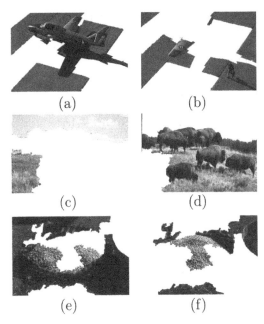

Figure 2. Segmentation using the NCut method proposed in Shi & Malik (2000). Images: (a) 86016; (b) 3096; (c) 42049; (d) 37073; (e) 38092; (f) 58060.

Figure 4. Segmentation using proposed method. Hierarchical Watershed with 15 regions and similarity graph modeled using region area as metric. Images: (a, b) 37073; (c, d) 38092; (e, f) 58060.

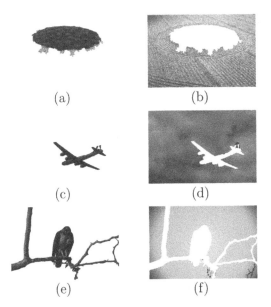

Figure 3. Segmentation using proposed method. Hierarchical Watershed with 5 regions and similarity graph modeled using region average grayscale as metric. Images: (a, b) 86016; (c, d) 3096; (e, f) 42049.

was to analyse the proposed method and compare the parameters used in the modeled graphs. Firstly, we modeled the images into graphs using hierarchical watershed, reducing the image into 5 regions and building a fully conected graph. The metric used to calculate the similarity matrix were the average grayscale between every pair of nodes. These results are given in Figure 3. Other experiments were done using the region's area as edge weight in the similarity matrix. The same process was done, but now using 15 regions in the hierarchical watershed, the results are in Figure 4.

The next step is to consider the other metrics proposed (volume and dynamics) to model the weighted graph generated by the watershed transform and compare the final results.

CONCLUSIONS AND FUTURE WORKS

In this paper our main goal is to propose a combination of segmentation methods with high relevance in the related literature, in order to generate and compare some segmentations results for images of general purposes from berkeley segmentation dataset. Our perspectives are that this method can achieve good results with reduced computation time (compared with the original techniques) and then use that for images of specific applications in future works. Also, we wish to evaluate the quality of results obtained, and compare them, through the implementation of a benchmark.

REFERENCES

BOCK, J. De.; SMET, P.D.; PHILIPS, W. Image segmentation using watersheds and normalized cuts. In: Proc. of the IS&T/SPIE Electronic Imaging, volume 5675, pp. 164–173, 2005.

CARVALHO, M.A.G.; FERREIRA, A.C.B.; COSTA, A.L.; CESAR-JR, R.M. Image segmentation using component tree and normalized cuts. In: Proc. of 23th Brazilian Symposium on computer graphics and image processing—SIBGRAPI, pp. 317–320, 2010.

FERREIRA, A.C.B. Um estudo comparativo de segmentacao de imagens por aplicacoes do Corte Normalizado em Grafos. 2010. 94 p. Dissertacao (Mestrado em Tecnologia e Inovacao)—Faculdade de Tecnologia, Universidade Estadual de Campinas, Limeira, 2010.

MARTIN, D.; FOWLKES, C.; TAL, D.; MALIK, J.A. Database of Human Segmented Natural Images and its Application to Evaluating Segmentation Algorithms and Measuring Ecological Statistics. In: Proc. of 8th Int'l Conf. Computer Vision, vol. 2, pp. 416–423, 2001.

MONTEIRO, F.C.; CAMPILHO, A. Watershed framework to region-based image segmentation. In: Proc. Of IEEE 19th International Conference on Pattern Recognition- ICPR, pp. 1–4, 2008.

SHI, J.; MALIK, J. Normalized cuts and image segmentation. In: IEEE Transactions on Pattern Analysis and Machine Intelligence PAMI, vol. 22, no. 8, pp. 888–905, 2000.

MEYER, F.; MARAGOS, P. The dynamics of minima and contours. In: P. Maragos, R.W. Schafer and M.A. Butt Editors, Mathematical Morphology and its Applications to Image and Signal Processing, pp. 329–336, 1996.

Computational Vision and Medical Image Processing – Tavares & Natal Jorge (eds)
© 2012 Taylor & Francis Group, London, ISBN 978-0-415-68395-1

A comparison between segmentation algorithms for urinary bladder on T2-weighted MR images

Zhen Ma, Renato Natal Jorge & João Manuel R.S. Tavares
Faculty of Engineering, University of Porto, Porto, Portugal

ABSTRACT: The urinary bladder on T2-weighted MR images has a high signal intensity appearance, which can be clearly identified from the neighboring structures. However, due to the complex imaging background, the appearance of the bladder is frequently influenced by noise and partial volume effect. Different algorithms have been proposed to segment the bladder. Nevertheless, these algorithms are at their beginning phases, and considerable improvements are needed to obtain an effective automatic segmentation algorithm. In this paper, the performances of four algorithms are evaluated using a case study, from which the effectiveness and the differences between the algorithms are discussed. Quantitative analysis of the segmentation results are presented to measure the deviations of the segmentation results and reflect the aspects that need to be improved.

1 INTRODUCTION

Magnetic resonance imaging (MRI) can provide a clear visualization of the urinary bladder (Cheng & Tempany 1998). However, the acquired image series are projections on two dimensional planes; therefore, the shape and geometry information of the bladder are not continuous. In order to study bladder-related conditions, critical indexes such as bladder wall thickness and bladder volume are needed. Accordingly, an accurate segmentation of the bladder on MR images is demanded.

T2-weighted MR images were chosen for this study because the bladder lumen has a high signal intensity appearance on these images and can be easily identified from the low-signal-intensity bladder wall and its neighboring structures. However, due to the influence of noise and partial volume effect, the intensity distribution of the bladder lumen is usually inhomogeneous. Various imaging clues have been adopted in different algorithms to segment this delicate organ. For example, the approach proposed in (Ma et al. 2011a) can achieve good performances using geometric deformable models with region-based external forces. Nevertheless, the current algorithms are in their incipient phases, and considerable works are needed to improve the aspects such as the reliability and automation of the algorithms. A comparison and discussion on the performances of these algorithms then become meaningful.

The algorithms to be evaluated in this study include a thresholding region growing algorithm, a C-means algorithm and two recent approaches proposed in (Ma et al. 2011a, Ma et al. 2011b). The four algorithms were selected because of their effectiveness to segment the bladder on T2-weighted MR images.

This paper is organized as follows: in Section 2, the segmentation algorithms are reviewed; then, in Section 3, the performances of the algorithms are evaluated and discussed; finally, in Section 4, the paper is concluded and the future works are indicated.

2 SEGMENTATION ALGORITHMS

2.1 *Region growing algorithm*

Region growing algorithms belong to the threshold-based algorithms (Ma et al. 2010), in which the threshold values play an important role for segmentation. The thresholds in the region growing algorithms can be defined empirically or by initial seeds; the latter way of definition was chosen in the first region growing algorithm proposed in (Adams & Bischof 1994). Given the complex imaging background on T2-weighted MR images and the intensity distributions of the bladder lumen, we adopted the rule to group the pixels with similar intensities into one class using pre-defined intensity thresholds. Hence, after the selection of the initial seeds, the region starts to merge the neighboring pixels of which the intensities are within the range defined by the thresholds. The merging stops when all the neighboring pixels at the front of the region have intensities that are outside the normal range. Therefore, all the pixels inside the segmented region have intensities within the range $[I_{min}, I_{max}]$, where I_{min} and I_{max} are two pre-defined thresholds. The initial seeds of this algorithm are required to be inside the bladder lumen.

A prior knowledge of the intensity distribution of the bladder lumen is needed to define the thresholds. Because of the large contrast between the appearances of the bladder lumen and the bladder wall, the selection of thresholds is not difficult, and the algorithm works well when the images are not severely affected by noise. Besides, this algorithm has high computational efficiency because of the simple merging criterion. However, if the influence of noise is considerable or the appearance of the bladder lumen is appreciably blurred by the partial volume effect, the segmentation result may contain unwanted inner boundaries or leak to the perivesical fat. Figures 1(a) and 1(b) illustrate two results obtained by using this algorithm, from which one can verify that its performance is sensitive to the threshold values.

2.2 C-means algorithm

C-means algorithm is an unsupervised classification technique, where C stands for the number of classes. The algorithm aims to minimize the intensity variation of each class. A pixel is assigned to the class of which the mean intensity has the minimal difference to the intensity of the pixel; then, the mean intensity of the class is updated and the pixels are re-assigned. The iteration stops when all the labels of the pixels remain unchanged. The initial assignments of the pixels affect the iteration times. To implement this algorithm, one only needs to define the value of C. A small value of C may cause over-segmentation, while a large one may cause many inner boundaries.

Nevertheless, in T2-weighted MR images, different structures may have similar appearances. The inhomogeneous intensity distribution can cause holes inside the segmented region. In order to eliminate the unwanted inner boundaries and make the algorithm more robust, spatial relationship between the pixels can be incorporated in the segmentation process. Hence, the Markov Random Field (MRF) (Kindermann & Snell 1980) was applied to smooth and post-process the results of the C-means algorithm. Figures 1(c) and 1(d) illustrate the segmentation result of the C-means algorithm and the result after being smoothed by using the MRF, respectively. One can see that the C-means algorithm result was considerably improved after incorporating the influences from the neighboring pixels by the MRF.

2.3 Coupling approach

The algorithm proposed in (Ma et al. 2011a) is a coupling system composed of three geometric

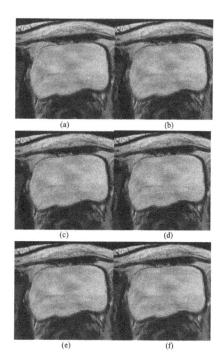

Figure 1. The segmentation results (white contours) of the four algorithms under comparison: (a) Leakage with the parameters $I_{min} = 130$ and $I_{max} = 255$ using thresholding region growing algorithm; (b) with parameter $I_{min} = 131$ and $I_{max} = 255$, overlapped with the ground truth (black contour); (c) the segmented boundary using C-means algorithm by classifying the image pixels as 4 clusters; (d) the segmented boundary using C-means algorithm after smoothed by the Markov random field and overlapped with the ground truth (red line); (e) the segmentation result of the coupling approach overlapped with the ground truth; (f) the segmentation result of the modified geodesic active contour overlapped with the ground truth.

deformable models. Segmentation of the bladder is based on the appearance comparisons with another two pelvic organs: the vagina and the rectum. The three models interact with each other through the intensity statistics of organs, and can segment the three organs simultaneously. The moving equation for the bladder was proposed as:

$$\frac{\partial \phi_1}{\partial t} = \delta(\phi_1) \left(\begin{array}{c} p_1 \left(e_1 - \max(e_2, e_3, e_1 - 1) \right) + \\ \alpha \nabla p_1 \cdot \nabla \phi_1 + \gamma_1 \mathrm{div} \left(\frac{\nabla \phi_1}{|\nabla \phi_1|} \right) \end{array} \right), \quad (1)$$

where $\phi_1 (X, t)$ is the level set function with X the coordinates and t the time; δ is the Dirac function; $e_i = \log (p_i)$, with the probability p_1 of a pixel belonging to the bladder, p_2 to the vagina, and p_3 to the rectum; γ is a parameter and controls the influence of curvature that can smooth the moving contours. The initial level set function $\phi_1(X,0)$ is normally defined as the signed distance function to the initial contours.

In this approach, the intensity statistics of the vagina and rectum are involved in the segmentation of the bladder. The contour movement is based on the comparisons between the logarithms of the probabilities of a pixel to the three pelvic organs. On T2-weighted MR images, the bladder wall has a similar appearance as the muscular layers of the vagina and rectum. Therefore, when the contour arrives at the bladder wall, it will stop moving forward according to the speed function defined in Eq. (1).

To exclude the influence from neighboring pelvic structures, the initial contours are required to be inside the bladder lumen. Based on the appearance comparison, the algorithm is not sensitive to noise and partial volume effect. The coupling approach requires the simultaneous presences of the three pelvic organs. However, when the vagina or the rectum does not appear on the image, the intensity statistics of the two organs can be set to the values obtained from other images. Although this algorithm was proposed for axial T2-wegihted images, it can be applied to segment the bladder on sagittal and coronal MR images given the fix of the intensity statistics of the vagina and rectum.

2.4 *Modified geodesic active model*

The approach proposed in (Ma et al. 2011b) contains two algorithms: one is a modified geodesic active contour to segment the inner boundary of the bladder wall; and the other is a shape guided model to segment the outer boundary of the bladder. The idea is to change the geodesic active contour (Caselles et al. 1997) from gradient-based to region-based, so as to handle the influence of noise and intensity variations. The moving equation was proposed as:

$$\frac{\partial \phi}{\partial t} = p(I)(1+\kappa)|\nabla \phi| + \lambda \nabla p(I) \cdot \nabla \phi, \qquad (2)$$

where ϕ is the level set function; λ is the weight; κ is the curvature; I is the intensity; p is a Gaussian distribution function defined as:
$p(I) = 1/\sqrt{2\pi}\sigma^* \exp(-(I-\mu)^2/2\sigma^{*2})$, in which the mean intensity μ and the variance σ^* are calculated as:

$$\mu = \frac{\int_\Omega H(\phi(x,y))I(x,y)dxdy}{\int_\Omega H(\phi(x,y))dxdy}, \quad \sigma^* = \max(\sigma,\sigma_0)$$

$$\text{with} \quad \sigma = \sqrt{\frac{\int_\Omega H(\phi(x,y))(I(x,y)-\mu)^2 dxdy}{\int_\Omega H(\phi(x,y))dxdy}},$$

$$\qquad (3)$$

where H is the Heaviside function and σ_0 is a predefined parameter.

The initial contours are required to be inside the bladder lumen. Unlike the original geodesic active contour, the external force of this algorithm is the expanding speed multiplied by the probability density. When the contour moves to the boundary of the bladder, where the intensity is beyond the normal range, it will slow down and attaches to the bladder wall. The modified calculation of intensity variance extends the range of intensity variation, which makes the algorithms flexible. Like the approach in Section 2.3, this algorithm can be used to segment the bladder on sagittal and coronal MR images.

3 SEGMENTATION & EVALUATION

A case study was used to evaluate the performances of the four segmentation algorithms. The image data were acquired from a 26-year-old woman under a field strength of 1.5T (TE: 103 ms, TR: 5440 ms, bandwidth: 130 Hz/pixel, FOV: 220×220 mm^2, acquisition matrix: 272×320 and flip angle: 150°). The spatial resolution of the image series is equal to $0.69 \times 0.69 \times 5.40$ mm^3. It contains 30 sagittal images, 26 axial images, and 25 coronal images; among them, the bladder can be clearly identified on 17 axial images, 23 sagittal images, and 7 coronal images.

3.1 *Segmentation*

For the thresholding region growing algorithm, the implementation is simple and the computation is efficient. The only requirement is to avoid defining the seeds as the pixels that have intensities beyond the normal range; then, the selections of the initial seeds have no influence to the final result. Given that the bladder wall has a large contrast appearance to the bladder lumen, the thresholding region growing algorithm can achieve good performance on most of the images, as illustrated in Figure 1(a). However, the threshold I_{min} needs to be adjusted frequently in order to obtain satisfied results. Additionally, when the appearance of the bladder wall is blurred, or the bladder lumen has large intensity variation, the boundary of the bladder cannot be correctly segmented by using this algorithm; an example is shown in Figure 2(a).

For the C-means algorithm, the number of pixel classes was chosen as 4, so that the bladder lumen can be identified from the bladder wall, and the segmented region contains few inner boundaries. As can be seen from Figure 1, the incorporation of neighborhood information can eliminate the inner boundaries caused by the inhomogeneous intensities of the bladder lumen. The accuracy and robustness of the C-means algorithm are considerably improved. However, when the area of the inhomogeneous region is large, using the MRF the inner boundary cannot be removed without over-segmentation. A case in point can be seen in Figure 2(b).

Due to the coupling of the three deformable models, the coupling approach in Section 2.3 requires longer computation time than the other three algorithms. When the vagina and the rectum cannot be clearly identified, the mean intensities of the vagina were fixed as 40.93 and 37.86, and the variances as 13.23 and 14.22, respectively, which were obtained from an axial image that was correctly segmented by the algorithm. Also, the intensity statistics of the two pelvic organs were set as those values when segmenting the sagittal and axial images. Although on some images those statistical values were not accurate, the segmentation results were not much influenced, due to the differences between the appearances of the pelvic organs. This strategy worked fine for the tested image series, as confirmed by the later quantitative analysis; however, the performance of this approach on some images was not as good as the modified geodesic active contour, especially when the bladder wall was blurred by the partial volume effect. The Gaussian functions were used as the intensity distribution functions of the pelvic organs, with the means and variances of the image intensity calculated as in Eq. (3). The region-based external forces make the algorithm less sensitive to the influence of noise and partial volume effect;

hence, one can see the boundary of the bladder was segmented successfully in Figure 2(c). An example of segmentation on sagittal images is shown in Figure 3(c).

The modified geodesic active contour proposed in Section 2.4 achieved satisfied results on the tested images. The modified calculation of the intensity variance makes the algorithm more flexible. Similar to the coupling approach, the region-based external force makes the algorithm less sensitive to noise. Besides, this algorithm does not rely on the information of other pelvic organs; and its computational time was less than the coupling approach, but higher than the first two algorithms. The overall performance of this algorithm was the best and most accurate among the four algorithms, as was verified in the later quantitative analysis.

3.2 Evaluation

If the influence of noise was moderate on the image, satisfied results could be obtained by the four algorithms; the obtained boundaries had little deviations from the ground truths. However, when the images suffered considerably influence of noise and partial volume effect, the approach proposed in (Ma et al. 2011a, Ma et al. 2011b) had much better performances; a case in point can be seen in Figure 2.

To evaluate the results of the four algorithms, the images were manually segmented by experienced technicians. The manual segmentations were regarded as the ground truths. The following

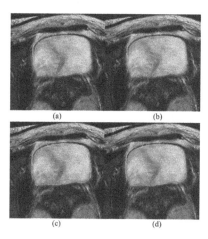

Figure 2. The segmentation results (white contours) of the four algorithms on an image with large intensity variance in the center region of the bladder lumen (mean intensity of the bladder region: 168.4; intensity variance: 19.5): (a) thresholding region growing algorithm; (b) C-means algorithm with MRF; (c) the coupling approach; (d) the modified geodesic active contour.

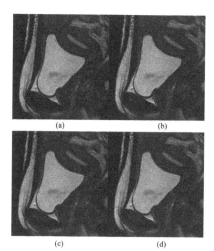

Figure 3. The segmentation results (white contours) of the four algorithms on a sagittal image overlapped with the ground truth (black contour): (a) thresholding region growing algorithm; (b) C-means algorithm with MRF; (c) the coupling approach; (d) the modified geodesic active contour.

indices were adopted to measure the deviations of the segmentation results:

$$PD(C_0, C_1) = \underset{p_1 \in C_0}{\text{Mean}} \left(\min_{p_1 \in C_1} d(p, p_1) \right),$$

$$CR(C_0, C_1) = \frac{\text{Area}\left(inside(C_0) \cap inside(C_1)\right)}{\text{Area}\left(inside(C_0) \cup inside(C_1)\right)},$$

$$AD = \frac{\left| \text{Area}\left(inside(C_0)\right) - \text{Area}\left(inside(C_1)\right) \right|}{\text{Area}\left(inside(C_0)\right)},$$

(4)

where C_0 is the ground truth and C_1 is the boundary segmented by algorithm.

The first index assesses the differences between C_0 and C_1 based on the mean distance of the points on C_0 to the points on C_1; it measures the average point-to-point matching between the two contours and indicates whether the segmented boundary matches the correct position. A satisfied segmentation should have a small value of this index. The second index reflects the region matching which checks the correctness of the segmented region. A satisfied segmentation should have a value near to 1.0. The first two indices are complementary and reflect different aspects on the deviations of the segmentation results. The third index is the error ratio of the cross-sectional area of the bladder, which can show the influence of the segmentation results to the quantitative analysis of the bladder lumen. A satisfied result should have a small error ratio.

Accordingly, we present in Table 1 the indices of the four algorithms on Figures 1 and 3, from which one can see the performances of the four algorithms were not much different on the two images, and all the four results were satisfied. To show the overall comparisons among the image series, the mean and variance of the indices on the 23 sagittal images and 15 axial images are presented in Tables 2 and 3, respectively; the axial images did not include the one illustrated in Figure 2, on which using the thresholding region growing algorithm and the C-means algorithm could not obtain a satisfied boundary of the bladder. Therefore, the comparisons were based on the results on the images in which all the four algorithms obtained qualitatively successful results.

3.3 Discussion

The indices in Table 2 are better than the ones in Table 3. The reason is mainly due to the fact that the sagittal images in the image series are less influenced by noise than the axial images. In both cases, the overall performances of the coupling approach and the modified geodesic active contour were satisfied, and were superior to the ones of the thresholding region growing algorithm and the C-means algorithm with MRF.

If the images were not severely influenced by noise and the bladder lumen could be clearly identified from the bladder wall through intensity, the first two algorithms could achieve satisfied results with easy implementation. However, the first algorithm was sensitive to the thresholds; therefore, in order to obtain a satisfied result, the thresholds needed to be adjusted frequently. For the C-means algorithm, the parameters to apply the MRF also needed to be adjusted so as to eliminate the inner boundaries. When handling images with considerable noise and partial volume effect, the performances of the two algorithms were not stable; and sometimes,

Table 1 Quantitative analysis of the image illustrated in Figs. 1 and 3 (1—thresholding region growing algorithm; 2—C-means algorithm with MRF; 3—Coupling approach; 4—Modified geodesic active contour; PD, CR, and AD are the indices defined in Eq. (4); a—Fig. 1; b—Fig. 3).

Methods	PD (mm)		CR		AD (%)	
	a	b	a	b	a	b
1	0.26	0.30	0.99	0.97	1.09	2.65
2	0.24	0.37	0.99	0.97	0.24	3.41
3	0.21	0.13	0.99	0.99	0.03	0.24
4	0.25	0.18	0.99	0.98	1.19	1.54

Table 2. Quantitative analysis of the sagittal images (1—thresholding region growing algorithm; 2—C-means algorithm with MRF; 3—Coupling approach; 4—Modified geodesic active contour; PD, CR, and AD are the indices defined in Eq. (4); Var. - variance).

Methods	PD (mm)		CR		AD (%)	
	Mean	Var.	Mean	Var.	Mean	Var.
1	0.36	0.17	0.96	0.03	3.43	3.79
2	0.44	0.19	0.95	0.04	4.79	5.93
3	0.21	0.16	0.98	0.03	2.29	3.73
4	0.17	0.19	0.98	0.02	1.31	1.96

Table 3 Quantitative analysis of the axial images (1—thresholding region growing algorithm; 2—C-means algorithm with MRF; 3—Coupling approach; 4—Modified geodesic active contour; PD, CR, and AD are the indices defined in Eq. (4); Var. - variance).

Methods	PD (mm)		CR		AD (%)	
	Mean	Var.	Mean	Var.	Mean	Var.
1	0.52	0.32	0.93	0.08	6.73	10.06
2	0.51	0.26	0.94	0.08	5.86	9.43
3	0.41	0.14	0.96	0.02	2.81	2.00
4	0.33	0.10	0.97	0.02	2.37	1.94

the boundary could not be segmented correctly by adjusting parameters when such influence was large, like in Figure 2. Another drawback is that the smoothness of the segmented boundary cannot be controlled in the two algorithms, which also contributed to the larger deviation from the ground truths.

On the other hand, due to the incorporation of various imaging clues, the performances of the last two algorithms were stable and less influenced by noise and partial volume effect. For the coupling approach, the appearance comparison assisted the segmentation of the bladder. The smoothing effect of the internal force and the modified variance enlarged its flexibility to handle intensity variations on T2-weighted MR images. The weakness of this algorithm is that the contour movement is related with the intensity statistics of the vagina and the rectum; hence, when the information of the two organs is unavailable or inaccurate, the performance of the algorithm is affected. Also, there are several parameters in the moving equations for segmenting the vagina and rectum, which need to be chosen carefully in order to obtain satisfied results, especially when the images are blurred appreciably by noise and partial volume effect. For the modified geodesic active contour, like the coupling approach, a smooth boundary of the bladder could be obtained; and the region-based external force made the algorithm less sensitive to noise and partial volume effect. The drawback of these two algorithms is that complicated computations are involved, which decreases their computational efficiency.

The differences between the four algorithms became larger when the level of noise and partial volume effect increased. The coupling approach and the modified geodesic active contour were more robust, and their performances were better than the ones of the thresholding region growing algorithm and the C-means algorithm. However, the implementations and the computational complexity of the latter two algorithms are simpler.

4 CONCLUSION

MR images of urinary bladder provide a clear visualization of this delicate organ. From this study, the current effective algorithms used to segment the bladder on T2-weighted MR images were discussed and compared.

With the quantitative analysis, one could confirm the effectiveness of each segmentation algorithm and identify the aspects that require further improvements. Three indices were used to quantitatively evaluate the performances of the four algorithms. From the experiments, we could verify that the segmentation algorithms could achieve satisfied results, but manual interventions were needed to achieve satisfied segmentations. For the tested image series, the coupling approach and the modified geodesic active contour proposed in (Ma et al. 2011a, Ma et al. 2011b) obtained better performances than the other two algorithms. However, the four algorithms had common problems, such as the sensitivity to parameter selections and less robustness to process images with severe influence of noise or partial volume effect. Hence, further works are needed to improve these aspects in order to attain more robust and fully automatic segmentation algorithms on T2-weighted axial MR images.

ACKNOWLEDGEMENTS

This work was partially done in the scope of the projects "Methodologies to Analyze Organs from Complex Medical Images—Applications to Female Pelvic Cavity", "Aberrant Crypt Foci and Human Colorectal Polyps: mathematical modeling and endoscopic image processing" and "Cardiovascular Imaging Modeling and Simulation—SIMCARD", with references PTDC/EEA-CRO/103320/2008, UTAustin/MAT/0009/2008 and UTAustin/CA/0047/2008, respectively, financially supported by FCT—Fundação para a Ciência e a Tecnologia, in Portugal.

The first author would like to thank FCT for his PhD grant with reference SFRH/BD/43768/2008.

REFERENCES

Adams, R. & Bischof, L. 1994. Seeded region growing. *IEEE Transaction on Pattern Analysis and Machine Intelligence* 16(6):641–647.

Caselles, V., Kimmel, R. & Sapiro, G. 1997. Geodesic active contours. *International Journal of Computer Vision* 22(1):61–79.

Cheng, D. & Tempany, C. 1998. MR imaging of the prostate and bladder. *Seminars in Ultrasound, CT, and MRI* 19(1):67–89.

Kindermann, R. & Snell, J.L. 1980. Markov random fields and their applications. Rhode Island: American Mathematical Society.

Ma, Z., Tavares, J., Jorge, R. & Mascarenhas, T. 2010. A review of algorithms for medical image segmentation and their applications to the female pelvic cavity. *Computer Methods in Biomechanics and Biomedical Engineering* 13(2):235–246.

Ma, Z., Jorge R., Mascarenhas, T. & Tavares, J. 2011a. Segmentation of Magnetic Resonance Images from Female Pelvic Cavity. *Proceedings of the 2nd International Conference on Mathematical and Computational Biomedical Engineering*. Washington, US.

Ma, Z., Jorge R., Mascarenhas, T. & Tavares, J. 2011b. Novel Approach to Segment the Inner and Outer Boundaries of the Bladder Wall in T2-weighted Magnetic Resonance Images. *Annals of Biomedical Engineering* 39(8):2287–2297.

Computational Vision and Medical Image Processing – Tavares & Natal Jorge (eds)
© 2012 Taylor & Francis Group, London, ISBN 978-0-415-68395-1

Computational algorithms for the segmentation of the human ear

E.M. Barroso, Zhen Ma & João Manuel R.S. Tavares
Faculdade de Engenharia da Universidade do Porto/Instituto de Engenharia Mecânica e Gestão Industrial, Porto, Portugal

Fernanda Gentil
Escola Superior de Tecnologia da Saúde do Porto/Clínica ORL—Dr. Eurico Almeida/IDMEC-Polo FEUP, Porto, Portugal

ABSTRACT: The main goal of this project is to identify an efficient segmentation algorithm for each anatomic structure of the ear. Therefore, in this paper, it is presented and analyzed computational algorithms that have been used to segment structures in images, especially of the human ear in Computed Tomography (CT) images.

1 INTRODUCTION

The organs of hearing and balance constitute the human auditory system, which can be divided into three main parts: external ear, middle ear and inner ear. The ear is by far the most complex organ of the human sensory system (Moller, 2006; Seeley, 2004).

A number of approaches have been presented for reconstructing and visualizing 3D models of the ear with diverse goals, such as with education purposes (Jun, 2005), to build customized biomechanical models (Deacraemer, 2003; Sim, 2008) and in the assessment of pre-operative procedures (Hussong, 2009; Rau, 2009). In order to attain these goals, different types of medical images have been used, acquired by several imaging techniques; for instance, Computerized Tomography (CT-standard, Micro-CT, Spiral-CT) (Christensen, 2003; Poznyakovskiy, 2008; Xianfen, 2005), Magnetic Resonance (MR-standard, Micro-MR) (Shi, 2010; Liu, 2007; Lane, 2005) and Histological processing (Liu, 2007). Using these imaging modalities, anatomical features of the ear have been studied in cats, guinea pigs, chinchillas and humans (Sim, 2008; Liu, 2007).

Solutions of image processing and analysis are essential to attain realistic geometric models for the anatomical structures of the ear. Particularly, the segmentation of the ear structures in images is crucial to build patient-customized biomechanical models to be successfully used in computational simulations. From this simulation, the understanding of the connections between the ear structures and their functions becomes easier as well as the optimization of prosthetic implants.

The study and optimization of cochlear implant systems can be an important application area of the realistic and accurate modeling of the ear. In fact, the position of the implanted electrodes has been identified as one of the most important variables in speech recognition, and the geometric modeling of the ear can facilitate the optimization of the electrode positions, which can be an important step towards efficient traumatic cochlear implant surgeries. Up to now, only manual insertion tools or insertion aids exist, providing the possibility to insert the electrode using a fixed insertion technique that is not adjustable to the patient (Hussong, 2010; Rau, 2010). Thus, based on accurate computational simulations the planning of surgical procedures can be enhanced (Tuck-Lee, 2008).

The biomechanical modeling of the ear also presents a key role in diagnosis and treatment of middle and inner ear diseases, because these two processes are hampered by the small size of the structures and by their hidden locations in the temporal bone (Seemann, 1999). In addition, through the computational modeling of the inner ear, anatomical abnormalities of the bony labyrinth can be easier identified. Therefore, it is possible to create templates that standardize the abnormal configurations (Melhem, 1998).

Image segmentation is a common task in Computational Vision and an important factor for the success of any efficient and accurate image analysis solution. Extracting the structures' contours in medical images, for example, by finding the image edges, can help doctors in detecting more efficient anomalies in visual inspections. However, the segmentation of structures in medical images is normally performed manually, requiring, for example, that medical technicians sketch the desired contours using pointing devices, such as a mouse or a trackball, which is very time-consuming and prone to errors. To overcome the disadvantages of manual segmentation, modern mathematical and physical techniques have been incorporated into the development of computational segmentation algorithms. These incorporations have greatly enhanced the accuracy of the segmentation results (Ma, 2010).

Segmentation is usually regarded as a task of image analysis and, based on the technique adopted, the current segmentation algorithms can be divided into three classes: thresholding, clustering and deformable models (Ma, 2010).

The objective of this work is to review image segmentation algorithms that have been used to segment the structures of the human ear. Hence, the identified algorithms will be analyzed, and their advantages and disadvantages will be pointed out, and some of their results will be presented and discussed.

The paper is organized as follows. In section 2, a review on the segmentation algorithms is made. Afterwards, the characteristics of the algorithms are illustrated through experiments on ear images. In section 4, the advantages and disadvantages of each type are summarized. In the last section, the conclusions are presented.

2 SEGMENTATION ALGORITHMS

In this section, three classes of segmentation algorithms are reviewed. Hence, the common features of each class are identified and discussed, and their advantages and disadvantages are summarized. Additionally, the applications of algorithms of each class on ear images are illustrated to further depict their main characteristics.

2.1 *Algorithms based on thresholding*

Thresholding is a common region segmentation method. In this technique, threshold values are defined, and the original image is divided into groups of pixels that have values within the ranges defined by the thresholds and groups of pixels with values beyond the ranges (Bankman, 2000). Thresholding is a simple, yet often an effective means to segment images in which the represented structures have distinct intensity levels, or other quantifiable feature. The algorithms are usually performed interactively, based on the visual assessment of the resulting segmentations (Pham, 2000).

There are several thresholding techniques, some of them are based on the image histogram, and others are based on local properties or local gradient.

The global thresholding is the most intuitive approach, and is termed "global" as just one threshold value is selected for the entire image, which is defined based on the image histogram. Instead, when the threshold value depends on local properties, it is classified as "local". Local thresholding algorithms can be further classified as edge-based, region-based or hybrid. The fundamental goal of edge detection algorithms is to identify the borders of the structures in an image that can be then used to extract features like corners, lines or curves. Canny, Sobel and Laplacian operators are examples of edge detectors (Ma, 2010).

The region based algorithms are another type of thresholding-based algorithms and their idea comes from the observation that quantifiable features inside a structure tend to be homogeneous (Ma, 2010). Therefore, these algorithms aim to search for the image pixels with similar feature values. Common examples of this type of algorithms are the region growing and the split and merge algorithms (Bankman, 2000).

Finally, hybrid algorithms combine different image cues to complete the segmentation and a typical example is the watershed algorithm (Ma, 2010).

Thresholding-based algorithms have been used to segment anatomic structures of the middle and inner ear (ossicles, cochlea, bone labyrinth), in Micro-CT, Magnetic Resonance and Spiral-CT images (Lee, 2010; Rodt, 2002; Xianfen, 2005; Melhem, 1998).

2.2 *Algorithms based on clustering*

Pattern recognition techniques can be used to perform the segmentation of structures in images, and clustering techniques have been very commonly applied in medical image segmentation (Ma, 2010). Clustering techniques have the same goal as classifier methods that seek to partition the feature space derived from the original image (Pham, 2000). These techniques can be divided into three main classes: supervised, unsupervised and semi-supervised (Sutton, 2000; Ma, 2010).

The supervised techniques are frequently used, and they include K-Nearest Neighbor (KNN) and Maximum Likelihood (ML) algorithms, supervised Artificial Neural Networks (ANN), Support Vector Machines (SVM), Active Shape Models (ASM) and Active Appearance Models (AAM) (Ma, 2010). A training data set is needed to perform supervised classification in order to extract the structure information, and the key issue of supervised clustering is the guidance provided by the labeled data (Zhu, 2010).

Unsupervised classification techniques extract the features of the structure to be segmented from the classified points, and examples of such techniques include Fuzzy C-Means (FCM) and Iterative Self-organizing Data Analysis Technique (ISODATA) algorithms and unsupervised neural networks (Ma, 2010). As already referred, the unsupervised methods explore the intrinsic structure data to segment the input image into regions with different statistics. However, these methods often fail to achieve the desired results, especially if the wanted segmentations include regions with very dissimilar characteristics. On the other hand, supervised image segmentation methods first build the classifier from a labeled training set. Although these methods are likely to perform better, labeling the training set is usually very time consuming.

Semi-supervised image segmentation is the last type of clustering technique and the methods overcome the problems of the traditional clustering techniques by inferring the segmentation from partially labeled images. For example, in Figueiredo (2007) a simple fully deterministic Generalized Expectation-Maximization algorithm (GEM) is described, which is a semi-supervised mixture-based clustering algorithm.

To conclude, the semi-supervised clustering is the recent type of clustering and takes advantage of the user's labels to attain the segmentation, while minimizing the labeling process; and this algorithm has been applied to problems of symptoms classification in medical image databases with promising results (Figueiredo, 2007).

Clustering technique was used by Shi (2010) in magnetic resonance images to segment the vestibular system. However, to overcome the limitations of the clustering techniques in the segmentation of the ear structures, the clustering algorithm was combined with a deformable model.

2.3 Algorithms based on deformable models

Algorithms based on deformable models are more flexible when compared to the types previously described, and have been successfully used in complex segmentations (Ma, 2010). According to the way that is used for tracking the moving contours, deformable models can be further classified into parametric or geometric models.

Parametric deformable models represent curves and surfaces explicitly in their parametric forms during the model deformation. This representation allows direct interaction with the model and can lead to a compact representation for fast real-time implementation. However, the adaptation of the model to new topologies, such in splitting or merging, during the model deformation, can hamper the use of parametric models. Parametric models include active contours (or snakes), active contours with statistical techniques integrated and Generalized Gradient Vector Flow snakes (GGVF).

On the other hand, geometric deformable models can handle topological changes more naturally. These models, based on the theory of curve evolution and the level set method, represent curves and surfaces implicitly as a level set of a higher-dimensional scalar function (McInerney, 1996). The geometric models include level set algorithms, Malladi's algorithm (Geodesic Active Contour—GAC) and Chan-Vese model.

Deformable models have been widely used in several Computational Vision applications, including the segmentation of the external and inner ear. Xie (2005) and Comunello (2009) applied the generalized gradient vector flow snake and active contours segmentation method of Mumford-Shah, respectively, to segment the tympanic membrane of the external ear. Xianfen (2005), Poznyakovskiy (2008) and Bradshaw (2010) used active contours and level set algorithms to segment the cochlea and the semi-circular canals of the inner ear.

3 RESULTS

In this section, it is described the pre-processing technique that was used to remove the noise in the original images and to decrease the computational cost, as well as the results of the tested segmentation algorithms.

3.1 Pre-processing

To enhance and smooth the original CT images of the temporal bone, an anisotropic diffusion Gaussian filter was used. The anisotropic diffusion filter blurs areas of low contrast and enhances the areas of high contrast (edges), as it works as a high pass filter. Thus, a band-pass filter, which initially performs a Gaussian filtering and then applies an anisotropic diffusion filter, was used to remove the noise presented in the input image, Figure 1.

To reduce the required computational time and also the computational cost, the region of the inner ear, i.e. Region of Interest (ROI), was first selected from the filtered image by searching for the pixels with highest intensity values, Figure 2.

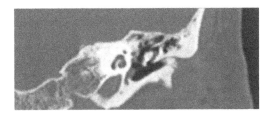

Figure 1. Computerized tomography image of a temporal bone.

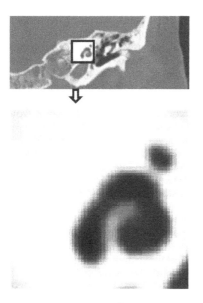

Figure 2. Selection of the ROI from the filtered image.

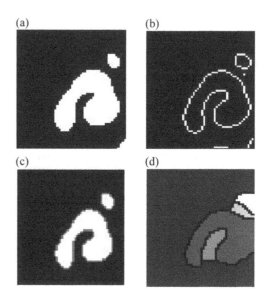

Figure 3. Results of Otsu method (a); Canny edge detection algorithm (b); region growing algorithm (c) and watershed algorithm (d) when is used the region of interest obtained from Figure 1, which is illustrated in Figure 2.

As illustrated in Figure 2, the membranous labyrinth of the inner ear is fully enclosed by the resultant ROI. Then, from the membranous labyrinth, it is possible to create a region that represents the boundary of the temporal bone. By this way, the image size is reduced and the structures of the interest are fully inside the ROI.

3.2 Segmentation

Figure 1 presents a CT image of the temporal bone, from which the appreciable influences of Partial Volume Effects (PVE) can be easily seen. The segmentation results of Otsu method, Canny edge detector, a region growing and a watershed algorithms are illustrated in Figures 3(a)–(d).

The boundaries obtained by the Canny edge detector are continuous, but this algorithm usually presents edges discontinuity due to the noises and PVE. Besides, the spatial relationships of the edge points are not reflected; as such, most of the detected boundaries are incomplete or wrongly connected. For the region growing algorithm, the boundaries of the cochlea and semicircular canal are well segmented. The watershed algorithm gives a complete segmentation of the image. However, over segmentation can be seen in the area between the cochlea and the temporal bone, because there are a lot of pixels with local maximum of gradient magnitude. Finally, the area of the segmented objects by the Otsu method is excessively large.

Figure 4 illustrates the segmentation results of the snake algorithm, Chan-Vese's model and algorithm proposed by Li & Xu.

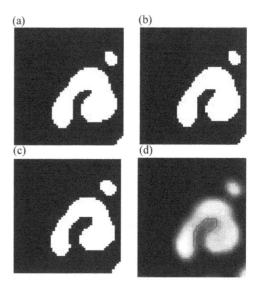

Figure 4. Illustration of the mask, which is obtained by the thresholding algorithm, (a) used to perform the snake algorithm (b), the results of the Chan Vese's model (c) and of the level set of Li and Xu (d).

Parametric deformable models are widely used in structure segmentation and 3D reconstruction. However, the computational complexity such as parameterization of the contours, handling of topological changes, and re-distribution of the contour points, considerably restricts their applications. The snake algorithm, Figure 4(b), has poor convergence to boundaries with larger curvatures. Additionally, the algorithm performance has a high dependence on the initial contour.

Figures 4(c) and 4(d) present the segmentation results of the Chan-Vese model and the algorithm proposed in the level set of Li and Xu. When these two results are compared with the results of the snake algorithm, Figure 4(b), one can see that the boundaries of the last two (deformable models) are more regular and less influenced by noise. The regulating effects of internal forces make the boundary shape more reasonable and less influenced by noise.

4 DISCUSSION

Thresholding is a simple, yet frequently effective means to segment images in which different structures have distinct intensities, or other quantifiable features; it is normally performed interactively, based on the operator's visual assessment of the resulting segmentation (Pham, 2000). Moreover, thresholding is often used as an initial step in a sequence of image processing operations. Its main limitations are that its performance is sensitive to the influence of noise and intensity inhomogeneity, and it typically does not take into account the spatial characteristics of the structure to be segmented. In addition, only two classes are generated by using the simplest form of thresholding. Also, artifacts may corrupt the histogram of the image and make the segmentation more difficult (Bankman, 2000).

Usually, the level set methods have slower speed of convergence than the parametric deformable models, due to their computational complexity, and parametric deformable models are sensitive to the initial conditions. On the other hand, geometric deformable models can automatically handle topology changes and allow multiple simultaneous boundary identifications. Specifically, algorithms based on geometric deformable models aim to eliminate noise influence, prevent leakage, enhance accuracy and efficiency, and make the algorithms more automatic and less dependent on the initial conditions (Tsai, 2001; Wang, 2007).

In conclusion, deformable models are promising to segment medical images, because these models can easily incorporate statistical information and other techniques, and the segmented boundaries have regular geometric properties. This way, they can provide contours with regular geometric properties.

5 CONCLUSIONS

In this paper, current segmentation algorithms were classified into three types and their respective characteristics were summarized. Applications of some of the present algorithms to segment ear structures were illustrated. The experimental examples were also used to further state the distinct characteristics of each type of algorithms.

Deformable models seem to be promising for the segmentation of the inner ear because they can easily incorporate statistical information in order to improve their performance/efficiency/ effectiveness.

ACKNOWLEDGEMENTS

This work was partially done in the scope of the projects "Methodologies to Analyze Organs from Complex Medical Images—Applications to Female Pelvic Cavity", "Aberrant Crypt Foci and Human Colorectal Polyps: mathematical modeling and endoscopic image processing", "Cardiovascular Imaging Modeling and Simulation—SIMCARD" and "Bio-computational study of tinnitus", with references PTDC/EEA-CRO/103320/2008, UTAustin/ MAT/0009/2008, UTAustin/CA/0047/2008 and PTDC/SAU-BEB/104992/2008, respectively, financially supported by Fundação para a Ciência e a Tecnologia (FCT), in Portugal.

The second author would like to thank FCT for his PhD grant with reference SFRH/ BD/43768/2008.

REFERENCES

Bankman, Isaac N. (2000). *Handbook of Medical Imaging Processing and Analysis*. San Diego: Academic Press, Reprint.

Bradshaw, Adrew P., Ian S. Curthoys, Michael J. Todd, John S. Magnussen, David S. Taubman, Swee T. Aw, and G. Michael Halmagyi. (2010). A Mathematical Model of Human Semicircular Canal Geometry: A New Basis for Interpreting Vestibular Physiology. *Journal of the Association for Research in Otolaryngology* 11: 145–59.

Christensen, Gray E., Jianchun He, John A. Dill, Jay T. Rubinstein, Michael W. Vannier, and Ge Wang. (2003). Automatic Measurement of the Labyrinth Using Image Registration and a Deformable Inner Ear Atlas. *Academic Radiology Journal* 10: 988–99.

Comunello, Eros, Aldo von Wangenheim, Vilson Heck Junior, Cristina Dornelles, and Sady Selamen Costa. (2009). A Computational Method for the Semi-Automated Quantitative Analysis of Tympanic Membrane Perforations and Tympanosclerosis. *Computers in Biology and Medicine* 39: 889–95.

Decraemer, W.F., J.J.J. Dirckx, and W.R.J. Funnell. (2003). Three-Dimensional Modelling of the Middle-Ear Ossicular Chain Using a Commercial High-Resolution X-Ray Ct Scanner. *Journal of the Association for Research in Otolaryngology* 4: 250–63.

Figueiredo, Mário A.T. 2007. Semi-Supervised Clustering: Application to Image Segmentation. In *Advances in Data Analysis* edited by Reinhold Decker and Hans -J. Lenz, 39–50. Berlin: Springer Berlin Heidelberg.

Hussong, Andreas, Thomas S. Rau, Tobias Ortmaier, Bodo Heimann, Thomas Lenarz, and Omid Majadani. (2009). An Automated Insertion Tool for Cochlear Implants: Another Step Towards Atraumetic Cochlear Implant Surgery. *Int Journal CARS* 5: 163–71.

Jun, Beom-Cho, Sun-Wha Song, Ju-Eun Cho, Chan-Soon Park, Dong-Hee Lee, Ki-Hong Chang, and Sang-Won Yeo. (2005). Three-Dimensional Reconstruction Based on Images from Spiral High-Resolution Computed Tomography of the Temporal Bone: Anatomy and Clinical Application. *The Journal of Laryngology & Otology* 119: 693–98.

Lane, John I., Robert J. Witte, Odell W. Henson, Colin L.W. Driscoll, John Camp, and Richard A. Robb. (2005). Imaging Microscopy of the Middle and Inner Ear Part Ii: Mr Microscopy. *Clinical Anatomy Wiley-Liss* 18: 409–15.

Lee, Dong H., Sonny Chan, Curt Salisbury, Namkeum Kim, Kenneth Salisbury, Sunil Puria, and Nikolas H. Blevins. (2010). Reconstruction and Exploration of Virtual Middle-Ear Models Derived from Micro-Ct Datasets. *Hearing Research* 263: 198–203.

Liu, Bo, Xiu L. Gao, Hong X. Yin, Shu Q. Luo, and Jing Lu. (2007). A Detailed 3d Model of the Guinea Pig Cochlea. *Brain Struct Funct* 212: 212–30.

Ma, Zhen, João Manuel R.S. Tavares, Renato Natal Jorge, and T. Mascarenhas. (2010). A Review of Algorithms for Medical Image Segmentation and Their Applications to the Female Pelvic Cavity. *Computer Methods in Biomechanics and Biomedical Engineering* 13: 235–46.

McInerney, Tim, and Demetri Terzopoulos. (1996). Deformable Models in Medical Image Analysis: A Survey. *Medical Image Analysis* 2: 91–108.

Melhem, Elias R., Huzeifa Shakir, Sivi Bakthavachalam, C. Bruce MacDonald, John Gira, Shelton D. Caruthers, and Hernan Jara. (1998). Inner Ear Volumetric Measurements Using High-Resolution 3d T2-Weighted Fast Spin-Echo Mr Imaging: Initial Experience in Healthy Subjects. *American Journal Of Neuroradiol* 19: 1819–22.

Moller, A.R. 2006. Hearing: *Anatomy, Physiology, and Disorders of the Auditory System, Second Edition*. San Diego: Academic Press, Reprint.

Pham, Dzung L., Chenyang Xu, and Jerry L. Prince. (2000). Current Methods in Medical Image Segmentation. *Annu. Rev. Biomed. Eng.* 2: 315–37.

Poznyakovskiy, Anton A., Thomas Zahnert, Yannis Kalaidzidis, Rolf Schmidt, Bjorn Fischer, Johannes Baumgart, and Yury M. Yarin. (2008). The Creation of Geometric Three-Dimensional Models of the Inner Ear Based on Micro Computer Tomography Data. *Hearing Research* 243: 95–104.

Rau, Thomas S., Andreas Hussong, Martin Leinung, Thomas Lenarz, and Omid Majdani. (2010). Automated Insertion of Performed Cochlear Implant Electrodes: Evaluation of Curling Behaviour and Insertion Forces on an Artificial Cochlear Model. *Int Journal CARS* 5: 173–81.

Rodt, T., P. Ratiu, H. Becker, S. Bartling, D.F. Kacher, M. Anderson, F.A. Jolesz, and R. Kikinis. (2002). 3d Visualisation of the Middle Ear and Adjacent Structures Using Reconstructed Multi-Slice Ct Datasets, Correlating 3d Images and Virtual Endoscopy Images. *Neuroradiology* 44: 783–90.

Seeley, Stephens, and Tate. (2004). *The Special Senses*, Anatomy and Physiology, Sixth Edition: The MacGraw-Hill Companies, Reprint.

Seemann, M.D., O. Seemann, H. Bonél, M. Suckfull, K.-H. Englmeier, A. Naumann, C.M. Allen, and M.F. Reiser. (1999). Evaluation of the Middle and Inner Ear Structures: Comparison of Hybrid Rendering, Virtual Endoscopy and Axial 2d Source Images. *European Radiology* 9: 1851–58.

Shi, Lin, Defeng Wang, Winnie C.W. Chu, Geoffrey R. Burwell, Tien-Tsin Wong, Pheng Ann Heng, and Jack C.Y. Cheng. (2010). Automatic Mri Segmentation and Morphoanatomy Analysis of the Vestibular System in Adolescent Idiopathic Scoliosis. *NeuroImage*: 9.

Sim, Jae Hoon, and Sunil Puria. (2008). Soft Tissue Morphometry of the Malleus-Incus Complex from Micro-Ct Imaging. *Journal of the Association for Research in Otolaryngology* 9: 5–21.

Sutton, Melanie A., James C. Bezdek, and Tobias C. Cahoon. 2000. Image Segmentation by Fuzzy Clustering: Methods and Issues. In *Handbook of Medical Imaging Processing and Analysis*. San Diego: Academic Press Series in Biomedical Engineering.

Tsai, Anthony Yezzi Andy, and Alan S. Willsky. (2001). Curve Evolution Implementation of the Mumford-Shah Functional for Image Segmentation, Denoising, Interpolation, and Magnification. *IEEE transactions on Image Processing* 10: 1169–86.

Tuck-Lee, James P., Peter M. Pinsky, Charles R. Steele, and Sunil Puria. (2008). Finite Element Modeling of Acoustical-Mechanical Coupling in the Cat Middle Ear. *Journal Acoustical Society of America* 124: 348–62.

Wang, Yonggang, Yun Zhu, and Qiang Guo. (2007). Medical Image Segmentation Based on Deformable Models and Its Applications. In *Deformable Models Theory and Biomaterial Applications*, 209–60: Springer New York.

Xianfen, Diao, Chen Siping, Liang Changhong, and Wang Yuanmei. 2005. 3d Semi-Automatic Segmentation of the Cochlea and Inner Ear. In *Engineering in Medicine and Biology 27th Annual Conference*, edited by IEEE. Shangai, China.

Xie, Xianghua, Majid Mirmehdi, Richard Maw, and Amanda Hall. (2005). Detecting Abnormalities in Tympanic Membrane Images. *Medical Image Understanding and Analysis*: 19–22.

Zhu, Yanping. (2010). An Efficient Supervised Clustering Algorithm Based on Neural Networks. In *3rd International Conference on Advanced Computer Theory and Engineering (ICACTE)*, edited by IEEE, 265–68.

Computational Vision and Medical Image Processing – Tavares & Natal Jorge (eds)
© *2012 Taylor & Francis Group, London, ISBN 978-0-415-68395-1*

Evaluation of wavelets in noise reduction of Electromyographic signals

F. Ballesteros & J. de Castro

Departamento de Matemática Aplicada a las Tecnologías de la Información, ETS de Ingenieros de
Telecomunicación, Universidad Politécnica de Madrid, Madrid, Spain

ABSTRACT: Our work analyzes the application of wavelets to Electromyography to eliminate the noise inherent to signals, prior to their classification. In particular, we study the behavior of several families of wavelets and hard and soft thresholding different methods in order to identify those that provide better Signal to Noise Ratio (SNR).

Keywords: Electromyography, Denoising, Wavelets, Thresholding, Signal to Noise Ratio

1 INTRODUCTION

Electromyography (EMG) is a technique for evaluating and recording the electrical activity produced by skeletal muscles in the diagnosis of neuromuscular diseases. The applications and diagnostic performance of electromyography have evolved, and nowadays there are systems controlled by microprocessors able to capture, represent, analyze and sort these signals. A challenge is the classification of these kind of signals and the automatic diagnostic, using expert systems.

The EMG checks the health of muscles and nerves that control muscles. It is used to diagnose muscle and nerve disorders and diseases of the spinal cord by recording the electrical activity of brain and spinal cord to a peripheral nerve root (found in arms and legs) that controls the muscles during contraction and at rest. During an EMG, assessing the changes in electrical voltage that occur during movement and when the muscle is at rest. Among the possible disorders are myopathy (muscle degeneration) and neuropathy (problems with the nerves that carry information to and from the brain and spinal cord, which can cause pain, loss of sensation and inability to control muscles). Figure 1 shows three EMG signals: a healthy patient, a patient with myopathy and a patient with neuropathy.

The new technological advances and investigations about EMG have improved the diagnosis, but a good diagnosis still depends heavily on the experience and knowledge of each professional. Quantitative methods aim to replace subjective assessment by precise measurements physiologically significant. Their performance is generally satisfactory when conditions are optimal (patient collaborator, fully established disease, low noise).

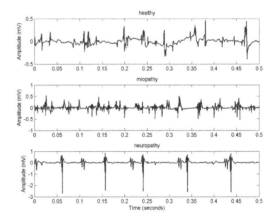

Figure 1. Three EMG signals: healthy, myopathy and neuropathy.

Unfortunatelly, these conditions are not usual, because there are still major constraints imposed by factors that can currently only be partially controlled, as is the case of noise (Gila et al. 2010). Noise, either technical or biological origin, always appears in registred signals.

In addition to the conventional Fourier transform analysis, there are other procedures that, unlike the former, are applicable to non-stationary signals (such as EMG) and provide information on frequency variation in time, known as time-frequency representation. Different types of time-frequency analysis, as wavelets or distribution of Choi-Williams, have been applied to the signal EMG during the muscle contraction for studying fatigue and relations between electrical and mechanical activity of the muscle (Karlsson et al. 2000).

The search for efficient signal denoising methods still is a valid challenge, at the crossing of functional analysis and statistics. The main methods (some of them with many variants) are: the Gaussian smoothing model (Lindenbaum et al. 1994), the anisotropic filtering model (Perona and Malik 1990), the Rudin-Osher-Fatemi total variation model (Guichard and Morel 2001), the Yaroslavsky (Yaroslavsky 1985), (Yaroslavsky and Eden 1996) neighborhood filters and a variant, the SUSAN filter (Smith and Brady 1995), the Wiener local empirical filter as implemented by (Yaroslavsky 1985), DUDE, the discrete universal denoiser (Ordentlich et al. 2003), and the translation invariant wavelet thresholding (Coifman and Donoho 1995), a simple and performing variant of the wavelet thresholding (Donoho and Johnstone 1994).

The Fourier transform can be used in denoising signals by filtering one or more frequencies. This strategy is simple, but has the disadvantage that it is possible to eliminate some relevant information when the signal has this information in the same frequency as the noise. In these cases it is better to use a wavelets based strategy, because wavelets allow to work with the frequency and time information at the same time, and this dual representation allows a better noise removal than Fourier analysis.

Wavelets have been applied successfully in data analysis. Specifically, are quite effective in denoising. The usual denoising strategy is to change to 0 the noise frequencies coefficients. Different ways to select that coefficients produce different denoising methods. In 1993, Donoho published the first method (Donoho 1993), and since then have been developed different methods and strategies for the elimination of signal noise (Hernández-Fajardo et al. 2008). In this work, we use some of the basic methods for denoising applied to the case of EMG signals. We assume that the signal is contaminated with additive Gaussian noise, and then we test several different methods. Finally, we show results and conclusions.

2 METHODOLOGY

Let $\{\psi_{j,k}: j,k \in \mathbb{Z}\}$ be an orthogonal basis of wavelets on the interval $I = [a,b]$, so that we can write any signal $u \in L^2(I)$ as the sum of the serie

$$u = \sum_{j,k \in \mathbb{Z}} <u, \psi_{j,k}> \psi_{j,k}$$

where

$$<u, \psi_{j,k}> = \int_I u(x)\psi_{j,k}(x)dx.$$

Let define the hard thresholding operator τ_h to be

$$\tau_h(x) = \begin{cases} x & \text{if } |x| \geq \lambda, \\ 0 & \text{if } |x| < \lambda. \end{cases}$$

And the soft thresholding operator τ_s to be

$$\tau_s(x) = \begin{cases} x + \lambda & \text{if } x \leq -\lambda, \\ 0 & \text{if } -\lambda < x < \lambda, \\ x - \lambda & \text{if } x \geq \lambda, \end{cases}$$

Figure 2 shows these operators.

The denoised signal using wavelet thresholding is

$$u_0 = \sum_{j,k \in \mathbb{Z}} \tau(<u, \psi_{j,k}>)\psi_{j,k}.$$

The hard thresholding technique introduces discontinuity, which makes it unstable and sensitive to small changes in the signal. On the other hand, applying soft thresholding, coefficients can be changed unnecessarily they are correct.

If the noisy signal can be written $u = \tilde{u} + w$, with $\tilde{u}$ the noiseless signal to estimate and w an additive Gaussian white noise of standard desviation σ, the threshold λ is often set to be $\sigma\sqrt{2\log N}$, known as *universal threshold*, where N is the number of samples of the digital signal. In that case, the estimator is the best in the min-max sense as N tends to infinity (Donoho and Johnstone 1994).

Thresholding techniques have been always very important in denoising methods with wavelets. We put in practice the wavelet transform and the multiresolution decomposition to denoise the signal. The method uses a single value thresholding (universal thresholding or Visu shrink) (Donoho and Johnstone 1994), (Jansen 2001), (Fodor and Kamath 2003), and eliminates the wavelet coefficients smaller than a threshold (using soft or hard thresholding). Then we construct a new signal (the denoised signal) with the new coefficients.

If we choose a very small threshold, then it is possible that we do not remove all possible noise

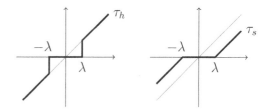

Figure 2. Hard thresholding operator τ_h (left) and soft thresholding operator τ_s (right).

of the signal. On the other hand, if we select a very big threshold, then we can lose relevant information from the signal. Consequence of this is the great importance of the choice of the thresholding value. This work assume the value proposed by Donoho (Donoho and Johnstone 1995) as a universal threshold

$$\lambda = \sigma\sqrt{\log 2N}$$

which depends on the size N of the signal and noise standard deviation σ. The size N of the signal is a known parameter, but σ needs to be estimated.

We improve the universal threshold method considering a different threshold value for each level of decomposition instead of the same threshold value for all the levels.

The multiresolution analysis uses families of wavelets. Each family has its own properties that allow a better or worse adjustment to one type of signal or another. So, it is very convenient to find the family of wavelets that best suits the signal, because after the multiresolution analysis is performed the thresholding stage which rejects coefficients close to 0. This results in a loss of information. Therefore, the smaller loss is the best suitable family to signal.

The first step of analysis is to decompose the signal into 3 levels, using several families of wavelets. After obtaining the approximation and detail coefficients at the next stage of the experiment to the coefficients of the decomposition into 3 levels are applied 4 different methods of denoising: Hard and soft thresholding with a single value for all coefficients, and hard and soft thresholding with a different value for the coefficients of each level of decomposition.

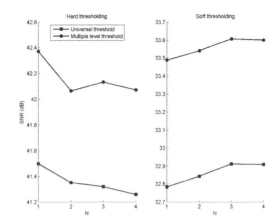

Figure 4. Coiflets family: SNR vs order N.

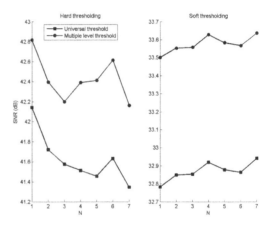

Figure 5. Symlets family: SNR vs order N.

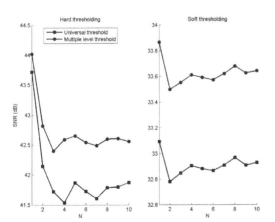

Figure 3. Daubechies family: SNR vs order N.

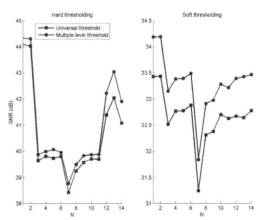

Figure 6. Biorthogonal family: SNR vs order N.

3 RESULTS AND CONCLUSIONS

We test four algorithms, two hard threshold and two soft thresholding, choosing one universal threshold value or a different threshold value for each level of decomposition. The results are obtained using the Daubechies family of wavelets, from db1 (Haar) to db10, the Coiflets family, from coif1 to coif4, the Symlets family, from sym2 to sym9, and 14 biorthogonal wavelets: bior1.3, bior1.5, bior2.2, bior2.4, bior2.6, bior2.8, bior3.1, bior3.3, bior3.5, bior3.7, bior3.9, bior4.4, bior5.5 and bior6.8. Based on the results obtained, as we can see in Figures 3, 4, 5 y 6 we can deduce that for any wavelet family applied, we always get better results using hard thresholding than soft thresholding. Moreover, for any wavelet family used there are better results using a threshold value for each level of decomposition that a single threshold for all coefficients of the decomposition. Also we concluded that one different threshold value for each level of decomposition has no significant influence on the algorithm execution time, while the results improve significantly.

REFERENCES

Coifman, R. and D. Donoho (1995, may). Translation invariant denoising. Technical Report 475, Dept. of Statistics, Stanford University.

Donoho, D.L. (1993). Unconditional bases are optimal bases for data compression and for statistical estimation. *Applied and Computational Harmonic Analysis 1*, 100–115.

Donoho, D.L. and I.M. Johnstone (1994). Ideal spatial adaptation by wavelet shrinkage. *Biometrika 81*, 425–455.

Donoho, D.L. and I.M. Johnstone (1995, December). Adapting to unknown smoothness via wavelet shrinkage. *Journal of the American Statistical Association 90*(432), 1200–1224.

Fodor, I.K. and C. Kamath (2003, December). Denoising through wavelet shrinkage: An empirical study. *Journal of Electronic Imaging 151*, 151–160.

Gila, L., A. Malanda, I. Rodríguez Carreño, J. Rodríguez Falces, and J. Navallas (2010). Métodos de procesamiento y análisis de señales electromiográficas. In *Anales del Sistema Sanitario de Navarra*, Volume 32, Supl. 3 of *Actualización en neurofisiología clínica*, pp. 22–43.

Guichard, F. and J.M. Morel (2001). *Image Analysis and P.D.E.s.* IPAM-UCLA.

Hernández-Fajardo, I., G. Evangelatos, I. Kougioumtzoglou, and X. Ming (2008, December). Signal denoising using wavelet-based methods. *Connexions.*

Jansen, M. (2001). *Noise reduction by wavelet thresholding*, Volume 161 of *Lecture notes in Statistics*. Springer-Verlag.

Karlsson, S., J. Yu, and M. Akay (2000, February). Time-frequency analysis of myoelectric signals during dynamic contractions: A comparative study. *IEEE Transactions on Biomedical Engineering 47*, 228–238.

Lindenbaum, M., M. Fischer, and A. Bruckstein (1994). On Gabor's contribution to image enhancement. *Pattern Recognition 27*(1), 1–8.

Ordentlich, E., G. Seroussi, S. Verdú, M. Weinberger, and T. Weissman (2003, September). A discrete universal denoiser and its application to binary images. *Proc. IEEE Int. Conf. on Image Processing 1*, 117–120.

Perona, P. and J. Malik (1990). Scale-space and edge detection using anisotropic diffusion. *IEEE Transactions on Pattern Analysis and Machine Intelligence 12*, 629–639.

Smith, S.M. and J.M. Brady (1995). Susan—a new approach to low level image processing. *International Journal of Computer Vision 23*, 45–78.

Yaroslavsky, L.P. (1985). *Digital Picture Processing. An Introduction*, Volume 67 of *Springer Series in Information Sciences*. WILEY-VCH Verlag.

Yaroslavsky, L.P. and M. Eden (1996). *Fundamentals of Digital Optics: Digital Signal Processing in Optics and Holography* (1st ed.). Secaucus, NJ, USA: Springer-Verlag New York, Inc.

Computational Vision and Medical Image Processing – Tavares & Natal Jorge (eds)
© 2012 Taylor & Francis Group, London, ISBN 978-0-415-68395-1

Assessing the detection of embolic signals using continuous wavelet transform

Ivo B. Gonçalves
DEEI/FCT, Universidade do Algarve, Campus de Gambelas, Faro, Portugal

Ana Leiria & M.M.M. Moura
DEEI/FCT & Centro de Investigação sobre o Espaço e as Organizações, Universidade do Algarve, Campus de Gambelas Faro, Portugal

ABSTRACT: Aiming the correct characterization of cerebral blood flow and emboli, embolic signals were added to simulated MCA Doppler signals and Short-Time Fourier Transform (STFT) and Continuous Wavelet Transform (CWT) were used in the evaluation. The power of the embolic signals added were 6, 7, 7.5 and 8 dB. The mother wavelets considered in the CWT analysis were Morlet, Meyer and Mexican Hat. The threshold values used for detection (equated in terms of false positive, false negative and sensitivity) were 2 dB and 3.5 dB for the CWT and STFT, respectively. The results indicate that although the STFT allows to accurately detect the emboli, better time localization can be achieved with the CWT. Among the CWT, the current best overall results were obtained with Mexican Hat-based CWT, better conveying energy conservation and optimal results for sensitivity (100% detection rate).

1 INTRODUCTION

Emboli presence in blood circulation is one of the main factors for the occurrence of a stroke, which may cause permanent damage or even death. A common type of embolus is a blood clot, which is a significant risk of a surgery and may occur in the intervened area or be caused by inactivity during recovery. Most post-operative patients are given medication to thinner the blood in order to prevent formation of blood clots. However, the effects of medication are not immediate or completely effective thus not absolutely preventing the development of blood clots which can become a critical complication if they travel through the bloodstream and lodge into the brain causing a stroke (Evans and McDicken 1992).

The use of clinical Doppler instrumentation is widely spread and a common practice in many clinical and hospital units for the assessment of blood flow. For the particular case of brain blood flow analysis, the Transcranial Doppler (TCD) enables the monitoring of the Middle Cerebral Artery (MCA), a critical channel for the detection of emboli. The monitoring phase is commonly done for periods of one hour or more (Evans and McDicken 1992).

Current best accepted embolus detection method consists in acoustic detection made by specialized medical personnel by hearing the Doppler shift sound. Human intervention in such complex and thorough analysis makes it difficult, expensive and eventually susceptible to errors where low relative intensity signals are concerned. Thus, it's important to develop and use methods which allow to detect, classify and quantify emboli and its characteristics.

Although signal acquisition by the TCD instrumentation is a requirement, and therefore takes a fundamental role in the system, it can be defined as the start point for the system. In fact the correct characterization of blood flow and cerebral emboli depends on the precision achieved by the spectral estimation process. Most TCD equipments use conventional spectral estimation methods based on Short-Time Fourier Transform (STFT). But STFT have well known limitations which lead to imprecise results, namely in quantitative estimations (e.g., size and speed of embolus) that are specially relevant in detection of small emboli.

Different authors use different criteria and that may hinder comparability. The work reported here aims to compare different approaches using a common set of comparison criteria. To that effect the assessment of emboli detection uses simulated embolic signals; the Continuous Wavelet Transform (CWT) analysis method using different mother wavelets (as suggested by the conclusions of an earlier study (Aydin and Markus 1999)) is evaluated as a possible alternative to the classical Short-Time Fourier Transform (STFT) spectral estimator.

Sets of signals were generated using the Wang Fish simulator (Wang and Fish 1995) using reference spectral parameters (Leiria 2005) to simulate blood flow signal in Middle Cerebral Artery (MCA) during a cardiac cycle. From each of the emboli free signals, new sets of signals were produced by adding simulated emboli with different Measured Emboli Power (MEP) values at four time intervals of the cardiac cycle.

After applying each of the methods to the generated signals, relevant spectral parameters were retrieved. These parameters are the maximum and mean frequencies, bandwidth and power variation over time and could be used to assess the quality of the estimation process. It should be noted however that in the present case emboli detection is signalled by the power variation over time crossing a threshold of the emboli to blood ratio.

The assessment of the CWT is quantified in terms of false positive and false negative events, sensitivity is analysed and the results are discussed.

2 SIMULATION

2.1 *Blood flow signals*

Characteristics of real blood flow TCD signals may vary depending on several factors as, for example, the targeted blood vessel. Thus, for a reliable simulated environment, it is important to guarantee that those characteristics are respected.

From different possibilities available in literature, the Wang and Fish simulator was chosen due to the demonstrated good MCA signals simulation for a low computational effort (Leiria 2005). The simulator is fed spectral parameters reference curves of mean frequency, power variation over time and bandwidth represented in Figure (1).

Each of the spectral parameters referred have a correspondence to a blood flow physical event. Frequencies (maximum or mean) hold information about blood flow velocities (maximum and mean, respectively) and bandwidth about the turbulence in the blood flow. Power variation over time allows to estimate the presence of abnormal events based on the variation of the backscattered power of the blood flow over time (Leiria et al. 2004).

A set of 100 signals were generated using a sampling frequency of 12.5 kHz, each representing a cardiac cycle of the duration of 923 ms.

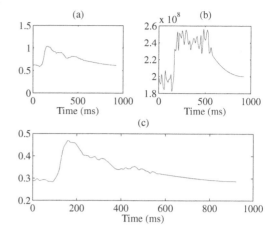

Figure 1. Reference curves for (a) mean frequency, (b) power variation over time and (c) bandwidth.

2.2 *Emboli*

Each simulated embolus is composed by a sinusoidal wave with a frequency obtained from the maximum frequency reference curve average value for the embolus duration period. The amplitude of the embolus signal is given by:

$$\sqrt{P_E} = \sqrt{\left(10^{\frac{MEP}{10}} - 1\right)P_B} \qquad (1)$$

where MEP is the desired simulated embolus power and P_B the power backscattered by blood without presence of emboli. The MEP values used, in dB, were:

$$p = \{6 \quad 7 \quad 7.5 \quad 8\} \qquad (2)$$

2.3 *Embolic blood flow signals*

The capability of detecting the presence of emboli in the blood flow varies along the cardiac cycle. An embolus in the blood flow probed during diastole has higher probability of being identified than during systole. Higher velocities and backscattered power occur during systole and, therefore, during diastole the evidence of the embolus will last longer giving higher relevance to the embolus (Leiria 2005).

To each simulated signal emboli were added at four delimited regions along the cardiac cycle. The first three areas are located around the systolic peak—rising curve (s_1), peak (s_2) and decaying curve (s_3)—and a fourth area located during the diastole (d_1). The four regions are centred in time at 72 ms, 140 ms, 260 ms and 660 ms having each a duration of 40 ms. In Figure (2) are the

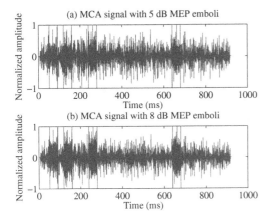

(a) MCA signal with 5 dB MEP emboli

(b) MCA signal with 8 dB MEP emboli

Figure 2. Time-domain MCA blood flow signals with (a) 5 dB and (b) 8 dB emboli added in the defined areas (limited in red).

time-domain representations of one simulated blood flow signal with emboli added of 5 dB and 8 dB. The emboli areas were the simulated emboli were added are delimited.

3 SIGNAL PROCESSING METHODS

3.1 STFT

By definition, the STFT consists of multiple Fourier transforms of windowed signals, that is, signals that were delimited by a "window" function $w(t)$ centred at time t in order to find frequency ω.

$$STFT(t,\omega) = |\int e^{-j\omega t'} x(t')w(t'-t)\partial t'|^2 \qquad (3)$$

In the present case, windowing is achieved with the rectangular function. The length of the window used is 360 bins using an overlapping of 359 (99.72%). The choice of such overlapping aims to achieve the best time resolution possible, whereas the window length is the one which provides best results for equally weighted estimation of power variation over time and mean frequency parameters for high overlapping percentage (Leiria 2005).

3.2 CWT

One of the most relevant characteristics of Wavelet Transforms (WT) is its ability to adjust the chosen analysis function ("mother-wavelet") to best match the signal under analysis. This adjustment consists in a scale factor which is applied to the analysis function, "compressing" or "stretching" it in each time instant. This allows a better perception of the different signal characteristics,

particularly frequencies, in each time instant. In a formal definition (Chui 1992), a wavelet series can be written as

$$x(t) = \sum_{j,k=-\infty}^{\infty} c_{j,k}\psi_{j,k}(t) \qquad (4)$$

where ψ is a wavelet function and the coefficients of the series is given by

$$c_{j,k} = \int_{-\infty}^{\infty} x(t)\psi^*(t)dt \qquad (5)$$

Thus, the Wavelet Transform, in its integral form is defined as

$$W_\psi(b,a) = 1/\sqrt{|a|}\int_{-\infty}^{\infty} x(t)\psi^*(t-b/a)dt \qquad (6)$$

where $x(t)$ is the time domain signal, $\psi^*(t)$ the wavelet function complex conjugate, and t and a the time and scale parameters, respectively. The factor $1/\sqrt{|a|}$ ensures energy preservation over the transformation. Thus, from (4) and (5), comes that

$$c_{j,k} = W_\psi(k2^{-j}, 2^{-j}) \qquad (7)$$

The transformation W_ψ is called the "Continuous Wavelet Transform" (CWT) relative to the "basic wavelet" function ψ. Thus, the $(j,k)th$ wavelet coefficient of f is given by the integral wavelet transformation of f at the translation (or dyadic position) $b = k2^{-j}$ with scaling (or binary dilation) $a = 2^{-j}$, where the same wavelet function ψ is used to generate the series (4) and to define the integral wavelet transform (6).

Wavelet transformation provides a time-scale decomposition, rather than a time-frequency. The relation between scale (a) and frequency (f) is given by $a = f_0/f$, where f_0 is the central frequency of the Fourier Transform of the wavelet function used (Matos et al. 2000).

A 180 points scale was applied to the WT configuration in order to achieve a scale resolution analogous to the STFT frequency resolution.

Although several "mother-wavelet" function families, namely Morlet, Mexican Hat, Meyer, Gaussian, and Daubechies (Daubechies 1992) wavelets were considered, in this paper Morlet, Mexican Hat and Meyer will be assessed.

4 EVALUATION METHODS AND CRITERIA

One hundred simulated signals were generated, the methods applied and average spectral parameters calculated. For each of the four MEP values considered, emboli were added to each of the simulated signals constituting four sets of 100 signals each. Aiming the detection of embolic events, attention was focused on the spectral parameter power variation over time.

A frequently referred parameter in emboli detection is embolic signal intensity to average background ratio (EBR) (Markus et al. 1993; Aydin 2007), translating the immediate human perception of an embolic event. In the scope of this work, the indicator used is given by

$$EBR(t) = 10log A_{total}(t)/A_{blood}(t) \qquad (8)$$

where A_{total} is the power of the embolic signal and A_{blood} the power of the blood signal, the latter being the average of the spectral parameter power variation over time from the 100 simulated signals before emboli were added.

When the integral of instantaneous EBR values under a running window exceeds a chosen threshold the detection of an embolus is signalled. Noting that each signal contains four emboli in pre-determined positions and fixed time duration, the detection is judged correct if the centre of the signalled area is within the time interval of the simulated embolus.

Supposing that two emboli are detected as one and the centre of the detected area is outside both emboli, the judgement would be a false positive and two false negatives.

5 RESULTS

The assessment of detection of embolic signals was quantified in terms of false positive and false negative event counting. Aiming to facilitate the comparison with other studies, sensitivity values were presented.

The performance of CWTs using Morlet, Mexican Hat and Meyer mother-wavelets and of STFT was evaluated for the four sets of 100 signals obtained by the addition of emboli.

Evaluation considered running windows of 20 ms with 50% overlap applied to $EBR(t)$ where an event is signalled when and while the integral of EBR exceeds the threshold of 2 dB and 3.5 dB for CWT and STFT, respectively. Each event is then judged according to added emboli intervals.

In order to illustrate the results, attention is first drawn to some particular cases. Figures 3, 4, 5 and 6 present the EBR of the same embolic simulated signal obtained with Morlet-based, Mexican Hat-based and Meyer-based CWTs and STFT, respectively.

The solid red lines delimit the emboli areas and the solid green lines delimit the area of the detected emboli. In black and white (B&W) printing, red

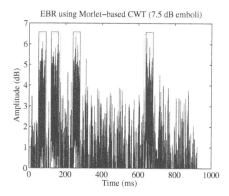

Figure 3. EBR measured using Morlet-based CWT with 20 ms window, 50% overlap and 2 dB threshold value for emboli added of 7.5 dB. Emboli areas signalled in red and emboli detection areas in green.

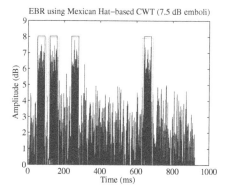

Figure 4. EBR measured using Mexican Hat-based CWT with 20 ms window, 50% overlap and 2 dB threshold value for emboli added of 7.5 dB. Emboli areas signalled in red and emboli detection areas in green.

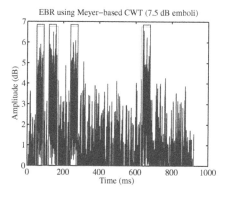

Figure 5. EBR measured using Meyer-based CWT with 20 ms window, 50% overlap and 2 dB threshold value for emboli added of 7.5 dB. Emboli areas signalled in red and emboli detection areas in green.

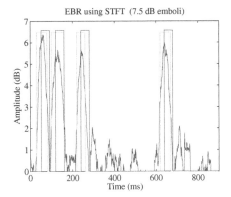

EBR using STFT (7.5 dB emboli)

Figure 6. EBR measured using STFT with 20 ms window, 50% overlap and 3.5 dB threshold value for emboli added of 7.5 dB. Emboli areas signalled in red and emboli detection areas in green.

and green will appear as dark grey and light grey, respectively.

It should be noted that in Figures 3, 4 and 5, a threshold of 2 dB was used, and in Figure 6 a threshold of 3.5 dB was applied. These figures illustrate two points that are worth mentioning, namely energy conservation and localization. Although both CWT based approaches correctly detect the presence of emboli, the EBR amplitude of the Mexican Hat-based CWT better conveys the amplitude of the added emboli. As far as localization is concerned, attention is drawn to the STFT: although visual inspection allows concluding that the emboli were indeed detected, intervals might be displaced in time.

For each set of signals with added emboli, the counts of false negative events and false positive events were noted, distinguishing the position of missed emboli and falsely detected emboli. The values of Morlet-based, Mexican Hat-based and Meyer-based CWTs and STFT are presented in Tables 1, 2, 3 and 4, respectively.

It is noted that using the Morlet-based CWT (Table 1) and Meyer-based CWT (Table 3) most of the emboli missed are located in the rising phase towards the systolic peak.

Most of the errors presented in Table 4 are due to the time displacement of the detection interval. This time displacement is also observed in the other emboli positions, although of no consequence to the final results.

The sensitivity, evaluated according to (9),

$$\text{sensitivity} = \frac{\text{true positives}}{\text{true positives} + \text{false negatives}} \quad (9)$$

is presented in Tables 5, 6, 7 and 8, being described per emboli area (s_1, s_2, s_3 and d_1) and globally along each cardiac cycle.

Table 1. False negative and false positive emboli detection counts for Morlet wavelet using a 2 dB threshold.

MEP (dB)	False negatives				False positives
	s_1	s_2	s_3	d_1	
6	21	0	3	11	1
7	4	0	0	0	1
7.5	0	0	0	0	1
8	0	0	0	0	1

Table 2. False negative and false positive emboli detection counts for Mexican Hat wavelet using a 2 dB threshold.

MEP (dB)	False negatives				False positives
	s_1	s_2	s_3	d_1	
6	0	0	0	0	2
7	0	0	0	0	2
7.5	0	0	0	0	2
8	0	0	0	0	2

Table 3. False negative and false positive emboli detection counts for Meyer wavelet using a 2 dB threshold.

MEP (dB)	False negatives				False positives
	s_1	s_2	s_3	d_1	
6	13	0	3	5	1
7	0	0	0	0	1
7.5	0	0	0	0	1
8	0	0	0	0	1

Table 4. False negatives and false positives emboli detection counts for STFT using a 3.5 dB threshold.

MEP (dB)	False negatives				False positives
	s_1	s_2	s_3	d_1	
6	37	10	54	26	20
7	19	0	3	1	9
7.5	6	0	0	0	6
8	5	1	0	0	5

Table 5. Sensitivity for Morlet wavelet results.

MEP (dB)	Per area (%)				Global (%)
	s_1	s_2	s_3	d_1	
6	79	100	97	89	91
7	96	100	100	100	99
7.5	100	100	100	100	100
8	100	100	100	100	100

Table 6. Sensitivity for Mexican Hat wavelet results.

MEP (dB)	Per area (%)				Global (%)
	s_1	s_2	s_3	d_1	
6	100	100	100	100	100
7	100	100	100	100	100
7.5	100	100	100	100	100
8	100	100	100	100	100

Table 7. Sensitivity for Meyer wavelet results.

MEP (dB)	Per area (%)				Global (%)
	s_1	s_2	s_3	d_1	
6	87	100	97	95	95
7	100	100	100	100	100
7.5	100	100	100	100	100
8	100	100	100	100	100

Table 8. Sensitivity for STFT results.

MEP (dB)	Per area (%)				Global (%)
	s_1	s_2	s_3	d_1	
6	63	90	46	74	68
7	90	100	97	99	97
7.5	94	100	100	100	99
8	95	99	100	100	99

6 CONCLUDING REMARKS

This paper describes some of the work done towards the assessment of different approaches to embolic blood flow signals. The setup of the experimental work included a simulator of MCA blood flow signals, the simulation and addition of embolic events of known characteristics to the simulated signals, a processing phase to extract relevant spectral parameters from the simulated embolic signals and, finally, the detection of emboli and its evaluation in terms of false positive and false negative counts and sensitivity rates.

Different cases of 6, 7, 7.5 and 8 dB were addressed where in each case four emboli per cardiac cycle signal were added, three emboli during the systole and one embolus during the diastolic phase of the cardiac cycle. The processing phase considered the STFT and three CWT using Morlet, Meyer and Mexican Hat mother-wavelets. The detection of emboli considered the integral of a windowed portion of the relative emboli to blood power ratio using 20 ms rectangular windows with 50% overlap, and a decision threshold value that,

aiming at the best performance, was set at 2 dB for the CWT approaches and at 3.5 dB for the STFT one. The detections were judged accurate if the middle of the detection interval coincided in the embolus duration interval. The results were analysed in terms of total count of false matches and in terms of sensitivity.

It was noted that the smaller total err count was achieved with the Mexican Hat-based CWT (100% detection rate) and that this approach also better conveyed the power amplitude of the added emboli. Meyer-based CWT was the second best, actually achieving better results for emboli above 6 dB. The STFT was strongly prejudiced by the shift in the time localization of the embolic events.

Further work will include expanding the evaluation criteria to encompass not only detection but also localization and characterization of the embolic events.

ACKNOWLEDGMENTS

This article was partially financed by Fundação para a Ciência e a Tecnologia.

REFERENCES

Aydin, N. (2007). Dwt based adaptive threshold determination in embolic signal detection. *Adaptive Hardware and Systems, NASA/ESA Conference on 0*, 214–219.

Aydin, N. and H.S. Markus (1999). Detection of embolic signals using wavelet transform. In *NSIP*, pp. 774–778.

Chui, C.K. (1992). *An Introduction to Wavelets*, Volume 1. Academic Press.

Daubechies, I. (1992). *Ten Lectures on Wavelets* (Sixth ed.). Society for Industrial and Applied Mathematics.

Evans, D.H. and W.N. McDicken (1992). *Doppler Ultrasound: Physics, Instrumentation, and Clinical Applications* (Second ed.). John Wiley and Sons.

Leiria, A. (2005). *Spectral Analysis of Embolic Signals*. Ph. D. thesis, University of Algarve, Portugal.

Leiria, A., M.M.M. Moura, J. Solano, D.H. Evans, and M.G. Ruano (2004, September). Middle cerebral artery blood flow: Accurate time-frequecy evaluation. In *Anais do III CLAEB'2004/XIX CBEB'2004—Conferência Latino-Americana de Engenharia Biomédica, João Pessoa, Brasil*, pp. 1095–1098.

Markus, H.S., A. Loh, and M.M. Brown (1993). Computerized detection of cerebral emboli and discrimination from artifact using doppler ultra-sound.

Matos, S., A. Leiria, and M.G. Ruano (2000, July). Blood flow parameters evaluation using wavelets transforms. In *Proceedings of World Congress on Medical Physics and Biomedical Engineering*.

Wang, Y. and P.J. Fish (1995, 20–23). Arterial doppler signal simulation by time domain processing. In *Engineering in Medicine and Biology Society, 1995., IEEE 17th Annual Conference*, Volume 2, pp. 999–1000 vol.2.

Computational Vision and Medical Image Processing – Tavares & Natal Jorge (eds)
© *2012 Taylor & Francis Group, London, ISBN 978-0-415-68395-1*

Comparison between some time-frequency analysis methods on electromyography (EMG) signal

H.A. Weiderpass
Santo André Foundation, Santo André, São Paulo, Brazil

C.G.F. Pachi & J.F. Yamamoto
ANSP—Academic Network at São Paulo, São Paulo, Brazil

I.C.N. Sacco, A. Hamamoto & A.N. Onodera
Department of Physical Therapy, Speech and Occupational Therapy, School of Medicine, USP, Brazil

ABSTRACT: There are several researches about an efficient method for the analysis and classification of electromyography (EMG) signals and using of wavelets is a promising approach for determining the spectral distribution of the signal intensity at any time. This study compared some time-frequency analysis methods for investigating the EMG activity of the thigh and calf muscles during gait among non-diabetic subjects and diabetic neuropathic patients and, using Adaptive Optimal Kernel (AOK) and Discrete Wavelet Transform (DWT) it also attempted to verify if there are EMG alterations in lower limbs muscles during gait related to the diabetic neuropathy.

1 BACKGROUND

The Fourier transform has revolutionized signal processing and its applications to various disciplines permitting its users to transcend the burdens of time series analyses and view energy content in terms of harmonics. Perhaps, its inability to handle no stationary phenomenon has proven problematic. As the Fourier transform decomposes a signal by a linear combination of projections onto an infinite-duration trigonometric basis, it is unable to capture local features, that is, as a result of the infinite extent of the Fourier integral, analysis give us time-averaged results (Kijewski-Correa and Kareem, 2006). Thus, it contains only globally averaged information and so has the potential to obscure transient or location specific features within the signal, challenging analysts to explore the use of time-frequency transformations with fixed windows or kernels, but it perform well only for a limited classes of signals. Representations with signal-dependent kernels can overcome this limitation (Jones and Baraniuk, 1995).

If $P(t,w)$ is a bilinear time-frequency representation, then

$$P(t,w) = \frac{1}{4\pi^2} \iint A(\theta,\tau)\Phi(\theta,\tau)e^{-j\theta t - j\tau w} d\theta d\tau. \quad (1)$$

$$A(\theta,\tau) = \int s\left(t + \frac{\tau}{2}\right)s^*\left(t - \frac{\tau}{2}\right)e^{j\theta t} dt. \quad (2)$$

where $A(\theta,\tau)$ is the ambiguity function and $\Phi(\theta,\tau)$ is the general kernel term.

An attractive kernel should have the following properties: a) it should permit low-pass frequencies to suppress cross-components and noise in the Discrete Fourier Transform (DFT); b) it should be smooth to reduce ringing artifacts in the DFT; c) it should take a functional form for which an optimization problem can be easily solved. A functional form that satisfies all of above requirements is a Radially Gaussian Kernel (RGK). A RGK is a two-dimensional function that is Gaussian along any radial profile:

$$\Phi(\theta,\tau) = e^{-\frac{\theta^2 + \tau^2}{2\sigma^2(\psi)}} \quad (3)$$

The function $\sigma(\psi)$ controls the 'spread' of the Gaussian at radial angle ψ. The term $\sigma(\psi)$ is the spread function. The angle ψ is determinate by:

$$\psi = \arctan(\tau/\theta). \quad (4)$$

The spread function determines the basic shape of the equal-energy contours of its corresponding kernel. If $\sigma(\psi)$ is smooth, then $\Phi(\theta,\tau)$ is also smooth. A RGK is a generalization of a two-dimensional lowpass Gaussian kernel. Since the shape of a RGK is completely parameterized by the one-dimensional function $\sigma(\psi)$, finding the optimal radially Gaussian kernel for a signal is equivalent to finding the optimal spread function $\sigma_{opt}(\psi)$ for the signal .

By controlling the volume under the optimal kernel, is controlled the tradeoff between cross-components suppression and smearing of the auto-components. An iterative step-project algorithm is used to compute the adaptive optimal kernel (Baraniuk and Jones, 1993).

Another possibility indicated nowadays is wavelet transform. It makes possible to detect small, transient signals, even if they are hidden in large waves (Grossmann et al, 1987). The continuous wavelet transform (CWT) of a signal $x(t) \in L^2(\mathbb{R})$ is defined as the inner product between the signal and the wavelet functions $\psi_{a,b}(t)$

$$W_\psi x(a,b) \equiv C_{a,b} = \langle x(t), \psi_{a,b}(t) \rangle \tag{5}$$

where $C_{a,b}$ are the wavelet coefficients and $\psi_{a,b}(t)$ are the dilated (contracted) and shifted versions of a unique wavelet function $\psi(t)$

$$\psi_{a,b}(t) = |a|^{-1/2} \psi\left(\frac{t-b}{a}\right) \tag{6}$$

(a,b are the scale and translations parameters, respectively). The CWT gives a decomposition of $x(t)$ in different scales, tending to maximum at those scales and time localizations where the wavelet best resembles $x(t)$ and on the other hand, dilated versions will match low frequency oscillations.

The CWT gives a decomposition of $x(t)$ in different scales, tending to maximum at those scales and time localizations where the wavelet best resembles $x(t)$ and on the other hand, dilated versions will match low frequency oscillations. This procedure is redundant and not efficient for algorithm implementation. In consequence, it is more practical to define the wavelet transform only at discrete scales a and discrete times b by choosing the set of parameters $\{a_j = 2^j, b_{j,k} = 2^j k\}$, with $j,k \in Z$.

2 METHODS

Thus, considering only the wavelet transform in discrete scales and discrete time units, we decided to investigate the behavior of the EMG signal using Discrete Wavelet Transform (DWT).

The discrete wavelet family (Quiroga, et al., 2001) (Wang and Gao, 2003) is defined as:

$$\psi_{j,k}(t) = 2^{-j/2} \psi(2^{-j} t - k) \quad j,k \in Z \tag{7}$$

In analogy with equation (5) the dyadic wavelet transform is defined as

$$W_\psi x(j,k) \equiv C_{j,k} = \langle x(t), \psi_{j,k}(t) \rangle \tag{8}$$

For well defined wavelets it can be inverted, thus giving the *reconstruction* of $x(t)$

$$x(t) = \sum_{j,k} C_{j,k}(t) \overset{\Lambda}{\psi}_{j,k}(t) \ j,k \in Z \tag{9}$$

The biological signal was decomposed into wavelet coefficients (Weiderpass, 2008). The information given by the dyadic wavelet transform can be organized according to a hierarchical scheme called multiresolution analysis (Mallat, 1989). Denoting by W_j the subspaces of L^2 generated by the wavelets $\psi_{j,k}$ for each level j, the space L^2 can be decomposed as a direct sum of subspaces W_j

$$L^2 = \sum_{j \in Z} W_j \tag{10}$$

Being defined the subspaces

$$V_j = W_{j+1} \oplus W_{j+2} \oplus ..., \quad j \in Z \tag{11}$$

The subspaces V_j are a multiresolution approximation of L^2 and they are generated by scalings and translations of a single function $\phi_{j,k} = \phi(2^{-j}n-k)$ called the scaling function. Then, for the subspaces V_j there are complementary subspaces W_j, namely:

$$V_{j-1} = V_j \oplus W_j, \quad j \in Z \tag{12}$$

A discretely sampled signal $x(n) \equiv a_0(n)$ with finite energy can be successively decomposed with the following recursive scheme:

$$a_{j-1}(n) = a_j(n) + d_j(n) \tag{13}$$

where the terms $a_j(n) = \sum_k a_{j-1}(k)\phi_{j,k}(n) \in V_j$ give the coarser representation of the signal and $d_j(n) = \sum_k a_{j-1}(k)\psi_{j,k}(n) \in W_j$ give details for each scale $j = 0,1,...,N$. For any resolution level $N > 0$ the decomposition level of the signal is

$$x(n) \equiv a_0(n) = d_1(n) + d_2(n) + \cdots + d_N(n) + a_N(n) \tag{14}$$

This method gives a decomposition of the signal that can be implemented with very efficient algorithms due to recursiveness of the decomposition. Moreover, Mallat (Mallat, 1989) showed that each detail (d_j) and approximation (a_j) signal can be obtained from the previous approximation (a_{j-1}) by convolution with FIR or truncated IIR high-pass and low-pass filters, respectively. A finite impulse response (FIR) filter is a type of a signal processing filter whose impulse response (or response to any finite length input) is of finite duration, because it settles to zero in finite time. This is in contrast to infinite impulse response (IIR) filters, which have internal feedback and may continue to respond indefinitely (usually decaying).

3 DATA

Frequency and energy were chosen for representing the biological signal and studying the electrical activity of the Vastus Lateralis (VL), Lateral Gastrocnemius (LG) and Tibialis Anterior (TA) muscles of diabetic patients and non-diabetic individuals (control) during the whole gait cycle. Figure 1, below, shows the position of electrodes and foot-switches for obtain the EMG signal for studying both groups of individuals. Peroneus Longus (PL) muscle was not considered in this study because had been detected interferences from other muscles in its signals of frequency and energy.

The electromyography (EMG) signals were decomposed using AOK and discrete wavelet transform. Initial evaluations show similar results in both the adaptive kernel analysis and by DWT (Figure 2). However, the computational processing times are very different. The adaptive kernel is up to 1000 times slower than the DWT. Thus, the choice fell on the latter.

The discrete wavelet transform was used for composing the EMG signal into six levels of details (d1–d6) and one residual (a6), choosing "gaus4" as mother function [MATLAB® Wavelet Toolbox]. Since the sampling rate is 2000 Hz, each scale covers the frequency band mentioned in Table 1.

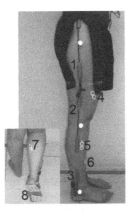

Figure 1. Position of EMG electrodes and footswitches on the patient: (1) electrogoniometer hip, (2) electrogoniometer knee, (3) electrogoniometer ankle, (4) electrode placed in the VL (5) electrode placed in PL, (6) electrode placed in the TA, (7) electrode placed in LG, (8) footswitches positioned in the rearfoot and forefoot.

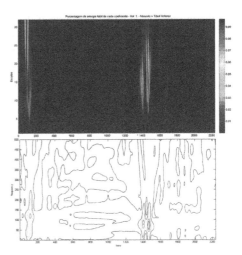

Figure 2. EMG signal decomposed via CWT (upper side) and AOK (lower side).

Table 1. Levels for multiresolution decomposition and their respective range frequency.

Scale denomination	Range frequency
First scale (d1)	500–1000 Hz
Second scale (d2)	250–500 Hz
Third scale (d3)	125–250 Hz
Fourth scale (d4)	62.5–125 Hz
Fifth scale (d5)	31.3–62.5 Hz
Sixth scale (d6)	15.6–31.3 Hz
Residual scale (a6)	0–15.6 Hz

After that, it was determined how the energy, $[W_\psi x(a,b)]^2$, is distributed in the various levels of the decomposed signal. Using this strategy, the signals "control" and "diabetic" was compared statistically.

4 RESULTS

The present study aimed at investigating the behavior of the variables frequency and energy to study the muscles VL, LG, TA in diabetic and non-diabetic group during gait and comparing these results with previous studies. The authors proposed by using discrete wavelet transform to obtain intensity patterns, which reflect the spectral distribution at any given time point.

Inter-group comparisons of the EMG data were performed using the t-test for independent samples and they showed evidences that the mean of energy of the VL muscle was statistically different and also, the LG muscle presented both energy and frequency significantly different between both groups ($p < 0.05$).

Furthermore, the Chi-square analysis of discrete signals in stance phase from LG muscle showed significant differences (p < 0.05) when comparing Propulsion phase and Non-Propulsion phases (weight acceptance, midstance and swing). Similarly, VL muscle showed significant differences (p < 0.05) when comparing stance (weight acceptance, midstance, propulsion phases) and swing phase.

These findings are important for a better understanding of the biomechanical changes that affect the gait function of diabetic neuropathic subjects. Nonetheless, further complementary studies using Principal Components Analysis (PCA) and Discriminant Analysis were proposed to classify variables into groups and to understand the underlying energy and frequency structure.

PCA was used from a multivariate perspective whose the objective is the analysis of the inter-subject variability of a set of continuous waveforms (Olney et al., 1998).

After the normalization, this set of variables can be defined one for each percentage of the gait cycle, obtaining a reduced set of principal components (PC's) that quantifies the differences between the analyzed time series across individuals and had made possible to compare diabetic and non-diabetic patients (Epifanio et al., 2008; Chester and Wrigley, 2008).

Therefore, considering only components with an eigenvalue greater than 1 (The Kaiser criterion), we analyzed the first two principal components that explain approximately 52% of the whole variance of the original data. (Fig. 3). Subsequently, these components were rotated to eliminate medium-range loading and obtain a clear pattern of loadings.

Varimax rotation was used and the component loadings larger than 0.55 had been taken into consideration. Factor loadings can be interpreted as correlations between the respective variables and

factors; thus they represent the most important information for the interpretation of factors (Tables 2a and 2b).

Based on the significant high loads we can see that the Factor 1 has higher loads to the frequencies, while the Factor 2 has higher loads to the energy. In addition, the factor loadings of the two groups of patients also present differences if compared.

In the diabetic group, the Factor 1 made three groups with positive factor loadings that indicate some variation in the same direction. Factor 2 has only two significant loads in opposite directions. In the control group, there are also three significant loads in Factor 1 but for another group of variables and the Factor 2 has only a significant and opposite load.

Patterns of variables are much clearer in Figure 4, as expected, the first factor is marked by high loadings on the frequency of the muscles and the second factor is marked by high loadings on the energy. We could thus conclude that, the signals of muscles measured by DWT are composed of those two aspects and it is useful for detecting differences between these groups of patients.

These results permits us to cluster variables that are related and, in this way, to simplify the complex

Table 2a. Factor loadings (Varimax normalized) for diabetic patients. Extraction: Principal components (marked loadings are >0,55).

Variables	Factor 1	Factor 2
VL_d_Hz	0,547110	0,220491
VL_d_Energ	−0,257705	−0,699488
LG_d_Hz	0,754386	−0,219501
LG_d_Energ	−0,247089	0,808755
TA_d_Hz	0,550789	−0,077828
TA_d_Energ	0,610670	0,338602
Expl.Var	1,672179	1,360873
Prp.Totl	0,278696	0,226812

Table 2b. Factor loadings (Varimax normalized) for non-diabetic patients. Extraction: Principal components (marked loadings are >0,55).

Variables	Factor 1	Factor 2
VL_c_Hz	0,610326	−0,170423
VL_c_Energ	0,556044	0,104834
LG_c_Hz	0,644845	0,271654
LG_c_Energ	−0,069240	−0,854561
TA_c_Hz	−0,007806	0,516597
TA_c_Energ	0,561587	−0,403715
Expl.Var	1,417742	1,273962
Prp.Totl	0,236290	0,212327

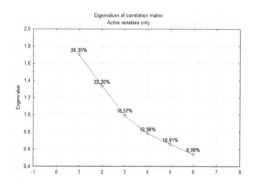

Figure 3. Screen graph can be used to distinguish PCs that explain large amounts of the variation seen in self the population from those that represent random effects and account for little of the variation.

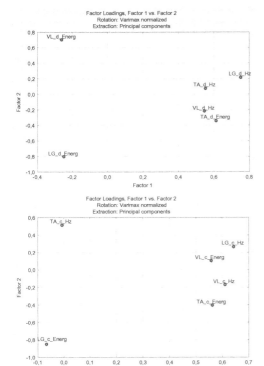

Figure 4. First factor (x-axis) represents high loadings on the frequency and the second factor (y-axis) is marked by high loadings on the energy. It is possible to observe different clusters between diabetics and non-diabetics group of patients.

picture presented by the main variables resulting from gait analysis.

5 DISCUSSION

Previous studies of EMG activity in diabetic neuropathic subjects found that the gastrocnemius, soleus, vastus lateralis muscles, and most importantly, of the tibialis anterior muscle present a delayed activation during gait, which may be associated with an earlier forefoot contact with the ground and higher loads to the lower limbs, especially at the foot (Abboud et al., 2000; Sacco and Amadio, 2003).

First, a delayed activation of the vastus lateralis was mentioned during the weight acceptance phase that may be indicative of the presence of a deficiency in the shock attenuation mechanisms and, furthermore, it had been found that there is a premature activation of the soleus and medial gastrocnemius, and a prolonged tibialis anterior

activity, leading to aco-contraction of these muscles during mid-stance in a possible attempt to improve foot stability (Akashi et al, 2008).

Principal Components Analysis confirmed that frequency and energy can represent important variables for studying the components of gait analysis.

Although it is still necessary to clarify the reasons for muscle activity patterns alterations and their relationship to diabetic neuropathy itself, we can see that differences into patterns of energy and frequency emerge among LG, VL and TA in diabetic and non diabetic patients.

In addition, Adaptive Optimal Kernel (AOK) and Discrete Wavelet Transform (DWT) showed both good methods for the analysis and classification of EMG signals. However, this study demonstrated that DWT provides significant advantage in computational timing which makes it the best choice for determining the spectral distribution of signal intensity.

REFERENCES

Abboud R.J., Rowley D.I., Newton R.W., 2000. Lower limb muscle dysfunction may contribute to foot ulceration in diabetic patients. Clin. Biomech. 15, 37–45.

Akashi P.M.H., Sacco I.C.N., Watari R., Henning E., 2008. Clinical Biomechanics 23, 584–592,.

Baraniuk R.G., Jones D.L., 1993. Signal-dependent time-frequency analysis using a radially Gaussian kernel, Signal Processing, vol. 32, pp. 263–284.

Chester V.L., Wrigley Allan T., 2008. The identification of age-related differences in kinetic gait parameters using principal component analysis. Clinical Biomechanics, 23; 212–220.

Epifanio I., Ávila C., Page A., Atienza C., 2008. Analysis of multiple waveforms by means of functional principal component analysis: normal versus pathological patterns in sit-to-stand movement. Med Biol Eng Comput, 46:551–561.

Grossmann A., Holschneider M., Kronald R.M., Morlet J., 1987. Detection of abrupt changes in sound signals with the help of wavelet transform, In: Inverse problems. An interdisciplinary study: Advances in electronics and electron physics Supplement, Academic Press, vol. 19, pp. 298–306.

Jones D.L., Baraniuk R.G., 1995. An Adaptive Optimal-Kernel Time-Frequency Representation, IEEE Transactions on Signal Processing, vol. 43, pp. 2361–2371, October.

Kijewski-Correa T., Kareem A., 2006. Efficacy of Hilbert And Wavelet Transforms for Time-Frequency Analysis, Journal on Engineering Mechanics, pp. 1037–1049, October.

Mallat S. 1989. A theory for multiresolution signal decomposition: the wavelet representation. IEEE Trans. Pattern Anal. Machine Intell,. 2 (7), 674–693.

Olney, S.J., Griffin, M.P., McBride, I.D., 1998. Multivariate examination of data from gait analysis of persons with stroke. Physical Therapy 78 (8), 814–828.

Quiroga R.Q., Sakowitz O.W., Basar E., 2001. Schürmann M. "Wavelet Transform in the analysis of the frequency composition of evoked potentials". Brain Research Protocols, 8, 16–24.

Sacco I.C.N., Amadio A.C., 2003. Influence of the diabetic neuropathy on the behavior of electromyographic and sensorial responses in treadmill gait. Clin. Biomech. 18 (5), 426–434.

Von Tscharner V., Goepfert B., Nigg N.B., 2003. Changes in EMG signals for the muscle tibialis anterior while running barefoot or with shoes resolved by non-linearly scaled wavelets. J. Biomechanics, 36, 1169–76.

Wang C, Gao R.X., 2003. Wavelet Transform with spectral post-processing for enhanced feature extraction. IEEE Trans. of Instrumentation and measurement. 52 (4), 1296–1301.

Weiderpass H.A., Yamamoto J.F., Salomão S.R., Berezowsky A., Pereira J.M., Costa M.A. & Burattini M.N., 2008. Steady-State sweep visual evoked potential processing denoised by wavelet transform. Progress in Biomedical Optics and Imaging—Proceedings of SPIE, 6917, paper 69171A.

Yavuzer G., Yetkin I., Toruner F.B., Koca N., Bolukbasi N., 2006. Gait deviations of patients with diabetes mellitus: looking beyond peripheral neuropathy. Eura. Medicophys. 42 (2), 127–133.

Computational Vision and Medical Image Processing – Tavares & Natal Jorge (eds)
© 2012 Taylor & Francis Group, London, ISBN 978-0-415-68395-1

A new interface for manual segmentation of dermoscopic images

P.M. Ferreira
Faculdade de Engenharia, Universidade do Porto, Portugal

T. Mendonça
Faculdade de Ciências, Universidade do Porto, Portugal

P. Rocha
Faculdade de Engenharia, Universidade do Porto, Portugal

J. Rozeira
Hospital Pedro Hispano, Matosinhos, Portugal

ABSTRACT: Dermoscopy (dermatoscopy, skin surface microscopy) is a non-invasive diagnostic technique for the *in vivo* observation of pigmented skin lesions, allowing a better visualization of the surface and subsurface structures. In the last few years, several computer-aided diagnosis systems of digital dermoscopic images have been introduced, since the interpretation of dermoscopic images is time consuming and subjective (even for trained dermatologists), and also to reduce the learning-curve of non-expert dermatologists. The validation of these algorithms requires a ground-truth database of manually segmented images. Therefore, this situation calls up for the development of new tools that can support the manual segmentation, making this task easier and faster to the dermatologists. In this paper, we present a graphical user interface for computer-aided manual segmentation of dermoscopic images that can easily be adapted to other medical images. This tools allows building up a reliable ground truth database of manually segmented images. Besides the manual segmentation of the lesion, this tool allows performing the segmentation of other specific regions of interest, which are essential for the development of newly computer-aided diagnosis systems.

1 INTRODUCTION

Currently, dermoscopy, also known to as dermatoscopy, epiluminescence microscopy, or skin surface microscopy, is clinically the most relevant *in vivo* imaging technique for melanoma diagnosis. Dermoscopy is a non-invasive technique for the observation of pigmented skin lesions, allowing a better visualization of the surface and subsurface structures, and the recognition of morphologic structures not visible by the naked eye (Argenziano 2000).

The dermoscopic diagnosis of pigmented skin lesions is currently performed by trained dermatologists based on a set on pattern analysis criteria such as the ABCD rule or the seven point check list. Both approaches involve a visual analysis of the skin lesion in which the lesions are evaluated according to several properties, such as the asymmetry, the border irregularity, the color, the diameter, and the presence of atypical vascular pattern or irregular diffuse pigmentation (Argenziano 1998).

The standard approach in dermoscopic image analysis has usually three stages: (i) image segmentation, (ii) feature extraction and feature selection, (iii) lesion classification (Mendonca 2007). The first step is one of the most important because the accuracy of the subsequent steps depends on image segmentation which permits the extraction of the lesion from the surrounding skin.

However, segmentation is a challenging task due to several reasons. Among these are the great variety of lesion shapes, sizes, and colors along with different skin types and textures. In addition, some lesions have irregular and fuzzy boundaries and in some case there is a low contrast between the lesion and the surrounding skin. Moreover, some images contain intrinsic cutaneous features such as black frames, skin lines, blood vessel hairs, and air bubbles (Celebi 2009) (Silveira 2009).

Nowadays some commercial applications are already available for the automatic (or semi-automatic) segmentation of dermoscopic images. However they are not yet widely used as they are not considered to be trustworthy. This situation calls up for the development of more sophisticated automatic technique, but also for the implementation of automatic tools to support manual segmentation.

The tool presented in this paper will allow building up a reliable ground truth database of manually segmented images to be used with multiple purposes. Among these are the assessment of the accuracy of newly developed automatic segmentation methods, as well as the use in medical training. Besides the identification of the lesion borders, this tool also allows marking other specific regions of interest, such as regions with typical or atypical vascular networks, dots, globules, star burst patterns, etc, whose recognition is crucial for further classification.

2 INTERFACE DESCRIPTION

This application allows performing the manual segmentation of dermoscopic images and storing the result of segmentation. For this, the user has a set of tools to be used sequentially to achieve the desired result.

The main functionalities of this interface are:

- Image upload and display
- Manual segmentation
- Boundary reshaping
- Storage of segmented image

The interface was implemented in a MATLAB environment (7.9.0 R2009b) because of its image processing toolbox and graphical facilities.

2.1 Image upload and display

With this application it is possible to open one image or several images at once. For this, it is necessary to select the option "Load images" in the "File" menu, or simply press the button 1 on the toolbar, Figure 1. Then a dialog box appears that enables the user to browse and select the image to be segmented. To open multiple images, simply press CTRL key and select the desired images.

The loaded image is displayed on the left side of the interface. If several images have been loaded, the user can easily change the image that is being displayed through the slider button, Figure 1.

2.2 Manual segmentation

In order to perform the manual segmentation, this application allows to draw a freehand region of interest on the loaded image. It is important to note that the manual segmentation can be performed using a pen tablet or a mouse. The user can choose between performing the manual segmentation of the lesion or other regions of interest through the radio buttons on the panel "Segmentation".

To achieve the manual segmentation it is necessary to select in the "Tools" menu the option

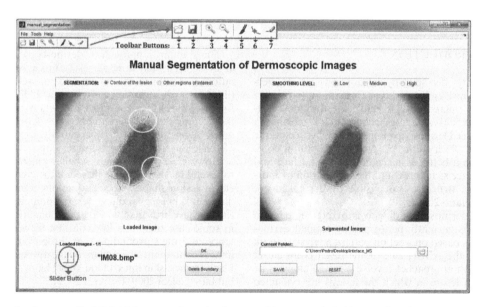

Figure 1. **Image on the left:** initial contour drawn by the user, with some undesirable extra lines (marked with circles). **Image on the right:** final contour after morphological filtering. Note that the final contour is smoother than the initial and without undesirable extra lines. **Toolbar Buttons:** 1-"Load Images"; 2-"Save as"; 3-"Zoom in"; 4-"Zoom out"; 5-"Manual segmentation"; 6-"Pointwise boundary reshaping"; 7-"Local boundary reshaping".

"Manual Segmentation", or simply press button 5 on the toolbar, Figure 1. Then, the user must click and drag the pen tablet to draw the contour of the lesion (or the contour of other regions of interest).

When the user confirms the segmentation, the image with the final contour is displayed on the right side of the interface, Figure 1. Note that the user can only confirm and complete the segmentation when a closed contour is drawn. When theuser lifts the pen from the tablet before closing the contour, the contour remains open. However, while the contour is open the user has the possibility of drawing until he/she completes and closes it.

To obtain the final contour from the initial one (drawn by user), a binary mask of the initial contour is first created, and then a morphological filtering is applied to this binary mask. The purpose of morphological filtering is smoothing and removing extra lines that not belong to the contour. These lines may arise when the contour is drawn by means of multiple segments, especially at the points of intersection of these segments, Figure 1.

Basically, morphological filtering is divided into three stages (i) morphological erosion; (ii) selection of the biggest binary object from the image and (iii) morphological dilation. The user also has the possibility to select the degree of smoothing between low, medium and high. In each of these morphological operations a flat disk-shaped structuring element is used, with a specific radius for each smoothing level (low: radius 1; medium: radius 3; high: radius 7).

The manual segmentation of other regions of interest can be done in a very similar way to the manual segmentation of the lesion. The main difference is that the contours of all segmented regions are shown on the same image with a different color. For thispurpose, the user must select the "Other regions of interest" radio button in the panel "Segmentation".

2.3 Boundary reshaping

Even after finishing the manual segmentation it is possible to make some adjustments in the contour, if necessary. Two distinct methods were implemented to reshape the contour previously done, namely "Pointwise boundary reshaping" and "Local boundary reshaping".

2.3.1 Pointwise boundary reshaping

This method must be used to make small adjustments in the contour, because the reshaping is done point-by-point. For this the user must select the option "Pointwise Boundary Reshaping" in the "Tools" menu, or simply press button 6 on the toolbar, Figure 1. Forthwith the boundary turns red with some control points. From these points it is possible to change the shape of the contour. For this, the user must click and drag the control points to their new positions, Figure 2.

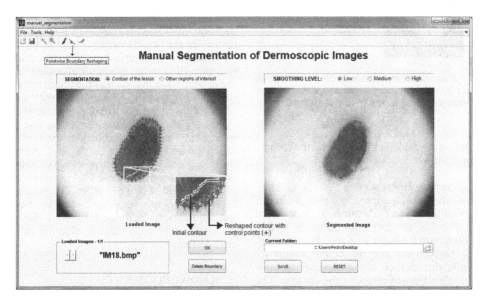

Figure 2. **Image on the left:** Initial contour (solid line) and the reshaped contour (with control points). **Image on the right:** final contour.

Table 1. Interactive behaviors supported by "reshaping the boundary" functionality.

Interactive behavior	Description
Boundary reshaping	Move the pointer over a control point. The pointer changes to a circle. Then, click and drag the control point to its new position.
Adding a new control point	Move the pointer over the boundary and press the **A** key. Click the left mouse button to create a new control point at that position on the boundary.

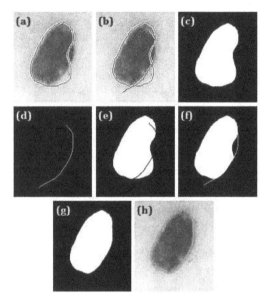

Figure 3. Local boundary reshaping: (a) Initial contour; (b) Initial contour and a new line to reshape the contour; (c)–(g): intermediate steps; and (h) Final contour.

The following table lists the interactive behaviors supported by this tool.

2.3.2 Local boundary reshaping

Local boundary reshaping must be used when it is necessary to make great adjustments to the initial contour. For this, the user must select the option "Local Boundary Reshaping" in the "Tools" menu, or simply press button 7 on the toolbar, Figure 1.

Basically, this method allows the user to draw a line to define the new shape of the contour. The line must intersect the initial contour at least in two points to form a closed contour. This can be used to increase or reduce the size of the initial contour.

Note that it is possible to increase and reduce the size of the contour with a single line, Figure 3.

The final contour Figure 3(h) is obtained through a set of logical, arithmetical, and morphological operations:

- First, a binary image from the initial contour and another binary image from the new line are created, Figure 3(c) and Figure 3(d) respectively;
- Image subtraction between image (c) and (d), Figure 3(e);
- Selection of the biggest binary object from image (e), and application of a logical OR operator between image (e) and (d), Figure 3(f);
- Application of a morphological filling in order to fill the image holes, and then a morphological close is used to remove the extra lines, Figure 3(g).

2.4 Storage of segmented image

Finally, this interface also allows storing the result of manual segmentation. The segmentation result is saved as a binary image, where the segmented object corresponds to the white pixels and the background to the black ones.

3 CONCLUSIONS

A graphical user interface was presented in this paper, for manual segmentation of dermoscopic images. This tool will allow constructing a ground truth database, in a very simple and fast way, to be used in the assessment of the automatic segmentation methods. Moreover, this tool also allows segmenting other specific regions of interest, and can be used in medical training.

The developed interface is very simple and intuitive, providing to the user a set of tools to achieve the desired objective, such as the image upload and display, the manual segmentation, the boundary reshaping, and the storage of segmented image.

Besides the manual segmentation, one of the most interesting tool is the boundary reshaping, with which the user can correct the shape of the contour previously done. For this purpose, two distinct methods were implemented, namely "Pointwise boundary reshaping" and "Local boundary reshaping".

This prototype version was set up based on the requirements and suggestions of dermatologists and is currently under evaluation in clinical environment.

ACKNOWLEDGMENTS

The authors would like to thank Fundação para a Ciência e Tecnologia who partially funded the research present on this paper through the project ADDI (reference PTDC/SAU-BEB/103471/2008) and to the project team.

REFERENCES

Argenziano, G. & Fabbrocini, G. (1998). Epilu-minescence microscopy for the diagnosis of doubtful melanocytic skin lesions: Comparison of the abcd rule of derma-toscopy and a new 7-point checklist based on pattern analysis. *Arch. Dermatol 134*(12), 1563–1570.

Argenziano, G. & Soyer, H. (2000). Dermoscopy, an interactive atlas. EDRA Medical Publishing. [ONLINE]. Available at: http://www. dermoscopy.org.

Celebi, M. & Schaefer, G. (2009, March). Lesion border detection in dermoscopy images. *Comput Med Imaging Graph 33*(2), 148–153.

Mendonca, T. & Marcal, A.R.S. (2007). Comparison of segmentation methods for automatic diagnosis of dermoscopy images. *Proc. IEEE Int. Conf. Engineering in Medicine and Biology Society*, 6572–6575.

Silveira, M. & Nascimento, J.C. (2009, February). Comparison of segmentation methods for melanoma diagnosis in dermoscopy images. *IEEE Journal of Selected Topics in Signal Processing 3(1)*.

InVesalius-An open-source imaging application

Thiago F. de Moraes, Paulo H.J. Amorim, Fábio S. Azevedo & Jorge V.L. da Silva
Center for Information Technology Renato Archer, Campinas—SP, Brazil

ABSTRACT: This work presents *InVesalius*, an open-source imaging. Initially, the historical context and motivation for its development are discussed. Then, the software structure and some development aspects are commented, as well as InVesalius main tools and applications. At the end, the results of a survey realized within the user community are presented.

1 INTRODUCTION

Medical imaging aims at providing physicians the capability of viewing the human body internally in a non-invasive way and also of making more accurate diagnoses. Even though the X-ray technique has been available since the early 20th century, three-dimensional medical images appeared only in 1972 with the invention of *Computerized Tomography* (CT) (Yoo 2004).

Besides X-ray, which is applied to conventional radiography and computerized tomography, another way of acquiring images from the body's interior is *Magnetic Resonance* (MRI). MRI applies a strong magnetic field in conjunction with radio-frequency waves. Nowadays, the mentioned techniques generate images in digital format. These images usually comply with the DICOM (*Digital Imaging and Communications in Medicine*) standard. A DICOM image contains voxels and meta-information such as the patient's name, equipment information and space-related image positioning (in the case of CT and MRI) (Pianykh 2007).

According to the DICOM standard, each CT or MRI image represents a body "slice". The 3D reconstruction is done by stacking these slices and interpolating the spaces among them to form a volume.

Most of the CT and MRI equipment manufacturers sell 3D reconstruction software separately, at prohibitive prices for the current reality of the Brazilian public health system. Even in the first years of the 21st century, free software for 3D reconstruction was not available. Nowadays, despite the existence of free software for this kind of application, various desirable aspects still lack. Some applications provide graphical interfaces that are not user-friendly. Others, despite being free software, require machines with high computational power to be executed. And there also are those that depend on a specific execution platform.

For more than a decade, Center for Information Technology Renato Archer (CTI) has rapid prototyping equipment (3D printers) and keeps as one of its goals the production of physical models to help medical professionals in surgery planning. Facing this scenario, in 2001 CTI started the development of the *InVesalius* software. Today in its third version, this medical image visualization and 3D reconstruction software is multi-platform and multi-language. Focusing on usability, it runs on conventional personal computers without the need for high computational power.

2 INVESALIUS DEVELOPMENT

InVesalius is free software based on the GNU Public License (GPL) version 2. This allows researchers and developers from universities and research centers from all over the world to cooperate in the software development and apply their work results and interests on it. Figure 1 shows a screenshot from InVesalius.

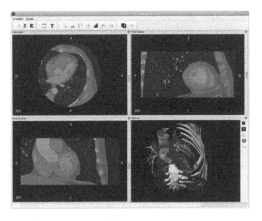

Figure 1. InVesalius software.

InVesalius code development is managed using the *Subversion* (Subversion 2011) version control tool. Basically, this tool allows to track and control code modifications and their authors. Within the InVesalius development team, the approach is to first document new features and bugs, and then to submit them to development or correction. This is done not only by developers, but by users as well, in a cooperative manner.

3 STRUCTURE

InVesalius has been developed using the *Python* programming language (Lutz 2009). Python is a multi-paradigm language, since it allows the use of Object Oriented, Procedural and Functional paradigms. In the particular case of InVesalius, Object Orientation was the most widely used paradigm; only in a few cases the functional and procedural paradigms were applied. Many different software libraries are also used and they will be mentioned in this text.

The use of InVesalius begins with the input data. First, the user selects the medical image files to work with, which can come in DICOM or *Analyze* formats. InVesalius currently supports Computerized Tomography (CT) files and Magnetic Resonance Imaging (MRI) files. The *GDCM* (GDCM 2011) (Nibabel 2011) library is used to support the DICOM (Pianykh 2007) format, and the *Nibabel* library is used for the Analyze files. It is important to mention that the use of the GDCM library allowed to support "non-standard" DICOM files and also compressed files, which are becoming common due to their reduced size.

The input images are converted to a three-dimensional matrix. This matrix is kept in a *memmap* structure in a disk file and mapped into physical memory (RAM) by a *mmap* system call, common to various operating systems. Thus, only the necessary matrix data are kept in memory at each time. Whenever other chunk of data is required, it is brought from the disk file to RAM on demand. This strategy enables physical examination files with a large number of slices to occupy less memory than if all their data were read into memory at once. The memmap structure is provided by the *Numpy* library (Oliphant 2006). Numpy is a numerical library for Python that provides matrices, vectors and mathematical operations on these structures. Powerful and easy to use, it allows the access to matrix data using indices instead of explicit method or function calls.

After opening the images, the user can visualize the examination and access a number of tools. It is possible to view the slices in the axial, sagittal or coronal orientations and also their corresponding three-dimensional reconstruction. It is worth mentioning that the use of a three-dimensional matrix made the access to different orientations easier because of the appropriate use of the matrix indices.

The *wxPython* library (Rappin and Dunn 2006), which is multi-platform, was used to build the InVesalius Graphical User Interface (GUI). wxPython uses the standard graphical interface provided by the platform it executes on. Thus, InVesalius GUI is usually able to keep the "look-and-feel" of a native application, requiring at most minor adjustments.

The *VTK* (Visualization ToolKit) (Schroeder, Martin, Martin, and Lorensen 1998) library was used for 2D and 3D visualization. Since the data are stored in a *memmap* matrix structure, it is necessary to convert them to the VTK structure. This is done only for the examination slices that are being viewed at the moment, i.e., on demand. The VTK library has also been useful in other features, and they will be mentioned in this work.

The importance of using the above mentioned libraries is that they are maintained updated and in the state-of-the-art of implementations.

4 TOOLS

The main tools of InVesalius 3 are described below and some of their applications are also discussed.

4.1 *Measurements*

InVesalius offers tools for linear and angular measurements, both available for 2D slices and for 3D reconstruction as well. The linear measurement tool allows to measure the distance between two points given by the user. Similarly, the angular measurement tool measures the angle between the two line segments determined by 3 points given by the user. These tools are useful, for example, to study modifications caused by a treatment or surgery, by comparing the measurements done before with those done after their execution. The tools may also be used to measure visible structures depicted in the examination images.

4.2 *Segmentation*

Nowadays, InVesalius provides two image segmentation techniques: *threshold* (González and Woods 2008) and *manual*. In the threshold technique, only the voxels with intensities between a minimum value and a maximum value are selected. Manual segmentation is a complement to the threshold technique. It allows the user to perform the interactive selection of voxels that were not selected by threshold, as well as to deselect voxels that were eventually selected by mistake.

4.3 *3D reconstruction*

After segmenting a region of interest from the image, the user is able to perform a 3D reconstruction. This operation is done by executing the *Marching Cubes* (Lorensen and Cline 1987) algorithm, using the implementation available from the VTK library. Using the voxels from the segmented images, the algorithm generates a polygonal surface constituted usually by triangles. This surface may be physically printed by rapid prototyping techniques and then be further applied to surgery planning or even to anatomy teaching.

4.4 *Volumetric visualization*

InVesalius provides an additional tool for 3D reconstruction: the volumetric visualization. This technique

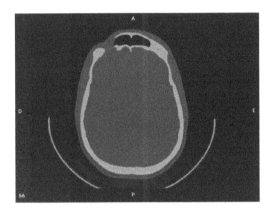

Figure 2.   Segmention.

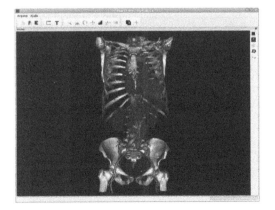

Figure 3.   Volumetric visualization in InVesalius.

allows the assignment of colors and transparency levels to the voxels' values. Thus, it is possible, for instance, to visualize the heart in 3D in shades of red, in conjunction with the bone structure in shades of gray, while the skin is hidden. The volumetric visualization technique used is *Raycasting*. For each pixel on the screen, the path of a light ray from this pixel to a light source is calculated. The final value of each pixel depends on the color and transparency values of the voxels that its light ray has intercepted. Together with the visualization of 2D slices, volumetric visualization is useful, for example, in the preparation of medical reports.

5   USER COMMUNITY

InVesalius, its user community and development are centralized at *Portal do Software Público Brasileiro* (*www.softwarepublico.gov.br*). Today, the community is composed by 4800 members in 71 countries. According to a survey done in February 2011, the community profile is composed in this way: 54% of the users are from the health field; 25% from computer science; 9% from engineering; and 12% from other areas (including veterinary, hospital management, paleontology and others).

6   CONCLUSION

This work presented InVesalius, a free option to proprietary medical visualization and three-dimensional software. Since its conception, InVesalius has been well accepted by its user community in Brazil and abroad. Additionally, a significant part of its community is from outside the medical field, which demonstrates the software versatility and its application to other knowledge domains.

The InVesalius development is a continuous effort. For the future, the main goals involve support to other physical examination formats, support to other image segmentation techniques, new user interaction features and network image transmission.

REFERENCES

GDCM (2011). Grassroots DICOM|download grassroots DICOM soft-ware for free at SourceForge.net. http://sourceforge.net/projects/gdcm/. accessed 29-March-2011.

González, R. and R. Woods (2008). *Digital Image Processing*. Pearson/Prentice Hall.

Lorensen, W.E. and H.E. Cline (1987, August). Marching cubes: A high resolution 3d surface construction algorithm. *SIGGRAPH Comput. Graph. 21*, 163–169.

Lutz, M. (2009). *Learning Python*. Learning Python. O'Reilly.

Nibabel (2011). Neuroimaging in python—NiBabel v1.1.0.dev documentation. http://nipy.sourceforge.net/nibabel/. accessed 29-March-2011.

Oliphant, T. (2006). *A guide to NumPy*. Trelgol Publishing.

Pianykh, O.S. (2007). *Digital Imaging and Communications in Medicine (DICOM)* (1th ed.). Springer Publising.

Rappin, N. and R. Dunn (2006). *wxPython in action*. Manning Pubs Co Series. Manning.

Schroeder, W., K. Martin, K. Martin, and B. Lorensen (1998). *The visualization toolkit*. Prentice Hall PTR.

Subversion (2011). Apache subversion. http://subversion.tigris.org/. accessed 29-March-2011.

Yoo, T.S. (2004). *Insight into Images* (1th ed.). A.K. Petters.

Computational Vision and Medical Image Processing – Tavares & Natal Jorge (eds)
© 2012 Taylor & Francis Group, London, ISBN 978-0-415-68395-1

GPU acceleration of legendre moments as biomarkers of bone tissue

José A. Lachiondo & Manuel Ujaldón
Computer Architecture Department, University of Malaga, Spain

ABSTRACT: Geometric moments are widely used within the image processing field for characterizing textural features aimed to a further clustering or image segmentation. In this paper, we propose Legendre moments as biomarkers for an efficient and accurate classification of bone tissue on images coming from a stem cell regeneration study. After validating their excellent properties in a wide set of vectors of features, we tackle its computational complexity, for this is the main disadvantage to be extensively used in real applications, overall when real-time constraints are imposed. Our solution introduces a novel approach to reduce the workload through a Principal Components Analysis (PCA), which is followed by the high-performance computation of Legendre moments on Graphics Processors (GPUs). The result is a powerful combination to develop a much faster response in contrast with solutions coming from conventional programming on multicore CPU platforms. With more than a six times faster code attained in our experimental studies versus similar methods run on CPU counterparts, our techniques offer a high performance alternative in clinical practice and, additionally, leave the door opened to real-time applications.

Keywords: GPU, CUDA programming, PCA, image classifier, Legendre moments

1 INTRODUCTION

A wide variety of histologically stained images in cell biology require deep analysis to determine both the phenotype and color for the tissue being analyzed. A typical example is cartilage and bone regeneration, where a specific microenvironment has been reported to induce the expression of skeletal matrix proteins, playing a regulatory role in the initiation of cartilage differentiation and the induction of bone-forming cells from pluripotent mesenchymal stem cells (Andrades et al. 2001).

The input data set is obtained from implants on 7 month old male rats. After 17 days of culture, in-vivo stem cells are implanted on animals into demineralized bone matrix or diffusion chambers. Four weeks later, rats are sacrificed, six chambers excised and tissues analyzed biochemically or processed for light microscopy after the appropriate fixation and sectioned at 7μm thickness. From each chamber, approximately 500 slices of tissue sample are obtained, each being a microscopic 1024×1024 RGB color image in TIFF format, for a total storage space of 10 Gbytes. Samples are stained with picrosirius to reveal features of either bone (intense red due to the presence of type I collagen) or cartilage (weak pink, which manifests the abundance of type II collagen), for which a single-color treatment suffices (see Figure 3). Other cases like X-ray images or images captured by an electronic microscope work with gray-scale images,

so our single color techniques may be applied to these areas too.

Our goal in this work analyzes the power of Legendre moments as new biomarkers for tracking such biomedical evolution at image level as a preliminary step for converting the complete analysis process to a semi-automatic task: the medical expert interacts with the computer to attain a number of descriptors and attributes about the images that help to understand the biomedical features.

The motivation of our work also entails two steps forward in performance since these algorithms are characterized by a heavy workload and a vast memory use. First, we apply Principal Components Analysis (PCA) to reduce computational complexity. Second, we exploit the capabilities of Graphics Processing Units (GPUs) with respect to GFLOPS (arithmetic intensity for a fast computation) and GB/sc. (memory bandwidth for a fast data retrieval) as our major keys for a significant reduction in the overall execution time.

2 CONCEPTUAL MODEL

Orthogonal moments of a digital image are useful in pattern recognition, object clustering and classification, motion estimate, coding and reconstruction (Teague 1980). A set of moments usually provides a compact representation for the global features of an image. Within them, Legendre moments offer advantages against other sets of orthogonal moments due to the lower complexity of their computational formulas and for being expressed within the same image space. They may also be useful on image reconstruction applications.

2.1 Legendre moments

In order to define Legendre moments, we first introduce its differential equation, which, in a canonical form, is defined as:

$$(1-x_2)\cdot y'' - 2\cdot x\cdot y' + \lambda\cdot y = 0 \qquad (1)$$

Its general solution is the linear combination of two solutions lineally independent:

$$y(x) = A\cdot y_1(x) + B\cdot y_2(x) \qquad (2)$$

As a particular case, if $\lambda = v\cdot(v+1)$ with $v = n \in N$, one of those two solutions is a Legendre polinomial of n order. In this case, the general solution takes the form:

$$y(x) = A\cdot P_n(x) + B\cdot Q_n(x) \qquad (3)$$

Legendre functions for certain values of v take a polinomial form, with the following expression:

$$P_n(x) = \sum_{k=0}^{\frac{n}{2}} (-1)\frac{(2n-2r)!}{2_n r!(n-2r)!(n-r)!}\cdot x^{n-2r} \qquad (4)$$

Legendre polynomials, $P_n(x)$ are a complete orthogonal set established inside the interval $[-1, 1]$

$$A_{pq} = \int_{-1} + 1 P_p(x)\cdot P_q(x)\cdot dx = \frac{2}{2p+1}\cdot \delta_{pq} \qquad (5)$$

where δ_{pq} is called the Kronecker function, being $\delta_{pq} = 1$, 0 otherwise.

Legendre moments are not invariant to linear transformations or rotation, which makes them less suitable than Zernike moments for certain image analysis applications, but when these drawbacks are overcome, they relax the computational cost against their counterparts (R. Mukundan and Ramakrishnan 1995).

2.2 Principal components analysis

Roughly speaking, we may say that using PCA we identify patterns within a data set in a manner that compiles their similarities and differences. For a large set of variables, p, with a high degree of relation, we may apply PCA to find a set of lower dimension, $r < p$, of linear combinations which describes a data matrix X with a minimal loss of useful information.

The contribution of PCA to the theory of Legendre moments lies in their orthogonality and computational complexity properties: Whereas each moment contributes individually to reconstruct and/or characterize an image, some moments retain better key image features, and PCA allows to identify the subset that better captures the essence of the image, thus minimizing the computational cost. For more details about the theory of PCA, see (Martínez and Avinash 2001).

3 USING GPUS TO COMPUTE LEGENDRE MOMENTS

Modern GPUs are powerful computing platforms that reside at the extreme end of the design spaces of throughput-oriented architectures, allowing hardware scheduling of a parallel computation to be practical. Their increased core counts and hardware multithreading are two appealing issues that CPU designs are adopting nowadays, but until both models converge, more than 100.000 software developers of many science fields enthusiastically embrace a programming model which enables using the GPU for tasks other than shading, texturing, interpolating/rasterizing and blending/coloring. Such programming model is CUDA (Compute Unified Device Architecture)(Nvidia 2010), recently devoted to general purpose computing (GPGPU 2009).

As a hardware interface, CUDA started by transforming the G80 microarchitecture related to the GeForce 8 series from Nvidia into a parallel SIMD architecture endowed with up to 128 cores, where a collection or threads run in parallel. Later, the GeForce GTX 280 would be released from the 9 series, the platform used during our experiments (see Figure 2 for the block diagram of this architecture and Table 2 for hardware features). From the CUDA perspective, cores are organized into a set of multiprocessors, each having a set of 32-bit registers, constants and texture caches, and 16 KB of on-chip shared memory as fast as local registers (one cycle latency). At any given cycle, each core executes the same instruction on different data (SIMD), and communication between multiprocessors is performed through global memory (the video memory tied to the graphics card, whose latency is around 400–600 cycles).

As a programming interface, CUDA consists of a set of C language library functions, and the CUDA-specific compiler generates the executable for the GPU from a source code where the following elements meet (see Figure 1):

- A program is decomposed into **blocks** that run *logically* in parallel (physically only if there are resources available). Assembled by the developer, a block is a group of threads that is mapped to a single multiprocessor, where they can share 16 KB of memory.
- All **threads** of concurrent blocks on a single multiprocessor divide the resources available equally amongst themselves. The data is also divided amongst all of the threads in a SIMD fashion with a decomposition explicitly managed by the developer.
- A **warp** is a collection of threads that can actually run concurrently (with no time sharing) on all of the multiprocessors. The developer has the freedom to determine the number of threads to be executed (up to a limit intrinsic to CUDA), but if there are more threads than the warp size, they are time-shared on the actual hardware resources.

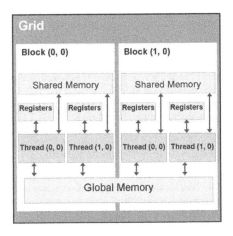

Figure 1. The CUDA programming model.

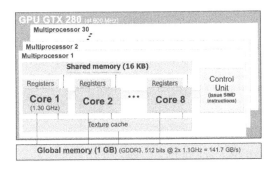

Figure 2. The CUDA hardware interface for the GTX 280 GPU used during our experimental analysis.

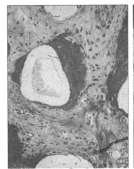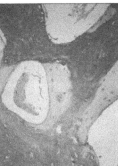

Figure 3. The input images to our experimental survey were taken from biomedical studies on stem cells to quantify the degree of cartilage and bone regeneration. On the left, a sample stained with picrosirius to reveal features of either bone (intense red due to type I collagen) or cartilage (weak pink thanks to type II collagen), for which a single-color treatment suffices. On the right, a sample stained with alcian blue, where cyan tones predominate in inverse intensities with respect to the presence of bone/cartilage as compared to the previous sample. This suggests that our analysis may be reduced to a single color channel, with similar classification accuracy than the luminance taken from grayscale images.

Table 1. G80 limitations for CUDA programming and its impact on performance.

Parameter	Limit	Impact
Multiprocessors per GPU	16	Low
Processors/Multiprocessor	8	Low
Threads/Warp	32	Low
Thread blocks/Multiproc.	8	Medium
Threads/Block	512	Medium
Threads/Multiprocessor	768	High
Registers/Multiprocessor	8192	High
Shared memory/Multiproc.	16 KB	Highest

- A **kernel** is the code to be executed by each thread. Conditional execution of different operations can be achieved based on a unique thread ID.

Hardware and software limitations in CUDA are listed in Figure 1 for the case of the G80 GPU, where we have ranked them according to their impact on the developer's implementation and overall performance based on our own experience.

All of the threads can access all of the GPU memory, but, as expected, there is a performance boost when threads access data resident in shared memory, which is explicitly managed by the programmer. In order to make the most efficient usage of the GPU's computational resources, large

411

Table 2. Summary of hardware features for the set of hardware processors used during our experimental survey.

Hardware feature	CPU	GPU
Commercial model	Intel Core 2 Kentsfield	Nvidia GeForce GTX 280
Number of cores and speed	Four @ 2.40 GHz	One @ 600 MHz
Streaming processors	Does not have	240 @ 1.30 GHz
Memory speed	2×400 MHz	2×1100 MHz
Memory bus width	128 bits	512 bits
Memory bandwidth	12.8 GB/sec.	141.7 GB/sec.
Memory size and type	4 GB DDR2	1 GBB GDDR3
Bus to video memory	–	PCI-e x16 2.0

data structures are stored in global memory and the shared memory should be prioritized for storing strategic, often-used data structures.

When developing applications for GPUs with CUDA, the management of registers becomes important as a limiting factor for the amount of parallelism we can exploit. Each multiprocessor contains 8,192 registers which will be split evenly among all the threads of the blocks assigned to that multiprocessor. Hence, the number of registers needed in the computation will affect the number of threads able to be executed simultaneously, given the constraints outlined in Table 1. For example, if a kernel (and therefore a thread) consumes 16 registers, only 512 threads can be assigned to a single multiprocessor, and this can be achieved by using 1 block with 512 threads, 2 blocks of 256 threads, and so on.

4 EXPERIMENTAL ANALYSIS

4.1 Input images

During our experimental analysis the source for our input data set consisted of real biomedical images used for cartilage and bone regeneration. They were taken with a Zeiss III phase inverted contrast microscope and a Nikon Microphot FXA camera, to produce an output of 2560×1920 pixels in RGB color TIFF format. We tried images with different stainings to study the influence of image contents over the execution time (see Figure 3). The workload of our image processing algorithms was strongly affected by image resolution and loosely affected by image contents, after which we selected image tiles of 64×64 pixels stained with picrosirius for the characterization of bone and cartilage regeneration. Figure 4 shows the decomposition process into 40×30 tiles for the 2560×1920 image, the regions of interest (new forming bone, existing bone and cartilage tissue), and the tiles used for training the image classifier. In our particular case, the luminance channel suffices for a successful classification, so we convert to grayscale images in a preprocessing stage prior to the actual computation of Legendre moments over the luminance channel to make our techniques also suitable for X-ray images or images captured by an electronic microscope.

4.2 Hardware resources

To demonstrate the effectiveness of our techniques, we have conducted a number of experiments on different CPU and GPU platforms (see Table 2 for hardware details). Stream processors (cores) outlined in Figure 2 are built on a hardwired design for a much faster clock frequency than the rest of the silicon area (1.30 GHz versus 600 MHz), leading to a peak processing power exceeding half of a TFLOP.

4.3 Implementation and optimizations

This section describes our implementation on a GPU and evaluates the performance of our image analysis algorithms on emerging architectures as compared to existing methods running on regular PCs.

The computation of Legendre moments was implemented up to and order $N = 16$, using only the repetition $r = 0$ for each order (that is, our list of moments include 17 instances: $A_{0,0}$, $A_{1,0}$, $A_{2,0}$, $A_{3,0}$, $A_{4,0}$, $A_{5,0}$, $A_{6,0}$, $A_{7,0}$, $A_{8,0}$, $A_{9,0}$, $A_{10,0}$, $A_{11,0}$, $A_{12,0}$, $A_{13,0}$, $A_{14,0}$, $A_{15,0}$, and $A_{16,0}$. In general, low order moments keep most of the image features for image analysis and classification, whereas moments of high order are used for image reconstruction, being more sensitive to noise and computationally demanding. This way, we maximize the significance to computational cost ratio.

For the calculation of autovectors, we use the NIPALS algorithm (a valid alternative is SVD), and then PCA within the eigenface recognition method to derive k eigenfaces down from the 17-dimensional space built from all Legendre moments considered.

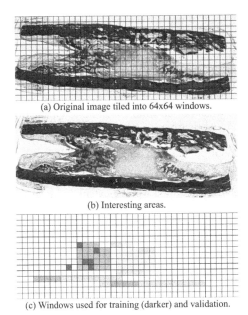

(a) Original image tiled into 64x64 windows.

(b) Interesting areas.

(c) Windows used for training (darker) and validation.

Figure 4. Biomedical tissue image stained with picrosirius, where the central region reveals the presence of cartilage tissue as spongy pink (marked in yellow), new forming bone as scattered red (marked in purple) and existing bone (marked as green). Within each area, 64×64 windows marked with stronger colors were used as samples for the training phase of the classifier. Legendre moments are computed for each of the 40×30 windows as result of the tiling process.

Table 3. Execution times (in milliseconds) for the different phases involved in our method for computing Legendre moments and characterizing the minimal subset which maximizes information gathering on a 64×64 image tile. Last column reflects the improvement factor attained on the GPU.

Computational phase	CPU	GPU	Acc.
Data input	0.60	0.59	1.01x
Legendre moments	4323.52	720.58	6.00x
Matrix average	0.06	0.07	0.85x
Matrix normalization	0.15	0.10	1.50x
Covariance	0.27	0.14	1.92x
PCA	199.97	24.99	8.00x
Image classification	1.78	2.09	0.85x
TOTAL	4526.35	748.56	6.04x

The ultimate goal for computing Legendre moments is to use them as features for characterizing every image tile of 64×64 pixels so that we can perform an accurate tile classification into the three types of bone tissue to be considered. The output from this classifier, when applied to the set of moments described above, classifies correctly 84% of new bone tissue, 90% of existing bone and 90% of cartilage for a whole set of 130 samples of each type, 30 of them used during the training phase.

Once our algorithms were ported to the CPU and the GPU, additional optimizations can be performed on both sides. Traditionally, the CPU exploits instruction-level parallelism using pipelining and superscalar executions, so does the GPU with data parallelism through a SIMD execution over 128/240 stream processors. Parallelism may be enhanced on both sides using a more novel approach based on task-level parallelism: On CPUs, using multiple cores (up to four in our platform); on GPUs, using multiple graphics cards (also limited to four in our case). In both cases, the code must be parallelized declaring four threads and partitioning input data into four symmetric chunks. With a similar programming effort, we expect the performance difference to be preserved after this optimization step.

Table 3 shows the execution times for our couple of implementations, the first one corresponds to a CPU using Microsoft Visual C++ 2005 and Windows XP, and the second one to our results on GPUs using CUDA. GPU execution times are significantly better on those phases characterized by arithmetic intensity. Due to its better scalability, we expect GPUs to evolve in a more favorable way in the near future, leading to a winner strategy by an order of magnitude and beyond.

5 CONCLUSIONS

In this work, we analyze the expressiveness of Legendre moments as descriptors of biomedical images for quantifying the degree of bone tissue regeneration from stem cells, and introduce a novel approach to the high-performance computation of Legendre moments on Graphics Processors (GPUs). The proposed method is compared against a similar implementation performed on CPUs, with factor gains exceeding 6× for a single 64×64 image tile. This is extraordinarily valuable in computational domains like real-time imaging or microscopic and biomedical imaging where large-scale images predominate.

In addition, methods on the GPU are rewarded with a higher scalability to become a solid alternative for computing Legendre moments in the years to come. Our subsequent PCA analysis is also more attractive in real-time or high-resolution imaging due to its inherent capability to limit the computation to a small number of selected moments which may retain the bulk of the information required for the successful classification of small tiles into image regions. In this respect, we have also identified those Legendre moments becoming more relevant for image segmentation into bone and cartilage regions within the context of our biomedical application, selecting moments of order $N \leq 16$ and a single repetition $r = 0$. This way, low order moments encapsulate most of the information and our vector of features may be greatly reduced without suffering a significant reduction in the segmentation accuracy.

GPUs are evolving towards general-purpose architectures (GPGPU 2009), where we envision image processing as one of the most exciting fields able to benefit from its impressive computational power. This work demonstrates that Legendre moments are a valid alternative for integrating the vector of features required to classify image tiles into regions characterizing bone and cartilage tissue, and distinguishes those relevant orders and repetitions for a reliable segmentation in computer-aided biomedical analysis.

6 FUTURE WORK

We pretend to make use of double-precision hardware for improving accuracy during the computation of Legendre moments, where this issue plays a critical role. In the current state of the GPU evolution, such implementation is not feasible because trigonometric functions are out of the scope of the double-precision operators, implemented commercially.

We also want to approach the implementation of Legendre moments using reduction formulas to save computations and develop faster algorithms on the GPU, but we believe this work represents a promising first step on a long road towards real-time processing of Legendre moments.

Overall, this effort is part of the developing of an image processing library oriented to biomedical applications and accelerated using the GPU as co-processor. Future achievements include the implementation of each step of our image analysis process so that it can be entirely executed on GPUs without incurring penalties from/to the CPU. Our plan also includes porting the code to TESLA nodes and CPU/GPU clusters.

At the same time frame in which this work was developed and written, the OpenCL 1.0 specification was built to provide a more general way for programming graphics cards of all type of vendors. The initiative, supported by all major GPU manufacturers, is expected to establish as a standard for general-purpose GPU programming. The first assignment we have in mind is to quantify the performance penalty that our implementation will have when ported from CUDA into OpenCL and run into other type of GPU platforms like those of ATI Radeon or later Intel Larrabee or AMD fussion. Given that each generation of GPU evolution adds flexibility to previous high-throughput GPU designs, software developers in many fields are likely to take interest in the extent to which CPU/GPU architectures and programming systems ultimately converge.

ACKNOWLEDGEMENTS

This work was supported by the Junta de Andalucía of Spain, under Project of Excellence P06-TIC-02109. We want to thank Silvia Claros, José Antonio Andrades and José Becerra from the Cell Biology Department at the University of Malaga for providing us the biomedical images used as input to our experimental analysis.

REFERENCES

Andrades, J.A., J. Santamaría, M. Nimni, and J. Becerra (2001). Selection, Amplification and Induction of a Bone Marrow Cell Population to the Chondroosteogenic Lineage by rhOP-1: An in vitro and in vivo Study. *International Journal Developmental Biology 45*, 683–693.

GPGPU (2009). General-Purpose Computation Using Graphics Hardware. http://www.gpgpu.org.

Martínez, A. and C. Avinash (2001, February). PCA versus LDA. *IEEE Transactions on Pattern Analysis and Machine Intelligence 23*(2), 228–233.

Nvidia (2010, October). CUDA Home Page. http://developer.nvidia.com/object/cuda.html.

R. Mukundan and K. Ramakrishnan (1995). Fast Computation of Legendre and Zernike Moments. *Pattern Recognition 28*(9), 1433–1442.

Teague, M. (1980). Image Analysis via the General Theory of Moments. *J. Optical Society of America 70*(8), 920–930.

Computational Vision and Medical Image Processing – Tavares & Natal Jorge (eds)
© 2012 Taylor & Francis Group, London, ISBN 978-0-415-68395-1

On the accurate classification of bone tissue images

J.E. Gil, J.P. Aranda & E. Mérida-Casermeiro
Applied Mathematics Department, University of Malaga, Spain

M. Ujaldón
Computer Architecture Department, University of Malaga, Spain

ABSTRACT: This work describes an expert system aimed to an accurate classification of cell tissue. We deal with phenotype and color analysis on a wide variety of microscopic images coming from studies of cartilage and bone tissue regeneration using stem cells. We investigate several trained and nonparametric classifiers based on neural networks, decision trees, bayesian classifiers and association rules, and analyze its effectiveness to distinguish several types of tissue existing in high-resolution biomedical images. The features selection includes texture, shape and color descriptors, among which we consider color histograms, Zernike moments and Fourier coefficients. Our study evaluates different selections for the feature vectors to compare accuracy and computational time as well as different stainings for revealing tissue properties. Overall, picrosirius reveals as the best staining and multilayer perceptron as the most effective classifier to distinguish between bone and cartilage tissue.

Keywords: Zernike Moments, Neural Network, Image Classification, Weka, Data Mining.

1 INTRODUCTION

A wide variety of histologically stained images in cell biology require deep analysis to determine both the phenotype and color for the tissue being analyzed. One example is cartilage and bone regeneration, where a specific microenvironment has been reported to induce the expression of skeletal matrix proteins, playing a regulatory role in the initiation of cartilage differentiation and the induction of bone-forming cells from pluripotent mesenchymal stem cells (Andrades et al., 2001). The skeletal data set is obtained from implants on 7 month old male rats. After 17 days of culture, in-vivo stem cells are implanted on animals into demineralized bone matrix or diffusion chambers. Four weeks later, rats are sacrificed, six chambers excised and tissues analyzed biochemically or processed for light microscopy after the appropriate fixation and sectioned at 7 μm thickness. From each chamber, approximately 500 slices of tissue sample are obtained, each being a microscopic 2560 × 1920 RGB color image in TIFF format.

Color analysis in our bone regeneration images is related to the staining of samples, which reveals the histogenic process that is taking place in the induction of cartilage and bone-forming cells from pluripotent mesenchymal stem cells. Thus, the shape of the image histogram for each of the red, green and blue color channels deducts key features

about tissue regeneration. For example, red channel is applied when using picrosirius staining, which reveals bone tissue by the presence of type I collagen; likewise, blue channel reveals cartilage tissue by the presence of type II collagen stained with alcian blue (see Fig. 1).

To assess the 3D change of the various tissue types from a medical image analysis perspective, the first technical step is to segment each image

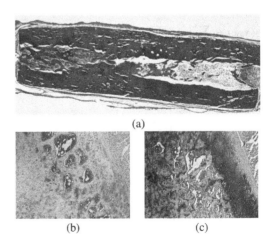

Figure 1. Tissue examples: (a) Picrosirius. (b) Alcian blue. (c) Safranin blue.

into regions corresponding to the tissue layers involved, namely, bone, cartilage, fibrous, muscle and spinal tissue. We are developing a computer-assisted system to assess the degree of regeneration of bone tissue to minimize the human role in this process.

2 CONCEPTUAL MODEL

The primary goal of our work is to segment bone tissue images into five different regions: bone, cartilage, fibrous, muscle and spinal. To accomplish this task, we have built a tool where the clinical expert selects samples for each tissue type through a list of tissue tiles or windows, indicating the percentage of each tissue type contained within each window.

The window size may vary from 32×32 to 128×128 pixels according to the input images size. For each window, a vector of parameters is built composed of mixed attributes, basically using RGB components as color descriptors and Zernike moments as phenotype descriptors. Once this sample is established, we apply Principal Component Analysis (PCA) to increase performance prior to the classifier analysis, which is primarily based on multilayer perceptron coming from the theory of neural networks as well as decision trees.

2.1 Multilayer perceptron

The core of our research has been conducted with the Multilayer Perceptron (MLP) neural network. This network contains a single layer of hidden neurons and is capable of making an approximation to whichever continuous function given a sufficient number of hidden neurons (Haykin, 1999).

$$g(x,w) = \sum_{j=0}^{N_s} w_{k,j} f(\sum_{i=0}^{N_e} w_{j,i} x_i) \qquad (1)$$

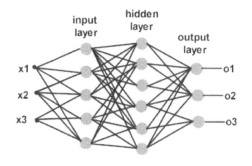

Figure 2. A typical topology for a multilayer perceptron neural network.

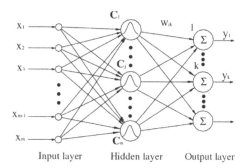

Figure 3. A radial base function neural network.

2.2 Radial basis functions

Radial Basis Functions (RBF) are designed with neurons in the hidden layer activated through radial non-linear functions with their own gravitational center and in the output layer through linear functions. Unlike MLP, RBF is built with a rigid architecture composed of three layers: input, hidden and output. This network is quite sensitive to the dispersion of the input parameters, so it is highly recommended to transform the input values to an specific scale in a preliminary stage.

$$y_i = g\left(\overline{x},\overline{w_i}\right) = \sum_{j=0} w_{i,j} \exp\left(-\frac{\left(\overline{x}-\overline{C}_j\right)^T\left(\overline{x}-\overline{C}_j\right)}{2\sigma_j^2}\right)$$

$$(2)$$

3 METHODS

We start building our tool in Matlab as a project decomposed into three main modules:

1. **Sample construction.** In this module, the user selects samples among our input images library, and, optionally, he may run a preliminar PCA (see Fig. 4).
2. **Window classification.** This module allows user to choose among a wide set of classifiers. We combine here Matlab and WEKA (Hall et al., 2009), an open source Java application which provides a rich set of classifiers such as decision trees, association rules and bayesian classifiers. The communication between Matlab and WEKA was established with the help of the Java virtual machine available in Matlab. Once the classifier is built, the user can display the results for a validation sample as Figure 5 shows.
3. **Image analysis** The image analysis process can be decomposed into four major tasks connected through a pipeline as Figure 6 shows. This module starts from an input image and a selected

416

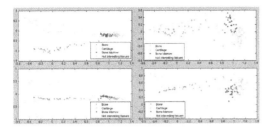

Figure 4. Our tool for PCA. On the X-axis, we set the first principal component, and on the Y-axis, we represent the second, third, fourth and fifth principal component on the upper left, upper right, lower left and lower right side, respectively.

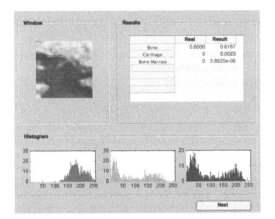

Figure 5. Displaying the results for a validation sample.

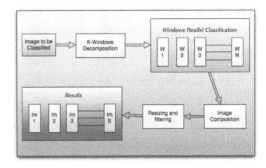

Figure 6. The image analysis pipeline implemented within our biomedical image processing application.

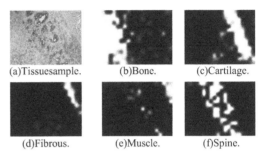

(a)Tissuesample.   (b)Bone.   (c)Cartilage.

(d)Fibrous.   (e)Muscle.   (f)Spine.

Figure 7. Image classification example. (a) Input biomedical image. (b-e) Regions classified as tissue classes (white areas).

4 EXPERIMENTAL ANALYSIS

To demonstrate the effectiveness of our techniques, we have conducted a number of experiments on a PC endowed with a Core 2 Duo P7550 CPU (45 nm., 2.26 GHz., 3 MB L2 Cache, 4 GB DDR3 memory) running under MacOS 10.6 and using Matlab R2009b.

4.1 Classifying 3 tissue classes

Our first experiment tries to classify tissue tiles of size 32×32 pixels into three different classes: Bone, cartilage and all the remaining types of tissue (muscle, fiber and spine) grouped into a third and heterogeneous class.

Our training sample is composed of 30 representative windows for every class plus 36 windows of non interesting areas and 40 random (mixed) windows. A total of 166 windows were selected manually, whose distribution is shown in Figure 8.

Among those 40 random windows, 20 were used for validation purposes, 10 were involved in the testing phase and 10 were used for training. The validation error was calculated using the k-cross-validation technique.

classifier. The first task decomposes the image into k windows (image tiles) and stores them in an array. The second task obtains the parameters vectors for each windows and classifies it. This is the bottleneck in our application, and because it is an embarrasingly parallel task, we have used the Parallel Computing Toolbox (Sharma et al., 2009) to classify windows simultaneously, so the execution time depends on the number of active workers active in Matlab. Once all windows have been classified, a third stage composes the output images, one for each type of tissue to distinguish. Therefore, this output is a matrix of elements where each element represents a tile. For example, for a 2560×1920 input image and a 32×32 window size, each output matrix contains 40×30 tiles. The last stage resizes images to the original size and applies a gaussian filter to smooth them. The final result is a set of images, one for every tissue type, with pixels replaced by its probability to belong to such tissue region (see Fig. 7).

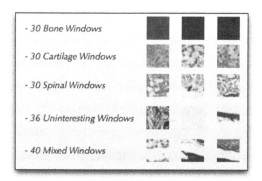

Figure 8. Samples and validation test used with a biomedical image stained with picrosirius to classify windows into three tissue classes: Bone, cartilage and all the others.

Each window is characterized by the following parameters to build a vector of 25 features used as input to the classifier, namely:

- Color histograms for the red, green and blue channel (H_R, H_G, H_B).
- Normalized color histograms (H_R^N, H_G^N, H_B^N).
- Histogram deciles by color (D_R, D_G, D_B).
- Normalized histograms deciles by color (D_R^N, D_G^N, D_B^N).
- Zernike moment of order 4 (Z_4). In a previous work (Ujaldón et al., 2011),, we demonstrate the lower computational complexity and higher significance of low order moments on biomedical images. The fact that lowest moments capture similar information than the histograms and the typical deviation, leads us to choose the moment of order 4 as the more convenient to be part of our set of parameters.
- Zernike moment of order 4 by color and normalized ($Z_{4R}^N, Z_{4G}^N, Z_{4B}^N$).
- Typical deviation by color and normalized ($\sigma_R, \sigma_G, \sigma_B$).
- Central moment ($\mu_{1,1,1}$).
- Components of the Fourier Transform by color and normalized (C_1, C_2, C_3, C_4, C_5).

The normalization process is performed by applying the following procedure: Given a set X of elements, and an element $x \in X$, be $M = \max(X)$ and $m = \min(X)$. Let it be $A = M - m$, $M_a = M + 0.2 \times A$ an estimation for the maximum and $M_i = m - 0.2 \times A$ an estimation for the minimum. The normalization function is then defined as follows:

$$f(x) = \frac{x - M_i}{M_a - M_i} \qquad (3)$$

And the central moment $\mu_{1,1,1}$ is defined by the following expression:

$$\mu_{1,1,1} = \sum_{i=0}^{N-1} \frac{(r_i - \bar{r}) \times (g_i - \bar{g}) \times (b_i - \bar{b})}{N} \qquad (4)$$

With all the 25 parameters listed above, we have created 7 different running tests, each with a different features vector, such as illustrated in Table 1.

4.1.1 Using the MLP classifier

This classifier was taken from the Neural Network Computing in Matlab, and samples were used to estimate the best configuration. To accomplish this task, we vary the number of neurons in layer one, ranging from 10 until 100, and using three learning algorithms:

- **traingda:** Gradient descent with adaptive learning rate backpropagation.
- **traingdx:** Gradient descent with momentum and adaptive learning rate backpropagation.
- **trainrp:** Resilient backpropagation.

Figure 9 shows the results obtained, where we can see that the last algorithm behaves better and reaches its peak (minimum error) when 30 neurons are used in the first layer. Consequently, we have chosen these parameters for building our MLP classifier, which later was applied to all seven running tests which proceeds similarly under different feature vectors.

Experimental results are shown in Table 2, where we can see the effect of performing a preliminary PCA: Execution times are reduced up to 50%, but at the expense of sacrificing accuracy

Table 1. Parameters selected for each running test performed to distinguish among three tissue classes.

	T1	T2	T3	T4	T5	T6	T7
H_R, H_G, H_B	•						
D_R, D_G, D_B	•						
H_R^N, H_G^N, H_B^N			•	•	•	•	•
D_R^N, D_G^N, D_B^N			•	•	•	•	•
Z_4	•						
$Z_{4R}^N, Z_{4G}^N, Z_{4B}^N$			•	•	•	•	•
$\sigma_R, \sigma_G, \sigma_B$				•	•	•	•
$\mu_{1,1,1}$				•	•	•	•
C_1					•		•
C_2, C_3					•	•	•
C_4, C_5						•	•

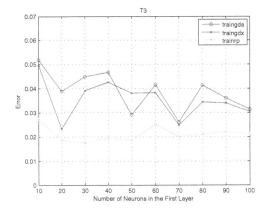

Figure 9. Classification error for our test run using the MLP classifier and three output tissue classes: Bone, cartilage and others.

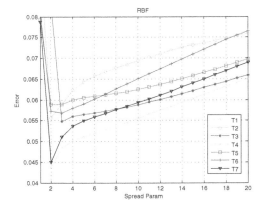

Figure 10. Classification error depending of the spread factor for our test run using the RBF classifier and three output tissue classes: Bone, cartilage and others.

(the error percentage goes up). We can also see how the error is reduced when input features are normalized, with the best results attained for the T3 test.

4.1.2 *Using the RBF classifier*

For this classifier we have used the newbr function provided by the Network Toolbox in Matlab. We repeat all runs already covered by the MLP in our benchmark, and experimental results are also shown in Table 2. This time, the normalization process improves accuracy by a wide margin, going down from 14% to just 5%. Accuracy remains better on the MLP side, but the execution is much faster on the RBF classifier. Therefore, precision comes along with MLP, but at the expense of computational performance.

4.1.3 *Using WEKA*

In our last experiment involving three classes, we use those classifiers provided by WEKA (Hall et al., 2009). Since this is a tool implemented in Java, computational times increase an average of 14 seconds for the sample and 9 seconds when PCA is used. In order to compare with previous analysis, we take only the T3 test which provides the best results so far, and the experimental results are shown in Table 3. The more accurate method implements base routines for generating M5 Model trees and rules.

4.2 *Classifying 5 tissue classes*

A more ambitious classification process entails to perform a distinction among all types of tissue grouped into the third class considered so far, namely, to separate muscle from fibrous and spine. This widens the number of classes up to five. Different stainings for the tissue are also tested here: Alcian blue and safranin blue (see Fig. 1).

Table 2. A comparison between MLP and RBF neural networks classifiers.

Classifier	T1	T2	T3	T4	T5	T6	T7
Error percentage (in %)							
MLP	3.25	1.86	1.83	1.94	1.98	2.28	1.85
MLP + PCA	3.74	2.91	2.95	3.22	2.69	2.45	3.66
RBF	14.26	5.58	8.31	4.38	5.89	5.73	4.50
RBF + PCA	14.26	11.25	9.67	5.52	6.58	6.55	5.62
Execution times (in seconds)							
MLP	21.89	6.83	5.92	7.63	6.09	8.19	7.18
MLP + PCA	21.05	3.10	3.61	3.54	3.14	3.58	2.91
RBF	0.11	0.11	0.11	0.11	0.11	0.11	0.12
RBF + PCA	0.08	0.08	0.08	0.08	0.08	0.08	0.08

Table 3. Error percentage for different WEKA classifiers when three tissue classes are distinguished. A rank has been built based on classification accuracy.

Classifier (Weka name)	No PCA	Rank	PCA	Rank
trees.M5P	3.23	3	0.0417	1
trees.DecisionStump	4.62	7	0.0483	3
trees.REPTree	3.08	2	0.0612	9
functions.IsotonicRegression	3.34	4	0.0531	6
functions.LeastMedSq	14.26	19	0.1426	20
functions.LinearRegression	91.87	20	0.0785	13
functions.PLSClassifier	5.25	11	0.0522	5
functions.SimpleLinearRegr.	4.79	8	0.0700	12
functions.SMOreg	12.23	18	0.0607	8
lazy.IBk	5.68	14	0.1208	19
lazy.LWL	3.65	5	0.0626	11
meta.AdditiveRegression	5.17	9	0.0785	14
meta.Bagging	2.36	1	0.0472	2
meta.CVParameterSelection	11.10	15	0.1110	16
meta.GridSearch	5.18	10	0.0514	4
meta.MultiScheme	11.10	16	0.1110	17
rules.ConjunctiveRule	5.39	12	0.0616	10
rules.DecisionTable	5.59	13	0.0838	15
rules.M5Rules	3.74	6	0.0593	7
rules.ZeroR	11.10	17	0.1110	18

Table 4. Error percentage incurred by each classifier when applied to two tissue staining for distinguishing among five different tissue classes.

Classifier	Alcian blue	Rank	Safranin blue	Rank
MLP	0.01	1	0.01	1
RBF	0.05	4	0.04	4
trees.M5P	0.13	9	0.10	12
trees.DecisionStump	0.16	12	0.08	6
trees.REPTree	0.16	13	0.11	14
functions.GaussianProcesses	0.17	16	0.15	18
functions.IsotonicRegression	0.15	11	0.08	7
functions.LinearRegression	0.05	3	0.08	10
functions.PLSClassifier	0.07	6	0.03	3
functions.SimpleLinearRegression	0.17	15	0.13	16
functions.SMOreg	0.05	2	0.07	5
lazy.LWL	0.13	10	0.08	9
meta.AdditiveRegression	0.16	14	0.08	8
meta.Bagging	0.12	8	0.09	11
meta.CVParameterSelection	0.18	17	0.16	19
meta.GridSearch	0.06	5	0.03	2
meta.MultiScheme	0.18	18	0.16	20
rules.ConjunctiveRule	0.18	20	0.12	15
rules.DecisionTable	0.12	7	0.14	17
rules.M5Rules	0.19	21	0.11	13
rules.ZeroR	0.18	19	0.16	21

4.2.1 Samples

Our samples were built by taking 10 windows for bone, cartilage and spine tissue, and 5 windows for muscle and fibrous tissue, for a total of 40 windows. Tile size is 128 × 128 pixels, and k-crossvalidation is used as technique to calculate the error.

4.2.2 Results

Input parameters for the MLP have been 65 neurons in the first layer together with the training algorithm trainrp. For the RBF case we have chosen a value of 0.83 for the spread parameter. In this case, parameters have been adjusted using a minimization algorithm (Kroon, 2010). The test used was again T3, this time without PCA.

Table 4 shows the results obtained, where we can see the error incurred for each classifier for each of the tissue standings. Overall, MLP performs best with a minimum error of barely one percent.

5 CONCLUSIONS

We have built a robust, multi-platform and easy to use application for an automatic classification of bone tissue which achieves a remarkable success in the process of segmenting biomedical images, mostly extracting the amount of bone and cartilage tissue. This allows to assess the degree of bone tissue regeneration starting from stem cells. Our tool exploits all computational power existing nowadays in multi-core CPUs thanks to a programming effort which leans on the Parallel Computing Toolbox provided by Matlab (Sharma et al., 2009).

The MLP classifier obtains the most accurate results, but at the expense of a higher computational complexity as compared to the RBF classifier. When a quick response is required, RBF may be used instead, and we have demonstrated how to reduce its error from a 14% to a 5% by using a normalization process for the feature vector and adjusting the spread parameter via an optimization algorithm.

We also study the influence of tissue staining, as our study considers picrosirius, alcian blue and safranin blue, to end up with clear signs that the first reveals better those features which may act as effective biomarkers.

With all this information provided by our tool, we contribute with a diverse, stable, reliable, fast and accurate computer-assisted system to assess the degree of regeneration of bone tissue, and therefore, aimed to minimize the amount of work required by clinical especialists.

ACKNOWLEDGEMENTS

This work was supported by the Junta de Andalucía of Spain, under Project of Excellence P06-TIC-02109. We want to thank Silvia Claros, José Antonio Andrades and José Becerra from the Cell Biology Department at the University of Malaga for providing us the biomedical images used as input to our experimental analysis.

REFERENCES

Andrades, J.A., J. Santamaría, M. Nimni and J. Becerra. Selection, Amplification and Induction of a Bone Marrow Cell Population to the Chondroosteogenic Lineage by rhOP-1: An in vitro and in vivo Study. *International Journal Developmental Biology*, vol. 45, pages 683–693.

Hall, M., E. Frank, G. Holmes, B. Pfahringer and I. H. Witten. The WEKA data mining software: An update. *SIGKDD Explorations*, vol. 11, number 1, pages 10–18.

Haykin. S. *Neural Networks: A Comprehensive Foundation*, pages 135–155. New York, USA: IEEE Press.

Kroon. D.J. Quasi newton limited memory BFGS and steepest, 2010.

Martín-Requena M.J. and M. Ujaldón. *Leveraging Graphics Hardware for and Automatic Classification of Bone Tissue*, Chapter 19, pages 209–228. Computational Methods in Applied Sciences. Computational Vision and Medical Image Processing - Recent Trends.

Piatetsky-Shapiro. G. Data mining and knowlledge discovery 1996 to 2005: Overcoming the hype and moving from university to business and analytics. *Data Mining and Knowledge Discovery*, vol. 15, number 1, pages 99–105.

Sharma G. and J. Martín. Matlab: A language for parallel computing. *Intl. Journal of Parallel Programming*, vol. 37, pages 3–36.

Tuceryan M. and A.K. Jain (1998). *Texture Analysis*. World Scientific Publishing Co.

Computational Vision and Medical Image Processing – Tavares & Natal Jorge (eds)
© *2012 Taylor & Francis Group, London, ISBN 978-0-415-68395-1*

Automated quantification of histone relocation in cell nuclei

T. Rieß
Interdisciplinary Center for Interactive Data Analysis, Modelling and Visual Exploration (INCIDE), University of Konstanz, Germany

C. Dietz
Interdisciplinary Center for Interactive Data Analysis, Modelling and Visual Exploration (INCIDE), University of Konstanz, Germany
Center for Applied Photonics (CAP), University of Konstanz, Germany

M. Horn
Interdisciplinary Center for Interactive Data Analysis, Modelling and Visual Exploration (INCIDE), University of Konstanz, Germany
Bioinformatics and Information Mining, University of Konstanz, Germany

O. Deussen
Interdisciplinary Center for Interactive Data Analysis, Modelling and Visual Exploration (INCIDE), University of Konstanz, Germany
Computer Graphics and Media Design, University of Konstanz, Germany

M. Leist & T. Waldmann
In-vitro Toxicology and Biomedicine, University of Konstanz, Germany

D. Merhof
Interdisciplinary Center for Interactive Data Analysis, Modelling and Visual Exploration (INCIDE), University of Konstanz, Germany
Visual Computing, University of Konstanz, Germany

ABSTRACT: Microscopy images of progenitor cells prepared with a specific epigenetic mark show its massive relocation during differentiation. We propose an image processing pipeline for the automated quantification of this relocation. A novel set of features which are extracted from polar representations of the microscopy images are used to construct a strong classifier via an adaptive boosting algorithm. In addition to the classification a measurement of the relocation in each nucleus is performed.

Keywords: biomedical image processing, feature extraction, image classification

1 INTRODUCTION

The last step during differentiation of mammalian tissues is the maturation phase when cell type specific gene expression are switched on to differentiate the progenitor cells into a specific cell type (Zimmer, Kuegler, Baudis, Genewsky, Tanavde, Koh, Tan, Waldmann, Kadereit, and Leist 2011). This switch is not only regulated by linear DNA sequence information, but also by the structural organization of DNA, called chromatin (Khorasanizadeh 2004). In this work we propose an image processing pipeline to quantify the chromatin structural changes during the maturation phase of the differentiation.

The microscopy images under consideration show immunostained progenitor cells at different days of differentiation with a well described repressive histone epigenetic mark (Kouzarides 2007). This mark is massively relocated during differentiation, from a relative homogenous and regular pattern toward a clear concentration at the nuclear periphery. To show that this relocation is not only occurring in a subset of cells, we quantify the amount of cells with ring structure at the nuclear periphery during differentiation for a large

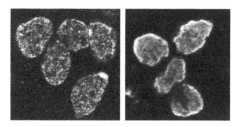

Figure 1. Cell nuclei after two days (left) and after seven days (right) of differentiation. The cells show a clear ring structure after seven days.

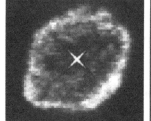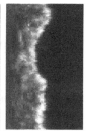

Figure 2. Polar image for a single cell nucleus. The microscopy image (left) is converted to a polar image (right). The center of the polar image is chosen close to the center of the nucleus.

number of microscopy images, see Figure 1 for two exemplary images.

Our image processing pipeline automatically classifies the microscopy images using a novel set of rotation-invariant features and an adaptive boosting algorithm. Moreover, for comparison the histone relocation is measured using an additional fluorescent marker. The methods are presented in detail in Section 2, the results of the automated classification and the measurement are summarized in Section 3, and finally in Section 4 conclusions are drawn and future research directions are given.

2 METHODS

In this section we present the technical details of the proposed image processing pipeline for the automated classification of microscopy images. In particular, we explain which features are extracted and used for the adaptive boosting algorithm.

2.1 Feature extraction

The features are extracted from polar representations (Kvarnström, Logg, Diez, Bodvard, and Käll 2008) created from the original microscopy image. These so-called polar images are determined by choosing a center point, a radius and a number of angles. Then rays originating at the center point and having the length of the chosen radius are collected and stacked for the chosen number of angles, see Figure 2 for an example. The polar images we use here are centered at seeding points that are distributed on a rectangular grid on the microscopy image. The distance between neighboured seeding points is chosen to be $r/5$, where r denotes the average nucleus radius in our test images. We use $4r$ angles and a radius of $6r/5$ for the construction of the polar images, thus each polar image has the width $W = 6r/5$ and the height $H = 4r$. Using our specific set of features on polar images yields rotational invariance, but not necessarily scaling invariance.

The features explained below are not only extracted from the complete polar image, but also from subwindows of the polar image. These subwindows cover the whole range of angles, meaning that their height is H. Hence, the rotational invariance of the features is preserved. We choose subwindows of width $W/2$ centered at x-positions $W/4$, $W/2$ and $3W/4$ within the polar image to extract the features. Note that the total number of features is proportional to the number of subwindows. In the following detailed explanation of the extracted features, let w and h denote the width and the height of the considered subwindow.

2.1.1 Histogram features
The histogram of the subwindow is computed and the following statistical values are used as features: mean, median, 20%-quantile, 80%-quantile, standard deviation and kurtosis. Histogram features describe global statistics of the pixel intensities.

2.1.2 Haar-like features
The response of a Haar-like feature (Lienhart, Kuranov, and Pisarevsky 2003) measures the difference of pixel intensities in distinct rectangles. Recall that the considered subwindow of the polar image is w pixels wide and h pixels high. Let (a, b, c, d) denote a rectangle that is defined by its upper left corner (a, b) and its lower right corner (c, d).

The first set of values are computed using two rectangles $(0, y, w/2 - 1, y)$ and $(w/2, y, w - 1, y)$ for $0 \leq y < h$. This means that the pixel intensity of the right half of each row y in the subwindow is subtracted from the pixel intensity of the left half, see Figure 3 (left) for a sketch.

The second set of values are computed using a rectangle $(0, y, w - 1, y + h/2)$ for $0 \leq y < h/2$. The pixel intensity within this rectangle is compared to the pixel intensity of the remaining area of the subwindow, see Figure 3 (right) for a sketch.

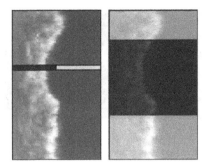

Figure 3. Sketch of the used rectangles for the Haar-like features. The left panel illustrates the per-row comparison of the left half and the right half, the right panel shows the comparison of a rectangle with full width and half height versus the remaining part.

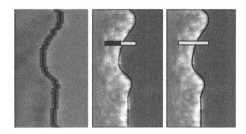

Figure 4. Haar-like filtered polar image (left), the computed contour is overlaid in red. The middle panel shows the original polar image overlaid with a sketch of the contour and the rectangles used for the Haar-like feature response in each row. The right panel shows a sketch of the rectangle used for the intensity measurements.

For both sets of computed values, we again use mean, median, 20%-quantile, 80%-quantile, standard deviation and kurtosis as the actual features. Both of these feature sets are a measure for how likely the seeding point is inside a cell nucleus, and how close this point is to the center of the nucleus. In particular, the second Haar-like feature is a measure for the symmetry.

2.1.3 Shape features

In order to extract the shape features, first a Gaussian filter with radius 3 is applied to the polar image. Then a Haar-like filter is applied to this image in the following manner: The value of the pixel at position (x, y) is computed as the difference of the pixel intensity of rectangle $(x - 4, y, x - 1, y)$ and the pixel intensity of rectangle $(x, y, x + 3, y)$. This value is then divided by $\ln x$. Afterwards, a dynamic programming approach is used to detect a vertical contour of maximum responses in this filtered image. The advantage of this contour detection algorithm over a standard gradient filter is that it is much more robust to noise. Moreover, it is possible to take the direction of the transition into account. Figure 4 shows a Haar-like filtered polar image and the resulting contour.

Let $c(y)$ denote the x-coordinate of the contour in the polar image. The response of a Haar-like feature comparing two rectangles $(c(y) - 4, y, c(y) - 1, y)$ and $(c(y), y, c(y) + 3)$ is computed for each row y in the original polar image. Similarly, the pixel intensity, its median, mean, sum, maximum and minimum within the rectangle $(c(y) - 4, y, c(y) + 3, y)$ is computed in the original polar image.

The actual extracted features are again the statistical values mean, median, 20%-quantile, 80%-quantile, standard deviation and kurtosis of the computed values. These features are measures for the shape and the intensity of the contour.

2.2 Boosting

We use an adaptive boosting algorithm Ada-Boost (Freund and Schapire 1999) to classify the polar images. The main idea of the AdaBoost algorithm is to use a linear combination of many weak classifiers in order to construct a strong classifier, where the weak classifiers are simple decision stumps using the extracted feature values, see (Smith, Carleton, and Lepetit 2009; He, Wang, Metaxas, Mathew, and White 2007; Viola and Jones 2004) approaches. At the beginning of the boosting process, all weak classifiers are equally weighted. The boosting algorithm uses training data to adjust the weights of the weak classifiers according to the distinctiveness for the class membership. This weight adjustment process is repeated iteratively until either a maximum number of iterations is reached, or the global classification error of the training data is below a given threshold.

For our classification of polar images, we use this algorithm twice. In a first boosting step, we construct a strong classifier for the decision between the two classes "nucleus" and "background", which distinguish if the seeding point of the polar image is inside or outside a cell nucleus. Only for some of the polar images classified as "nucleus", a second boosting step is performed, which constructs a strong classifier for the distinction of the classes "ring" and "no ring". This classifier determines if the seeding point belongs to a nucleus with or without a visible ring structure which is due to the histone relocation. To further improve the performance in the first boosting step "nucleus" versus "background", we also use features extracted from a second channel of the microscopy images, which only shows the DAPI stained nuclei.

2.3 Classification

Using the strong classifiers constructed by the boosting phase explained above, unlabelled microscopy images can be classified. Prior to the classification, all features of all polar images are extracted. Similar to the two steps of the boosting algorithm, the classification consists of two stages: First, the classification of "background" versus "nucleus" is performed, which also uses the DAPI channel as mentioned above. The seeding points classified as "nucleus" are then pruned by keeping only those that have maximum response within a circle of radius r (this means that only one seeding point per nucleus is kept). The polar images corresponding to those seeding points are then classified into the two classes "ring" and "no ring". Note that the whole process does not involve any segmentation, it is a pure classification of polar images created from the original microscopy image. In order to improve the classification performance, we use additional images: The images are acquired via confocal microscopy, thus there is a complete image stack available. Using a combination of the classification results of the three images in the middle of the stack yields our final classification result.

2.4 Direct measurement of the histone relocation

In addition to the classification explained above, the histone relocation per nucleus can be measured directly. For this measurement, an additional fluorescent marker (lamin) is applied to the experiment, which marks the periphery of the cell nuclei. This information is then extracted from a third channel in the microscopy images, see Figures 5, 6 and 7 for the three channels of an example image. The image processing pipeline for the measurement then consists of the following steps.

2.4.1 Nucleus segmentation
On the DAPI channel, single cell nuclei are segmented using a standard thresholding algorithms in conjunction with a connected components algorithm and basic morphological operations (erode, dilate). See Figure 6 for the DAPI channel of an example image.

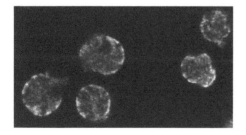

Figure 5. The histone channel of an example image (here: after 4 days of differentiation). The intensities are measured (per nucleus) in this channel.

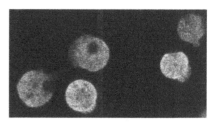

Figure 6. The DAPI channel of an example image. This channel is used to segment the nuclei.

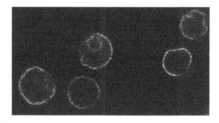

Figure 7. The lamin channel of an example image. This channel is used to segment the periphery of the nuclei.

2.4.2 Periphery segmentation
On the lamin channel, again standard thresholding, connected components and morphological operations are used to segment the periphery of the cell nucleus. See Figure 7 for the lamin channel of an example image and Figures 8 and 9 for the resulting segmentations of the periphery and the inner part.

2.4.3 Intensity measurement
On the histone channel, the actual intensity on a ring along the periphery and in the inner part of each nucleus is measured. The ratio of the intensity of the inner part of each nucleus and the periphery is recorded. See Figure 5 for the histone channel of an example image.

2.5 Implementation

Both image processing pipelines, for classification of histone relocation and for the direct measurement, are implemented in the data processing framework KNIME (Berthold, Cebron, Dill, Gabriel Kötter, Meinl, Ohi, Sieb, Thiel, and Wiswedel 2008), which is a general tool to algorithmically process data in a very convenient way. A KNIME-workflow consists of interconnected nodes, each of which can either load data, process data or output data, while the data is passed from one node to another via interactively defined connections. Recent extensions provide all necessary image processing algorithms that can readily be applied to microscopy images as presented in this work.

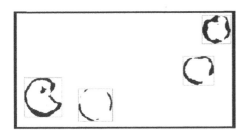

Figure 8. Segmentation of the nucleus periphery from the lamin channel of the example image, see Figure 7. The intensity along this periphery is measured in the histone channel, see Figure 5.

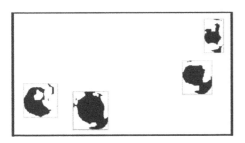

Figure 9. Segmentation of inner part from the lamin channel, see Figure 7. The intensity in the inner part is measured in the histone channel, see Figure 5.

3 RESULTS

We use a set of 46 images with a total of 1990 classified seeding points as ground truth (1150 "background", 840 "nucleus"—250 "ring", 590 "no ring"). For the first boosting "nucleus" versus "background", we use 300 random seeding points for each class as training data, for the second boosting "ring" versus "no ring", we use 250 random seeding points for each class. The linear combination of weak classifiers is slightly biased towards "background" in order to avoid too many false positives in the first boosting step, and it is slightly biased towards "ring" in the second boosting step to improve the recognition rate for weak rings.

The global classification error in the boosting phase is shown in Figure 10. The boosting "nucleus" versus "background" only uses 17 features and reaches a global error of 0.01, while the boosting "ring" versus "no ring" uses 50 features and reaches a global classification error of 0.054. Table 1 shows which features are actually used in each boosting.

The final classification result of 29 microscopy images of progenitor cells and at different days of differentiation are shown in Table 2, Figure 11 shows an exemplary image. The first classification step

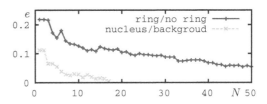

Figure 10. Number of used features N versus global classification error e in the boosting phase. The stop criterion is $e < 0.01$ or $N > 50$.

Table 1. Number of histogram (hst), Haar-like and contour features used in the two boosting steps.

Boosting	# hst	# Haar-l.	# cont.
Nucleus/background	1	8	8
Ring/no ring	11	12	27

Table 2. Results for images of progenitor cells. Shown are the number of nuclei classified as "ring" and "no ring" on the days of differentiation, and the number of false positives (fp) for both classes.

#	Day 2	Day 4	Day 7
no r.	467 (95.7%)	134 (67.3%)	13 (8.0%)
ring	21 (4.3%)	65 (32.7%)	149 (92.0%)
fp n.r.	2 (0.4%)	20 (14.9%)	2 (15.4%)
fp r.	12 (57.1%)	19 (29.2%)	1 (0.7%)

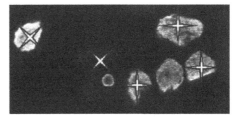

Figure 11. Example classification result. Nuclei classified as "ring" are marked by "X", nuclei classified as "no ring" are marked by "+". Note that the algorithm misses one nucleus and there is one false positive "ring" in this image.

(nucleus detection) has a total detection rate of 97.0%. The classification results are as expected, the ring structure is detected in almost all cells after 7 days. Note that the poor classification result on day 4 is due to the fact that at this stage the histone relocation is not yet completed, which yields a very difficult classification.

For comparison, the direct measurement results are presented in Figure 12. Shown are the mean of

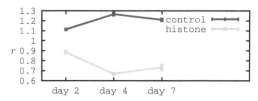

Figure 12. Direct measurement results using the ring segmentation and intensity measurement per cell. The day of the experiment is plotted versus the mean of the intensity ration r (the intensity of the inner part of the nucleus divided by the intensity along the periphery per cell). Shown are the results for histone and for a control marker, which is known not to accumulate at the nucleus periphery. Note that for the histone measurement of day 7 only a small subset of the images were usable due to degrading of the marker.

the ratios of the intensities of the histone signal along the periphery and in the inner part of the nucleus along with the standard error bars. Note that the measurement are very sensitive to the image quality, and in the presented experiments the degradation of the lamin marker was an issue, hence the measurement results for day 7 only use a subset of the original image set in which the marker is still present (but this decreases the measurement accuracy).

4 CONCLUSIONS

We presented an image processing pipeline for an automated classification of cell nuclei in microscopy images. The classification is based on features extracted from polar images that are weighted using an adaptive boosting algorithm. In addition to the classification, we presented a second image processing pipeline for direct measurement of the histone relocation per cell nucleus. Both approaches have clear advantages and disadvantages: The classification works very well for clearly visible relocation or non-relocation, for example at the beginning or at the end of the experiment, and it is relatively robust to poor image quality. However, it does not perform optimal in the middle of the experiment, where the relocation is not yet distinct. On the other hand, the direct measurement works well in each stage of the experiment, but it is very dependent on the correct segmentation and on the image quality, in particular the degrading of the lamin marker decreases the percentage of correct measurements.

Future research directions involve a reduction of the number of labelled training images necessary for a robust classification, and the usage of extended AdaBoost variants for multi-class classification, in particular to improve the classification results of images showing cells without a clearly

visible ring structure. Moreover, an improvement of the direct measurement method using more advanced segmentation methods is desirable.

ACKNOWLEDGEMENTS

The Interdisciplinary Center for Interactive Data Analysis, Modelling and Visual Exploration INCIDE (C. Dietz, T. Rieß, M. Horn, O. Deussen, D. Merhof) is funded via a grant of the German Excellence Initiative by the German Research Foundation (DFG) and the German Council of Science and Humanities awarded to the University of Konstanz. The Center for Applied Photonics CAP (C. Dietz) is supported by the Ministry of Science, Research and the Arts Baden-Württemberg.

REFERENCES

Berthold, M., N. Cebron, F. Dill, T. Gabriel, T. Kötter, T. Meinl, P. Ohl, C. Sieb, K. Thiel, and B. Wiswedel (2008). KNIME: The Konstanz Information Miner. In *Proc. Data Analysis, Machine Learning and Applications*, pp. 319–326.

Freund, Y. and R. Schapire (1999). A short introduction to boosting. In *Proceedings of the Sixteenth International Joint Conference on Artificial Intelligence*, pp. 1401–1406. Morgan Kaufmann.

He, W., X. Wang, D. Metaxas, R. Mathew, and E. White (2007). Cell segmentation for division rate estimation in computerized video timelapse microscopy. In *Society of Photo-Optical Instrumentation Engineers (SPIE) Conference Series*, Volume 6431.

Khorasanizadeh, S. (2004). The nucleosome: from genomic organization to genomic regulation. *Cell* (116), 259–272.

Kouzarides, T. (2007). Chromatin modifications and their function. *Cell* (128), 693–705.

Kvarnström, M., K. Logg, A. Diez, K. Bodvard, and M. Käll (2008). Image analysis algorithms for cell contour recognition in budding yeast. *Optics Express* 16(17), 12943–1257.

Lienhart, R., E. Kuranov, and V. Pisarevsky (2003). Empirical analysis of detection cascades of boosted classifiers for rapid object detection. In *DAGM 25th Pattern Recognition Symposium*, pp. 297–304.

Smith, K., A. Carleton, and V. Lepetit (2009). Fast Ray features for learning irregular shapes. In *IEEE 12th International Conference on Computer Vision*, pp. 397–404.

Viola, P. and M. Jones (2004). Robust real-time face detection. *International Journal of Computer Vision* 57, 137–154.

Zimmer, B., P. Kuegler, B. Baudis, A. Genewsky, V. Tanavde, W. Koh, B. Tan, T. Waldmann, S. Kadereit, and M. Leist (2011). Coordinated waves of gene expression during neuronal differentiation of embryonic stem cells as basis for novel approaches to developmental neurotoxicity testing. *Cell Death and Differentiation* (18), 383–395.

Computational Vision and Medical Image Processing – Tavares & Natal Jorge (eds)
© 2012 Taylor & Francis Group, London, ISBN 978-0-415-68395-1

An automated vehicle counting system from UAV images

Antonio M. Rodrigues Neto & Elcio H. Shiguemori
IEAv—Institute for Advanced Studies, São José dos Campos, SP, Brazil
UNIP—Universidade Paulista, São José dos Campos, SP, Brazil

Ana Paula A. de Castro
IEAv—Institute for Advanced Studies, São José dos Campos, SP, Brazil

ABSTRACT: This work addresses the problem of movement identification from aerial video. Characteristic points information have been used to estimate of the aircraft displacement. The moving objects have been identified employing operations on video frames. The results show that the approach is indicated for the application, since it is desired automated vehicle identification.

1 INTRODUCTION

The use of Unmanned Aerial Vehicles (UAVs) has grown in recent years and has shown several advantages in the process of obtaining information on remote sensing. The low cost in the manufacturing and maintenance processes, large autonomy and versatility, are some of the motivations in the employment of UAVs. Applications such as monitoring of power lines (Jones, 2007), search and rescue (Rudol & Doherty, 2008), natural disasters and emergencies (Rao et al., 2005), are some examples of its use. Most of these applications consider images taken by onboard cameras for information extraction about UAV flight region. The process of extracting information from images can be done in different ways. The image processing can be done in ground stations where, using a datalink, the images are downloaded and processed in computers (Tristancho et al., 2009). However, processing can also be done in embedded systems. This paper aims to present the use of images and data mining techniques for extracting information of roads and highways in regions flown by UAVs, presenting information to decision making. Aerial video of regions containing images of highways and roads are used in the tests. Algorithms for detecting feature points present in the sequence of video images are applied, and then the vehicle detection is performed applying image translation and differentiation. Lastly, the number of moving vehicles is estimated.

2 COUNTING OF VEHICLES FROM THE IMAGE PROCESSING

The identification of moving vehicles from images can be used in several applications, including traffic monitoring and security. The problems caused by the excess of vehicles on roads and highways has been enormous in recent years (Zhuang et al., 2009). The counting of vehicles is an important input to the traffic problem (Hsieh et al., 2006) and has been approached by different methodologies. Zhuang (2009) present the main approaches for counting vehicles. Among them, considering static cameras and vehicle detection using image differentiation. Pang (2007) proposed a method for counting vehicles considering occlusions in traffic images. Fixed cameras are used with different perspectives to the identification of vehicles present in the image sequence. Wang (2007) presents a system for automatic counting of vehicles for traffic controlling. The system considers DSP devices for image processing.

3 VEHICLES DETECTION FROM VIDEOS OF UAV

Most applications of automatic vehicle detection from images is carried with the use of static cameras. These applications are extremely important, but for monitoring large areas, require a large number of cameras or need to be positioned at strategic points. By employing images from UAVs need to consider that the UAV is moving. This approach takes advantage of the UAV to move quickly and at low cost to analyze an area of interest. In this context, Videos of flown regions are considered. The stream of images is used to detect moving vehicles. Previous work to address the detection of moving vehicles from images of UAVs was presented by Kaaniche (2005).

4 COUNTING OF VEHICLES FROM IMAGES OF UAV

The identification and counting of vehicles is an important process for the extraction of information and decision making. In this study, the vehicle identification has been performed in the sequence of aerial images. Moving vehicles have been identified by applying the difference between images at different instants of time. The technique of image subtraction has been successfully used in systems that make use of static cameras and when changes in lighting and scenery are not critical for accuracy. When images from UAVs are employed for identification and counting of vehicles in motion, moving the camera should be compensated. For this

reason, in this work, characteristic points of the images were extracted using the SIFT algorithm proposed by Lowe (Lowe, 1999). The SIFT has been used to identify these characteristic points in images obtained by different positions (Lowe, 2004). Thus, it is possible to make the matching between the descriptors of the feature points of sequences of images (Lowe, 2004) and then estimate the displacement of the camera. Then the translation and the cutting of images can be applied to compensate the UAV displacement, it is possible to highlight moving objects in the scene. However, the resulting images can be noisy and contain distortions caused by instabilities of the UAV and situations such as trees moved by the wind. Morphological operations, erosion and dilation, are applied for image filtering (Maragos & Schafer, 1986) in order to facilitate the identification of moving vehicles.

To apply morphological operations is required prior knowledge of characteristics such as shape and size of objects to be identified and the choice of a structuring element that represents these characteristics (Maragos & Schafer, 1986). In the examples used were considered the size of objects to be detected and the amount of noise.

A square mask with dimensions of 3×3 points has shown satisfactory results in the elimination of noise and highlight the desired objects to detect. Figure 1 shows the sequence of operations applied to images.

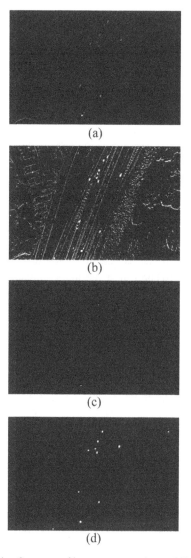

(a)

(b)

(c)

(d)

Figure 1. Sequence of image segmentation and filtering, (a) result of subtraction of images, (b) thresholded image, (c) image after application of erosion and (d) image after application of the dilation.

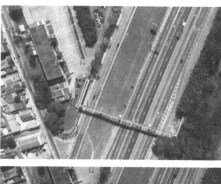

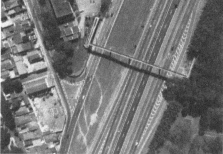

Figure 2. Example of video sequence.

430

To perform the test phase, images obtained by a videography of a flight over the city of São José dos Campos, São Paulo, Brazil, have been used. Sequence of images containing roads and streets have been selected, in which the methodology is applied to automatic counting of moving vehicles from aerial images. In Figure 2 are presented examples of images taken from aerial videography.

5 RESULTS

Preliminary tests were conducted to evaluate the performance of the methodology. To measure the accuracy and sensitivity (Fawcett, 2006) of the algorithm, the situations: True Positives (TP): number of vehicles identified correctly by the system; False Positives (FP): misclassification as a vehicle in motion; and False Negatives (FN): not identified moving vehicles.

A first experiment was performed considering the first 5 seconds of videography and images were taken at intervals of 0.16 seconds. Table 1 shows the results.

Figure 3 shows a sequence of images where the moving vehicles that are correctly identified are highlighted.

The results presented in Table 1 show a good accuracy in most cases and a good average precision indicating the effectiveness of using morphological operations in image filtering even in the presence of trees moving and outdoor lighting, which are critical in systems that make use of image subtraction for motion detection. In some images, the system has presented low sensitivity. The main reasons were failure to detect small objects, objects

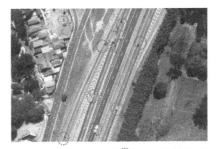
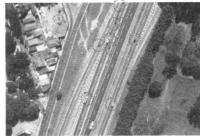
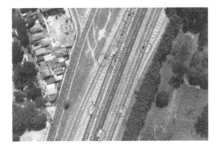

Figure 3. Example of vehicle identification.

Table 1. Accuracy and sensitivity rates.

Frame	Objects in motion	Sensibility	Accuracy
1	10	80,00%	80,00%
2	10	80,00%	80,00%
3	10	90,00%	81,82%
4	11	72,73%	88,89%
5	12	75,00%	90,00%
6	11	81,82%	75,00%
7	13	69,23%	90,00%
8	13	61,54%	100,00%
9	11	63,64%	100,00%
10	12	41,67%	100,00%
11	12	41,67%	100,00%
12	12	50,00%	100,00%
13	13	30,77%	80,00%
14	11	63,64%	70,00%
15	10	80,00%	100,00%
Average	11,40	65,45%	89,05%

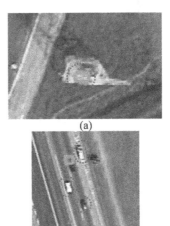

(a)

(b)

Figure 4. Examples of false positives and false negatives (a) object height above the ground falsely accused as a moving object by the system and (b) objects in motion is not detected by the system to be of small size and present themselves in similar colors the background color.

at low speeds and in similar color to the background color. The system also accused some false positives in the case of objects at much above the ground, see Figure 4.

6 CONCLUSIONS

This study discussed the use of aerial images obtained during the flight to detect and count vehicles. Extracted frames are used for video detection and counting of vehicles. Characteristic points are used to make corrections to the translation then do the subtraction and detection of vehicles. The results show that the approach is appropriate and can be used to extract information for traffic and safety problems.

REFERENCES

Fawcett, T. (2006). An introduction to ROC analysis. Pattern Recognition Letters. v27, n. 8, p. 861–874.

Hsieh, J.W., S.H. Yu, Y.S. Chen, and W.F. Hu (2006). Automatic traffic surveillance system for vehicle tracking and classification. *IEEE Transactions on Intelligent Transportation Systems 7(2)*.

Jones, D.I. (2007). An experimental power pickup mechanism for an electrically driven uav. In *IEEE Int. Symp. Ind. Electron, pp. 2033–2038.*

Kaaniche, K., B. Champion, C. Pegard, and P. Vasseur (2005). A vision algorithm for dynamic detection of moving vehicles with a uav. pp. 1878–1883.

Lowe, D.G. (1999). Object recognition from local scale-invariant features. In *Proceedings of the Seventh International Conference on Computer Vision (ICCV'99), pp. 1150–1157.*

Lowe, D.G. (2004). Distinctive image features from scale-invariant keypoints. In *International Journal of Computer Vision, 60, 2, pp. 91–110.*

Maragos, P., and R.W. Schafer (1986). Applications of morphological filtering to image analysis and processing. In *Proc. IEEE Int. Conf. Acoust., Speech, Signal Processing, pp. 2063–2066.*

Pang, C.C.C., W.W.L. Lam, and N.H.C.A. Yung (2007). A method for vehicle count in the presence of multiple-vehicle occlusions in traffic images. In *IEEE Transactions on Intelligent Transportation Systems, pp. 441–459.*

Rao, J., Z. Gong, J. Luo, and S. Xie (2005). Unmanned airships for emergency management. In *Safety, Security and Rescue Robotics, Workshop, pp. 125–130.*

Rudol, P. and P. Doherty (2008). Human body detection and geolocalization for uav search and rescue missions using color and thermal imagery. In *IEEE Aerospace Conference, pp. 1–8.*

Tristancho, J., C. Barrado, S.P. Mansilla, and E. Pastor (2009). A telemetry modeling for intelligent uav monitoring. In *IEEE/AIAA Digital Avionics Systems Conference, pp. 7.C.1–1–7.C.1–4.*

Wang, K., Z. Li, Q. Yao, W. Huang, and F. (2007). An automated vehicle counting system for traffic surveillance. In *IEEE International Conference on Vehicular Electronics and Safety, pp. 1–6.*

Zhuang, P., Y. Shang, and B. Hua (2009). Statistical methods to estimate vehicle count using traffic cameras. Multidimensional Systems and Signal Processing 20, 121–133. 10.1007/s11045-008-0068-x.

Computational Vision and Medical Image Processing – Tavares & Natal Jorge (eds)
© 2012 Taylor & Francis Group, London, ISBN 978-0-415-68395-1

Tracking rural and urban landmarks for UAV autonomous navigation

Ruan M. Andrade & Elcio H. Shiguemori
IEAv—Institute for Advanced Studies, São José dos Campos, SP, Brazil
UNIP—Universidade Paulista, São José dos Campos, SP, Brazil

Ana Paula A. de Castro
IEAv—Institute for Advanced Studies, São José dos Campos, SP, Brazil

ABSTRACT: This work addresses the problem of movement identification from aerial video. Characteristic points information have been used to estimate of the aircraft displacement. The moving objects have been identified employing operations on video frames. The results show that the approach is indicated for the application, since it is desired real-time processing.

1 INTRODUCTION

There are several researches that focus the problem of solving the aerial, terrestrial or nautical vehicle autonomous navigation based on vision (Kundur and Raviv 1998; Azinheira et al., 2002).

When dealing with vision-based autonomous navigation systems several challenges have to be dealt with (Shiguemori et al., 2007; Rodrigues et al., 2009). The vision system captures a huge amount of data that must be processed in real time so that relevant information can be extracted from frames to feed controlling and navigation systems, in some of these applications following a point of interest can increase the accuracy and to provide more information about the object under study. A mobile camera can be used to follow these points of interest and increase the limits of observation. For Unmanned Aerial Vehicles (UAV), this information is fundamental for the safe and efficient accomplishment of the preplanned mission by the UAV. Landmark recognition systems for UAV (Canhoto et al., 2009; Shiguemori et al., 2007) have strict requirements of high processing speed, limited payload for navigation systems and significant landmark variations due to factors such as humankind actions, the seasons landscape changes and Sun illumination. This work presents a landmark tracking using a mobile camera to support the autonomous navigation based on images. Techniques are used for image processing and computer vision (OpenCV Intel, 2001). The computational vision system is composed by characteristic points of images and attributes of landmarks. The image processing techniques (Gonzales and Woods, 2008) are used to emphasize points of interest, while the techniques of computer vision (OpenCV Intel, 2001) are applied to extract information about a known landmark.

Based on this information, the tracking of the landmarks is done using a mobile camera with vertical and horizontal. Thus, it is possible to extract more environment information to increase the accuracy of the navigation of an Unmanned Air Vehicle.

2 LANDMARK RECOGNITION

The aim of the landmark recognition system is to recognize landmarks captured by the on-board UAV vision system in real-time when flying over specific locations, thus supporting the navigation system to accomplish a planned mission. UAVs onboard landmarks recognition systems are complex and require low cost and high performance techniques employment.

The use of remote sensing images, like satellite or aerial images also brings significant challenges to the recognition system. High resolution remote sensing images usually are large volume data to onboard recognition system deal with. This system was conceived in two major sets of threads, the first set is accomplished in the UAV ground control station and the second one onboard, to accomplish the flight mission.

In the UAV ground control station the user needs to plan the flight mission on high resolution satellite images and select the landmarks to be recognized (Canhoto et al., 2009; Shiguemori et al., 2007). Before extracting, each frame is pre-processed to gray levels (no color information was used in this work), rotated and scaled to be as similar as possible to the parameters of the satellite image. In real flights, information for rotating and scaling the frames could be obtained from UAV onboard instruments, like electrical compass and radio-altimeter.

Table 1. Representation of the seed and its neighbors in region growing.

a(x−1, y−1)	a(x−1, y)	a(x−1, y+1)
a(x, y−1)	a(x, y)	a(x, y+1)
a(x+1, y−1)	a(x+1, y)	a(x+1, y+1)

3   REGION GROWING

Region growing is a technique that captures the largest number of pixels with similar data within a certain region of an image (Gonzales and Woods, 2008). Usually the data of one or more original pixels (seeds) are the benchmarks for growth. From there, the comparison is made between the seed and their neighbors. If they are within the pre-established criteria such as color intensity scale, the neighboring pixel will be part of this region and can be used as seed for the next comparison. Otherwise, it will not be part of the region. The procedure continues checking all the neighboring pixels until there is no one with characteristics in common with the current seed. At this time, the region is closed (Gonzales and Woods, 2008). The estimation of area information is given by the sum of pixels similar to the seed (Gonzales and Woods, 2008). In Table 1 shows the representation of region growing.

4   SPEEDED UP ROBUST FEATURES (SURF)

Due to the invariance of some features present in images, such as lighting, rotation and scale, the SURF (Bay et al., 2006) algorithm has been used as one of the approaches surveyed, since aerial images considered in this work may have variations in lighting, rotation and scale. SURF is a robust method to extract and describe key points of an image (Bay et al., 2006). Basically the algorithm is divided into three steps, creating the integral of image, determination of points of interest through the Fast Hessian and creation of descriptors of each key point. The algorithm has been used successfully in many applications such as object recognition (Zhao and Qin, 2009), remote sensing (Song and Zhang, 2010), satellite images (Teke and Temizel, 2010), among others.

5   RURAL AND URBAN LANDMARKS TRACKING

In the work, aerial images were employed to simulate the flight of a UAV over the city containing urban and rural areas. Relevant landmarks have been considered in the images tests containing buildings, houses and ground landmarks to get different view angles. An example of image building used is shown the Figure 1. Figure 1 shows the sequences of images used at time t, at time $t +1$ and at time $t +2$. It can be noted that with the displacement of the aircraft, the angle of view of the buildings is modified, thus, only some features present in the image at time t are not the same at time $t +1$ and $t +2$, difficulty in tracking based on images.

Initially, an algorithm has been developed to simulate the tracking of a reference point using sequential aerial images. The tracking process has been done with data collected of the source image and searching them in the next image. With use of pixel information are obtained position data (x, y) and intensity in grayscale (Gonzales and Woods, 2008). With these data, the region growing technique is applied, and then the area is calculated

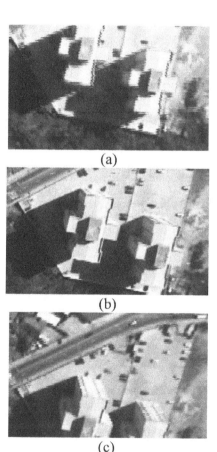

(a)

(b)

(c)

Figure 1. Sequence of images containing buildings. (a) obtained at time t, (b) obtained at time $t +1$ and (c) obtained at time $t +2$.

(Gonzales and Woods, 2008). These data are stored and located in the following image, comparing the pixels of the same intensity and region.

Examples of selection regions are shown in Figure 2 and Figure 3, highlighted with the dotted line.

One outstanding problem with this method considering the application exists when there is another element in the image scanned with the same intensity of color and the same area as the target of interest.

In a second approach, the detection of the landmarks has been done using the SURF algorithm (Bay et al., 2006). With information of characteristic points of reference image, the detection of the landmark is made in the image of videography. Figure 4 shows results with rural landmarks at ground level. Figures 5 and 6 shows results with landmark just above the ground. Note that in Figure 7(b) that some false positives are detected, which can be eliminated by applying filters.

In the testing phase, a set of twelve images was used, considering landmarks of different sizes and view angles of approach. It has showed approximately 80% accuracy. It was found that at main cause of errors is related to inappropriate selection of the landmark to be tracked. When the landmarks are well defined, as the top of a hangar, highlighted in Figure 5, or top of buildings such as those shown in Figures 6 and 7, the percentage of accuracy is approximately 100%.

Tables 2–6 present the results, considering the same images in the two methodologies applied.

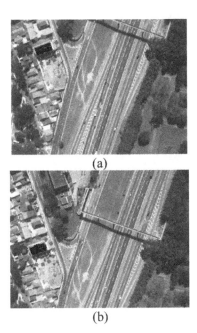

(a)

(b)

Figure 2. Example of implementing the approach. (a) reference image, (b) tracking the landmark.

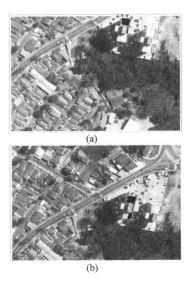

(a)

(b)

Figure 3. Example of application of the approach. (a) reference image, (b) tracking the landmark.

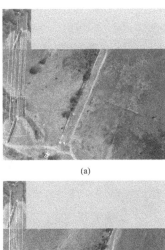

(a)

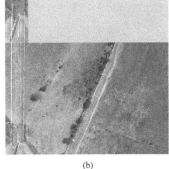

(b)

Figure 4. Implementation of the SURF algorithm in aerial images with ground landmarks.

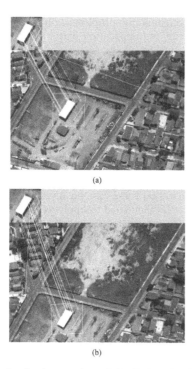

(a)

(b)

Figure 5. Implementation of the SURF algorithm in aerial images with landmark just above the ground.

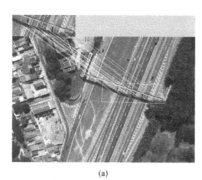

(a)

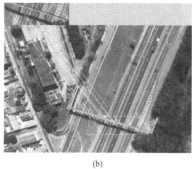

(b)

Figure 6. Implementation of the SURF algorithm in aerial images with landmark just above the ground.

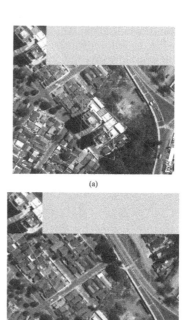

(a)

(b)

Figure 7. Application of the SURF algorithm in aerial images with landmark above the ground.

Table 2. Results considering rural landmarks on the ground.

Instant	Region growing	SURF algorithm
1	100%—1930 pixels	100%—25 key points
2	100%—2000 pixels	100%—14 key points
3	0%—0 pixels	67%—3 key points

Table 3. Results considering rural landmarks above the ground.

Instant	Region growing	SURF algorithm
1	100%—1700 pixels	100%—42 key points
2	50%—1533 pixels	95%—19 key points
3	0%—0 pixels	93%—14 key points

Table 4. Results considering urban landmarks on the ground.

Instant	Region growing	SURF algorithm
1	100%—2496 pixels	100%—21 key points
2	100%—2610 pixels	88%—16 key points
3	100%—2497 pixels	93%—14 key points

436

Table 5. Results considering urban landmarks above the ground.

Instant	Region growing	SURF algorithm
1	100%—1890 pixels	100%—29 key points
2	100%—1798 pixels	100%—23 key points
3	0%—0 pixels	91%—11 key points

Table 6. Results with images of urban areas. Mark high above the ground.

Instant	Region growing	SURF algorithm
1	100%—3068pixels	100%—26 key points
2	50%—1030 pixels	91%—11 key points
3	0%—0 pixels	50%—2 key points

6 CONCLUSIONS

In the present work a landmark recognition system for UAV autonomous navigation is presented. Approaches were applied to automatically track landmarks present in the flown region with the objective of assisting an autonomous navigation system based on images. The results show that the approaches are promising for aerial image landmark recognition from frames obtained by a video camera attached to a helicopter.

REFERENCES

Azinheira, J.R.; Rives, P.; Carvalho, J.R.H.; Silveira, G.F.; Paiva, E.C.D.; Bueno, S.S.; (2002). Visual servo for the hovering of an outdoor robotic airship. *in IEEE International Conference on Robotics and Automation*, 2782–2792.

Bay, H.; Tuytelaars, T.; Gool, L.V. Surf: Speeded up robust features. In *European Conference on Computer Vision, pages 404–417, 2006*.

Canhoto, A.; Shiguemori, E.H.; Domiciano, Marco A. Pizani. Image Sequence Processing Applied to Autonomous Aerial Navigation. In: IEEE International Conference on Signal and Image Processing Applications (ICSIPA), 2009, Kuala Lumpur. Procedings IEEE International Conference on Signal and Image Processing Applications (ICSIPA). Kuala Lumpur: IEEE Signal Processing Society Malaysia, 2009. v. 1.

Chuang, C.H.; Lie, W.N.; Region Growing based on extended gradient vector flow field model for multiple objects segmentation. In: *Image Processing, 2001. Proceedings. 2001 International Conference on, pages 74–77*.

Gonzales, R.C.; Woods, R.E. Digital Image Processing. Third Edition, 2008.

OpenCV Intel, Open Source Computer Vision Library Reference Manual, 2001. Available in: http://www.cs.unc.edu/Research/str/FAQs/OpenCV/OpenCVReference Manual.pdf. Accessed: March 12th, 2010.

Kundur, S.R. and Raviv, D. (1998). A vision-based pragmatic strategy for autonomous navigation. *Pattern Recognition* 31, 1221–1239.

Rodrigues, R.C.B.; Shiguemori, E.H.; Forster, C.H.Q.; Pellegrino, S.R.M.; Color and Texture Features for Landmarks Recognition on UAV Navigation. In: *Simpósio Brasileiro de Sensoriamento Remoto, 2009, Natal – RN. São José dos Campos: INPE, 2009. v. XIV. pages 7111–7118*.

Shiguemori, E.H.; Monteiro, M.V.T.; Martins, M.P.; Landmarks Recognition for Autonomous Aerial Navigation by Neural Network and Gabor Transform. In: *IS&T/SPIE 19th Annual Symposium Eletronic Imaging Science and Technology, 2007, San Jose, CA, USA. Image Processing: Algorithms and Systems V, 2007. v. 6497*.

Song, Z.L.; Zhang, J., Remote Sensing Image Registration Based on Retrofitted SURF Algorithm and Trajectories Generated From Lissajous Figures. In: *IEEE Geoscience and Remote Sensing Letters, Vol. 7, No. 3, July 2010, pages 491–495*.

Teke M.; Temizel A., Multi-Spectral Satellite Image Registration Using Scale-Restricted SURF. In: *2010 International Conference on Pattern Recognition, pages 2310–2313, 2010*.

Zhao, M.; Qin, S., Socket Connector Recognition Based on SVM with Speeded Up Robust Feature (SURF). In: *The Ninth International Conference on Electronic Measurement & Instruments, pages 827–831, 2009*.

Author index

Abdel-Dayem, A.R. 267
Ablavsky, V. 15
Acosta, O. 245
Albuquerque, V.H.C. 161
Alegre, E. 199
Almeida, D. 355
Almeida, G. 155
Alves, S. 89
Ambrósio, P.E. 143
Amorim, B.S.R. 37
Amorim, P.H.J. 405
Andrade, R.M. 329, 433
Antonov, V.A. 97
Aranda, J.P. 415
Araujo, A.F. 183, 193
Araújo, M. 315
Aubrecht, C. 347
Azevedo, F.S. 405

Balbi, S. 251
Ballesteros, F. 383
Barbosa, J.G. 19
Barros, F.M. 343
Barroso, E.M. 377
Baugh, K.E. 347
Bělohlávek, O. 279
Bento, D. 189
Bernardes, A.A. 193
Binaghi, E. 251
Boldyš, J. 279
Bornemann, L. 173
Bourgeat, P. 245

Canale, S. 323
Cardoso, A.S. 19
Chitiboi, T. 173
Cohen, L.D. 239, 245
Correia, A. 93, 101

Da Roza, T.H. 319
da Silva, J.V.L. 405
Dawid, M.S. 291
de Aquino, L.C.M. 23
De Benedictis, A. 251
De Beule, M. 57
de Carvalho, M.A.G. 367

de Castro, A.P.A. 429, 433
de Castro, J. 383
de Moraes, T.F. 405
de Posada, N.G. 89
De Santis, A. 323
Deriu, M.A. 205
Deussen, O. 423
Dias, L.A.V. 69
Dias, R. 209
Dietz, C. 423
Domiciano, M.A.P. 69
Duarte, S. 319
Dvořák, J. 279
Dzielicki, J. 307

Elvidge, C.D. 347
Eskola, H. 261

Fernandes, A.A. 233, 297
Fernandes, C. 209
Fernandes, P.R. 355
Fernandez, C. 3
Ferreira, P.M. 399
Figueiral, M.H. 85, 101
Figueiredo, R. 93
Fiot, J.-B. 239, 245
Folgado, J. 355
Fonseca, A. 333
Fonseca, J. 155
Fonseca, P. 85
Frąckiewicz, M. 131
Freire, S. 333, 337
Freitas, D.R. 225
Fripp, J. 239, 245

Gambaruto, A.M. 179
Garbe, C. 27, 311
García-Olalla, O. 199
García-Ordás, M.T. 199
Gavidia, G. 51
Gayubo, F. 221
Gentil, F. 27, 311, 377
Geraldes, M.J. 315
Gil, J.E. 415
Giraldi, G.A. 23
Gonçalves, I.B. 387

Gonçalves, P.J.S. 79
Gonzàlez, J. 3
González-Castro, V. 199
González-Hidalgo, M. 167
Grosmann, M.H. 97
Gzik, M. 43, 47, 307
Gzik-Zroska, B. 307

Habermann, M. 329
Hahn, H.K. 173
Hahn, S. 347
Hamamoto, A. 393
Hes, L. 315
Horn, M. 423

Iacoviello, D. 323
Imai, Y. 209
Isabel, A. 221
Ishikawa, T. 209, 217

Jaguegivane, S.D. 233
Janardo, J.C. 233
João, A.J. 179
Jorge, R.N. 27, 297, 311, 319, 371
Joutsen, A. 261

Kähler, C.J. 205
Kawlewska, E. 43, 47
Kawlewski, K. 47
Kordolaimi, S.D. 107

Lachiondo, J.A. 409
Larkin, A.I. 97
Larysz, D. 43, 47
Larysz, P. 43
Leble, V. 209
Leiria, A. 387
Leist, M. 423
Lima, R. 209, 217, 221
Lopes, G. 31
López, M.A.G. 89
López, R. 51
Loureiro, J. 319
Lyra, M.E. 107

Ma, Z. 111, 117, 371, 377
Marcal, A.R.S. 37
Marques, J.S. 37
Marques, T. 93
Marranghello, N. 183, 193
Martin, G.B. 123
Martins, J.M.M. 79
Martins, P. 27, 311
Mascarenhas, T. 319
Massanet, S. 167
Mastrangelo, F. 205
Mauricio, J. 303
Melício, F. 155
Mellouli, N. 257
Mendonça, T. 37, 399
Merhof, D. 423
Mérida-Casermeiro, E. 415
Minotto, R. 251
Mir, A. 167
Monteiro, F.C. 189
Monteiro, J.M. 101
Montevecchi, F.M. 205
Monti, E. 251
Morbiducci, U. 205
Moreira, P.M. 73
Moura, D.C. 19
Moura, M.M.M. 387

Nakamura, M. 213
Nakamura, R.Y.M. 161
Nava, E. 291
Neto, A.M.R. 329, 429
Neto, B.A. 273
Neves, L.A.P. 23
Nicolau, C.P. 273
Nogueira-Silva, C. 285
Nunes, J.F. 73

Oliveira, C.M. 149
Oliveira, M.S.N. 217
O'Neill, J. 303
Onodera, A.N. 393
Osintsev, A.V. 97

Pachi, C.G.F. 393
Paço, J. 27, 311
Paes, R.L. 329, 343
Palus, H. 131
Papa, J.P. 161
Parente, M. 27, 297, 311, 319
Pariente, C.A.B. 143
Pedoia, V. 251
Pedrana, G. 123

Pennella, F. 205
Pereira, A.I. 189, 217
Pereira, A.S. 183, 193
Pereira, M.E. 233
Pinão, J. 149
Pinho, A.J. 9
Pinho, D. 221
Pinto, T.W. 367
Pirri, F. 323
Pontes, M.A. 183
Porcides, G.M. 23

Quintero, J.L. 291

Ramos, I.M. 225
Raniga, P. 239, 245
Rasponi, M. 205
Reis, L.P. 361
Reis-Campos, J. 85
Ribeiro, C.H.L. 343
Ribeiro, F. 31
Ribeiro, M.B. 233, 303
Ricordeau, A. 257
Ridolfi, L. 205
Rieß, T. 423
Ripandelli, S. 205
Roberty, N.C. 137
Robles, L.F. 199
Roca, X. 3
Rocha, P. 399
Rodrigues, A.T. 273
Rodrigues, P.J. 217
Rogeri, J.G. 183, 193
Rossi, M. 205
Rozeira, J. 37, 399
Ruben, R.B. 355

Sacco, I.C.N. 393
Sagratella, S. 323
Salenius, J. 261
Salvado, O. 245
Salvara, A.-L.N. 107
Santiago, C.B. 361
Santos, F. 261
Santos, M.J. 101
Santos, T. 333, 337
Schepinov, V.P. 97
Schwier, M. 173
Sclaroff, S. 15
Sequeira, A. 179
Shiguemori, E.H. 69, 329, 429, 433
Silva, C.C. 161

Silva, P.F. 111
Silva, T.D.C.A. 117
Simões, A.F. 93
Simões, R. 285
Skopalová, M. 279
Sloboda, D. 123
Soudah, E. 51
Sousa, A. 361
Souza, E. 123
Spann, M. 63

Talaia, P. 297
Tavares, J.M.R.S. 73, 111, 117, 161, 183, 193, 225, 371, 377
Teixeira, A.R. 137
Tenedório, J.A. 333, 337
Thangali, A. 15
Torres, P.M.B. 79
Trigueiros, P. 31
Trouche, C. 123

Ujaldón, M. 409, 415
Ujir, H. 63

Van Cauter, S. 57
Van Haver, A. 57
Vasconcelos, M.J.M. 225
Vaz, M.A.P. 85, 101
Ventura, S.R. 225
Verdonk, P. 57
Verhegghe, B. 57
Villemagne, V. 245
Viotti, M.H. 123
Viriato, N. 85

Wada, S. 213
Waldmann, T. 423
Weiderpass, H.A. 393
Wolański, W. 43, 47, 307

Yaginuma, T. 217
Yamaguchi, T. 209, 217
Yamamoto, J.F. 393
Yuan, Q. 15

Zaloti Jr., O.D. 69, 343

COMPUTATIONAL VISION AND MEDICAL IMAGE PROCESSING